rar

D1338040

Cardiovascular Critical Care

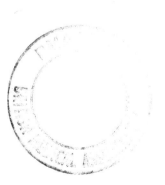

To our teachers and colleagues, many of whom are contributors to this book.

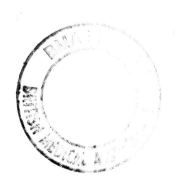

Cardiovascular Critical Care

EDITED BY

Mark J.D. Griffiths MRCP PhD EDICM BDICM
Consultant in Intensive Care Medicine
Royal Brompton & Harefield NHS Foundation Trust
London, UK

Jeremy J. Cordingley MRCP FRCA EDICM
Consultant in Intensive Care Medicine and Anaesthesia
Royal Brompton & Harefield NHS Foundation Trust
London, UK

Susanna Price MRCP PhD EDICM FESC
Consultant in Intensive Care Medicine and Cardiology
Royal Brompton & Harefield NHS Foundation Trust
London, UK

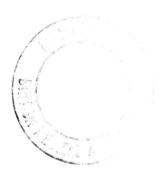

⊛WILEY-BLACKWELL BMJ|Books

A John Wiley & Sons, Inc., Publication

This edition first published 2010, © 2010 by Blackwell Publishing Ltd

BMJ Books is an imprint of BMJ Publishing Group Limited, used under licence by Blackwell Publishing which was acquired by John Wiley & Sons in February 2007. Blackwell's publishing programme has been merged with Wiley's global Scientific, Technical and Medical business to form Wiley-Blackwell.

Registered office: John Wiley & Sons Ltd, The Atrium, Southern Gate, Chichester, West Sussex, PO19 8SQ, UK

Editorial offices: 9600 Garsington Road, Oxford, OX4 2DQ, UK
The Atrium, Southern Gate, Chichester, West Sussex, PO19 8SQ, UK
111 River Street, Hoboken, NJ 07030-5774, USA

For details of our global editorial offices, for customer services and for information about how to apply for permission to reuse the copyright material in this book please see our website at www.wiley.com/wiley-blackwell

The right of the author to be identified as the author of this work has been asserted in accordance with the Copyright, Designs and Patents Act 1988.

Library of Congress Cataloging-in-Publication Data

Cardiovascular critical care / edited by Mark J.D. Griffiths . . . [et al.].
    p. ; cm.
  Includes bibliographical references.
  ISBN 978-1-4051-4857-3
  1. Cardiac intensive care.   I. Griffiths, M. J. D.
  [DNLM: 1. Cardiovascular Diseases.   2. Critical Care. WG 120 C26716 2010]

  RC684.C36C377 2010
  616.1'2028 – dc22
                                                                    2009029876

ISBN: 978-1-4051-4857-3

A catalogue record for this book is available from the British Library.

Set in 9.25/11.5pt Minion by Graphicraft Limited, Hong Kong
Printed and bound in Singapore by Fabulous Printers Pte Ltd

1   2010

Contents

The colour plate section can be found facing p. 82

Contributors

David Alexander MBChB, FRCA
Consultant Anaesthetist, Department of Anaesthesia and Critical Care,
Royal Brompton & Harefield NHS Foundation Trust, London, UK

Joseph E. Arrowsmith MB BS, MD, FRCP, FRCA, FHEA
Consultant in Cardiothoracic Anaesthesia & Intensive Care, Papworth
Hospital, Cambridge, UK

Nicole Assmann MD, FRCA
Consultant Anaesthetist, Royal Free Hospital, London, UK

Robert S. Bonser MD, FRCP (Lon), FRCS (Eng), FRCS (C/Th), FESC
Consultant Cardiothoracic Surgeon, University Hospital Birmingham
NHS Trust, Birmigham, UK

Ronald Bradley FRCP
Emeritus Professor, Intensive Care Medicine, St Thomas' Hospital,
London, UK

Gerald S. Carr-White MD
Department of Cardiology, Guys' and St Thomas' NHS Foundation
Trust, London, UK

Katerina Chamaidi MD
Adult Congenital Heart Centre and Centre for Pulmonary Hypertension,
Royal Brompton & Harefield NHS Foundation Trust, London, UK and
General Hospital of Trikala, Greece

Nick Curzen PhD, FRCP, FESC
Wessex Cardiac Unit, Southampton University Hospitals NHS Trust,
Southampton, UK and Southampton University Medical School,
Southampton, UK

Barbara J. Deal MD
M.E. Wodika Professor of Cardiology, Feinberg School of Medicine,
Northwestern University, Children's Memorial Hospital, Chicago,
IL, USA

Antonia Pijuan Domènech MD
Adult Congenital Heart Centre and Centre for Pulmonary Hypertension,
Royal Brompton & Harefield NHS Foundation Trust, London, UK and
Adult Congenital Heart Disease Unit, Hospital Vall d'Hebron, Barcelona,
Spain, UK

Vamsidhar B. Dronavalli MRCS (Edin)
Research Fellow Cardiothoracic Surgery, Department of Cardiothoracic
Surgery, University Hospital Birmingham NHS Trust, Birmingham, UK

John Dunning MD
Papworth Hospital, Cambridge, UK

Florian Falter MD, FRCA, PhD
Consultant in Cardiothoracic Anaesthesia & Intensive Care, Department
of Anaesthesia, Papworth Hospital, Cambridge, UK

Simon J. Finney PhD, MSc, MRCP, FRCA
Consultant in Intensive Care and Anaesthesia, Adult Intensive Care Unit,
Royal Brompton & Harefield NHS Foundation Trust, London, UK

Michael Gatzoulis MD
Adult Congenital Heart Centre and Centre for Pulmonary Hypertension,
Royal Brompton & Harefield NHS Foundation Trust, London, UK and
National Heart & Lung Institute, Imperial College, London, UK

Derek Gibson MD
Department of Cardiology, Royal Brompton & Harefield NHS Foundation
Trust, London, UK

Alex Hobson PhD, FRCP, FESC
Wessex Cardiac Unit, Southampton University Hospitals NHS Trust,
Southampton, UK and Southampton University Medical School,
Southampton, UK

David Hunter MD, MBBS, FRCA
Consultant Anaesthetist & Intensivist, Anaesthetic Department, Royal
Brompton & Harefield NHS Foundation Trust, London, UK

Maninder S. Kalkat FRCS (Cardiothoracic)
Consultant Cardiothoracic Surgeon, Department of Cardiothoracic
Surgery, Birmingham Heartlands Hospital, Birmingham, UK

Brian Keogh MD
Consultant Anaesthetist and Intensivist, Department of Intensive Care and
Anaesthesia, Royal Brompton & Harefield NHS Foundation Trust,
London, UK

Philip Marino BSc (Hons), MRCP (UK)
Specialist Registrar in Respiratory & Intensive Care Medicine, Kingston
Hospital, Kingston-upon-Thames, UK

Keith McNeil MB, BS, FRACP
Head of Transplant Services, The Prince Charles Hospital, Brisbane,
Australia

Mark Messent MD
Consultant Anaesthetist & Intensivist, Intensive Care Unit, St
Bartholomew's Hospital, London, UK

Hugh Montgomery MB BS, BSc, FRCP, MD
Director, Institute for Human Health and Performance, University
College London, London, UK

James Napier MBChB, FRCS, FCEM, EDICM
Intensive Care Unit, St Bartholomew's Hospital, London, UK

John Pepper M.Chir, FRCS
Professor of Cardiothoracic Surgery, Department of Surgery, Royal
Brompton & Harefield NHS Foundation Trust, London, UK

Divaka Perera MD
Department of Cardiology, Guys' and St Thomas' NHS Foundation Trust,
London, UK

Liao Pinhu MD, PhD
Unit of Critical Care, National Heart and Lung Institute, Imperial
College London, London, UK and Youjiang Medical University for
Nationalities, Baise, PR, China

Michael R. Pinksy MD, CM, DM, MC
Professor of Critical Care Medicine, Department of Critical Care
Medicine, Bioengineering and Anesthesiology, Univerity of Pittsburgh
School of Medicine, Pittsburgh, PA, USA

Kanchan Rege MA, MRCP, FRCPath
Consultant Haematologist, Papworth Hospital, Cambridge, UK

Andrew Rhodes MD
Consultant in Intensive Care Medicine, Department of Anaesthesia and
Intensive Care Medicine, St George's Hospital, London, UK

Vivek Sivaraman MBBS, MRCP, MD
Specialty Trainee, Anaesthetics and Critical Care, Central London School
of Anaesthesia, London, UK

Lorna Swan MB ChB, MRCP, MD
Consultant Cardiologist, Adult Congenital Heart Disease Unit, Royal
Brompton & Harefield NHS Foundation Trust, London, UK

Marius Terblanche MBChB, FRCA, EDIC, Dip(Epid)
Consultant in Critical Care Medicine, Guy's & St Thomas' Hospital,
London, UK

Richard Trimlett MD
Consultant Cardiac Surgeon, Royal Brompton & Harefield NHS
Foundation Trust, London, UK

Jean-Louis Vincent MD, PhD
Professor of Intensive Care Medicine;
Head, Department of Intensive Care, Erasme University Hospital,
University of Brussels, Belgium

Alain Vuylsteke MD, FRCA
Consultant Anaesthesia and Intensive Care, Royal Brompton
& Harefield NHS Foundation Trust, London and Cardiothoracic
Anaesthesia and Intensive Care, Papworth Hospital, Cambridge, UK

Justin Woods FRCA
Clinical Research Fellow in Intensive Care Medicine, Department of
Anaesthesia and Intensive Care Medicine, St George's Hospital,
London, UK

David A. Zideman MD
Chief of Service, Department of Anaesthetics, Imperial College Healthcare
NHS Trust and Hammersmith Hospital, London, UK

Introduction

More than 850,000 people in the United Kingdom suffer from heart failure, at a cost to the NHS of an estimated £625 million per year. Approximately 2.65 million people have coronary artery disease, accounting for 13% of all deaths in England, many of them premature. It has been calculated that the cost of heart disease in the UK today is over £7 billion, a sum that includes the financial burden of informal care provided by more than 400,000 families and friends. Cardiac pathology is also no respecter of age. Thus, the increasing success of surgery provided to children born with heart defects in the 1980s and 1990s has delivered a generation of young adults who require on-going monitoring and treatment. There are approximately 250,000 such adults in the UK.

The burden of disease is therefore significant. The common thread that binds together individuals who suffer from these conditions is both the adverse quality of life that it brings, and the need to design, validate and apply effective therapeutic interventions to extend both life and quality of life. The successes in this area have been legion and include cardiopulmonary bypass surgery, conducted successfully for the first time only in the 1950s; a large and increasing variety of percutaneous interventions both for coronary artery disease and valvular pathologies; the management of arrhythmias both malignant and benign; and novel cardiopulmonary support systems up to and including ventricular assist devices and extracorporeal membrane oxygenation. The development and application of these support systems and therapeutic interventions necessitates the provision of intensive care of the highest quality.

On the Department of Health's Census Day (15 January 2008), there were 3473 Level 2 and Level 3 intensive care unit (ICU) beds occupied in NHS Trusts in England. Sixteen percent (552) of these beds were in cardiothoracic units, although it is almost certain that significant numbers of patients not requiring surgical interventions, but with cardiovascular pathologies, were being cared for in general intensive care or high dependency areas. In certain respects, cardiovascular ICU might be regarded as routine. Thus, for the year ending March 2007, 35,487 cardiac operations were performed with a 96.6% survival rate in over 40 centres in the UK as a whole [1]. These remarkable survival results, comparable to those achieved by the best healthcare systems across the world, are a reflection of the skill not only of surgical and anaesthetic practitioners but also of those involved in the provision of intensive care.

Rapid advances in research and clinical practice in this arena mandate the development of first-rate educational resources for those involved in clinical practice. I am delighted therefore to be able to introduce this volume, edited by three of my colleagues, which provides a superb overview of contemporary cardiovascular critical care. The clinical field involved is broad. Effective pre-operative assessment of patients by intensivists is a skill that all should possess. A working knowledge of the haematological complications of cardiovascular surgery and critical care is mandatory. Care of the medical patient with ischaemic heart disease or in acute cardiogenic shock has progressed in leaps and bounds, and now spills over into the use of adjunct support such as non-invasive respiratory support [2]. The particular problems associated with the management of the patient with adult congenital heart disease are recognised in this volume, together with those consequent upon pregnancy, eclampsia and the hypertensive crisis. Mark Griffiths and colleagues have recruited authors with recognised expertise in their subject, who together have produced a volume that should assist greatly those practising in cardiovascular critical care to the benefit of their patients.

References

1. UK Healthcare Commission statistics, 2008.
2. *New Engl J Med* 2008; 259: 142–51.

Timothy W. Evans DSc FRCP FRCA FMedSci
Professor of Intensive Care Medicine, Imperial College School of Medicine;
Consultant in Intensive Care Medicine, Royal Brompton Hospital, London

1 Shock

Marius Terblanche[1] and Nicole Assmann[2]
[1]Guy's & St Thomas' Hospital, London, UK
[2]Royal Free Hospital, London, UK

Take home messages

- Human survival is absolutely dependent on oxygen for respiration, the process by which cells derive energy in the form of adenosine triphosphate (ATP).
- Mitochondrial respiration is compromised by a reduction in oxygen delivery due to circulatory failure (e.g. hypovolaemic shock) and/or an inability to appropriately utilise delivered oxygen (e.g. during sepsis).
- Circulatory failure of any cause activates a systemic immune/inflammatory response.
- Inflammatory signalling and gene expression of inflammatory mediators starts a cascade of downstream effects often culminating in organ dysfunction or failure.

1.1 Introduction

Oxygen is the most supply-limited metabolic substrate. Under normal physiological conditions oxygen (O_2) supply is closely matched to mitochondrial consumption. Shock is caused by an imbalance between the supply and demand of oxygen. Depending on the aetiology, either the delivery of oxygen and other metabolic substrate is reduced or increased metabolic requirements are unmet despite increased delivery. The inability of peripheral tissues to utilise substrate may contribute to this imbalance.

A number of different conditions can cause shock (Table 1.1). The original Hinshaw and Cox classification differentiated between four main categories [1]. More recently, endocrine shock, caused by thyroid disease or adrenal insufficiency, was recognised as another aetiological category but will not be discussed here [2].

To unravel the often complex clinical scenarios associated with shock, we find it useful to start by differentiating between low versus high cardiac output states. We therefore divide this overview of shock into three parts:

Cardiovascular Critical Care. Edited by M. Griffiths, J. Cordingley and S. Price.
© 2010 Blackwell Publishing Ltd.

Table 1.1 Classification of shock.

Category	Cause of shock
Hypovolaemic	Loss of circulating volume
Cardiogenic	Myocardial or endocardial disease
Obstructive	Mechanical extra-cardiac obstruction of blood flow
Distributive	Vasodilatation and altered distribution of blood flow
Endocrine	Thyroid disease, adrenal insufficiency

- low cardiac output states,
- high output states, and
- the pathway to multi-organ failure.

1.2 Low output states

Low cardiac output and systemic hypoperfusion leads to oxygen supply failure. This situation is exacerbated by anaemia in haemorrhagic shock – oxygen delivery (DO_2I) is determined by the cardiac output (CO) and blood O_2 content (C_aO_2), with the latter predominantly a function of haemoglobin concentration and arterial oxygen saturations.

$$DO_2I = CO \times C_aO_2$$
$$CO \quad = [HR \times SV]$$
$$C_aO_2 = \text{Hb-bound } O_2 + \text{dissolved } O_2$$
$$= [1.39^* \times \text{Hb concentration} \times \text{arterial } O_2 \text{ saturation}] + [0.02^{\ddagger} \times p_aO_2]$$

HR: heart rate; SV: stroke volume; Hb: haemoglobin.
*Each gram of normal haemoglobin contains 1.39 of O_2 when fully saturated. A figure of 1.34 is usually used due to the presence of inactive haemoglobin derivatives.
‡The amount of dissolved O_2 is linearly related to the partial pressure of oxygen (p_aO_2).

Initially, peripheral tissues compensate for the reduced DO_2I through increased O_2 extraction, thus maintaining normal levels of O_2 consumption (VO_2) [3]. This mechanism cannot compensate for DO_2I reductions below a critical level, beyond which VO_2 declines to become 'supply-limited'. Anaerobic metabolism and hyperlactataemia follows while organ function deteriorates in the face of adenosine triphosphate (ATP) depletion and a failure of ion pumps to maintain trans-membrane gradients and cell integrity.

Cellular and tissue hypoxia form a central element in development of multiple organ failure and activate the immune system through a number of mechanisms (see below) [4, 5]. Irrespective of initial cause, continued hypoperfusion and cellular ischaemia triggers complex cascades resulting in the production of pro-inflammatory mediators and leukocyte activation with the release of reactive oxygen species (ROS) and proteolytic enzymes. Nuclear factor kappa-β (NF-kB), hypoxia inducible factor (HIF)-1 and inducible nitric oxide synthase (iNOS) play critical roles [6–10]. As a consequence, the vascular endothelium becomes permeable and expresses cellular adhesion molecules (CAM) and other inflammatory mediators [11, 12].

Low cardiac output-associated oxygen debt is associated with multiple organ failure (MOF) and mortality in post-operative patients [13]. The degree of tissue oxygen debt is similarly related to enhanced inflammatory responses, increased risk of acute lung injury and increased mortality [14]. Clinical studies demonstrate a causal relationship between traumatic injury and/or shock and a predisposition to sepsis/MOF, probably due to an excessive inflammatory response coupled with failure of cell-mediated immunity [15–17].

Hypovolaemic shock

Hypovolaemic shock is caused by a loss of circulating volume and/or non-haemorrhagic causes [2]. The latter include absolute loss of fluid (vomiting, diarrhoea, high-output fistulas or evaporative losses: fever, surgery, burns), or third space fluid sequestration through shifts between the intravascular and extravascular space (trauma, ileus, small bowel obstruction). The resulting decrease in intravascular volume reduces venous return, stroke volume and ultimately cardiac output causing tissue hypoperfusion.

Acute volume loss leads to the activation of compensatory mechanisms involving [18, 19]:
- volume and pressure receptors,
- the sympathetic nervous system (SNS),
- the renin-angiotensin (RAAS) system, and
- anti-diuretic hormone (ADH).

The earliest response arises from mainly atrial and pulmonary pressure receptors. The baroreceptor response and activation of the SNS produces arterial and venous vasoconstriction, and tachycardia. Venous vasoconstriction aims to restore preload and cardiac output, while arterial vasoconstriction increases mean arterial pressure (MAP). Blood flow is also diverted to vital organs (brain, heart, kidneys). Interstitium-to-intravascular space fluid shift (facilitated by reduced capillary pressures) also occurs and expands intravascular volume by as much as 1 litre in the first hour and a further 1 litre during the first 48 hours [20].

The RAAS is activated by the SNS and by a reduction in renal blood flow. Renin, released by the juxtaglomerular cells, leads to an increase in angiotensin II (AT-II). AT-II, a potent vasoconstrictor, stimulates the adrenal production of aldosterone, which in turn promotes renal sodium and water retention. ADH/vasopressin, a hormone secreted by the posterior pituitary, is a potent vasoconstrictor and increases water retention by the kidneys. These events increase circulating volume. During the later stages, erythropoietin is secreted to increase red cell volume and plasma protein synthesis is increased.

Table 1.2 Estimated fluid loss in haemorrhagic shock*.

	Class I	Class II	Class III	Class IV
Blood loss (ml)	Up to 750	750–1500	1500–2000	>2000
Percentage blood volume	Up to 15%	15–30%	30–40%	>40%
Pulse rate (bpm)	<100	>100	>120	>140
Systolic blood pressure	Normal	Normal	Decreased	Decreased
Diastolic blood pressure	Normal	Decreased	Decreased	Decreased
Respiratory rate (per min)	14–20	20–30	30–40	>35
Urine output (ml/hour)	>30	20–30	5–15	<5
Mental status	Slightly anxious	Mildly anxious	Anxious, confused	Confused, lethargic

* For a 70-kg man.
Adapted from Committee on Trauma of the American College of Surgeons [23].

Healthy individuals can compensate for fluid losses of up to 30% of the circulating volume (Table 1.2). However, compensatory responses are highly variable and the ability to tolerate a reduction in cardiac output is greatly influenced by coexisting cardiovascular disease, autonomic neuropathy and medication such as beta-receptor antagonists.

Clinical features
The amount of volume loss chiefly determines the clinical picture. The presentation of hypovolaemic shock is that of a low cardiac output state. SNS activation causes vasoconstriction of cutaneous vessels and activation of sympathetic innervated sweat glands. Tachycardia, and pale, cold, clammy skin, or diaphoresis is clinically seen while capillary refill is reduced. Oliguria reflects a decreased renal perfusion pressure and insufficient compensatory mechanisms to minimise renal fluid losses. Similarly, cerebral hypoperfusion leads to agitation and later to coma. Respiratory compensation for the developing metabolic acidosis is evident as tachypnoea, often without a subjective feeling of shortness of breath.

Management
Managing a patient with shock requires a robust and organised team approach. The sequence of interventions is dictated by the presenting picture. As a general rule the aims of management are to maintain oxygenation, control bleeding and substitute circulating volume sufficiently to avoid significant cellular hypoxia, but without aiming for a normal blood pressure.

Resuscitation should be guided by clinical and laboratory makers of tissue perfusion (such as pH, lactate and base excess). Importantly, clinicians should remember that all of these markers share the disadvantage of being global indicators which show delayed normalisation during resuscitation. A trend towards improvement rather than full normalisation of these parameters is an appropriate short-term goal.

Although securing the airway and maintaining oxygenation is a priority in any critical condition, controlling the source of bleeding is the crucial first step in the management of haemorrhagic shock. This may have to be achieved by direct compression or rapid surgical intervention, occasionally prior to the restoration of circulating volume. Fluid resuscitation should, however, be commenced concurrently. Large bore intravenous access must be established rapidly and rapid infusing devices may be needed to keep up with losses. The source of bleeding may be external and obvious, but source identification may require investigations such as ultrasound scan, computed tomography (CT) or angiography.

In less severe bleeding or after the initial control of bleeding, at least partial restoration of circulating volume is the major management component. Aggressive restoration of circulating volume and mean arterial pressure before surgical treatment may worsen the outcome, possibly by promoting clot dissolution and rebleeding [21]. Clinicians must therefore find a balance between these complications and maintaining a DO_2I sufficient to avoid multiple organ failure.

Blood loss up to 20–30% of circulating volume may be replaced with balanced crystalloid or colloid solutions; beyond that, red cell transfusion is usually required. Whether crystalloids or colloids are superior for fluid resuscitation is still under debate. Crystalloids distribute in the extracellular space, with about 20% of the infused volume remaining in the circulation. This necessitates infusion of large volumes, with the potential for causing oedema and subsequent impaired oxygen and substrate diffusion into cells. Activation of neutrophils, which contribute to organ dysfunction, and dilution of plasma proteins are further disadvantages [22]. To avoid hyperchloraemic acidosis, balanced solutions such as Hartmann's should be used instead of normal saline.

Colloids expand the intravascular space more and for longer than crystalloids. If endothelial integrity becomes compromised, however, leakage into the interstitium may occur and worsen oedema. Colloids also affect clotting and impair renal function. Gelatins are currently considered to have the least detrimental effect on the kidneys and may be the colloid of choice. In analogy to the finding with crystalloids, solutions with a balanced electrolyte composition could be advantageous. The Advanced Trauma Life Support guidelines currently recommend crystalloids as the fluid of choice in haemorrhagic shock, but since the question is not clearly settled many clinicians continue to use a combination of colloids and crystalloids [23].

Severe bleeding is associated with consumption and dilution of clotting factors and platelets. Platelets and clotting factors (fresh frozen plasma, cryoprecipitate) are therefore commonly replaced. Other pro-coagulant agents, such as recombinant factor VIIa or prothrombin complex, have been successfully used in severe haemorrhage, but their effectiveness remains unconfirmed by randomised trials. Point of care testing is increasingly used and is in the authors' experience very helpful, giving accurate results within minutes.

Clotting products and platelets should ideally be administered after obtaining appropriate laboratory results (prothrombin time, PT; activated partial thromboplastin time, APTT; fibrinogen levels, platelet count). Fresh frozen plasma (FFP) is usually administered if clotting times are more than 1.5 times normal, particularly if bleeding is ongoing. Fibrinogen levels should be checked and cryoprecipitate given if levels are less than 1.0 mg/dl. The threshold for platelet transfusion is less clearly defined. Platelet counts of less than 50 000 μ/l with ongoing bleeding may warrant substitution. In patients on antiplatelet medication higher thresholds may be appropriate.

Cardiogenic shock

In cardiogenic shock, primary cardiac dysfunction in the presence of an adequate circulating volume causes tissue hypoperfusion and hypoxia. Haemodynamic criteria for diagnosis include hypotension (systolic blood pressure < 90 mmHg), reduced cardiac index (cardiac output related to body surface area; CI < 2.2 l/min/m²) and elevated pulmonary capillary wedge pressure (a reflection of left ventricular end-diastolic pressure; PCWP > 15 mmHg).

Myocardial infarction is the commonest cause. Other causes include myocarditis, end-stage cardiomyopathy, myocardial contusion after chest trauma and endocardial pathology (e.g. acute endocarditis or papillary muscle rupture causing acute regurgitant valvular defects).

Myocardial perfusion is critically dependent on the perfusion window, determined by perfusion *pressure* (diastolic pressure in proximal aorta minus ventricular wall pressure) and perfusion *time* (diastolic time). Myocardial relaxation (diastolic) and contractility (systolic) dysfunction due to ischaemia reduce myocardial compliance, and hence filling. As a consequence, stroke volume, cardiac output and proximal aortic blood pressure fall. Simultaneous increases in ventricular end-diastolic pressures increase wall tension. Furthermore, tachycardia reduces perfusion time. Together, these changes cause a further decrease in coronary perfusion and further aggravate the situation.

Compensatory mechanisms (SNS, RAAS) resulting in tachycardia, higher afterload and fluid retention increase myocardial oxygen demand at a time when supply is already significantly impaired. Arrhythmias and valvular dysfunction sometimes associated with ventricular dilatation often make a bad situation worse.

The clinical features and management options are discussed in detail in Chapters 13 and 14.

Obstructive shock

Mechanical obstruction of cardiac output can be caused by impaired ventricular filling due to cardiac tamponade, tension pneumothorax, pulmonary embolus or uncommonly haemothorax and ascites.

Cardiac tamponade occurs as a complication of acute myocardial infarction with rupture of the free ventricular wall, after cardiac surgery or following chest trauma. A relatively small but rapidly expanding accumulation of blood within the pericardium (less than 200 ml) impairs ventricular filling to such a degree that cardiac output is compromised. A slowly accumulating effusion can also eventually lead to significant filling impairment, but much higher amounts of pericardial fluid are necessary as the pericardial sack has sufficient time to stretch.

Typical clinical features of tamponade are tachycardia, jugular venous distension, muffled heart sounds and pulsus paradoxus. Hypotension, largely resistant to fluid administration, is present. The diagnosis is usually made or confirmed by echocardiography. Drainage of the accumulated pericardial blood or fluid is the definitive treatment. Following cardiac surgery, anecdotal evidence suggests that oliguria and a worsening base deficit in the context of rising central venous pressures should prompt urgent echocardiography to exclude tamponade.

Tension pneumothorax presents with a very similar picture, but absent breath sounds and hyperresonance of the affected side suggest pneumothorax. It develops when air entering the pleural space cannot escape due to a flap-valve mechanism. Intrapleural accumulation of air leads to a rise in intrathoracic pressure, collapse of the affected lung, and mediastinal shift to the opposite side, which severely reduces cardiac filling and output. Immediate release of the intrathoracic pressure by placement of a large bore needle in the second intercostal space in the mid-clavicular line on the affected side is the appropriate treatment.

Obstruction of the pulmonary vasculature by *pulmonary emboli* (thrombus or air) may cause a clinical picture similar to that described above. Large pulmonary emboli lead to a sudden increase in right ventricular afterload and right ventricular failure. It is not clear whether mechanical outflow obstruction alone causes this picture of acute pulmonary hypertension and subsequent circulatory failure; the release of vasoactive mediators has also been implicated [24]. The clinical features and management options of thromboembolic disease are discussed in detail in Chapter 21.

1.3 High output states

Sepsis

Sepsis is an overwhelming response to infection characterised by systemic inflammation and widespread tissue injury [25, 26]. Clinical diagnosis requires evidence of infection plus, traditionally, at least two signs of systemic inflammatory response syndrome (SIRS). However, expanded diagnostic criteria for SIRS in response to infection were recently proposed (Table 1.3) [27]. Severe sepsis is defined as sepsis with new onset organ failure. Septic shock represents a state of persistent arterial hypotension despite adequate volume resuscitation, and which is unexplained by other causes.

Epidemiology

Sepsis occurs in approximately 25% of ICU patients, and bacteraemic sepsis in 10% [28]. Furthermore, approximately 27% of patients admitted to ICU in the United Kingdom meet the criteria for severe sepsis within 24 hours following ICU admission [29]. Mortality rates range between 19 and 96%

Table 1.3 Diagnostic criteria for sepsis and severe sepsis.

Infection

Documented or suspected *and* some of the signs of systemic inflammation

Signs of systemic inflammation

General parameters	Fever or hypothermia; heart rate; tachypnoea; altered mental state; significant oedema or positive fluid balance; hyperglycaemia
Inflammatory parameters	Leukocytosis or leukopaenia; increase in immature white cell bands; elevated CRP or procalcitonin
Haemodynamic parameters	Arterial hypotension; elevated mixed venous oxygen saturation or cardiac index; arterial hypoxaemia; acute oliguria; increased creatinine; coagulation abnormalities; ileus; thrombocytopenia; hyperbilirubinaemia
Tissue perfusion parameters	Hyperlactataemia; decreased capillary refill or mottling

Organ dysfunction and failure

Organ failure can be diagnosed by using the MODS or SOFA score [63, 64].

Septic shock

A state characterised by persistent arterial hypotension despite adequate volume resuscitation, and unexplained by other causes.

Hypotension is defined by	systolic arterial pressure below 90 mmHg, or mean arterial pressure lower than 60 mmHg, or reduction in systolic blood pressure of more than 40 mmHg from baseline

Adapted from Levy et al. [27].

MODS, multiple organ dysfunction score; SOFA, sequential organ failure assessment.

[28]. Note, patients still categorised as having severe sepsis at the end of the 30-day follow-up period had a 96% mortality rate [30]. In the same study, progression to severe sepsis and septic shock in patients with infection/sepsis occurred in 10.9 and 13.1%, respectively.

Pathophysiology

The receptors of the innate immune system recognise pathogen-associated molecular patterns. Pattern recognition receptors (PRRs) (Table 1.4) have a number of functions, including opsonisation, activation of complement, activation of the coagulation cascades, phagocytosis, activation of proinflammatory signal pathways, and the induction of apoptosis. Cells bearing PRRs – macrophages, dendritic cells, mast cells, neutrophils, eosinophils, natural killer (NK) cells – are activated by inflammation and rapidly differentiate into short-lived effector cells to eradicate the infection.

Toll-like receptors (TLRs) are cell surface-based PRRs. TLRs are potent initiators of the host response to infection and have been termed the 'light and the fire' of septic shock [31]. TLRs have a wide range of specificity, being activated by bacterial, fungal and yeast proteins. For example, host cell activation following exposure to lipopolysaccharide (LPS), originating from Gram-negative bacteria, is dependent on LPS-binding protein (LBP)

Table 1.4 Pattern recognition receptors (PRR).

PRRs in the extracellular compartment
- Mannan-binding lection (MBL)
- C-reactive protein (CRP)
- Serum amyloid protein (SAP)

PRRs based on cell surfaces
- Toll-like receptors (TLRs)
- Peptidoglycan-recognition proteins (PGRPs)
- Triggering receptor expressed on myeloid cells (TREM-1)
- Myeloid DAP12-associating lectin (MDL-1)
- Macrophage mannose receptor (MMR)
- Macrophage scavenging receptor (MSR)

PRRs in the intracellular compartment
- Protein kinase (PKR)
- Nucleotide-binding oligomerisation domain (NOD-1, NOD-2)
- 2′–5′-oligoadenylate synthase (OAS)/ RNaseL pathway (OAS/RNaseL)

and the opsonic receptor CD14. The LPS/LBP-CD14 complex binds TLR4, leading to the activation of inflammatory signalling.

Clinical picture
Patients with septic shock by definition have an infection, show signs of systemic inflammation, and will be hypotensive with concomitant symptoms and signs of inadequate tissue perfusion. Patients may have fever or be hypothermic. Heart and respiratory rates are elevated. Further signs of SIRS, such as leukocytosis or leukopaenia, hyperglycaemia and peripheral oedema, are often present. CRP and procalcitonin levels are usually increased. Unless the patient is also hypovolaemic, the typical picture is one of a high cardiac output and reduced systemic vascular resistance.

Systolic blood pressures below 90 mmHg or mean arterial pressures below 70 mmHg in the absence of vasopressors are commonly seen. Signs of inadequate tissue perfusion, such as hyperlactataemia and decreased capillary refill time or mottled skin, are also often present. Mixed or central venous oxygen saturation is often elevated due to reduced peripheral extraction. However, low saturations imply an inadequate cardiac output for the existing metabolic demand. This finding is especially important when associated with a raised lactate level since it highlights potentially correctable cellular hypoxia.

Due to the combination of a dysregulated circulation (at systemic and microcirculatory level) and the inflammatory response, the function of other organs is often disturbed and arterial hypoxaemia, acute oliguria and an increased creatinine, hyperbilirubinaemia, and alterations in mental state or coma are frequently encountered.

Management
Critical care and infectious disease experts representing 11 international organisations recently developed management guidelines for severe sepsis

and septic shock [32]. These guidelines, presented in the form of a Resuscitation Bundle and a Management Bundle, integrate evidence-based interventions with process-of-care measures (Table 1.4). The haemodynamic management of septic shock is referred to here but is discussed in detail in Chapter 12.

Other high output shock states

Neurogenic shock resulting from spinal cord damage at or above the upper thoracic level is commonly seen after trauma. The central nervous system injury causes autonomic dysfunction. Disruption of the sympathetic innervation leads to vasodilatation and bradycardia. It is characterised by severe hypotension, slow or normal heart rate and warm skin, indicating the inability to respond to the reduced systemic vascular resistance, with vasoconstriction and an increased heart rate. The relative hypovolaemia is treated with cautious fluid resuscitation, taking into account that coexisting injuries with blood loss may aggravate the picture and warrant a more aggressive approach. Vasoconstrictors are indicated when hypotension persists despite euvolaemia. Bradycardia is treated with anticholinergic agents.

Anaphylactic shock occurs when a sensitised individual with pre-existing IgE antibodies is exposed to an antigen. The binding of the antigen to its corresponding IgE antibody on the surface of mast cells causes a type I immune response with mast cell degranulation and release of vasoactive substances such as histamine.

The clinical picture reflects the resulting vasodilatation, increased vascular permeability, bronchospasm and in severe cases myocardial depression: urticaria or generalised erythema, breathing difficulties and hypotension or cardiovascular collapse characterise the condition. Treatment consists of stopping exposure to the antigen, ensuring oxygenation and use of adrenaline as primary therapy, followed by fluid resuscitation. Corticosteroids and antihistamine agents are also administered [33].

1.4 The pathway to organ failure

Shock and resuscitation produce inflammation. Irrespective of the initiating trigger, similar inflammatory pathways are activated which leads to similar downstream effects on organ function (Figure 1.1).

Intracellular signal pathways and inflammatory gene expression

Signals from the extracellular space are transmitted through the cell membrane and subsequently propagated via a number of serial or parallel proteins serving as transducers or regulators. The main pathways are the protein kinase system activating the transcription factor nuclear factor-κB (NF-κB), and three mitogen-activated protein kinase (MAPK) cascades which lead to the activation of other transcription factors including the activator protein-1 (AP-1) family [34].

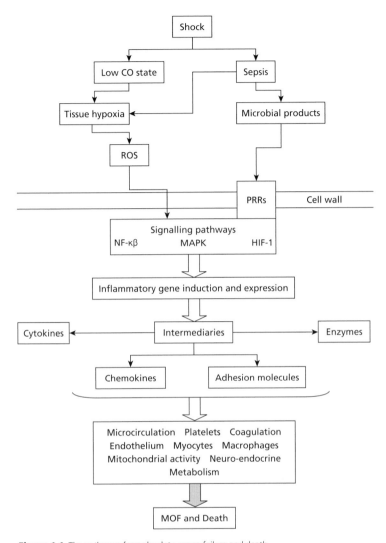

Figure 1.1 The pathways from shock to organ failure and death.

Effects of gene induction and the role of intermediaries

Gene induction and expression generate a variety of inflammatory mediators, which include cytokines, chemokines, adhesion molecules and enzymes.

Cytokines

Numerous cytokines are produced with pro- and anti-inflammatory actions (Table 1.5). The primary proinflammatory cytokines are interleukin (IL)-1 and tissue necrosis factor (TNF)-α. Both further activate inflammatory signalling pathways, leading to an amplification of the response. TNF-α additionally activates apoptosis via a 'death' pathway.

Table 1.5 Main actions and effects of inflammatory cytokines [50, 62, 65–67].

Pro-inflammatory cytokines	Anti-inflammatory cytokines
TNF-α ● regulates cell proliferation and apoptosis ● recruits and activate neutrophils, macrophages and lymphocytes **IL-1β** ● similar biological effects to TNF-α but produces less severe response ● causes hypotension, increased cardiac output, leuko- and thrombocytopenia, pulmonary oedema and lactic acidosis **IL-6** ● stimulates release of acute-phase proteins (e.g. CRP, SAA) by hepatocytes **IL-12** ● hepato- and splenomegaly, leukopaenia, anaemia, myelodepression, pulmonary oedema ● interstitial macrophage infiltration **IFN-γ** ● tachycardia, myalgia, malaise and leukopaenia ● enhances mortality and levels of circulating TNF-α induced by LPS **LIF/OSM** ● LIF: activates other cytokines ● OSM: enhances expression of chemokines **MIF** ● enhances lethality of LPS ● counter-regulates the inhibitory effects of glucocorticoids on cytokine production ● activates lymphocytes and stimulates antibody production ● causes the release of IL-2 and IFN-γ ● increases the production of pro-inflammatory cytokines and chemokines by macrophages **HMGB1** ● phagocytic cell activation ● evokes intracellular signalling with increased expression of RAGE, adhesion molecules, TNF-α, chemokines, PAI-1 and tPA ● increases activity of iNOS in enterocytes **G-CSF** ● proliferation, differentiation and activation of lymphocytes	**IL-4** ● reduces LPS-induced cytokine production by monocytes and macrophages **IL-10** ● inhibits release of TNF-α, IL-1 and IL-6 by endotoxin-stimulated macrophages **IL-13** ● downregulates monocyte and macrophage function **IL-6** ● inhibits release of IL-1 and TNF-α **TGF-β** ● deactivates monocytes and macrophages ● decreases expression of MHC class II ● inhibits synthesis of TNF-α and IL-1 **IL-1ra** ● competitive inhibitor of IL-1 receptor **Soluble receptors** ● TNFR: binds TNF-α to prevent ligand–receptor interaction ● IL-6R: prolongs half-life of IL-6

TNF-α, tissue necrosis factor; IL, interleukin; CRP, C-reactive protein; SAA, serum amyloid A; IFN, interferon; LIF, leukaemia inhibitory factor; OSM, oncostatin M; MIF, macrophage migration factor; LPS, lipopolysaccharide; HMGB1, high mobility group B1; PAI, platelet activator inhibitor; tPA, tissue plasminogen activator; G-CSF, granulocyte-colony stimulating factor; TGF, transforming growth factor; TNF-α/IL-ra, interleukin receptor antagonist; RAGE, receptor of advanced glycation end-products.

Chemokines

Chemokines affect leukocyte function and trafficking. IL-8, a major neutrophil chemotactic factor, is expressed under the influence of TNF-α and IL-1. Its actions include the proliferation, differentiation and activation of leukocytes. RANTES (regulated upon activation, normal T-cells expressed and secreted) are mainly produced by activated T-cells and are stimulated by IL-1 and TNF-α. RANTES recruits and activates monocytes, lymphocytes and eosinophils. Lastly, monocyte-chemoattractant protein (MCP)-1 contributes to the recruitment of inflammatory macrophages.

Adhesion molecules

Activated endothelial and epithelial cells express adhesion receptors which control leukocyte adhesion and trafficking at the site of inflammation. Selectins (P-, E- and L-selectin) mediate leukocyte rolling along the vessel wall, simultaneously sensing the presence of activating factors on endothelial cell surface (EC) surface. Stimulated neutrophils express beta-2 integrins, which mediate firm adhesion to ECs by binding to intercellular adhesion molecules (ICAM-1, 2) and vascular cell adhesion molecule (VCAM-1). These firm associations with neutrophils precede their transmigration through the EC layer into inflamed tissues. Soluble forms of various adhesion molecules, such as the selectins, are released into plasma during an inflammatory response and therefore have been used as markers of endothelial activation.

Enzymes

The two main enzyme systems activated as part of the inflammatory process involve eiconasoids and nitric oxide synthase [35–37].

1. *Eiconasoids*: IL-1 and TNF-α stimulate membrane lipid metabolism by phospholipase A to form arachidonic acid and lyso-platelet activating factor (PAF). Arachidonic acid is subsequently metabolised via the cyclo-oxygenase and lipoxygenase pathways to form prostaglandins and leukotrienes, respectively, while lyso-PAF is transformed by acetyltransferase to platelet activating factor (PAF). The effects of eiconasoid induction are multiple (Table 1.6).

2. *Nitric oxide synthase*: Nitric oxide (NO) is physiologically produced by the constitutive enzyme endothelial NO synthase (eNOS) in response to local blood flow. NO regulates vasomotor tone and microvascular blood flow, and inhibits leukocyte and platelet adhesion.

   During inflammation, expression of an inducible form of NOS (iNOS) is increased predominantly in vascular smooth muscle. NO production by iNOS is unregulated and an order of magnitude greater than that of eNOS. The subsequent overproduction of NO is associated with a decrease in blood pressure, impaired vascular reactivity, abnormal RBC deformability and reduced oxygen consumption. Although inhibiting NO during sepsis increases blood pressure, it also reduces microvascular blood flow and exacerbates abnormal oxygen transport.

Effects of activation of the pro-inflammatory system

The expression of cytokines, chemokines, enzymes and adhesion molecules sets the scene for the development of organ failure by affecting the microcirculation, endothelium, coagulation system, mitochondrial respiration, white blood cells, neuro-endocrine system, hepatocytes and the complement system.

Table 1.6 Clinical effects of eiconasoids [35, 67].

Prostaglandins
- Smooth muscle contraction
- Mucosal oedema
- Increased vascular permeability
- Cellular infiltration
- Mucus secretion

Prostaglandin E2
- Inhibits TNF-α secretion
- Enhances IL-6 secretion

Thomboxane A2
- Stimulates TNF-α and IL-1 secretion

Leukotrienes
- Increased vascular permeability
- Vasodilation
- Smooth muscle contraction

Platelet activating factor
- Activates and aggregates platelets
- Stimulates release of vasoactive mediators

Microcirculation

Inflammation induces changes in microvascular geometry, haemodynamics and oxygen transport [36]. Increased microvascular stopped-flow (the stopping of flow through capillaries seen during sepsis) results in a maldistribution of blood flow within the microcirculation and a consequent loss of matching between local oxygen demand and delivery. Increased oxygen flow heterogeneity possibly further impairs oxygen extraction.

Endothelium

The pro-inflammatory response causes endothelial cell (EC) injury, activation and dysfunction [37]. The physical disruption associated with *endothelial injury* allows inflammatory fluid and cells to shift from the blood into the interstitial space [38]. ECs also interfere directly with the initiation and regulation of fibrin formation and removal during severe infection, and may also play a prominent role in all three major pathogenic pathways associated with coagulopathy in sepsis (see below).

Endothelial dysfunction refers to decreased endothelial-dependent vascular relaxation and decreased expression or activity of eNOS. In healthy volunteers, even brief exposure to endotoxin or certain cytokines impairs endothelium-dependent relaxation for many days [39, 40]. This effect has been termed 'endothelial stunning'. Furthermore, failure of an EC's ability to sense changes in its environment may further contribute to a failure in matching oxygen supply to demand [41].

Platelets and the coagulation system

Nearly all patients with shock have coagulation abnormalities ranging from a small decrease in the platelet count and a subclinical prolongation of global clotting times, to fulminant disseminated intravascular coagulation (DIC) [42]. Under normal circumstances, haemostasis is a balance between opposing systems. The prothrombotic system attempts to form thrombin and a fibrin clot. Tissue factor (TF) is the main activator of coagulation. On the other hand, thrombin generation is limited by antithrombin (AT), the protein C system and tissue factor pathway inhibitor (TFPI), while ECs express various membrane-associated components with anticoagulant properties.

Pro-inflammatory mediators induce TF expression on the surface of activated mononuclear cells and vascular ECs, while the antithrombotic and fibrinolytic regulatory systems become defective due to endothelial dysfunction. This activation of coagulation and impaired fibrinolysis is associated with fibrin deposition and tissue ischaemia and necrosis, and in critically ill patients with an increased risk for death [43]. Conversely, inhibition of coagulation is associated with prevention of organ dysfunction [44].

Monocytes/macrophages

Macrophages are possibly the most important source of cytokines and are responsible for the primary response to microorganisms in most tissues [45]. Macrophages remove endotoxin and bacteria from the lymph and blood circulation. Macrophage activation also induces the production of intracellular O_2 radicals, hydrogen peroxide, NO and other microbicidal products, thus killing phagocytosed organisms. However, these products can cause extensive tissue damage.

Neutrophils

Neutrophil activation by opsonins and soluble stimuli (cytokines and chemokines) is crucial for host defence against bacterial or fungal infection. They are the principal phagocytes delivered to inflammatory sites. The neutrophil's destructive capacity leads to host injury in numerous disease states [46, 47].

Neutrophil-mediated tissue injury is dependent upon a balance of competing protective and destructive pathways. Host protection is normally achieved through a number of mechanisms. Antioxidants and powerful protease inhibitors within the extracellular matrix inactivate destructive enzymes and oxidants. These anti-proteases are in return inactivated by hypochlorous acid produced by neutrophil myeloperoxidase. Secondly, neutrophils contain antioxidants to protect themselves and surrounding tissue. Lastly, neutrophils are cleared without releasing their toxic contents as they would after necrotic cell death, through the process of apoptosis and removal by tissue macrophages. While TNF-α increases neutrophil apoptosis rates in healthy human controls, numerous inflammatory agents inhibit neutrophil apoptosis in disease states [48, 49].

Mitochondrial activity

Although mitochondrial respiration increases during the early phase of acute critical illness, it invariably falls after 12–16 hours [50]. This decrease appears to be an acquired intrinsic defect in cellular respiration, a phenomenon termed 'cytopathic hypoxia' [51].

Although the exact mechanism for these changes remains unclear, inhibition of cytochrome *a, a3* and one or more mitochondrial respiratory complexes may play a role. Furthermore, recent data have highlighted the importance of nicotinamide adenine dinucleotide (NAD+/NADH) depletion through the activation of the enzyme poly(ADP-ribose) polymerase-1 (PARP) [52]. PARP is a nuclear enzyme activated in response to DNA injury. Through a number of mechanisms, PARP causes acute cell dysfunction and necrotic cell death. In addition, PARP activation plays an important role in the up-regulation of inflammatory cascades through interaction with several transcription factors.

Metabolism

Profound metabolic alterations, including hypermetabolism, enhanced energy expenditure and insulin resistance, occur during shock and critical illness [53]. Alterations in carbohydrate metabolism and muscle tissue protein catabolism follow. These changes are exacerbated by cytokine release. During sepsis, glycaemic control is further disturbed due to insulin resistance and the loss of feedback control [54]. Although low cardiac output states are associated with hyperlactataemia due to tissue hypoxia, the elevated lactate levels seen in stable septic patients appear to be mainly a result of impaired clearance [55].

Neuro-endocrine system

The acute-phase response is associated with the release of stress hormones, including catecholamines, vasopressin, adrenocorticotropic hormone (and cortisol), glucagons and growth hormone. In this way an effective circulation is maintained and energy substrate levels are increased.

A number of endocrine changes are seen during critical illness and shock [56]. These include insulin resistance, reductions in vasopressin concentration, the sick euthyroid syndrome, reduced adrenal responsiveness and inhibition of anabolism. The underlying mechanisms for these changes are unclear, but increased secretions of stress hormones, cytokines and NO have been implicated [54, 57, 58]. Importantly, the magnitude of these changes has prognostic implications [59, 60].

Hormones, reactive nitrogen and oxygen species also affect mitochondrial function. Since mitochondria have receptors for glucocorticoids and thyroid hormones, increased thyroid hormone levels increase the maximum rate of ATP synthesis while reducing production efficiency [61]. All these changes combine to reduce energy production. The fall in ATP supply exerts a further negative effect on metabolic pathways.

Complement system

The complement system supports both innate and humoral immunity by depositing complement components on immune targets, and by promoting inflammation.[62] Activation of this enzyme cascade results in a rapid amplification of the system, causing enhanced production of inflammatory mediators, increased recruitment of leukocytes to sites of infection, enhanced neutrophil–EC interaction, and increased local blood flow and capillary permeability.

1.5 Conclusion

Cell stress, in the form of inadequate tissue perfusion during low output states or direct contact with microorganisms, activates signalling pathways leading to induction and expression of inflammatory mediators. Endothelial abnormalities and associated dysregulated coagulation, coupled with the local toxic effects of immune cell activation contribute to failure of oxygen delivery and consumption at the level of the microcirculation. Meanwhile, mitochondrial dysfunction results in cellular hypoxia and decreased oxygen consumption. The end result is catastrophic destabilisation of organ function, often leading to death.

Case study

A 67-year-old female smoker presented to the emergency department with community-acquired pneumonia. She was clammy, confused and oliguric. Arterial blood gases, taken while receiving oxygen at high flow via a face mask, showed severe hypoxia (p_aO_2 6.8 kPa, p_aCO_2 4.5 kPa) and lactic acidosis (pH 7.12, lactate 7.5 mmol/l). Her mean arterial blood pressure (MAP) was 45 mmHg, white cell count $28 \times 10^9/l$ and C-reactive protein level 452 mg/l.

Appropriate antibiotic therapy was administered, invasive ventilation initiated, and a central venous catheter inserted. The cardiac index and central venous oxygen saturations ($S_{cv}O_2$) at this stage were 1.8 l/min/m^2 and 52%, respectively. Rapid volume resuscitation increased her cardiac index to 2.5 l/min/m^2 and $S_{cv}O_2$ to 71%. The serum lactate decreased to 2.2 mmol/l. Despite these improvements her MAP remained low and vasopressor therapy (noradrenaline) was started, causing her MAP to increase to 65–70 mmHg.

Over the next 24 hours she was mechanically ventilated using a protective ventilatory strategy, her blood glucose level was normalised, and a low-dose hydrocortisone infusion was started pending the results of an adrenocorticotrophic hormone (ACTH) test. Continuous renal replacement therapy was also started.

Over the next 2 weeks she gradually improved. A percutaneous tracheostomy was performed on day 4 and antibiotic coverage was stopped on day 5. Her oxygenation improved and renal function recovered. On day 11 she was liberated from mechanical ventilation and was finally discharged from the ICU after 15 days.

References

1. Hinshaw L, Cox B. *The Fundamental Mechanisms of Shock*. New York: Plenum Press, 1972:13.
2. Cheatham M, Block E, Promes J, HG S. Shock: an overview. In: Irwin R, Rippe J, eds. *Intensive Care Medicine*. Philadelphia: Lippincot Williams & Wilkins, 2003:1761–78.
3. McLuckie A. Shock: an overview. In: Bersten A, Soni N, Oh T, eds. *Oh's Intensive Care Manual*. Butterworth Heineman, 2003:71–8.
4. Villavicencio R, Billiar T. *The Role of Nitric Oxide in the Initiation of Inflammation in Shock. Immune Response in the Critically Ill*. Berlin Heidelberg: Springer-Verlag, 2002:182–9.
5. Vincent J-L, Lopes Ferreira F. Multiple organ failure: clinical syndrome. In: Evans T, Fink MP, eds. *Mechanisms of Organ Dysfunction in Critical Illness*. Berlin Heidelberg: Springer-Verlag, 2002:394–403.
6. Schumacher P. Cellular response to hypoxia: role of oxidant signal transduction. In: Evans T, Fink MP, eds. *Mechanisms of Organ Failure in Critical Illness*. Berlin Heidelberg: Springer-Verlag, 2002:3–16.
7. Hierholzer C, Harbrecht B, Menezes JM, et al. Essential role of induced nitric oxide in the initiation of the inflammatory response after hemorrhagic shock. *J Exp Med* 1998; 187:917–28.
8. Guillemin K, Krasnow MA. The hypoxic response: huffing and HIFing. *Cell* 1997; 89:9–12.
9. LaRocco MT, Rodriguez LF, Chen CY, et al. Reevaluation of the linkage between acute hemorrhagic shock and bacterial translocation in the rat. *Circ Shock* 1993; 40:212–20.
10. Szabo C, Thiemermann C. Invited opinion: role of nitric oxide in hemorrhagic, traumatic, and anaphylactic shock and thermal injury. *Shock* 1994; 2:145–55.
11. Ali MH, Schlidt SA, Chandel NS, et al. Endothelial permeability and IL-6 production during hypoxia: role of ROS in signal transduction. *Am J Physiol* 1999; 277:L1057–65.
12. Chandel NS, Trzyna WC, McClintock DS, et al. Role of oxidants in NF-kappa B activation and TNF-α gene transcription induced by hypoxia and endotoxin. *J Immunol* 2000; 165:1013–21.
13. Shoemaker WC, Appel PL, Kram HB. Tissue oxygen debt as a determinant of lethal and nonlethal postoperative organ failure. *Crit Care Med* 1988; 16:1117–20.
14. Rixen D, Siegel JH. Metabolic correlates of oxygen debt predict posttrauma early acute respiratory distress syndrome and the related cytokine response. *J Trauma* 2000; 49:392–403.
15. Faist E, Angele M, Zedler S. Immunoregulation in shock, trauma and sepsis. In: Marshall J, Cohen J, eds. *Immune Response in the Critically Ill*. Berlin Heidelberg: Springer-Verlag, 2002:312–35.
16. Chaudry I, Ayala A. *Immunological Aspects of Hemorrhage*. Austin: RG Landes Company, 1992:1–132.
17. Faist E, Baue AE, Dittmer H, et al. Multiple organ failure in polytrauma patients. *J Trauma* 1983; 23:775–87.
18. Ganong W. Cardiovascular homeostasis in health & disease. In: Ganong W, ed. *Review of Medical Physiology*. Vol. 18. Stamford: Appleton & Lange, 1997:586–601.
19. Ganong W. Cardiovascular regulatory mechanisms. In: Ganong W, ed. *Review of Medical Physiology*. Vol. 18. Stamford: Appleton & Lange, 1997:553–66.

20. Drucker WR, Chadwick CD, Gann DS. Transcapillary refill in hemorrhage and shock. *Arch Surg* 1981; 116:1344–53.

21. Bickell WH, Wall MJ, Jr, Pepe PE, et al. Immediate versus delayed fluid resuscitation for hypotensive patients with penetrating torso injuries. *N Engl J Med* 1994; 331:1105–9.

22. Rhee P, Burris D, Kaufmann C, et al. Lactated Ringer's solution resuscitation causes neutrophil activation after hemorrhagic shock. *J Trauma* 1998; 44:313–9.

23. Committee on Trauma of the American College of Surgeons. *Advanced Trauma Life Support for Doctors*. Chicago, 1997:98.

24. Almog Y, Avnon LS. The pressure is rising. *Crit Care Med* 2007; 35:323–4.

25. Terblanche M, Almog Y, Rosenson R, Smith T, Hackam D. Statins: panacea for sepsis? *Lancet Infect Dis* 2006; 6:242–8.

26. Terblanche M, Brett SJ. SIRS and the postoperative stress response. *J Crit Care* 2006; 21:53–5.

27. Levy MM, Fink MP, Marshall JC, et al. 2001 SCCM/ESICM/ACCP/ATS/SIS International Sepsis Definitions Conference. *Crit Care Med* 2003; 31:1250–6.

28. Brun-Buisson C. The epidemiology of the systemic inflammatory response. *Intensive Care Med* 2000; 26 Suppl 1:S64–74.

29. Padkin A, Goldfrad C, Brady AR, et al. Epidemiology of severe sepsis occurring in the first 24 hrs in intensive care units in England, Wales, and Northern Ireland. *Crit Care Med* 2003; 31:2332–8.

30. Alberti C, Brun-Buisson C, Chevret S, et al. Systemic inflammatory response and progression to severe sepsis in critically ill infected patients. *Am J Respir Crit Care Med* 2005; 171:461–8.

31. Beutler B. Science review: key inflammatory and stress pathways in critical illness – the central role of the Toll-like receptors. *Crit Care* 2003; 7:39–46.

32. Dellinger RP, Carlet JM, Masur H, et al. Surviving Sepsis Campaign guidelines for management of severe sepsis and septic shock. *Crit Care Med* 2008; 36:297–327.

33. Pongracic JA, Kim JS. Update on epinephrine for the treatment of anaphylaxis. *Curr Opin Pediatr* 2007; 19:94–8.

34. Saklatvala J, Clark A, Dean J. The intracellular signaling pathways in inflammatory stress. In: Evans T, Fink M, eds. *Mechanisms of Organ Dysfunction in Critical Illness*. Berlin Heidelberg: Springer-Verlag, 2002:137–45.

35. Cook JA. Eicosanoids. *Crit Care Med* 2005; 33:S488–91.

36. Bateman RM, Sharpe MD, Ellis CG. Bench-to-bedside review: microvascular dysfunction in sepsis – hemodynamics, oxygen transport, and nitric oxide. *Crit Care* 2003; 7:359–73.

37. Vallet B. Bench-to-bedside review: endothelial cell dysfunction in severe sepsis: a role in organ dysfunction? *Crit Care* 2003; 7:130–8.

38. Stefanec T. Endothelial apoptosis: could it have a role in the pathogenesis and treatment of disease? *Chest* 2000; 117:841–54.

39. Bhagat K, Collier J, Vallance P. Local venous responses to endotoxin in humans. *Circulation* 1996; 94:490–7.

40. Bhagat K, Moss R, Collier J, et al. Endothelial 'stunning' following a brief exposure to endotoxin: a mechanism to link infection and infarction? *Cardiovasc Res* 1996; 32:822–9.

41. Curtis SE, Vallet B, Winn MJ, et al. Role of the vascular endothelium in O2 extraction during progressive ischemia in canine skeletal muscle. *J Appl Physiol* 1995; 79:1351–60.

42. Levi M. Sepsis and the coagulation cascade. *Adv Sepsis* 2000; 1:16–22.

43. van der Poll T, Buller HR, ten Cate H, et al. Activation of coagulation after administration of tumor necrosis factor to normal subjects. *N Engl J Med* 1990; 322:1622–7.

44. Bernard GR, Vincent JL, Laterre PF, et al. Efficacy and safety of recombinant human activated protein C for severe sepsis. *N Engl J Med* 2001; 344:699–709.

45. Cavaillon JM, Adib-Conquy M. Monocytes/macrophages and sepsis. *Crit Care Med* 2005; 33:S506–9.

46. Seely AJ, Pascual JL, Christou NV. Science review: cell membrane expression (connectivity) regulates neutrophil delivery, function and clearance. *Crit Care* 2003; 7:291–307.

47. Weiss SJ. Tissue destruction by neutrophils. *N Engl J Med* 1989; 320:365–76.

48. Takeda Y, Watanabe H, Yonehara S, et al. Rapid acceleration of neutrophil apoptosis by tumor necrosis factor-alpha. *Int Immunol* 1993; 5:691–4.

49. Watson RW, Redmond HP, Wang JH, et al. Bacterial ingestion, tumor necrosis factor-alpha, and heat induce programmed cell death in activated neutrophils. *Shock* 1996; 5:47–51.

50. Hasibeder W, Germann R, Wolf HJ, et al. Effects of short-term endotoxemia and dopamine on mucosal oxygenation in porcine jejunum. *Am J Physiol* 1996; 270:G667–75.

51. Fink MP. Bench-to-bedside review: cytopathic hypoxia. *Crit Care* 2002; 6:491–9.

52. Liaudet L. Poly (adenosine 5'-diphosphate) ribose polymerase activation as a cause of metabolic dysfunction in critical illness. *Curr Opin Clin Nutr Metab Care* 2002; 5:175–84.

53. Trager K, Leverve X, Radermacher P. Metabolism in sepsis and effects of drug therapy. *Adv Sepsis* 2004; 2:118–26.

54. Agwunobi AO, Reid C, Maycock P, et al. Insulin resistance and substrate utilization in human endotoxemia. *J Clin Endocrinol Metab* 2000; 85:3770–8.

55. Levraut J, Ciebiera JP, Chave S, et al. Mild hyperlactatemia in stable septic patients is due to impaired lactate clearance rather than overproduction. *Am J Respir Crit Care Med* 1998; 157:1021–6.

56. Singer M, De Santis V, Vitale D, et al. Multiorgan failure is an adaptive, endocrine-mediated, metabolic response to overwhelming systemic inflammation. *Lancet* 2004; 364:545–8.

57. Sugita H, Kaneki M, Tokunaga E, et al. Inducible nitric oxide synthase plays a role in LPS-induced hyperglycemia and insulin resistance. *Am J Physiol Endocrinol Metab* 2002; 282:E386–94.

58. Van den Berghe G, de Zegher F, Bouillon R. Clinical review 95: acute and prolonged critical illness as different neuroendocrine paradigms. *J Clin Endocrinol Metab* 1998; 83:1827–34.

59. Annane D, Sebille V, Troche G, et al. A 3-level prognostic classification in septic shock based on cortisol levels and cortisol response to corticotropin. *JAMA* 2000; 283:1038–45.

60. Rothwell PM, Lawler PG. Prediction of outcome in intensive care patients using endocrine parameters. *Crit Care Med* 1995; 23:78–83.

61. Scheller K, Seibel P, Sekeris CE. Glucocorticoid and thyroid hormone receptors in mitochondria of animal cells. *Int Rev Cytol* 2003; 222:1–61.

62. Riedemann NC, Guo RF, Ward PA. Novel strategies for the treatment of sepsis. *Nat Med* 2003; 9:517–24.

63. Marshall JC, Cook DJ, Christou NV, et al. Multiple organ dysfunction score: a reliable descriptor of a complex clinical outcome. *Crit Care Med* 1995; 23:1638–52.

64. Vincent JL, de Mendonca A, Cantraine F, et al. Use of the SOFA score to assess the incidence of organ dysfunction/failure in intensive care units: results of a multicenter, prospective study. Working group on 'sepsis-related problems' of the European Society of Intensive Care Medicine. *Crit Care Med* 1998; 26:1793–800.

65. Vincent J-L, De Backer D. Pathophysiology of sepsis. *Adv Sepsis* 2001; 1:87–92.

66. Cavaillon JM, Adib-Conquy M. The pro-inflammatory cytokine cascade. In: Marshall J, Cohen J, eds. *Immune Response in the Critically Ill.* Berlin Heidelberg: Springer-Verlag, 2002:37–66.

67. Dinarello CA. Proinflammatory and anti-inflammatory cytokines as mediators in the pathogenesis of septic shock. *Chest* 1997; 112:321S–9S.

2 Resuscitation in Intensive Care

David A. Zideman

Imperial College Healthcare NHS Trust and Hammersmith Hospital, London, UK

Take Home Messages

- The use of strategies to prevent cardiac arrest is an important part of the resuscitation programme. The regular monitoring of standard physiologic parameters using selected warning criteria together with an active management plan can prevent deterioration into cardiac arrest.
- The national guidelines for resuscitation are universally applicable, but they may require individual tailoring to local staff and available equipment. These modifications should be pre-planned, reviewed and practised regularly.
- Intensive care units should train in and practise resuscitation procedures regularly. ICU staff should be pre-allocated resuscitation team roles to ensure maximum efficiency.
- The rapid diagnosis and treatment of ventricular fibrillation in intensive care can have spectacular results. However, it does require the immediate availability of equipment and the empowerment of nurses to defibrillate without reference to resident medical staff.
- Pulseless electrical activity and asystole should be managed aggressively. Chest compressions should be started immediately and continued without interruption. Active diagnosis of the cause of the arrest plus aggressive treatment of this cause can result in a return of spontaneous circulation.
- Post cardiac arrest patients must be evaluated as to the cause of the arrest and any presenting factors aggressively treated to prevent re-arrest.
- Post resuscitation care is essential to the overall recovery of the patient. The use of post-arrest induced mild hypothermia and the prevention of hyperthermia have been shown to improve patient outcome.
- Clinical governance procedures must be applied to all resuscitation events.
- Current European resuscitation guidelines together with any update statements can be sourced at www.erc.edu.

Cardiovascular Critical Care. Edited by M. Griffiths, J. Cordingley and S. Price.
© 2010 Blackwell Publishing Ltd.

2.1 Introduction

In December 2005 the European Resuscitation Council (ERC) published its latest international guidelines [1] based on the International Liaison Committee on Resuscitation (ILCOR) Consensus on Science statements [2, 3]. The 2005 process followed the 5-year review cycle, coordinated by ILCOR, which was commenced in 2003 and reviewed over 400 topics and some 20,000 references. The reviews were brought together for a Consensus Conference in January 2005 with publication of the proceedings in November 2005 [2, 3].

The Guidelines provide a series of protocols for the management of cardiac arrest, but these do require careful consideration when being applied to specific circumstances or highly sophisticated treatment areas, such as intensive care. The 2005 guidelines have specific recommendations for in-hospital resuscitation that recognise the blurring of the boundaries between basic and advanced life support when resuscitation is carried out in a healthcare environment. They also contain a section on 'resuscitation in special circumstances' that contains many measures that can only be undertaken in an intensive care area or may closely reflect intensive care practice, for example the management of cardiac arrest following cardiac surgery. However, despite the 'hi tech' environment of intensive care, the basic principles of resuscitation still pertain.

The 2005 guidelines can be summarised as the ERC Chain of Survival (Figure 2.1). The chain starts with 'early recognition and call for help to prevent a cardiac arrest' (*Link one*). This link recognises the importance of monitoring and observation in the pre-arrest period and the avoidance of progression to a cardiac arrest by effective pre-arrest management. When cardiac arrest occurs, early cardio-pulmonary resuscitation (CPR) is performed (*Link two*), to 'buy time', followed by early defibrillation (*Link three*) if the rhythm is appropriate, to 'restart the heart'. Finally there is post-resuscitation care (*Link four*) to 'restore quality of life'.

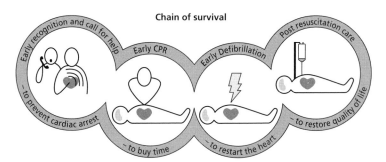

Figure 2.1 European Resuscitation Council Chain of Survival. Copyright European Resuscitation Council (www.erc.edu).

2.2 Recognition of an imminent cardiac arrest

The recognition and prevention of an imminent cardiac arrest are key to the successful management of seriously ill patients. Serious measurable pre-event physiological abnormalities have been recorded in 79% of cardiac arrests, 55% of deaths and 54% of unexpected intensive care unit (ICU) admissions [4]. Others have reported serious respiratory and cardiovascular problems that have remained untreated and resulted in cardiac arrest, death or unexpected admission to an ICU [5–7]. The introduction of a simple vigilance mechanism using Early Warning Scores or 'critical care calling criteria' has assisted in alerting staff at an early stage to the imminent deterioration in a patient's condition [8–10]. The response to an alert by a Medical Emergency Team (MET) or a critical care outreach service using established standard operating procedures may well prevent further deterioration in the patient's condition and even ICU admission [11–15].

The ICU provides the ideal setting for the early recognition and management of a patient who is in imminent danger of progressing to a cardiac arrest. In the ICU environment, where patients are fully monitored, the healthcare professional has a major advantage; none-the-less this should not lead to complacency. All too often intensive care charts show a steady and progressive decline in physiological parameters that do not trigger a change in treatment or the appropriate supportive response. This may be prevented by the careful individual setting of maximum and minimum physiological values to initiate interventions, but even these cannot replace clinical vigilance.

2.3 In-hospital resuscitation

The algorithm for the management of in-hospital cardiac arrest is shown in Figure 2.2. It depends on the rapid recognition of cardiac arrest and the ability of the healthcare professional to determine the presence of 'Signs of Life'. Although ICU staff may use bedside monitoring as their primary trigger it is still important that they check the airway, breathing and circulation at the earliest detection of cardiac arrest.

Call for help

It is essential that there is a call for help immediately cardiac arrest is detected. This call must summon local help initially, but how extensive this activation call is will depend on local protocols and in some units may not call the hospital cardiac arrest team. However, it is important that these protocols are not compromised by individual preferences and that cardiac arrest calls do summon appropriately trained and skilled staff.

Begin resuscitation

The 2005 protocols emphasise the importance of beginning chest compressions as soon as cardiac arrest is detected. In the monitored patient

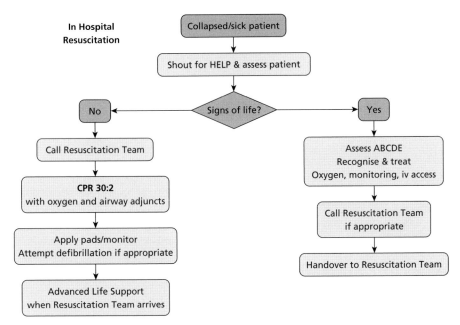

In Hospital Resuscitation

- Collapsed/sick patient
- Shout for HELP & assess patient
- Signs of life?
  - No → Call Resuscitation Team → CPR 30:2 with oxygen and airway adjuncts → Apply pads/monitor Attempt defibrillation if appropriate → Advanced Life Support when Resuscitation Team arrives
  - Yes → Assess ABCDE Recognise & treat Oxygen, monitoring, iv access → Call Resuscitation Team if appropriate → Handover to Resuscitation Team

Figure 2.2 Algorithm for the treatment of in-hospital cardiac arrest. Copyright European Resuscitation Council (www.erc.edu).

there should be no delay between the monitor showing a cardiac arrest rhythm, the absence of a pressure wave on the arterial line trace or the cessation of expired carbon dioxide. It is important to establish that none of these monitored signs is as a result of monitor malfunction or sensor disconnection, but this should not delay commencing resuscitation. Thirty chest compressions should be commenced, followed by two ventilations (see below), and both compressions and ventilations continued with minimal interruptions throughout the whole of the resuscitation event.

The only exception to beginning chest compressions immediately may be where the patient is in monitored ventricular fibrillation (VF) or ventricular tachycardia (VT) and a defibrillator is immediately available. In this case the defibrillation pads should be applied and the first defibrillation attempted as soon as possible. To enable rapid defibrillation without preliminary chest compressions, all staff, including nursing staff, must be trained and empowered to use the defibrillator. If immediate defibrillation fails then chest compressions and ventilations (ratio of 30:2) must be commenced immediately before further attempts at defibrillation are made (see Figure 2.3).

Airway

The majority of patients in ICU have undergone advanced airway management by tracheal intubation through the mouth, nose or directly into the trachea. It is essential to check that the tracheal tube has not been dislodged, displaced or become blocked. It may be necessary to reposition

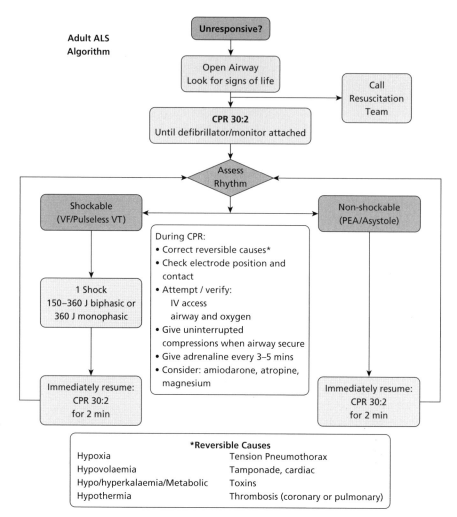

Figure 2.3 Advanced life support (ALS) cardiac arrest algorithm. Copyright European Resuscitation Council (www.erc.edu).

the tracheal tube or to remove and replace the tube if it has become obstructed. In either case the maintenance of a clear airway must be the priority and this may require advanced airway skills. Any adjustment to the airway device or its replacement must be carried out by those fully trained in advanced airway skills using the full array of advanced alternative airway adjuncts, including a range of supraglottic airways (laryngeal mask airways) and an emergency tracheostomy kit. It must be remembered that the usual guide of an expired carbon dioxide trace for the correct position of the tracheal tube in the airway cannot be used during resuscitation as there is no circulation delivering carbon dioxide to the lungs. There will be some patients on ICU who are not intubated. These patients must be managed skilfully and initially the airway maintenance should be by manual chin-lift and jaw-thrust, with airway suction if necessary.

Breathing

As with the airway, the majority of patients on ICU will be ventilated. Following cardiac arrest it is not necessary to remove the patient from the ventilator. It is important that once resuscitation has been started one of the team checks the ventilator is working correctly and that the inspired oxygen is raised to 100%. If the patient is being effectively mechanically ventilated then chest compressions should be performed without interruptions for ventilation.

If the ventilator has failed, the tracheal tube becomes displaced or the patient is not being ventilated then ventilation must be established using a self-inflating bag-valve-mask, with supplemental oxygen supplied through a reservoir bag. Recent studies have demonstrated that healthcare professionals tend towards hyperventilation when performing manual ventilation techniques [16]. Hyperventilation must be avoided as it increases intrathoracic pressure and decreases venous return, resulting in a diminishing cardiac output and poor outcome [17].

Circulation

During CPR the circulation is totally dependent on the provision of adequate and effective chest compressions, the emphasis now being to minimise interruptions to compressions. Chest compressions should be delivered by the healthcare professional placing his or her hands in the centre of the chest [18], compressing at a rate of approximately 100 compressions per minute [19–21] to a depth of 4–5 cm [16, 22]. The effectiveness of compressions can be gauged by observing the arterial pressure and the expired air carbon dioxide traces, and the rate and depth of compressions suitably modified to provide the best results. If ventilation cannot be established or maintained then compression-only resuscitation should be undertaken [23].

Rhythm

The next stage is to assess the cardiac rhythm. The incidence of the three main cardiac arrest rhythms in ICU is determined by the hospital population and the specialties the ICU serves. However, an incidence of VF/VT has been quoted as high as 43.5%, with pulseless electrical activity (PEA) at 38.8% and asystole at 36.5% in a European University Hospital [24], and 32.4% for VF/VT and 35.1% for asystole in a General Hospital [25].

2.4 Management of arrest rhythms

Ventricular fibrillation and ventricular tachycardia

Both of these rhythms are treatable by electrical defibrillation. In the normal course of events the defibrillator in an ICU should be immediately available. There are two major types of defibrillation waveform. Defibrillators delivering a monophasic waveform are no longer manufactured but may still be in service. Most modern defibrillators deliver a biphasic electrical current – a positive followed by a negative current flow. Biphasic defibrillators have a higher first shock efficacy (86–98%) than those delivering monophasic shocks (54–91%), but there is little difference between the two types of biphasic waveforms (biphasic truncated exponential and rectilinear biphasic) [26–29].

If the change in rhythm is recognised quickly then defibrillation should be delivered without delay, even before starting chest compressions. An initial shock of 150–200 J biphasic or 360 J monophasic should be delivered immediately, followed by 2 minutes of chest compressions. Delaying the commencement of chest compressions to establish the effectiveness of the defibrillation attempt may compromise the myocardium if a perfusing rhythm has not been restored [30]. Chest compressions should continue for 2 minutes before they are briefly stopped to assess the rhythm and the arterial pressure trace. If VF/VT is still present then a second shock (150–200 J biphasic or 360 J monophasic) should be delivered and chest compressions recommenced. The sequence of single defibrillation attempts followed by 2 minutes of chest compressions should be continued until there is successful conversion or there is a change to a non-shockable rhythm. There are a number of factors that affect the efficacy of defibrillation and these are summarised in Table 2.1. These should be optimised whenever possible.

If VF or VT is refractory to defibrillation, defined as a continuation after the third cycle, amiodarone 300 mg (diluted in 20 ml of 5% dextrose) intravenously (IV) should be administered. Alternatively lidocaine 100 mg IV can be given if amiodarone is unavailable. Using a different pad or paddle position (Table 2.1) may also be successful in the treatment of refractory rhythms.

Cardiac arrest in ICU is considered to be a witnessed event. Therefore, if there is a delay in acquiring a defibrillator then a single precordial thump should be attempted using the ulnar edge of a clenched fist delivered

Table 2.1 Factors affecting the success of defibrillation.

Transthoracic impedence
- Shaving the chest – remove hair from the place where the electrodes will be placed
- Electrode size – minimum size 150 cm^2
- Coupling agent – use pre-gelled pads or specific coupling agents. Do not use bare electrodes
- Paddle force – apply paddles firmly to the chest wall (optimal force = 8 kg)

Electrode position
- Conventional – place one electrode in the mid-axillary line in the position of the V6 electrode. Place the other electrode to the right of the upper sternum below the clavicle
- Bi-axillary – place one electrode on the right and the other on the left lateral chest walls
- Anterior–posterior – place one electrode over the left precordium and the other on the back behind the heart but below the scapula

Table 2.2 Causes of pulseless electrical activity.

Hypoxia	Tension pneumothorax
Hypovolaemia	Tamponade
Hypo/hyperkalaemia/metabolic	Toxins
Hypothermia	Thrombus (coronary/pulmonary)

sharply to the chest wall from a height of about 20 cm. The success of this method has been recorded when administered in the first 10 seconds of ventricular fibrillation [31].

Asystole and pulseless electrical activity

These rhythms usually have an underlying cause that can be summarised as '4Hs and 4Ts' (Table 2.2). In all cases resuscitation should commence immediately with chest compressions together with ventilations. Each diagnosis should then be considered and the appropriate treatment administered to correct the cause.

- *Hypoxia* – check the airway and correct displacement or blockage (see above). Check the effectiveness of ventilation. Administer 100% inspired oxygen and consider changing from a machine ventilator to a self-inflating manual ventilation bag if the machine is malfunctioning.
- *Hypovolaemia* – arrest haemorrhage where possible and restore the circulating intravascular volume. Where hypovolaemia has resulted from a redistribution of the circulating volume, the use of an alpha-adrenergic agonist (noradrenaline or metaraminol) may be useful to support the intravascular volume expansion.
- *Hypo/hyperkalaemia and metabolic causes* – can be detected by biochemical tests and should be treated empirically.
- *Hypothermia* – core temperature readings should be carefully monitored and maintained. (See – 'Post-resuscitation care' below).
- *Tension pneumothorax* – this is not an uncommon event in patients being mechanically ventilated. Diagnosis can be made clinically, by a plain radiograph or with an ultrasound device. Immediate decompression using either needle decompression, open thoracostomy (ventilated) or tube thoracic drain (non-ventilated) will often restore cardiac output.
- *Cardiac tamponade* – this is more difficult to diagnose, but patients may show classic clinical pre-arrest signs of distended neck veins and hypotension. Treatment is by needle pericardiocentesis, best carried out under ultrasound control, or by thoracotomy ideally performed by a cardiothoracic surgeon.
- *Toxins* – these may be therapeutic agents or the accidental/deliberate ingestion of toxic substances. Specific antidotes, where available, should be used, but most of the treatment is supportive in these circumstances.

- *Thromboembolic* – pulmonary embolism may cause cardiac arrest by mechanical circulatory obstruction. Management is by vigorous chest compressions, which may help to relieve the obstruction, and immediate administration of thrombolytic drugs.

All of the above should be considered as potentially reversible causes. Unlike VF/VT there is no definitive treatment of asystole or PEA, so chest compressions and ventilation must be maintained whilst correction of these causes is attempted.

2.5 Drugs

There are very few drugs recommended for routine use during resuscitation.

Vasopressors

Adrenaline has remained the primary vasopressor for use in cardiac arrest for many years. It is a sympathomimetic drug used for its alpha- and beta-adrenergic agonist effects. The alpha-agonist effects cause peripheral vasoconstriction, raising coronary blood flow and cerebral perfusion pressure. The beta-agonist effects increase rate and force of ventricular contraction, but this increases myocardial oxygen consumption and can induce ventricular arrhythmias. Adrenaline 1 mg (10 ml of 1 in 10,000 solution or 1 ml of 1 in 1000 solution) should be administered IV every 3–5 minutes during resuscitation. If no IV access is available the same dose can be given via the intraosseous route or, when venous access is delayed, in a dose of 2–3 mg down the endotracheal tube.

Vasopressin is an alternative to adrenaline. Although preliminary research looked promising [32] a meta-analysis of five randomised trials did not show any statistically significant difference between adrenaline and vasopressin in restoring spontaneous circulation, death within 24 hours or death before hospital discharge [33]. Current guidance states that 'there is insufficient evidence to support or refute the use of vasopressin as an alternative to, or in combination with, adrenaline in any cardiac arrest rhythm'.[2]

Anti-arrhythmics

Amiodarone increases the duration of the action potential and refractory period in the atrial and the ventricular myocardium. It is recommended for refractory VF/VT (see above) and in haemodynamically stable VT. Administration often results in bradycardia and hypotension. The cause is the release of histamine by the drug solvent, but this can be limited by administering the dose slowly.

Lidocaine should only be used in refractory VF or pulseless VT when amiodarone is not available [34]. Magnesium sulphate is indicated in shock-refractory VF in the presence of possible hypomagnesaemia [35]. The initial intravenous does is 2 g (4 ml of 50% magnesium sulphate) administered over 1–2 minutes and repeated after 10 minutes.

Magnesium is specifically recommended for torsades de pointes and digoxin toxicity.

Other drugs

Atropine is a parasympathetic blocker and therefore blocks the action of the vagus nerve on both the sinoatrial node and the atrioventricular node. It is indicated in asystole or PEA with a heart rate of less than 60 beats per minute. The recommended dose is 3 mg as a single bolus.

Calcium should only be given in resuscitation when PEA is caused by hyperkalaemia, hypocalcaemia or an overdose of calcium channel blocking drugs. The recommended initial dose is 10 ml of 10% calcium chloride solution.

Buffers have remained controversial during resuscitation as the arterial blood gas values may not truly reflect the real tissue acid-base status [37]. The recommended treatment for the acidosis that develops during cardiac arrest is improved chest compression provided that effective ventilation is maintained. However, when the pH falls below 7.1 there may be additional benefit from small titrated doses of 8.4% sodium bicarbonate solution.

Thrombolysis has been shown in one study to improve ICU survival [38] and two studies have shown possible benefits when given to patients in cardiac arrest with suspected or proven pulmonary embolus [39, 40]. It is recommended that following thrombolysis in resuscitation CPR be continued for 60–90 minutes before terminating resuscitation attempts [41].

Theophylline (aminophylline) has been used in cardiac arrest but has failed to demonstrate any increase in return of spontaneous circulation (ROSC) or survival to hospital discharge [36]. It may be considered in asystolic cardiac arrest in a dose of 5 $mg.kg^{-1}$ given by slow intravenous injection.

2.6 Peri-arrest arrhythmias

Changes in rhythm that occur immediately before or after resuscitation need expert and expeditious management if the outcome of the resuscitation event is to be satisfactory. The ICU provides the ideal environment for the management of these arrhythmias. Both algorithms start with the need to give oxygen, establish venous access, record a 12-lead ECG and identify and treat reversible causes. The management of these rhythms are best summarised in two algorithms: bradycardia and tachycardia (Figures 2.4 and 2.5). Bradycardias are usually defined as a heart rate of below 60 beats min^{-1}. However, it is more useful to describe a bradycardia in terms of haemodynamic status and their clinical effects: heart rate < 40 beats min^{-1}, systolic blood pressure < 90 mmHg, ventricular arrhythmias requiring suppression and heart failure. Similarly, the entry point for all three tachycardias is again by physiological status, and the management will depend on the answer to the question 'Is the patient stable?' Signs of instability include reduced conscious level, chest pain, systolic blood pressure < 90 mmHg and heart failure.

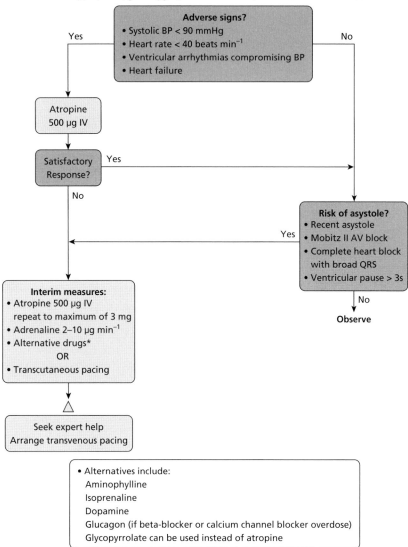

Figure 2.4 Bradycardia algorithm. Copyright European Resuscitation Council (www.erc.edu).

2.7 Other interventions

The practice of resuscitation is continuously evolving. A number of interventions have been described but as yet have not reached the status of full recommendation for routine use in standard resuscitation practice. Those relevant to resuscitation in ICU include open-chest CPR [42],

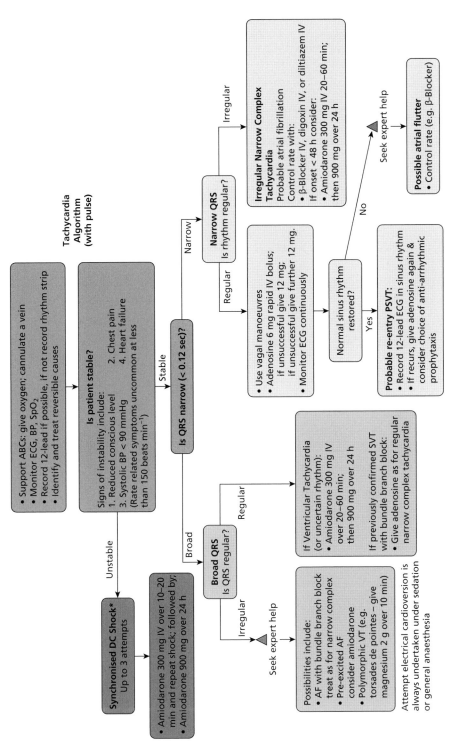

Tachycardia Algorithm (with pulse)

- Support ABCs: give oxygen; cannulate a vein
- Monitor ECG, BP, SpO_2
- Record 12-lead if possible, if not record rhythm strip
- Identify and treat reversible causes

Is patient stable?

Signs of instability include:
1. Reduced conscious level   2. Chest pain
3. Systolic BP < 90 mmHg   4. Heart failure
(Rate related symptoms uncommon at less than 150 beats min^{-1})

Unstable →

Synchronised DC Shock*
Up to 3 attempts

- Amiodarone 300 mg IV over 10–20 min and repeat shock; followed by;
- Amiodarone 900 mg over 24 h

Stable →

Is QRS narrow (< 0.12 sec)?

Broad →

Broad QRS
Is QRS regular?

Irregular →

Seek expert help

Possibilities include:
- AF with bundle branch block treat as for narrow complex
- Pre-excited AF consider amiodarone
- Polymorphic VT (e.g. torsades de pointes – give magnesium 2 g over 10 min)

Attempt electrical cardioversion is always undertaken under sedation or general anaesthesia

Regular →

If Ventricular Tachycardia (or uncertain rhythm):
- Amiodarone 300 mg IV over 20–60 min; then 900 mg over 24 h

If previously confirmed SVT with bundle branch block:
- Give adenosine as for regular narrow complex tachycardia

Narrow →

Narrow QRS
Is rhythm regular?

Irregular →

Irregular Narrow Complex Tachycardia
Probable atrial fibrillation
Control rate with:
- β-Blocker IV, digoxin IV, or diltiazem IV
If onset < 48 h consider:
- Amiodarone 300 mg IV 20–60 min; then 900 mg over 24 h

Seek expert help →

Possible atrial flutter
- Control rate (e.g. β-Blocker)

Regular →

- Use vagal manoeuvres
- Adenosine 6 mg rapid IV bolus; if unsuccessful give 12 mg; if unsuccessful give further 12 mg.
- Monitor ECG continuously

Normal sinus rhythm restored?

No → Seek expert help

Yes →

Probable re-entry PSVT:
- Record 12-lead ECG in sinus rhythm
- If recurs, give adenosine again & consider choice of anti-arrhythmic prophylaxis

Figure 2.5 Tachycardia algorithm. Copyright European Resuscitation Council (www.erc.edu).

interposed abdominal compression CPR (IAC-CPR) [43], active compression-decompression CPR (ACD-CPR) [44], impedence threshold device (ITD) [45], Lund University cardiac arrest system (LUCAS) [46] and load-distributing band CPR [47].

2.8 Post-resuscitation care

The 2005 guidelines included full and detailed recommendations for post-resuscitation care in an effort to improve the outcome of patients who survive the initial cardiac arrest but then continue to deteriorate because of poor or ineffective management in the post-resuscitation period [48]. There is no doubt that as early resuscitation becomes more successful then the management of patients after cardiac arrest becomes increasingly important. The Intensive Care National Audit and Research Centre (ICNARC) database for the years 1995 to 2005 has shown that of the 24,132 patients admitted to intensive care following cardiac arrest, 28.6% survived to discharge, with 79.9% of ICU survivors returning to their normal place of residence. The highest hospital mortality (60.6%) was for in-hospital non-perioperative events [49].

Many factors affect the survival and physical status of patients following the severe physiological trauma of a cardiac arrest. In many ways the ICU is the ideal environment for the management of the post-resuscitation patient; however, it may not be appropriate for everyone. For example, in the patient with a brief cardiac arrest, where defibrillation from ventricular fibrillation was rapid and there was an immediate return of cardiac function, that patient may not require intensive care. At the other end of the scale are those expected to die, where intensive care may also not be appropriate.

The following criteria should be considered for the post-resuscitation patient.

Airway and breathing
Unconscious patients require tracheal intubation with controlled ventilation. It will be necessary to exchange a supra-glottic airway device inserted during the resuscitation for an endotracheal tube to enable formal airway control. This will have to be carried out with extreme care considering the potentially unstable cardiac condition of the patient. There are no defined target blood gas values for ventilation following cardiac arrest, so normocarbia should be aimed for. Hypocarbia from hyperventilation causes cerebral vasoconstriction and decreased blood flow [50].

Circulation
Haemodynamic instability following successful resuscitation is not uncommon and every effort must be made to treat arrhythmias effectively as described above. Hypotension must be managed and hypertension controlled; however, there is no established target mean arterial blood pressure. Both hyper- and hypokalaemia must be controlled as both can cause ventricular arrhythmias.

Cerebral function

There are a number of post-resuscitation management issues that can aid the recovery of cerebral function and the outcome from cardiac arrest. Most of these require intensive care management. Seizures occur in 40% of patients who remain comatose after cardiac arrest. Seizures may be controlled using benzodiazepines, phenytoin, propofol or a barbiturate, but care must be taken not to induce hypotension. Status epilepticus and status myoclonus are associated with a poor outcome [51]. The control of body temperature using antipyretics or active cooling is essential in the post-arrest period because the risk of neurological disability increases for each degree rise in body temperature above 37°C [52]. Therapeutic hypothermia, cooling to 32–34°C for 12–24 hours, improved the neurological outcome of adults who remained comatose after out-of-hospital cardiac arrest [53, 54]. ILCOR published a statement recommending therapeutic cooling of out-of-hospital cardiac arrest survivors for 12–24 hours [55, 56]. As yet there is no evidence to support or refute the use of hypothermia for in-hospital events. Cooling can be achieved using either external or internal techniques [54]. An infusion of 30 ml.kg^{-1} of saline at 4°C will decrease core temperature by 1.5°C [57, 58]. However, controlled intravascular cooling methods, using external cooling devices, may control induced hypothermia more precisely [59]. Shivering can be effectively controlled with conventional sedation and neuromuscular paralysis. Close control of rewarming is critical and should be slow (0.25–0.5°C.h^{-1}) and hyperthermia must be avoided. Again intravascular devices provide a more accurate and controlled rewarm.

Tight control of blood glucose to between 4.4 and 6.1 mmol.l^{-1} using insulin reduced mortality in critically ill patients, mainly surgical adult patients [60]. There is a need for studies of the effects of this tight control following cardiac arrest.

Prognosis

There are no specific neurological tests that can predict outcome within the first few hours of the post-arrest period. Of those who remain comatose, half will have died within 3 days. Day 3 is also the time marker to predict a poor outcome for those without a pupillary response to light or an absent response to pain [61, 62]. There is insufficient evidence to support the use of any individual clinical marker as a predictor of outcome. There is, however, a 100% predictive specificity for median nerve somatosensory evoked potentials for patients comatose for 72 hours who are normothermic [63]. Electroenencephalographs (EEGs) that are either normal or grossly abnormal are also predictive of outcome.

2.9 Ethical issues

The ethical principles behind the procedures for do not attempt resuscitation (DNAR) decisions are: beneficence (providing benefit and balancing this against risk), non-maleficence (do no harm), justice (spreading benefits and risks evenly throughout society) and autonomy (the patient's right to make his or her own informed decisions). The decision should be made bearing in mind that over 70% of resuscitation events are unsuccessful and that patients should be allowed to die with dignity.

The decision to withhold resuscitation in the intensive care environment may seem anachronistic. However, there will be occasions when further medical interventions of a seriously ill patient may be considered futile. This is a difficult decision and must be made with the full multi-disciplinary team caring for the patient and, if possible, in conjunction with the relatives so that they understand the logical progression of care. The decision, once made, should be carefully recorded in the patient's notes, together with the reasons [64].

DNAR does not mean withdrawal of medical or nursing care. It is specific to the end-of-life event. As such it should be reviewed at regular intervals, taking any change in the patient's medical status into account. It is essential to review the DNAR order when the patient is moved from the ICU so that it is not continued inappropriately.

2.10 Summary

Prevention of an impending cardiac arrest is as important as the cardiac arrest event itself. Intensive care units provide the ideal environment for the monitoring and preventative measures needed to halt the progress of an individual towards cardiac arrest. If cardiac arrest does occur the staff should adhere to the recognised national guidelines and should function as a trained cohesive team to attain the best results. Regular resuscitation practice is therefore an essential part of the intensive care training programme.

Case study

Mrs A was a 56-year-old lady who was admitted to intensive care as a level 2 patient requiring post-operative care following an extensive gynaecological pelvic exenteration. She did not have any notable medical history or investigations prior to surgery. Her time in intensive care progressed well and she was due to be discharged on the morning of day 3.

One hour prior to her planned discharge her cardiac monitor alarmed and the ECG showed ventricular fibrillation. Her supervising nurse called for help. The automated external defibrillator (AED) was immediately available and the self-adhesive pads were placed on the patient's chest. The AED confirmed ventricular fibrillation and advised defibrillation. The supervising nurse checked 'all clear' and pressed the 'shock' button. The defibrillator administered a 150-J biphasic shock;

Continued

re-analysis of the rhythm showed a return to sinus rhythm together with a return of a palpable pulse and measurable blood pressure. No chest compressions had been performed due to the rapid defibrillation.

Mrs A had a virtually immediate return of consciousness. She was transferred immediately to the cardiac catheter laboratory where two stenotic lesions in her coronary circulation were successfully stented. She was discharged to the ward the following day and then to home some weeks later.

Commentary:

1. Ventricular fibrillation can occur at any time and may not have any relevant previous history.
2. Rapid diagnosis and defibrillation precluded the need for chest compression.
3. Rapid defibrillation can result in a virtually immediate return of spontaneous circulation, spontaneous respiration and consciousness.

References

1. European Resuscitation Council. European Resuscitation Council Guidelines for Resuscitation 2005. *Resuscitation* 2005;67 S1:S1–89.
2. 2005 International Consensus on Cardiopulmonary Resuscitation and Emergency Cardiovascular Care Science with Treatment Recommendations. *Resuscitation* 2005;67(2–3):157–342.
3. 2005 International Consensus on Cardiopulmonary Resuscitation and Emergency Cardiovascular Care Science with Treatment Recommendations. *Circulation* 2005;112(22 Supplement):1–136.
4. Kause J, Smith G, Prytherch D, et al. A comparison of antecedents to cardiac arrests, deaths and emergency intensive care admissions in Australia and New Zealand, and the United Kingdom – the ACADEMIA study. *Resuscitation* 2004 Sep;62(3):275–82.
5. Hodgetts TJ, Kenward G, Vlackonikolis I, et al. Incidence, location and reasons for avoidable in-hospital cardiac arrest in a district general hospital. *Resuscitation* 2002;54(2):115–23.
6. Franklin C, Mathew J. Developing strategies to prevent inhospital cardiac arrest: analyzing responses of physicians and nurses in the hours before the event. *Crit Care Med* 1994;22(2):244–7.
7. McQuillan P, Pilkington S, Allan A, et al. Confidential inquiry into quality of care before admission to intensive care. *BMJ* 1998;316(7148):1853–8.
8. Goldhill DR, Worthington L, Mulcahy A, et al. The patient-at-risk team: identifying and managing seriously ill ward patients. *Anaesthesia* 1999;54(9):853–60.
9. Hodgetts TJ, Kenward G, Vlachonikolis IG, et al. The identification of risk factors for cardiac arrest and formulation of activation criteria to alert a medical emergency team. *Resuscitation* 2002;54(2):125–31.
10. Subbe CP, Davies RG, Williams E, et al. Effect of introducing the Modified Early Warning score on clinical outcomes, cardio-pulmonary arrests and intensive care utilisation in acute medical admissions. *Anaesthesia* 2003;58(8):797–802.

11. The MERIT study investigators. Introduction of the medical emergency team (MET) system: a cluster-randomised controlled trial. *Lancet* 2005;365(9477): 2091–7.

12. Bellomo R, Goldsmith D, Uchino S, et al. A prospective before-and-after trial of a medical emergency team. *Med J Aust* 2003;179(6):283–7.

13. Buist MD, Moore GE, Bernard SA, et al. Effects of a medical emergency team on reduction of incidence of and mortality from unexpected cardiac arrests in hospital: preliminary study. *BMJ* 2002;324(7334):387–90.

14. Ball C, Kirkby M, Williams S. Effect of the critical care outreach team on patient survival to discharge from hospital and readmission to critical care: non-randomised population based study. *BMJ* 2003;327(7422):1014.

15. Priestley G, Watson W, Rashidian A, et al. Introducing Critical Care Outreach: a ward-randomised trial of phased introduction in a general hospital. *Intensive Care Med* 2004;30(7):1398–404.

16. Abella BS, Alvarado JP, Myklebust H, et al. Quality of cardiopulmonary resuscitation during in-hospital cardiac arrest. *JAMA* 2005;293(3):305–10.

17. Aufderheide TP, Sigurdsson G, Pirrallo RG, et al. Hyperventilation-induced hypotension during cardiopulmonary resuscitation. *Circulation* 2004; 109(16):1960–5.

18. Handley AJ. Teaching hand placement for chest compression – a simpler technique. *Resuscitation* 2002;53(1):29–36.

19. Yu T, Weil MH, Tang W, et al. Adverse outcomes of interrupted precordial compression during automated defibrillation. *Circulation* 2002;106(3): 368–72.

20. Swenson RD, Weaver WD, Niskanen RA, et al. Hemodynamics in humans during conventional and experimental methods of cardiopulmonary resuscitation. *Circulation* 1988;78(3):630–9.

21. Kern KB, Sanders AB, Raife J, et al. A study of chest compression rates during cardiopulmonary resuscitation in humans: the importance of rate-directed chest compressions. *Arch Intern Med* 1992;152(1):145–9.

22. Wik L, Kramer-Johansen J, Myklebust H, et al. Quality of cardiopulmonary resuscitation during out-of-hospital cardiac arrest. *JAMA* 2005;293(3):299–304.

23. Becker LB, Berg RA, Pepe PE, et al. A reappraisal of mouth-to-mouth ventilation during bystander-initiated cardiopulmonary resuscitation. A statement for healthcare professionals from the Ventilation Working Group of the Basic Life Support and Pediatric Life Support Subcommittees, American Heart Association. *Resuscitation* 1997;35(3):189–201.

24. Enohumah KO, Moerer O, Kirmse C, et al. Outcome of cardiopulmonary resuscitation in intensive care units in a university hospital. *Resuscitation* 2006;71:161–70.

25. Myrianthefs P, Kalafati M, Lemonidou C, et al. Efficay of CPR in a general, adult ICU. *Resuscitation* 2003;57:43–8.

26. Van Alem AP, Chapman FW, Lank P, et al. A prospective, randomised and blinded comparison of first shock success of monophasic and biphasic waveforms in out-of-hospital cardiac arrest. *Resuscitation* 2003;58(1):17–24.

27. Carpenter J, Rea TD, Murray JA, et al. Defibrillation waveform and post-shock rhythm in out-of-hospital ventricular fibrillation cardiac arrest. *Resuscitation* 2003;59(2):189–96.

28. Morrison LJ, Dorian P, Long J, et al. Out-of-hospital cardiac arrest rectilinear biphasic to monophasic damped sine defibrillation waveforms with advanced life support intervention trial (ORBIT). *Resuscitation* 2005;66(2):149–57.

29. Martens PR, Russell JK, Wolcke B, et al. Optimal Response to Cardiac Arrest study: defibrillation waveform effects. *Resuscitation* 2001;49(3):233–43.

30. Van Alem AP, Sanou BT, Koster RW. Interruption of cardiopulmonary resuscitation with the use of the automated external defibrillator in out-of-hospital cardiac arrest. *Ann Emerg Med* 2003;42(4):449–57.

31. Kohl P, King A, Boulin C. Antiarrhythmic effects of acute mechanical stimulation. In: Kohl P, Sachs F, Franz M, eds. *Cardiac Mechano-Electric Feedback and Arrhythmias: From Pipette to Patient*. Philadelphia: Elsevier Saunders; 2005. pp 304–14.

32. Lindner KH, Prengel AW, Brinkmann A, et al. Vasopressin administration in refractory cardiac arrest. *Ann Intern Med* 1996;124(12):1061–4.

33. Aung K, Htay T. Vasopressin for cardiac arrest: a systematic review and meta-analysis. *Arch Intern Med* 2005;165(1):17–24.

34. Dorian P, Cass D, Schwartz B, et al. Amiodarone as compared with lidocaine for shock-resistant ventricular fibrillation. *N Engl J Med* 2002;346(12):884–90.

35. Baraka A, Ayoub C, Kawkabani N. Magnesium therapy for refractory ventricular fibrillation. *J Cardiothorac Vasc Anesth* 2000;14(2):196–9.

36. Mader TJ, Smithline HA, Durkin L, et al. A randomized controlled trial of intravenous aminophylline for atropine-resistant out-of-hospital asystolic cardiac arrest. *Acad Emerg Med* 2003;10(3):192–7.

37. Weil MH, Rackow EC, Trevino R, et al. Difference in acid-base state between venous and arterial blood during cardiopulmonary resuscitation. *N Engl J Med* 1986;315(3):153–6.

38. Ruiz-Bailen M, Aguayo de Hoyos E, Serrano-Corcoles MC, et al. Efficacy of thrombolysis in patients with acute myocardial infarction requiring cardiopulmonary resuscitation. *Intensive Care Med* 2001;27(6):1050–7.

39. Janata K, Holzer M, Kurkciyan I, et al. Major bleeding complications in cardiopulmonary resuscitation: the place of thrombolytic therapy in cardiac arrest due to massive pulmonary embolism. *Resuscitation*. 2003;57(1):49–55.

40. Scholz KH, Hilmer T, Schuster S, et al. Thrombolysis in resuscitated patients with pulmonary embolism. *Dtsch Med Wochenschr* 1990;115(24):930–5.

41. Böttiger BW, Martin E. Thrombolytic therapy during cardiopulmonary resuscitation and the role of coagulation activation after cardiac arrest. *Curr Opin Crit Care* 2001;7(3):176–83.

42. Boczar ME, Howard MA, Rivers EP, et al. A technique revisited: hemodynamic comparison of closed- and open-chest cardiac massage during human cardiopulmonary resuscitation. *Crit Care Med* 1995;23(3):498–503.

43. Babbs CF. Interposed abdominal compression CPR: a comprehensive evidence based review. *Resuscitation* 2003;59(1):71–82.

44. Lafuente-Lafuente C, Melero-Bascones M. Active chest compression-decompression for cardiopulmonary resuscitation. *Cochrane Database Syst Rev* 2004(2):CD002751.

45. Plaisance P, Lurie KG, Vicaut E, et al. Evaluation of an impedance threshold device in patients receiving active compression-decompression

cardiopulmonary resuscitation for out of hospital cardiac arrest. *Resuscitation* 2004;61(3):265–71.

46. Steen S, Liao Q, Pierre L, et al. Evaluation of LUCAS, a new device for automatic mechanical compression and active decompression resuscitation. *Resuscitation* 2002;55(3):285–99.

47. Casner M, Anderson D. Preliminary report of the impact of a new CPR assist device on the rate of return of spontaneous circulation in out of hospital cardiac arrest. *PreHospital Emerg Med* 2005;9:61–7.

48. Langhelle A, Nolan J, Herlitz J, et al. Recommended guidelines for reviewing, reporting, and conducting research on post-resuscitation care: the Utstein style. *Resuscitation* 2005;66(3):271–83.

49. Nolan J, Laver S, Welch C, et al. Case mix, outcome and activity for admissions to adult general ICUs following a cardiac arrest: a secondary analysis of the ICNARC Case Mix Programme Database (Abstract). *J Intensive Care Soc* 2007;8(1):38.

50. Menon DK, Coles JP, Gupta AK, et al. Diffusion limited oxygen delivery following head injury. *Crit Care Med* 2004;32(6):1384–90.

51. Wijdicks EF, Parisi JE, Sharbrough FW. Prognostic value of myoclonus status in comatose survivors of cardiac arrest. *Ann Neurol* 1994;35(2):239–43.

52. Zeiner A, Holzer M, Sterz F, et al. Hyperthermia after cardiac arrest is associated with an unfavorable neurologic outcome. *Arch Intern Med* 2001;161(16):2007–12.

53. Hypothermia After Cardiac Arrest Study Group. Mild therapeutic hypothermia to improve the neurologic outcome after cardiac arrest. *N Engl J Med* 2002;346(8):549–56.

54. Bernard SA, Gray TW, Buist MD, et al. Treatment of comatose survivors of out-of-hospital cardiac arrest with induced hypothermia. *N Engl J Med* 2002;346(8):557–63.

55. Nolan JP, Morley PT, Vanden Hoek TL, et al. Therapeutic hypothermia after cardiac arrest. An advisory statement by the Advancement Life Support Task Force of the International Liaison Committee on Resuscitation. *Resuscitation* 2003;57(3):231–5.

56. Nolan JP, Morley PT, Vanden Hoek TL, et al. Therapeutic hypothermia after cardiac arrest: an advisory statement by the Advanced Life Support Task Force of the International Liaison Committee on Resuscitation. *Circulation* 2003;108(1):118–21.

57. Bernard S, Buist M, Monteiro O, et al. Induced hypothermia using large volume, ice-cold intravenous fluid in comatose survivors of out-of-hospital cardiac arrest: a preliminary report. *Resuscitation* 2003;56(1):9–13.

58. Kliegel A, Losert H, Sterz F, et al. Cold simple intravenous infusions preceding special endovascular cooling for faster induction of mild hypothermia after cardiac arrest – a feasibility study. *Resuscitation* 2005;64(3):347–51.

59. Al-Senani FM, Graffagnino C, Grotta JC, et al. A prospective, multicenter pilot study to evaluate the feasibility and safety of using the CoolGard System and Icy catheter following cardiac arrest. *Resuscitation* 2004;62(2):143–50.

60. Krinsley JS. Effect of an intensive glucose management protocol on the mortality of critically ill adult patients. *Mayo Clin Proc* 2004;79(8):992–1000.

61. Booth CM, Boone RH, Tomlinson G, et al. Is this patient dead, vegetative, or severely neurologically impaired? Assessing outcome for comatose survivors of cardiac arrest. *JAMA* 2004;291(7):870–9.

62. Edgren E. Prediction of prognosis following cardiac arrest. *Acta Anaesth Belg* 1988;39, Suppl. 2:121–6.

63. Zandbergen EG, de Haan RJ, Hijdra A. Systematic review of prediction of poor outcome in anoxic-ischaemic coma with biochemical markers of brain damage. *Intensive Care Med* 2001;27(10):1661–7.

64. Decisions relating to cardiopulmonary resuscitation: a joint statement from the British Medical Association, the Resuscitation Council (UK) and the Royal College of Nursing. *J Med Ethics* 2001;27(5):310–6.

3 Cardiovascular Monitoring in Critical Care

Michael R. Pinsky

University of Pittsburgh School of Medicine, Pittsburgh, PA, USA

Take Home Messages

- No monitoring device will improve patient-centered outcomes unless coupled to a treatment that improves outcome.
- Specific patterns of haemodynamic variables are often diagnostic of hypovolaemic, cardiogenic and distributive shock.
- Single static haemodynamic measures are of limited utility in predicting response to therapy.
- Dynamic measures of cardiac output created by a fluid challenge or stroke volume and pulse pressure variation created by positive-pressure breathing accurately predict volume responsiveness.

3.1 Introduction

Haemodynamic monitoring is a crucial part of bedside care of the critically ill patient. One of the main reasons for monitoring haemodynamic variables is to detect an impending cardiovascular crisis before organ damage occurs. Another goal of haemodynamic monitoring is to allow clinicians to monitor the response to cardiovascular therapy. Many treatments have to be titrated to specific cardiovascular responses, thus making their use dependent on such monitoring. Finally, the pattern of haemodynamic values often helps differentiate causes of haemodynamic instability and circulatory shock. Traditionally circulatory shock has been grouped into disease processes broadly related to decreased blood volume (hypovolaemic), impaired ventricular pump function (cardiogenic), obstruction to blood flow (obstructive) or impaired vascular autoregulation (distributive). Since these processes often have quite different and often opposite treatment, making these aetiological distinctions is important in defining therapy.

Cardiovascular Critical Care. Edited by M. Griffiths, J. Cordingley and S. Price.
© 2010 Blackwell Publishing Ltd.

Most intensive care units monitor and display, as they have done for the last 20 years, only electrocardiography (ECG), heart rate (HR), blood pressure and pulse oximetry O_2 saturation (SpO_2). Furthermore, with few exceptions, such monitoring does not drive treatment protocols but rather serves as an automated record of vital signs used to trigger further attention. Since no monitoring device, no matter how accurate, can improve patient outcomes unless it is coupled to a treatment that itself improves outcome, haemodynamic monitoring must be applied within the context of therapeutic interventions that are effective in reversing the identified disease process, and improving outcome in terms of patient survival and/or quality of life [1]. The effectiveness of haemodynamic monitoring therefore depends not only on the accuracy and validity of the available technology but also on the healthcare professional's ability to diagnose and effectively treat the underlying diseases for which the monitoring is used. With rapidly developing technology and improvement in our understanding of the pathophysiology of diseases, the utility of haemodynamic monitoring has changed significantly over time. Thus, haemodynamic monitoring represents a functional tool that may be used to derive estimates of performance and physiological reserve that may in turn direct treatment.

Much of the monitoring is used to identify single haemodynamic values, such as blood pressure, HR or SpO_2 (see above), and assess treatments specifically aimed to restore these values to normal ranges. This approach may seem reasonable but might be inappropriate under conditions commonly occurring in the intensive care unit. One would not be remiss to give beta adrenergic blockers to reduce heart rate, vasodilators to decrease hypertension, and supplemental O_2 to improve SpO_2. Although effective temporising treatment of single variable abnormalities may be indicted, tachycardia, hypertension and hypoxaemia are important signposts of more severe underlying disease states that may require aggressive and quite different treatments from those listed above. For example, occult haemorrhage in a patient with baseline impaired gas exchange but intact sympathetic response often manifests itself as tachycardia and hypertension with decreasing SpO_2. Neither beta adrenergic blockade nor vasodilators are indicated in the initial management of such patients and may be quite detrimental. Thus, it is not enough to monitor the patient closely; one needs to also interpret all the haemodynamic data in the context of the pathophysiology and stage of the patient's disease.

Finally, recent data suggest that pre-emptive resuscitation in high risk surgery patients [2] and even aggressive early resuscitation following presentation of haemodynamic instability in sepsis [3] using haemodynamic monitoring to define treatment and goals of resuscitation improve survival. However, application of these same treatments following the establishment of organ failure not only does not improve survival but also may increase mortality due to the increased risks associated with invasive monitoring and aggressive therapies [4–6].

3.2 Static haemodynamic monitoring of single variables

Although their utility as a single absolute haemodynamic value is questionable, a few haemodynamic variables are commonly measured at the bedside and their values are used in clinical decision making. The most common variables used in clinical settings are arterial blood pressure (BP), HR, SpO_2, central venous pressure (CVP), pulmonary artery occlusion pressure (Ppao), cardiac output (CO) and mixed venous oxygen saturation (SvO_2). Although BP, HR and SpO_2 can all be measured non-invasively, the other measures require some degree of invasive haemodynamic monitoring. Threshold values for individual haemodynamic variables exist such that values above or below them may reflect cardiovascular compromise. Clearly, bradycardia (HR < 45/min) and tachycardia (HR > 130/min), hypotension (mean BP < 65 mm Hg) and hypertension (mean BP > 180 mm Hg) are usually not tolerated for prolonged intervals without resulting in end-organ dysfunction and/or death.

These values are often used as threshold single variable triggers to activate medical response teams. However, they represent the extreme of cardiovascular decompensation, whereas most patients can be in circulatory shock with sympathetic compensation with haemodynamic values within these broad limits. Furthermore, specific constellations of specific haemodynamic values reflect autonomic response to specific disease processes. Since the primary determinant of cardiac and cerebral perfusion is perfusion pressure, the body tries to prevent hypotension by increasing vasomotor tone in the face of reduced venous return or impaired cardiac performance. Thus, patients may be in overt shock with mean BP values > 65 mm Hg [7]. These same subjects will also have evidence of increased sympathetic tone. Thus, tachycardia and cool extremities represent co-travelers in the haemodynamic profile of low CO shock. Similarly, an elevated central venous pressure (i.e. > 10 mm Hg) indicates right ventricular pressure overload usually due to an expanded effective circulating blood volume, even though this information says nothing about the exact cause of the process. Also, CO can only be interpreted relative to metabolic demand as blood flow varies to match these needs. It is difficult to define normal CO or oxygen delivery (DO_2I); more important is whether they are adequate to meet metabolic requirements. Since O_2 extraction is increased to sustain O_2 consumption in the face of decreasing DO_2I, low venous O_2 saturation is a sine qua non of inadequate DO_2I, and SvO_2 values < 70% reflect metabolic stress [8].

An overly simplistic yet accurate description of some good rules that can be applied to specific single haemodynamic variables is summarised in Table 3.1. The rationale for these simplistic statements is described more fully below.

Systemic arterial blood pressure

After pulse rate, arterial pressure is the most common haemodynamic variable monitored and recorded. Blood pressure is not a single pressure

Table 3.1 Haemodynamic monitoring truths for single variables.

Tachycardia is never a good thing.
Hypotension is always pathological.
There is no such thing as a normal cardiac output.
CVP is only elevated in disease.
Peripheral oedema is of cosmetic concern.

Reproduced with permission from Pinsky MR. Hemodynamic evaluation and monitoring in the ICU. *Chest* 2007; 132(6):2020–9.

value but a range of pressure values from systole to diastole. Therefore, for tissues other than the heart, if the back or venous pressure is not elevated, mean arterial pressure (MAP) is the best approximation of the organ perfusion pressure. Continuous invasive arterial blood pressure monitoring also allows one to quantify arterial pulse pressure (systole minus diastole).

Blood pressure is usually measured non-invasively using a sphygmomanometer and the auscultation technique [9]. Importantly, very large and obese subjects in whom the upper arm circumference exceeds the width limitations of a normal blood pressure cuff will record pressures that are higher than they actually are. In such patients, using the large thigh blood pressure cuff usually resolves this problem. Blood pressure can be measured automatically using computer-driven devices (e.g. Dynamat®). Sphygmomanometer-derived blood pressure measures display slightly higher systolic and lower diastolic pressures than simultaneously measured indwelling arterial catheters, but the MAP is usually similar and the actual systolic and diastolic pressure differences are often small except in the setting of increased peripheral vasomotor tone. If perfusion pressure of the finger is similar to arterial pressure, then both blood pressure and the pressure profile may be recorded non-invasively and continuously using the optical finger probe (e.g. Fenapres®). However, finger perfusion is often compromised during hypovolaemic shock and hypothermia, limiting this technique.

Accurate and continuous measurements of arterial pressure can be done through arterial catheterisation of easily accessible arterial sites in the arm (axillary, brachial or radial artery) or groin (femoral artery). Upper extremity sites other than the radial artery are rarely used because of fear of vascular compromise distal to the catheter insertion site, although data supporting these fears are limited. Arterial catheterisation displaying continuous arterial pressure waveforms allows arterial waveform analysis, essential in the calculation of pulse pressure and pulse pressure variations and CO by pulse contour analysis [10]. The overall accuracy of these techniques varies based on the quality of the arterial pressure signal and the method used to calculate flow [11–13].

Blood pressure is physiologically regulated through baroreceptor reflex arcs that keep it constant despite changing CO, whereas CO varies with changing tissue metabolic demands. Thus, a normal blood pressure does not necessarily reflect haemodynamic stability [7], since different organs may have markedly different intra-organ vascular resistances and global blood flow may vary as baseline vasomotor tone varies. Therefore, there is no threshold blood pressure value that can define adequate organ perfusion among organs, between different patients or in the same patient over time [14]. Arterial pressure is a primary determinant of organ blood flow because increased intra-organ flow only occurs because local vasodilation allows a high organ input pressure to increase local blood flow. Hypotension (MAP < 65 mm Hg) should be considered as a pathological state of organ hypoperfusion and loss of autoregulation of blood flow.

The relation between specific haemodynamic variables is complex in health and even more complex in disease. If disease causes CO and DO_2I to decrease, MAP decreases as well. Baroreceptors in the aortic arch and carotid body alter vasomotor tone through modulation of sympathetic tone to maintain cerebral perfusion pressure (e.g. MAP > 65 mm Hg) [9]. The haemodynamic effects of this increased sympathetic tone are tachycardia and restoration of MAP toward normal values by reducing unstressed circulatory blood volume and increased arterial vasomotor tone.

The blood circulating in the blood vessels can be considered as having two different physiological components. The first component is the initial volume needed to distend the vessels enough to cause an increase in vascular pressure. This vascular volume is called unstressed volume and comprises approximately 60% of the total circulating blood volume of a normal subject. Once the vasculature is distended enough to cause its vessels to stretch, further increases in blood volume cause a marked increase in vascular pressure. This additional volume is called the stressed blood volume. One of the primary means by which the body maintains an adequate upstream pressure driving venous return to the heart is by varying unstressed volume. Increasing sympathetic tone in response to stress decreases the unstressed volume by diverting blood flow away from vascular beds with high unstressed volume, like the splanchnic circulation, and also increasing general vasomotor tone. Both these processes function to maintain a constant arterial pressure despite hypovolaemia and reduced CO. Thus, hypotension reflects a failure of the sympathetic nervous system to compensate for circulatory shock, while normotension does not ensure adequate tissue perfusion. Since regulation of blood flow distribution occurs by regional vasodilation of arterial resistance vessels, hypotension impairs blood flow distribution by autoregulation [15, 16].

Central venous pressure (CVP) or right atrial pressure

CVP is also called right atrial pressure. CVP is the pressure in the large central veins proximal to the right atrium relative to atmosphere. CVP is usually measured using a fluid-filled catheter (central venous line or pulmonary artery catheter), with the distal tip located in the superior vena cava connected to a manometer or more often to a pressure transducer of a monitor, displaying the waveform in a continuous fashion. CVP can also be measured non-invasively as jugular venous pressure by the height of the column of blood distending the internal and external jugular veins, when the subject is sitting in a semi-reclined position, such that the small elevations in CVP will be reflected in a persistent jugular venous distention. However, the accuracy of jugular venous distention to assess absolute CVP values has not been substantiated.

Blood flows back to the heart from the peripheral venous reservoirs. The driving pressure for that flow is the difference in pressure between those venous reservoirs, called mean systemic pressure, and CVP, which is the back-pressure to systemic venous return. Although CVP rises with increases in intravascular volume, the relationship is not linear or consistent. Still, if CVP is 10 mm Hg or less it has some physiological significance. For example, Jellenik *et al.* showed that if CVP is 10 mm Hg or less, then CO will uniformly decrease in ventilated patients in whom 10 cm H_2O positive end-expiratory pressure (PEEP) is applied [17]. However, if CVP is > 10 mm Hg, CO may increase, remain the same or decrease. There is no threshold value of CVP that identifies patients whose CO will increase in response to fluid challenge [18]. From a static variable perspective, an elevated CVP only occurs in disease processes, but the clinical utility of CVP as a guide for diagnosing which disease is causing it or what the individual patient's response to treatment will be cannot be identified from measures of CVP.

Haemodynamic values measured by pulmonary artery catheter

The pulmonary artery catheter (PAC) is designed to estimate LV filling pressures by measuring Ppao [19, 20]. It can also measure pulmonary artery pressure (Ppa), CVP, SvO_2, CO and right ventricular ejection fraction. Just as CVP is the back-pressure for system venous return to the right ventricle, Ppao is the back-pressure to pulmonary blood flow to the left ventricle. Ppao can be used to identify the presence of a hydrostatic component to pulmonary oedema and to assess pulmonary vascular resistance. However, Ppao values do not correlate with LV end-diastolic volume, and neither do they predict preload responsiveness [21]. PAC can also be used to monitor RV end-diastolic volume, which, in turn, can be used in differentiating different causes of circulatory shock such as right-sided cardiac failure [22]. However, the utility of any static single-point measurement in predicting preload responsiveness or in improving outcome in unstable patients has not been demonstrated [23–25].

Cardiac output can be calculated by measuring blood flow using dilution techniques with a thermal [26] or lithium indicator via PAC or CVP. As mentioned before, because there is no normal CO and because an accurate measurement of CO is less important than accurate documentation of trends in blood flow, these measures may have profound clinical utility if the trends are accurate and stable over time.

However, SvO_2 measurements may be a better assessment of DO_2I adequacy. The normal value for SvO_2 is 70–75%. Muscle activity, anaemia, hypoxaemia and decreased CO all independently decrease SvO_2, whereas hyperdynamic sepsis, hypothermia and muscle relaxation increase SvO_2.

Although SvO_2 above 70% does not necessarily reflect adequate tissue oxygenation (for example, in sepsis), a persistently low SvO_2 ($< 50\%$) is associated with tissue ischaemia [27]. Although central venous oxygen saturation ($ScvO_2$) and SvO_2 are not equivalent, measures of $ScvO_2$ tend to track SvO_2. Therefore, $ScvO_2$ may be used to monitor resuscitation efforts if special attention is paid to related clinical variables [28]. Unfortunately, the variance of $ScvO_2$ relative to SvO_2 makes its use in clinical practice guidelines questionable at best. At present, using $ScvO_2$ as a tight surrogate marker of SvO_2 is not recommended.

Since intrathoracic structures are acted upon by pleural pressure (Ppl) but measured relative to atmosphere, measures of Ppao may not accurately measure Ppao relative to Ppl. Ventilation causes significant swings in Ppl. Pulmonary vascular pressures, when measured relative to atmospheric pressure, will reflect these respiratory changes in Ppl. To minimize this 'respiratory artifact' on intrathoracic vascular pressure recordings, measures are usually made at end-expiration. During quiet spontaneous breathing, end-expiration occurs at the highest vascular pressure values, whereas during passive positive-pressure breathing, end-expiration occurs at the lowest vascular pressure values. With assisted ventilation or with forced spontaneous ventilation, it is often difficult to define end-expiration [29]. These limitations are the primary reasons for inaccuracies in estimating Ppao at the bedside.

Pulmonary artery pressure

The pulmonary vascular bed is a low resistance circuit with a large reserve that normally allows increases of CO with minor changes in the pulmonary artery pressure (Ppa). However, increases in the downstream venous pressure (e.g. left ventricular failure) or in the flow resistance (e.g. lung diseases and hypoxic pulmonary vasoconstriction) all cause Ppa to increase if flow or CO remains constant. Although increases in CO alone do not normally cause pulmonary hypertension, with an increased pulmonary vascular resistance the Ppa can be increased due to changes in CO. The normal range of values for Ppa is: systolic 15–30 mm Hg, diastolic 4–12 mm Hg and mean 9–18 mm Hg [30]. A list of the normal range of various measured and derived haemodynamic variables is given in Table 3.2.

Pulmonary artery occlusion pressure

Pulmonary artery occlusion pressure (Ppao) is measured as the stop flow (balloon occlusion) end-expiratory Ppa pressure. Unfortunately, the ability of healthcare professionals to accurately measure Ppao from either a strip chart recording or a freeze frame snapshot of the monitor screen is poor. Thus, it is difficult to assess the utility of Ppao as a therapeutic guide with any degree of confidence. Ppao is thought to reflect LV filling because of the unique characteristics of the pulmonary circulation. Balloon inflation of the pulmonary artery catheter forces the tip to migrate distally into smaller vessels until the tip occludes a medium-sized (1.2 cm diameter) pulmonary artery. This occlusion stops all blood flow in that vascular tree distal to the occlusion site until such time as other venous branches reconnect

Table 3.2 Primary and derived haemodynamic parameters from haemodynamic monitoring*.

	Normal range
Primary haemodynamic variables	
Heart rate (HR)	60–85/min
Mean arterial pressure (MAP)	80–95 mm Hg
Central venous pressure (CVP)	–2 to +6 mm Hg
Mean pulmonary arterial pressure (MPAP)	12–22 mm Hg
Pulmonary artery occlusion pressure (Ppao)	4–8 mm Hg
Cardiac output (CO)	4–8 l/min
Mixed venous oxygen saturation (SvO_2)	70–75%
Derived haemodynamic variables	
Stroke volume (SV) = CO/HR × 1000	70 ± 5 ml
Height and weight to calculate body surface area (BSA)	
Cardiac index (CI) = CO/BSA	$3.2 ± 0.6$ l/min/m^2
Stroke index (SI) = SV/BSA	$45 ± 6$ ml/m^2
LV stroke work (LVSW) = SV × (MAP – Ppao) × 0.144 g m/m^2	$56 ± 6$ g m/m^2
LV stroke work index (LVSWI) = LVSW/BSA	
Total peripheral resistance (TPR) = [(MAP)/CO] × 80 dynes/sec/cm^5	900–1400 dynes/sec/cm^5
Systemic vascular resistance (SVR) = [(MAP – PAOP)/CO] × 80 dynes/sec/cm^5	900–1400 dynes/sec/cm^5
Systemic vascular resistance index (SVRI) = SVR/BSA	
RV stroke work (RVSW) = SV × (MPAP – CVP) × 0.144	$8.8 ± 0.9$ g m/m^2
RV stroke work index (RVSWI) = RVSW/BSA	
Pulmonary vascular resistance (PVR) = [(MPAP – PAOP)/CO] × 80 dynes/sec/cm^5	150–250 dynes/sec/cm^5
Pulmonary vascular resistance index (PVRI) = PVR/BSA	

*Normal values only serve as a reference in normal subjects and may not reflect appropriate levels in stress states. To calculate indexed values, calculate the unadjusted value, then divide by BSI.

downstream to this venous draining bed about 1.5 cm from the left atrium. Thus, if a continuous column of blood is present from the catheter tip to the left heart, then Ppao measures pulmonary venous pressure at this first junction, or J-1 point, of the pulmonary veins [31]. As downstream pulmonary blood flow ceases, distal pulmonary arterial pressure falls in a double exponential fashion to a minimal value, reflecting the pressure downstream in the pulmonary vasculature from the point of occlusion first through the alveolar capillaries and then through the pulmonary veins. Thus, the Ppa value where the first exponential pressure decay is overtaken by the second longer exponential pressure decay reflects pulmonary capillary pressure (Pcap), useful in calculating pulmonary arterial and venous resistances (Figure 3.1).

Validation of balloon occlusion can be made by sampling distal blood from the occlusion tip for blood gas analysis. Since the sampled blood will be from the stagnant pool of blood, its removal will make it be pulled back

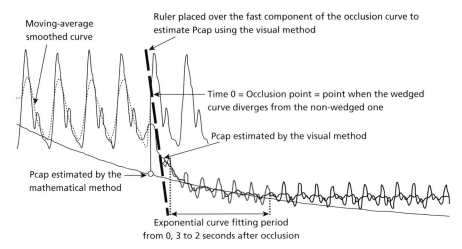

Figure 3.1 Calculation of pulmonary capillary pressure (Pcap) from the pulmonary arterial waveform during a distal balloon occlusion manoeuvre. (Reproduced with permission from Takala. *Intensive Care Med* 2003; 29:890–3.)

into the pulmonary artery catheter from the pulmonary veins which means it crosses the alveolar capillaries twice; thus pCO_2 will be lower than arterial pCO_2 and its pO_2 higher, due to this increased gas exchange. Ppao is used most often in the bedside assessment of pulmonary oedema, pulmonary vasomotor tone, intravascular volume status, and LV preload and performance [32].

Pulmonary oedema can be caused by either Pcap elevations, referred to as hydrostatic or secondary pulmonary oedema, or increased alveolar capillary or epithelial permeability, referred to as primary pulmonary oedema. Usually hydrostatic pulmonary oedema requires Pcap values in excess of approximately 18 mm Hg. However, if alveolar endothelial or epithelial cell injury is present, alveolar flooding can occur at much lower pulmonary capillary pressures. Furthermore, in the setting of chronic pulmonary vascular congestion, increased pulmonary lymphatic flow and increased respiratory excursions promote a rapid clearance of lung interstitial fluid, minimising oedema formation. Still, when pulmonary oedema Pcap < 18 mm Hg a non-hydrostatic cause is implicated, whereas values > 20 mm Hg suggest a hydrostatic cause of pulmonary oedema [31]. Ppao may be > 20 mm Hg without any evidence of hydrostatic pulmonary oedema, either because Ppl is also elevated or because of increased pulmonary lymphatic flow or when Ppao is chronically elevated leading to remodeling of the alveolar–capillary membrane.

The pulmonary circulation normally has a low resistance, with pulmonary arterial diastolic pressure only slightly higher than Ppao and mean pulmonary arterial pressure a few mm Hg higher than Ppao. Pulmonary vascular resistance (PVR) can be estimated as the ratio of the pulmonary vascular pressure gradient (mean pulmonary artery pressure minus Ppao) and CO (i.e. PVR = (mean Ppa – Ppao)/CO). Normal pulmonary vascular resistance index is between 2 and 4 mm Hg/l/min/m^2. Usually these values are multiplied by 80 to give a normal pulmonary vascular resistance range in dynes per second per cm^5 of 150–250. Either an increased pulmonary vascular resistance or a passive pressure buildup from the pulmonary veins can induce pulmonary hypertension. If pulmonary hypertension is caused by an increased PVR then the causes are primarily within the lung, including pulmonary embolism, pulmonary fibrosis, essential pulmonary hypertension, hyperinflation and pulmonary veno-occlusive disease. The one exception to this rule is chronic left-sided pressure overload, as occurs with mitral stenosis. If PVR is normal then LV dysfunction is the more likely cause of pulmonary hypertension [33].

Ppao is often taken to reflect LV filling pressure and, by inference, LV end-diastolic volume. Patients with cardiovascular insufficiency and a low Ppao are presumed to be hypovolaemic and initially treated with fluid resuscitation, whereas patients with similar presentations but an elevated Ppao are presumed to have impaired contractile function. Although there is no accepted high and low Ppao values for which LV underfilling is presumed to occur or not, Ppao values < 10 mm Hg are usually used as presumed evidence of a low LV end-diastolic volume, whereas values > 18 mm Hg suggest a distended LV [34]. Unfortunately, there are very little data to support this approach and almost no data to defend this logic. In fact, most studies document that absolute Ppao values do not predict fluid responsiveness.

There are multiple documented reasons for this observed inaccuracy that relate to individual differences in LV diastolic compliance and contractile function [35]. First, the relationship between Ppao and LV end-diastolic volume is not linear and can be different among subjects and within subjects over time. Thus, neither absolute values of Ppao nor changes in Ppao will define a specific LV end-diastolic volume or its change [36]. Second, Ppao is not the distending pressure for LV filling. It is only the internal pressure of the pulmonary veins relative to atmospheric pressure. It is directly altered by changes in Ppl. Although we can estimate Ppl using oesophageal balloon catheters, pericardial pressure is often different. Changes in pericardial pressure will alter LV end-diastolic volume independent of Ppao. Finally, LV diastolic compliance can very rapidly change the relationship between LV filling pressure and LV end-diastolic volume because of myocardial ischaemia, arrhythmias and acute RV dilation (ventricular interdependence).

A major use of the pulmonary artery catheter is to assess LV performance. Ppao is often used as a substitute for LV end-diastolic volume when constructing Starling curves, which show the relationship between changing LV preload and ejection phase indices such as LV stroke work (LV stroke volume × developed pressure). Using this construct, patients with heart failure can be divided into four groups depending on their Ppao (> or < 18 mm Hg) and cardiac index values (> or < 2.2 l/min/m^2) [34]. Those patients with low cardiac indices and high Ppao are presumed to have primary heart failure, and a low CO and low Ppao, on the other hand, reflect hypovolaemia. Those with high cardiac indices and high Ppao are presumed to be volume overloaded, and having a high CO and low Ppao reflects increased sympathetic tone. Although this may be a useful construct for determining diagnosis, treatment and prognosis of patients with acute coronary syndrome, it poorly predicts the cardiovascular status of individual subjects.

3.3 Haemodynamic profile analysis: grouping of static variables

Except in the face of severe hypoxaemia and anaemia, the primary means by which DO_2I is increased to match metabolic requirements is by varying CO and tissue O_2 extraction. Since metabolic demands can vary widely, there is no normal CO or DO_2I value, but rather minimal thresholds for resting conditions and potentially adequate higher levels during stress. Operationally, it is better to access CO as being either adequate or inadequate to meet the metabolic demands of the body. Inadequate DO_2I is presumed to occur if tissue O_2 extraction is markedly increased, as manifest by a decrease in a $SvO_2 < 70\%$.

Of the four categories of shock listed above, only distributive shock states following intravascular volume resuscitation are associated with an increased CO but decreased vasomotor tone [37]. Thus, CO, stroke work, DO_2I and SvO_2 are decreased in cardiogenic, hypovolaemic and obstructive shock but may be normal or even increased in distributive shock. Cardiogenic shock can be caused by impaired contractility, pump function or impaired diastolic compliance. The cardinal signs of cardiogenic shock are increased back pressure to cardiac filling (CVP and Ppao) and upstream oedema (peripheral and pulmonary). Hypovolaemic shock represents a decrease in effective circulating blood volume and venous return. It can be caused by primary or secondary intravascular volume loss and increased unstressed vascular volume. The specific findings of hypovolaemic shock are decreased filling pressures. The specific findings of obstructive shock are often less specific but include decreased LV diastolic compliance and signs of cor pulmonale. Distributive shock represents loss of normal sympathetic responsiveness resulting in decreased vasomotor tone. In the non-resuscitated subject this presents as hypovolaemic shock, but with fluid resuscitation blood pressure does not increase despite an increase in CO. It is due to loss of vascular responsiveness. The specific findings of distributive shock are an increased CO, DO_2I and SvO_2 despite persistent hypotension. Haemodynamic monitoring can aid in determining the aetiology of circulatory shock (Table 3.3).

3.4 Functional haemodynamic monitoring: response to therapy

A primary goal of resuscitation is to increase DO_2I and to restore regional DO_2I to those tissues that are hypoperfused. Thus, the primary functional

Table 3.3 Classification of different haemodynamic profiles based on two primary and one derived variable.

	Pulmonary artery occlusion pressure (mm Hg)	Cardiac index (l/min/m²)	Systemic vascular resistance index (dynes/sec/cm⁵/m²)
Normal	6–15	2.5–4.0	1900–2400
Hypovolaemia	< 6	< 2.5	> 2400
Fluid overload	> 15	> 2.5	< 2400
Septic shock	< 15	> 4.0	< 1900
Left heart failure	> 15	< 2.5	> 1900
Mixed	< 15	2.5–4.0	< 1900
Pulmonary hypertension	< 15	< 2.5	PRVI > 300

Adapted from data originally described in Minoz et al. *Crit Care Med* 1994; 22:573–9.

question usually asked of the haemodynamically unstable patient is will CO increase with fluid resuscitation and, if so, by how much? Physiologically speaking this equates to defining whether the patient's CO increases with preload, provided by a volume challenge. Although specific patterns of haemodynamic values, as described above, reflect specific types of disease, they do not predict individual patient response to therapy.

Haemodynamic monitoring to evaluate the effect of therapy is known as functional monitoring, because it implies a therapeutic application [1]. Because a rapid change in trends of measured values in response to a specific therapy has a greater clinical utility, the most common type of functional monitoring is a therapeutic trial.

The volume challenge

One of the methods used in assessing preload responsiveness is to infuse a small fluid bolus rapidly and evaluate the haemodynamic response by observing changes in arterial blood pressure, heart rate, CO, SvO_2 and/or other relevant measures. A patient is considered to be a 'responder' if there is an improvement in circulatory status, such as increasing MAP, stroke volume and CO or a decreasing heart rate. Other indicators of preload responsiveness are increasing SvO_2 or decreasing blood lactate, which reflect improved effective blood flow. A fluid challenge must be conducted within the context of known or suspected tissue hypoperfusion [38]. Importantly, a volume challenge is only a diagnostic test to identify those who are preload responsive, and it should not be considered as a completion of fluid resuscitation [39]. If clinical evidence of hypoperfusion persists, then volume responders should be given additional fluid resuscitation with minimal risk for worsening right ventricular failure or inducing pulmonary oedema.

One of the primary disadvantages of this diagnostic approach in haemodynamically unstable patients is that it is only positive in half of hypotensive patients [40]. Thus, it will delay primary treatment in half of the patients who are not responders to a volume challenge. This is of special importance when a delayed appropriate therapy can be associated with negative consequences on patient survival. Furthermore, a volume challenge in a non-responder may worsen or precipitate pulmonary oedema and CO. Fortunately, there are several validated alternative methods that mimic a reversible or transient volume challenge without any volume actually being administered, which are discussed in the following paragraphs.

Preload responsiveness in positive pressure ventilated patients

Positive pressure ventilation cyclically alters the pressure gradient for systemic venous return, proportionally altering right ventricular output on the next beat during inspiration. After about 2–4 beats, left ventricular filling and output are also proportionally altered. Thus, in patients whose ventricles are preload responsive, positive pressure ventilation will induce cyclical changes in stroke volume. Since the critical physiological determinant is the tidal volume induced change in intrathoracic pressure, the greater the increase in tidal volume for the same lung compliance, the greater the transient decrease in venous return and subsequently greater the decrease in LV output [41]. The degree of changes in either arterial pulse pressure or systolic blood pressure in response to a series of increasing tidal breaths quantifies the degree of preload responsiveness [42, 43]. On the other hand, when a fixed tidal volume is delivered during positive pressure ventilation, the degrees of variation in systolic pressure [44], pulse pressure [45–47], stroke volume [48–51] and aortic flow [52–54] accurately reflect preload responsiveness. These dynamic predictors of preload responsiveness are often referred to as systolic pressure variation (SPV), pulse pressure variation (PPV) and stroke volume variation (SVV) and are calculated as the maximal difference in their respective values of 3–10 breaths divided by their mean values. A systolic pressure or a pulse pressure variation of 13% or more in septic patients breathing with a tidal volume of 8 ml/kg is highly sensitive and specific for detecting preload responsiveness [45] (Figure 3.2).

Arterial pressure pulse contour analysis has been used to estimate stroke volume variation and preload responsiveness [55]. Unfortunately, there are controversial results regarding the accuracy of the pulse contour algorithm used to calculate stroke volume using commercially available devices, and studies are limited [11–13, 56]. Similarly, recent studies suggest that the pulse oximetry plethysmographic waveform amplitude co-varies with arterial pulse pressure [60–62]. Like PPV, plethysmographic signal variation predicts fluid responsiveness in hypotensive patients [63, 64]. If validated to predict preload responsiveness in a broader group of haemodynamically unstable patients, such non-invasive techniques could expand the application of this applied physiological approach at the bedside. Finally, more than 36% superior vena cava collapse assessed by echocardiography during positive pressure ventilation identifies individuals whose CVP is < 10 mm Hg [57–59]. Since a CVP < 10 mm Hg

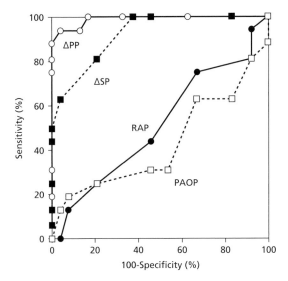

Figure 3.2 Receiver operator characteristics of the ability of pulse pressure variation (ΔPP), systolic pressure variation (ΔSP), right atrial pressure (RAP) and pulmonary artery occlusion pressure (PAOP) to predict a 15% increase in cardiac output in response to a 500 ml fluid bolus in septic patients receiving mechanical ventilation. (Reproduced from Michard et al. [21], with permission from *Am J Respir Crit Care Med*.)

is associated with a decrease in CO if PEEP is increased, this finding has some clinical relevance. However, these methods to date have been more of a curiosity than a clinical tool.

Preload responsiveness during spontaneous breathing

During spontaneous inspiration, venous return normally increases owing to a fall in intrathoracic pressure [65]. A normal right ventricle pumps this increased blood flow into the pulmonary circulation. Therefore CVP will decrease with decreasing intrathoracic pressure with each spontaneous inspiratory effort. An inspiratory decrease in CVP of more than 1 mm Hg when intrathoracic pressure decreases more than 2 mm Hg accurately predicts preload responsiveness, whereas those patients whose CVP does not decrease in such a setting do not increase their CO in response to fluid challenge [66], but this approach requires central venous catheterisation. A change in inferior vena cava diameter during positive pressure ventilation can be also interpreted as CVP changes [67], but it requires complex echocardiographic technology and has minimal diagnostic utility at the bedside.

Passive leg raising

Passive leg raising to 30° transiently increases venous return [68] in patients who are preload responsive. Since this only transiently increases CO and blood pressure [69] in responders, it is only a diagnostic test and cannot be considered as a treatment for hypovolaemia. The main advantage of this approach is that it is reversible and easy to perform [70]. It also can be repeated many times to reassess preload responsiveness without any risk of inducing pulmonary oedema in potential non-responders. One of the major limitations of this technique is that in severely hypovolaemic patients the blood volume mobilised by leg raising which is dependent on total blood volume could be small, which in turn can show minimal to no increase in CO and blood pressure, even in responders.

3.5 Conclusion

A systematic approach to functional haemodynamic monitoring is the cornerstone of an effective resuscitation effort. If a patient responds to volume challenge or any equivalent preload responsiveness tests, then volume resuscitation should be initiated. In preload responsive patients who, despite increase in CO in response to fluid resuscitation, cannot maintain an adequate perfusion, a decrease in vascular tone should be suspected and vasopressors should be given in addition to fluids. If a hypotensive patient is neither preload responsive nor exhibiting reduced vasomotor tone, then the problem is the heart or an obstruction in blood flow such as thromboembolic events. In which case, both diagnostic and therapeutic actions must be taken simultaneously (e.g. echocardiography, dobutamine or thrombolytic therapy). This systematic approach can be incorporated in a protocolised cardiovascular management algorithm based on functional haemodynamic monitoring [71, 72], which in turn can improve patient-centred outcomes and cost of the healthcare system, by faster and more effectively response in order to diagnose and treat haemodynamically unstable patients both inside and outside of intensive care units.

Case study

A 45-year-old white male sustained multiple trauma following a motor vehicle accident, including multiple right-sided rib fractures and lung contusion, pelvic fracture and ruptured spleen. This was initially treated by endotracheal intubation, mechanical ventilation and emergent splenectomy. Post-operatively the patient did well, but at 12 hours following surgery he developed progressive tachycardia (HR 120 sinus), low urine output (< 10 ml/hour, specific gravity 1.024) and hypoxaemia (SpO$_2$ 88% on FiO$_2$ 0.4). Central venous pressure (CVP) was 14 mm Hg and blood pressure was 110/80 with a mean of 95 mm Hg. Initially the treating physicians were reticent about giving a volume challenge because of the hypoxaemia and elevated CVP. A pulmonary artery catheter was inserted revealing a mixed venous O$_2$ saturation (SvO$_2$) of 45%, a pulmonary artery pressure (Ppa) of 55/20 with a mean of 25 mm Hg, a pulmonary artery occlusion pressure (Ppao) of

Continued

18 mm Hg, a cardiac index of 2.0 l/min/m^2 and a haemoglobin of 10.6 gm%. Because of the low SvO$_2$ and CO and high Ppao, dobutamine was started at 5 μg/kg/min. This resulted in worsening tachycardia and hypotension, with a MAP of 50 mm Hg. Dobutamine was stopped and noradrenaline started, with an increase in MAP (65 mm Hg) but with no change in SvO$_2$, CO or urine output.

Since the patient was on mechanical ventilation and fully controlled, the physicians monitored arterial pulse pressure variation (PPV) throughout the respiratory cycle, revealing a PPV of 45%. Intra-abdominal pressure was measured, as the fluid level of the Foley urinary catheter urine column height, as 25 cm urine. Based on these data, aggressive fluid resuscitation was initiated and the patient received approximately 3000 ml of combined colloid and crystalloid infusion over 1 hour, with an increasing cardiac index (3.5 l/min/m^2), SvO$_2$ (68%) and MAP (70 mm Hg) but no increase in urine output or change in CVP or Ppao. Intra-abdominal pressure remained elevated and an abdominal CT revealed a massive retroperitoneal haemorrhage. The patient was returned to the operating room where an undiagnosed ruptured right psoas artery was repaired and the associated retroperitoneal blood collection drained and four units of packed red blood cells infused. The patient did well in the immediate operative state and was extubated the next day, being discharged from the hospital by the 8th day.

Comment

This case illustrates many of the insights underscored in this chapter. First, that volume status and volume responsiveness cannot be determined by either CVP or Ppao values. Dynamic measures of volume responsiveness, such as PPV, need to be used. Second, a 'normal' CO and MAP can co-exist with severe haemorrhagic shock as evidenced by the low SvO$_2$ and tachycardia. Finally, organ perfusion pressure determines blood flow, such that the increased intra-abdominal pressure prevented the noradrenaline-induced increase in MAP from increasing renal blood flow and urine output.

Acknowledgement

This work was supported in part by the NIH grants HL67181, HL07820 and HL073198.

References

1. Pinsky MR, Payen D. Functional hemodynamic monitoring. *Crit Care* 2005, 9(6):566–72.
2. Bland RD, Shoemaker WC, Abraham E, et al. Hemodynamic and oxygen transport patterns in surviving and nonsurviving postoperative patients. *Crit Care Med* 1985, 13:85–90.

3. Rivers E, Nguyen B, Havstad S, et al. Early goal-directed therapy in the treatment of severe sepsis and septic shock. *N Engl J Med* 2001, 345:1368–77.

4. Gattinoni L, Brazzi L, Pelosi P, et al. A trial of goal-oriented hemodynamic therapy in critically ill patients. SvO_2 Collaborative Group. *N Engl J Med* 1995, 333:1025–32.

5. Heyland DK, Cook DJ, King D, et al. Maximizing oxygen delivery in critically ill patients: a methodologic appraisal of the evidence. *Crit Care Med* 1996, 24:517–24.

6. Kern JW, Shoemaker WC. Meta-analysis of hemodynamic optimization in high-risk patients. *Crit Care Med* 2002, 30:1686–92.

7. Partrick DA, Bensard DD, Janik JS, et al. Is hypotension a reliable indicator of blood loss from traumatic injury in children? *Am J Surg* 2002, 184:555–9.

8. Pinsky MR, Vincent JL. Let us use the pulmonary artery catheter correctly and only when we need it. *Crit Care Med* 2005, 33:1119–22.

9. Bur A, Hirschl MM, Herkner H, et al. Accuracy of oscillometric blood pressure measurement according to the relation between cuff size and upper-arm circumference in critically ill patients. *Crit Care Med* 2000, 28:371–6.

10. Wesseling KH, Jansen JRC, Settels JJ, et al. Computation of aortic flow from pressure in humans using a nonlinear, three-element model. *J Appl Physiol* 1993, 74:2566–73.

11. Opdam HI, Wan L, Bellomo R. A pilot assessment of the Flotrac TM cardiac output monitoring system. *Intensive Care Med* 2006, DOI 10.1007/s00134-006-0410-4.

12. Pittman J, Bar-Yosef S, SumPing J, et al. Continuous cardiac output monitoring with pulse contour analysis: a comparison with lithium indicator dilution cardiac output measurement. *Crit Care Med* 2005, 33:2015–21.

13. Headley JM. Arterial pressure-based technologies: a new trend in cardiac output monitoring. *Crit Care Nurs Clin North Am* 2006, 18(2):179–87.

14. LeDoux D, Astix ME, Carpati C, et al. Effects of perfusion pressure on tissue perfusion in septic shock. *Crit Care Med* 2000, 28:2729–32.

15. Ruokonen E, Takala J, Uusaro A. Effect of vasoactive treatment on the relationship between mixed venous and regional oxygen saturation. *Crit Care Med* 1991, 19:1365–9.

16. Bellomo R, Kellum JA, Wisniewski SR, et al. Effects of norepinephrine on the renal vasculature in normal and endotoxemic dogs. *Am J Respir Crit Care Med* 1999, 159:1186–92.

17. Jellinek H, Krafft P, Fitzgerald RD, et al. Right atrial pressure predicts hemodynamic response to apneic positive airway pressure. *Crit Care Med* 2000, 28:672–8.

18. Kumar A, Anel R, Bunnell E, et al. Pulmonary artery occlusion pressure and central venous pressure fail to predict ventricular filling volume, cardiac performance, or the response to volume infusion in normal subjects. *Crit Care Med* 2004, 32:691–9.

19. Pinsky MR, Vincent JL, DeSmet JM. Estimating left ventricular filling pressure during positive end-expiratory pressure in humans. *Am Rev Respir Dis* 1991, 143:25–31.

20. Teboul JL, Pinsky MR, Mercat A, et al. Estimating cardiac filling pressure in mechanically ventilated patients with hyperinflation. *Crit Care Med* 2000, 28:3631–6.

21. Michard F, Boussat S, Chemla D, et al. Relation between respiratory changes in arterial pulse pressure and fluid responsiveness in septic patients with acute circulatory failure. *Am J Respir Crit Care Med* 2000, 162:134–8.

22. Hines R, Rafferty T. Right ventricular ejection fraction catheter: toy or tool? Pro: a useful monitor. *J Cardiothorac Vasc Anesth* 1993, 7:236–40.

23. Monnet X, Teboul JL. Invasive measures of left ventricular preload. *Curr Opin Crit Care* 2006, 12(3):235–40.

24. Osman D, Ridel C, Ray P, et al. Cardiac filling pressures are not appropriate to predict hemodynamic response to volume challenge. *Crit Care Med* 2007, 35:64–8.

25. The National Heart, Lung, and Blood Institute Acute Respiratory Distress Syndrome (ARDS) Clinical Trials Network. Pulmonary artery versus central venous catheter to guide treatment of acute lung injury. *N Engl J Med* 2006, 354:2213–24.

26. Snyder JV, Powner DJ. Effects of mechanical ventilation on the measurement of cardiac output by thermodilution. *Crit Care Med* 1982, 10:677–82.

27. Rady MY, Rivers EP, Martin GB, et al. Continuous central venous oximetry and shock index in the emergency department: use in the evaluation of clinical shock. *Am J Emerg Med* 1992, 10:538–43.

28. Scheinman MM, Brown MA, Rapaport E. Critical assessment of use of central venous oxygen saturation as a mirror of mixed venous oxygen in severely ill cardiac patients. *Circulation* 1969, 40:165–72.

29. Hoyt JD, Leatherman JW. Interpretation of the pulmonary artery occlusion pressure in mechanically ventilated patients with large respiratory excursions in intrathoracic pressure. *Intensive Care Med* 1997, 23:1125–31.

30. Sharkey SW. Beyond the wedge: clinical physiology and the Swan-Ganz catheter. *Am J Med* 1987, 83:111–22.

31. Swan HJ, Ganz W, Forrester J, et al. Catheterization of the heart in man with use of a flow-directed balloon-tipped catheter. *N Engl J Med* 1970, 283:447–51.

32. Pinsky MR. Clinical significance of pulmonary artery occlusion pressure. *Intensive Care Med* 2003, 29:175–8.

33. Abraham AS, Cole RB, Green ID, et al. Factors contributing to the reversible pulmonary hypertension of patients with acute respiratory failure studies by serial observations during recovery. *Circ Res* 1969, 24:51–60.

34. Forrester JS, Diamond G, Chatterjee K, et al. Medical therapy of acute myocardial infarction by application of hemodynamic subsets (first of two parts). *N Engl J Med* 1976, 295:1356–62.

35. Raper R, Sibbald WJ. Misled by the wedge? The Swan-Ganz catheter and left ventricular preload. *Chest* 1986, 89:427–34.

36. Kumar A, Anel R, Bunnell E, et al. Pulmonary artery occlusion pressure and central venous pressure fail to predict ventricular filling volume, cardiac performance, or the response to volume infusion in normal subjects. *Crit Care Med* 2004, 32:691–9.

37. Carroll GC, Snyder JV. Hyperdynamic severe intravascular sepsis depends on fluid administration in cynomolgus monkey. *Am J Physiol* 1982, 243:R131–41.

38. Dellinger RP, Carlet JM, Masur H, et al., for the Surviving Sepsis Campaign Management Guidelines Committee. Surviving Sepsis Campaign Management Guidelines. *Crit Care Med* 2004, 32:858–73.

39. Pinsky MR: Using ventilation-induced aortic pressure and flow variation to diagnose preload responsiveness. *Intensive Care Med* 2004, 30:1008–10.

40. Michard F, Teboul JL. Predicting fluid responsiveness in ICU patients. A critical analysis of the evidence. *Chest* 2002, 121:2000–8.

41. Reuter DA, Bayerlein J, Goepfert MS, et al. Influence of tidal volume on left ventricular stroke volume variation measured by pulse contour analysis in mechanically ventilated patients. *Intensive Care Med* 2003, 29:476–80.

42. Perel A: Analogue values from invasive hemodynamic monitoring. In: Pinsky MR, ed. *Applied Cardiovascular Physiology*. Berlin, Germany: Springer-Verlag; 1997:129–40.

43. Charron C, Fessenmeyer C, Cosson C, et al. The influence of tidal volume on the dynamic variables of fluid responsiveness in critically ill patients. *Anesth Analg* 2006, 102:1511–17.

44. Perel A: Assessing fluid responsiveness by the systolic pressure variation in mechanically ventilated patients. Systolic pressure variation as a guide to fluid therapy in patients with sepsis-induced hypotension. *Anesthesiology* 1998, 89:1309–10.

45. Michard F, Boussat S, Chemla D, et al. Relation between respiratory changes in arterial pulse pressure and fluid responsiveness in septic patients with acute circulatory failure. *Am J Respir Crit Care Med* 2000, 162:134–8.

46. De Backer D, Heenen S, Piagnerelli M, et al. Pulse pressure variations to predict fluid responsiveness: influence of tidal volume. *Intensive Care Med* 2005, 31:517–23.

47. Solus-Biguenet H, Fleyfel M, Tavernier B, et al. Non-invasive prediction of fluid responsiveness during major hepatic surgery. *Brit J Anesth* 2006, 97(6):808–16.

48. Slama M, Masson H, Teboul JL, et al. Respiratory variations of aortic VTI: a new index of hypovolemia and fluid responsiveness. *Am J Physiol Heart Circ Physiol* 2002, 283:H1729–33.

49. Reuter D, Felbinger TW, Schmidt C, et al. Stroke volume variation for assessment of cardiac responsiveness to volume loading in mechanically ventilated patients after cardiac surgery. *Intensive Care Med* 2002, 28:392–8.

50. Hofer CK, Muller SM, Furrer L, et al. Stroke volume and pulse pressure variation for prediction of fluid responsiveness in patients undergoing off-pump coronary artery bypass grafting. *Chest* 2005, 128(2):848–54.

51. Wiesenack C, Fiegl C, Keyser A, et al. Assessment of fluid responsiveness in mechanically ventilated cardiac surgical patients. *Eur J Anaesthesiol* 2005, 22(9):658–65.

52. Feissel M, Michard F, Mangin I, et al. Respiratory changes in aortic blood velocity as an indicator of fluid responsiveness in ventilated patients with septic shock. *Chest* 2001, 119:867–73.

53. Monnet X, Rienzo M, Osman D, et al. Esophageal Doppler monitoring predicts fluid responsiveness in critically ill ventilated patients. *Intensive Care Med* 2005, 31:1195–201.

54. Slama M, Masson H, Teboul JL, et al. Monitoring of respiratory variations of aortic blood flow velocity using esophageal Doppler. *Intensive Care Med* 2004, 30:1181–7.

55. Berkenstadt H, Margalit N, Hadani M, et al. Stroke volume variation as a predictor of fluid responsiveness in patients undergoing brain surgery. *Anesth Analg* 2001, 92:984–9.

56. Pinsky MR. Probing the limits of arterial pulse contour analysis to predict preload responsiveness. *Anesth Analg* 2003, 96:1245–7.

57. Vieillard-Baron A, Chergui K, Rabiller A, et al. Superior vena caval collapsibility as a gauge of volume status in ventilated septic patients. *Intensive Care Med* 2004, 30:1734–9.

58. Vieillard-Baron A, Augarde R, Prin S, et al. Influence of superior vena caval zone condition on cyclic changes in right ventricular outflow during respiratory support. *Anesthesiology* 2001, 95:1083–8.

59. Barbier C, Loubieres Y, Schmit C, et al. Respiratory changes in inferior vena cava diameter are helpful in predicting fluid responsiveness in ventilated septic patients. *Intensive Care Med* 2004, 30:1740–6.

60. Cassesson M, Besnard C, Durand PG, et al. Relation between respiratory variations in pulse oximetry plethysmographic waveform amplitude and arterial pulse pressure in ventilated patients. *Crit Care* 2005, 9:R562–8.

61. Monnet X, Lamia B, Teboul JL. Pulse oximeter as a sensor of fluid responsiveness: do we have our finger on the best solution? *Crit Care* 2005, 9(5):429–30.

62. Cannesson M, Desebbe O, Hachemi M, et al. Respiratory variation in pulse oximeter waveform amplitude are influenced by venous return in mechanically ventilated patients under general anaesthesia. *Eur J Anaesthesiol* 2006, 23:1–7.

63. Natalini G, Rosano A, Taranto M, et al. Arterial versus plethysmographic dynamic indices to test responsiveness for testing fluid administration in hypotensive patients: a clinical trial. *Anesth Analg* 2006, 103:1478–84.

64. Feissel M, Badie J, Merlani PG, et al. Pre-ejection period variation in fluid responsiveness of septic ventilated patients. *Crit Care Med* 2005, 33(11):2534–9.

65. Pinsky MR. Determinants of pulmonary artery flow variation during respiration. *J Appl Physiol* 1984, 56:1237–45.

66. Magder SA, Georgiadis G, Tuck C. Respiratory variations in right atrial pressure predict response to fluid challenge. *J Crit Care* 1992, 7:76–85.

67. Feissel M, Michard F, Faller JP, et al. The respiratory variation in the inferior vena cava diameter as a guide to fluid therapy. *Intensive Care Med* 2004, 30:1834–7.

68. Thomas M, Shillingford J: The circulatory response to a standard postural change in ischaemic heart disease. *Brit Heart J* 1965, 27:17–27.

69. Boulain T, Achard JM, Teboul JL, et al. Changes in blood pressure induced by passive leg raising predict response to fluid loading in critically ill patients. *Chest* 2002, 121:1245–52.

70. Monnet X, Rienzo M, Osman D, et al. Response to leg raising predicts fluid responsiveness during spontaneous breathing or with arrhythmia. *Crit Care Med* 2006, 34:1402–7.

71. McKendry M, McGloin H, Saberi D, et al. Randomised controlled trial assessing the impact of a nurse delivered, flow monitored protocol for optimisation of circulatory status after cardiac surgery. *Brit Med J* 2004, 329:438–44.

72. Pearse R, Dawson D, Fawcett J, et al. Early goal-directed therapy after major surgery reduces complications and duration of hospital stay. A randomised, controlled trial. *Crit Care* 2005, 9:R687–93.

4 Cardiovascular Investigation of the Critically Ill

Susanna Price and Jeremy J. Cordingley
Royal Brompton & Harefield NHS Foundation Trust, London, UK

Take Home Messages

- Basic investigations are still valuable in the management of critically ill patients.
- Many investigations have not been well validated in the critically ill.
- The risk:benefit ratio should be considered for each investigation.
- The greatest risk to the patient is misinterpretation of investigations – expert opinion is often warranted.

4.1 Introduction

Investigation of the critically ill patient with cardiac disease requires a broad knowledge of cardiovascular pathophysiology, the range of investigations available, and their specificity and sensitivity. In addition, knowledge of what is normal for the patient population being dealt with is essential, as what is regarded as normal in some may be abnormal in others (e.g. haemoglobin concentration and saturations in some patients with complex congenital heart disease). Certain investigations, for example transoesophageal echocardiography (TOE), carry a risk to the patient and the potential benefits must be balanced against these risks. In others, the greatest risk is misinterpretation – particularly where the investigation requires significant expertise on the part of the reporter or operator. Here, the presence of an experienced investigator is crucial. In the intensive care unit (ICU) many investigations are not as well validated as in the out-patient setting, so that application of first principles and an understanding of the abnormalities in the context of the clinical status of the patient is crucial.

Cardiovascular Critical Care. Edited by M. Griffiths, J. Cordingley and S. Price.
© 2010 Blackwell Publishing Ltd.

4.2 Electrocardiography (ECG)

Basic ECG
Whilst continuous recordings to obtain signal-averaged ECG, QT
dispersion, ST segment changes and heart rate variability are available,
standard 3- or 5-lead ECG recording is the most commonly used, widely
available and well-validated method for detecting the presence of
arrhythmia and myocardial ischaemia in the ICU. Every patient should
undergo a 12-lead ECG on first arrival in the ICU, and comparison with
previous ECGs is desirable where possible. A repeated 12-lead ECG should
be performed with the onset of any new or recurrent symptoms, where
there is haemodynamic instability, with the development of arrhythmia,
following any cardiovascular intervention, or daily in some instances,
for example aortic root endocarditis. In patients with temporary pacing
wires (endocardial or epicardial), daily assessment of the underlying heart
rhythm and of the thresholds (output and sensitivity) is essential.

Diagnosis of myocardial ischaemia
Silent myocardial ischaemia in the ICU is probably underdiagnosed,
occurring in up to 21% of patients in one study [1]. Certainly, symptoms of
ischaemia in critically ill patients may be hidden by the use of sedative and
analgesic medication, and communication of symptoms may be hindered
further by endotracheal intubation. Here, the diagnosis may depend upon
12-lead ECG recording (on and off pacing) and ST segment monitoring,
although the latter is not as extensively validated in the critically ill [2].
These investigations should be used in conjunction with the measurement
of troponin (section 4.9) and echocardiography (section 4.5). Markers of
ischaemia should be requested at rest where there is a high index of
suspicion for ischaemia. New haemodynamic instability either at rest or
upon attempting weaning from respiratory support should trigger
investigation for myocardial ischaemia.

Arrhythmia
Arrhythmia are common in cardiac ICU patients, with atrial fibrillation
(AF) occurring in 10–65% of patients following cardiac surgery, and is
associated with increased mortality, morbidity and length of stay [3]. In
patients with poor ventricular function, the loss of atrial transport can be
associated with up to a 30% reduction in cardiac output (CO). Where there
is reliance on telemetry for diagnosis, particularly where the patient is
paced, the change in rhythm may be missed and only be signified by a fall in
CO. Careful analysis of a 12-lead ECG should suggest the diagnosis of AF,
flutter or other atrial tachycardia. If the diagnosis is unclear, or there is
inadequate information regarding rhythm disturbance, 24-hour Holter(s)
may be useful. Where the diagnosis remains uncertain, discussion with an
electrophysiologist is often useful, enabling targeted pharmacological or
interventional therapies to be instituted. Following cardiac surgery, if
atrial depolarisation is unclear on the surface ECG, an atrial ECG may be
performed using the temporary atrial pacing wires (Figure 4.1). This can be

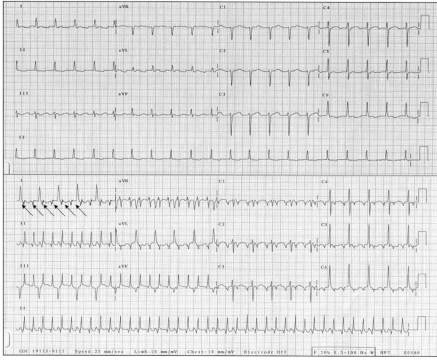

Figure 4.1 Twelve-lead electrocardiogram in a patient in atrial flutter. In the upper part of the figure is shown a standard surface ECG. In the lower part of the figure, an atrial electrode has been connected, revealing regular atrial flutter waves in all 12 leads (arrowed in lead I).

particularly useful in patients with congenital heart disease, where atrial tachycardia may mimic sinus tachycardia. This subject is discussed in depth in Chapter 17.

Right ventricular dysfunction

ECG markers of right ventricular (RV) dysfunction (RV 'strain') are 8–69% sensitive and 70–98% specific for the diagnosis of RV dysfunction in the context of pulmonary embolism [4]. The diagnostic sensitivity and specificity are improved where the ECG is used in conjunction with transthoracic echocardiography (TTE). In the context of acute myocardial infarction (AMI), performance of a right-sided ECG is useful in the diagnosis of RV infarction in the context of inferior infarction as it will alter management significantly [5]. This is particularly important where there is RV hypertrophy, as any impairment of RV function will cause significant haemodynamic compromise. The management of RV failure and infarction is discussed in Chapters 13 and 14.

ECG in pericardial disease

Pericardial disease is an unusual primary indication for admission to the cardiac ICU, but not an uncommon associated finding. There are findings in the ECG that may suggest the presence of pericardial disease – either pericardial collection or pericarditis. Where a large pericardial collection results in tamponade, ECG complexes may be small, with voltages that change with a phase more rapidly than with respiration due to the heart swinging in the pericardial fluid. There is commonly a pericardial element to the ECG changes associated with acute myocardial infarction, although these may be difficult to differentiate [6]. The ECG in acute pericarditis has four defined stages; however, the differentiation between this and AMI may still be challenging [7].

4.3 Critically ill patient with device implanted

Pacemaker

In ICU patients with permanent pacemaker implantation, the incidence of cardiovascular disease is high (40% coronary artery disease, 56% hypertension, 20% diabetes). Where a permanent pacemaker is implanted, it is essential to know the make and type of device, and how it is programmed. Many pacemakers may be used to facilitate investigation of the patient by interrogation to determine previous and ongoing rhythm disturbance, using anti-tachycardia pacing modes, and alteration of programming to optimise the patient's cardiovascular status. After defibrillation or surgical intervention, a permanent pacemaker or automatic implantable cardioverter defibrillator (AICD) should be interrogated by a cardiac physiologist to ensure that no damage has occurred to the unit or leads, and that pacemaker programming is still optimal.

Mechanical circulatory support

It may prove difficult to diagnose arrhythmias in patients with implanted ventricular assist devices (VAD), particularly where a permanent pacemaker is also implanted, as CO, blood pressure and VAD flows may be unchanged despite significant rhythm abnormalities. This is particularly apparent where blood flow in the systemic circulation is non-pulsatile. A high threshold of suspicion is required, and where necessary echocardiography (in addition to 12-lead ECG) or pacemaker interrogation may be required to detect and diagnose underlying rhythm abnormalities.

4.4 Haemodynamic investigations

The measurement of CO and other haemodynamic parameters in the intensive care setting is usually regarded as patient monitoring (Chapter 3); however, on occasion, it may be used to assist diagnosis.

Haemodynamic instability

The approach to a patient with sudden acute severe haemodynamic instability should follow standard resuscitation ABCDE guidelines.

Complete examination is important particularly to look for evidence of haemorrhage, sites of infection and peripheral ischaemia. The diagnosis is usually evident from the history, clinical examination and basic investigations but may require transfer for other studies, such as CT scanning or cardiac catheterisation.

Low cardiac output

A low CO state is usually evident from clinical examination. Low CO may result in increased blood lactate concentration, alterations in venous oxygen saturation of haemoglobin and metabolic acidosis. However, a raised lactate concentration is usually a late indicator of low cardiac output, unless hepatic function is also significantly impaired. Lactate is produced by skeletal muscle, brain, skin, gastrointestinal tract and red blood cells and is metabolised in the liver and kidneys. Lactate production is increased both during tissue ischaemia and by increased glycolysis primarily in skeletal muscle. Increased lactate concentrations in patients with hyperdynamic sepsis are related to both increased production and decreased lactate clearance. Raised blood lactate concentrations (> 2 mmol/l) are associated with a worse prognosis and should trigger investigation and management of the underlying cause.

Inadequate CO is associated with reduced mixed venous oxygen saturation (SvO_2) of haemoglobin ($< 70\%$). Increased SvO_2 is seen in patients with volume resuscitated hyperdynamic sepsis syndrome or septic shock. Central venous oxygen saturation ($ScvO_2$) does not have a constant relationship to SvO_2 and varies according to position of the line tip, coma, use of sedative or anaesthetic drugs, and the presence of an increased metabolic rate. However, trends in $ScvO_2$ tend to follow those of SvO_2 and have been used successfully to target early goal-directed therapy in patients with severe sepsis [8]. Oximetric catheters are available for continuous measurement of SvO_2 and $ScvO_2$. In addition to use as an indicator of adequacy of total perfusion, an unexpected saturation (either high or low) should prompt further investigation of the underlying problem.

CO should be measured if there is any concern that it is inadequate. The choice of measurement technique will depend on availability of equipment and skills and the particular requirements of the patient. For example, pulse contour analysis-based CO monitors will not provide accurate data if an intra-aortic balloon pump (IABP) is in use (Chapter 3) and pulmonary artery catheterisation may not be possible in some patients with congenital heart disease.

Post cardiac surgery

Following cardiac surgery, estimation of CO by clinical examination may be unreliable even by experienced practitioners [9]. If clinical status suggests catastrophically low CO, resuscitation should be carried out in conjunction with early consideration of re-exploration and echocardiography (see section 4.5) when time allows. In a high-risk patient or when there is clinical suspicion that CO may be low, it should be measured. The finding of low CO (cardiac index < 2.5 l/min/m^2) should then be further investigated to determine the underlying cause, first by echocardiography. Measurement of CO and echocardiography should not be seen as mutually exclusive and are best used in tandem. In circumstances where measured CO is low and initial echocardiography does not reveal the cause, further review by an expert in critical care echocardiography should be sought.

Cardiac tamponade is a common cause of haemodynamic instability and may be difficult to diagnose, particularly with TTE, as images are often suboptimal and collections may be small and localised [10]. If TTE is unhelpful TOE should be performed to exclude a pericardial collection. Where doubt still exists, it is important to note that tamponade is a clinical diagnosis and there should be a low threshold for surgical re-exploration. As in paediatric cardiac surgical patients impaired cardiac filling may occur in the absence of a demonstrable pericardial collection (tight pericardium) from restriction due to pressure from surrounding tissues [11]. In the presence of low CO without apparent cause, resternotomy should be the investigation of choice.

Coronary artery bypass graft (or native artery) obstruction may present in the immediate post-operative period as arrhythmias, ECG changes or a low CO syndrome. Echocardiography may reveal new regional wall motion abnormalities, but the definitive investigation is coronary angiography or re-exploration.

Diagnosis of arrhythmias

AF is common after cardiac surgery and may cause significant haemodynamic instability, particularly in patients with impaired left ventricular function. AF is usually easy to recognise but may go unnoticed in patients receiving ventricular or dual chamber pacing, particularly if the unpaced ventricular rate remains below the pacing rate. Atrial flutter and other atrial arrhythmias can be difficult to diagnose from a standard 12-lead ECG but are considerably easier from an atrial ECG.

Prediction of fluid responsiveness

A number of methods have been proposed to predict fluid responsiveness in mechanically ventilated patients (Chapter 3). Techniques that involve assessment of the magnitude of changes in stroke volume, systemic systolic and pulse pressure induced by inspiration have the best performance [12]. However, stroke volume and arterial blood pressure variation may also be altered by impaired right ventricular function, obstructive airways diseases and spontaneous breathing, common in cardiothoracic intensive care patients.

4.5 Ultrasound

Ultrasound is widely used in the diagnosis, monitoring and management of critically ill cardiac patients. The real-time diagnostic capabilities, together with the progressive miniaturisation of devices, and increasing ease of use are leading to a rapid expansion of its applications in the ICU [13]. Vascular ultrasound can be used for insertion of central venous catheters, and may be of use in peripheral venous and arterial cannulation, particularly where the anatomy may be abnormal, where multiple previous interventions have been performed, or where the patient is markedly obese or oedematous. The full scope of ultrasound investigation of the critically ill is beyond the scope of this chapter; however, two applications warrant specific discussion – echocardiography and lung ultrasound.

Echocardiography

Echocardiography has many roles in the cardiothoracic ICU, ranging from its use during cardiac arrest, to more sophisticated and complex diagnostic applications. In general, the first imaging mode of choice should be TTE (fast, non-invasive), although its use may be limited by image quality, where TOE may be required. Intra-cardiac echocardiography is a mode well known in the cardiac catheter laboratory, providing high-resolution images with the positioning of an intra-cardiac ultrasound probe. It has been proposed as a potential cardiac monitoring device for the ICU; however, the cost of such technology currently prohibits its routine use in ICU.

Peri-arrest echocardiography

Limited or focused echocardiography may be used as a supplement to Acute Life Support in order to determine the diagnosis of the underlying electrical vs mechanical cardiac activity and as a clue to the underlying diagnosis leading to cardiac arrest, or the peri-arrest state, including detection of pericardial fluid, acute pulmonary embolism, hypovolaemia, right and/or left ventricular failure, and severe valvular pathology [15].

Echocardiography as a monitoring device

Echocardiography is widely used in the ICU as a non-invasive measure of the filling status of the right and left heart (Figure 4.2), to measure CO and pulmonary arterial pressures [16], and may therefore be used as a measure of response to therapeutic interventions. Where the patient is ventilated, echocardiography may be used to alter ventilatory settings to minimise the potentially detrimental effect of positive pressure ventilation on right ventricular performance and cardiac filling. Although not ideal as a monitoring device (requiring multiple, repeated studies), there is evidence that useful haemodynamic information may be obtained rapidly and reliably, in addition to suggesting either primary or secondary cardiovascular pathology as a cause of haemodynamic collapse [17].

Echocardiography as a diagnostic tool

Echocardiography may be used in the diagnosis of pathology commonly seen in the general ICU, as well as to confirm the diagnosis and direct management of known cardiac pathology in the cardiothoracic ICU. Common clinical scenarios, the potential echocardiographic findings and the likely underlying cause in the critically ill are shown in Table 4.1 [18].

Table 4.1 Echocardiographic findings in the ICU.

Clinical finding	Cardiac cause	Echocardiographic finding	Notes
Low cardiac output (unresponsive to inotropes)	Valvular disease	Any severe stenotic or regurgitant lesion	Difficult to assess in ICU. Sequential stenotic lesions may mask severity of individual lesions (see text)
	Intrinsic cardiac disease	HOCM/LVH with LVOTO Large VSD/ASD Severe LV/RV dysfunction	
	Extrinsic cardiac disease	Tamponade, pericardial effusion, pericardial disease	NB. Post-operative cardiac surgical patients (see text)
Oliguria	Hypovolaemia	Low trans-mitral/tricuspid velocities Small ventricular volumes Apposition of LV papillary muscles in systole	If severe LVH papillary apposition may be an unreliable sign
	Intrinsic cardiac disease	Poor LV function, severe AS	High LA pressure demonstrated
	Pericardial disease	Pericardial effusion, pericardial tamponade, pericardial constriction	NB. Post-operative cardiac surgical patients (see text)
Increased filling pressures (left-sided)	Impaired LV	Increased E > A ratio (corrected for age), short IVRT	See text for detailed explanation
	Mitral valve disease	Significant MS or MR	MR: dynamic ventricle, increased forward velocities (> 1 m/sec), short duration and low velocity (< 3 m/sec) regurgitant jet
Increased filling pressures (right-sided)	Secondary to left-sided disease	Significant AS, AR, MS, MR or LV disease	
	Impaired RV	Reduced RV LAX function	Any reduction in association with PHT is significant. Mild impairment after CABG is normal
	Tricuspid regurgitation	Annular dilatation or endocarditis	If severe, RV dynamic with increased forward velocities (> 1 m/sec), short duration and low velocity regurgitant jet
Sepsis/SIRS	LV/RV dysfunction	Ventricular dilatation, systolic/diastolic dysfunction	Changes controversial and may be masked by inotropes
Endocarditis[†]	Source of sepsis Native/prosthetic valve, pacemaker wires, extra-cardiac 'endocarditis'	Endocarditis[†] Vegetations, paraprosthetic leaks, aortic root abscess	Vegetations rare in prosthetic valve endocarditis
Pulmonary hypertension	Acute PE	Dilated RV, severe TR	May rarely demonstrate intra-cardiac thrombus
	Post-pneumonectomy Mitral valve disease	Displaced heart, increased pulmonary acceleration time Significant MS or MR (2D, PW, CW and colour Doppler)	Views often difficult even with TOE Severe MR in ITU may be difficult to diagnose (see text)
Failure to wean from ventilator	Intrinsic cardiac disease	Ischaemia, severe MR, HOCM, LV/RV dysfunction	Stress echo may be necessary to make diagnosis
CVA/embolic event	Intra-cardiac thrombus	LA appendage, RA, apical LV thrombus Endocarditis	Exclude intra-cardiac shunt with contrast study
Cyanosis	Intra-cardiac shunting	Positive contrast study	Use agitated blood/saline. Perform Valsalva manoeuvre

HOCM, hypertrophic obstructive cardiomyopathy; LVH, left ventricular hypertrophy; LVOTO, left ventricular outflow tract obstruction; VSD, ventricular septal defect; ASD, atrial septal defect; LV, left ventricle; RV, right ventricle; AS, aortic stenosis; LA, left atrium; IVRT, isovolumic relaxation time; E:A ratio, early:late atrial filling; MS, mitral stenosis; MR, mitral regurgitation; AR, aortic regurgitation; LAX function, long axis function; PHT, pulmonary hypertension; CABG, coronary artery bypass graft; PE, pulmonary embolism; TR, tricuspid regurgitation; PW/CW Doppler, pulse wave/continuous wave Doppler; TOEE, trans-esophageal echocardiography. (Reproduced from Price et al. [18], with permission from *Intensive Care Medicine*.)

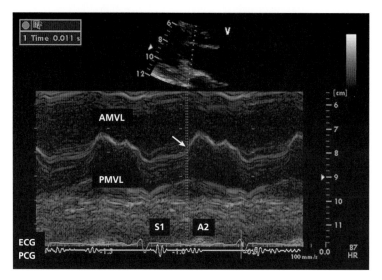

Figure 4.2 Trans-thoracic echocardiogram, parasternal long axis view, demonstrating a short isovolumic relaxation time (IVRT, arrowed) consistent with significantly elevated left atrial pressure. AMVL, Anterior mitral valve leaflet; PMVL, posterior mitral valve leaflet; ECG, electrocardiogram; PCG, phonocardiogram; S1, first heart sound; A2, aortic component of second heart sound.

Lung ultrasound

The practice of lung ultrasound in the ICU is generally limited to detection of pleural collections and facilitation of their drainage; however, the potential application in the critically ill cardiac patient expands beyond this [13]. Lung ultrasound may be used for the diagnosis and delineation of pneumothorax, particularly anteriorly in the supine position, lung abscess, the detection of interstitial fluid and alveolar consolidation. Unlike other modes of ultrasound, many diagnoses depend upon the presence and interpretation of artefacts produced by the lung–air interface. In some units, the use of lung ultrasound has largely replaced the performance of routine chest radiography; however, this practice is not widespread.

4.6 Radiography

Chest X-ray

Despite debate in general ICU about the utility of daily portable anterior-posterior (AP) chest X-ray (CXR), this is carried out in most patients in cardiothoracic intensive care, with the exception of those not requiring respiratory support and those who are haemodynamically stable. Studies have shown variable rates of new clinically important findings on routine CXRs, with almost 20% in some reports [14]. Routine CXR should be timed to occur after placement or removal of indwelling catheters and drains to minimise exposure to ionising radiation. Quality of imaging is improved by careful patient positioning and removing radio-opaque objects from the field.

Haemodynamics

Portable AP CXR may be helpful in diagnosing causes of haemodynamic instability and in excluding associated complications of indwelling catheters. The central venous catheter (CVC) tip should lie in the superior vena cava, but up to 30% have been found to be in an incorrect position following initial insertion. Atypical position of a central venous catheter may reveal abnormal venous connections, such as persistent left superior vena cava, knowledge of which may be useful in choosing the site of insertion of a pulmonary artery catheter or pacing wire.

CXR evidence of elevated left atrial pressure includes upper lobe blood vessel dilatation, increased cardiothoracic ratio, thickened interlobular septae and alveolar oedema. The finding of alveolar oedema alone does not help to distinguish between elevated left atrial pressure and increased permeability oedema. Vascular pedicle width has been correlated with pulmonary artery occlusion pressure [19]. Pulmonary vascular markings provide information about the magnitude and distribution of pulmonary blood flow, but CXR is not useful in excluding pulmonary embolus.

Anatomical

Cardiothoracic ratio is increased on AP compared to PA CXR. Abnormalities or enlargement of cardiac chambers and valvular calcification or prostheses may be seen but are better investigated using echocardiography. Pericardial collections are difficult to diagnose from portable CXR but can be suspected from an increase in cardiac diameter or apparent lateral migration of venous lines and pacing wires in serial films. Pericardial calcification may indicate tuberculosis and/or constrictive pericarditis. The presence of a widened mediastinum, pleural effusion and displacement of the oesophagus and left main bronchus should raise suspicion of aortic injury in patients with chest trauma.

Pneumothorax is usually evident on portable CXR. Anterior pneumothoraces may not be easy to see and a high index of suspicion is required, particularly in patients with severe obstructive lung disease (asthma or COPD) or ARDS. In these patients a small pneumothorax may cause significant haemodynamic compromise. CT scanning or lung ultrasound may be required to confirm the diagnosis.

Pleural fluid collections rarely cause haemodynamic compromise except when adjacent to a pericardial collection. Tension haemothorax can cause cardiovascular collapse but is usually obvious on portable CXR. Lung collapse or severe atelectasis can cause haemodynamic instability in patients with poor right ventricular function or Fontan-type circulation.

CT pulmonary angiography

There are few studies of imaging for the diagnosis of pulmonary embolism in patients with critical illness, particularly in the presence of underlying pulmonary disease. Here, the diagnosis should be suspected in patients with hypoxaemia and disproportionate pulmonary hypertension. D-dimers are often detected in critically ill patients without PE and isotope scans are logistically difficult and often unhelpful in the critically ill [20]. CT pulmonary angiography with modern multidetector scanners allows emboli in subsegmental branches of the pulmonary arteries to be visualised, resulting in a sensitivity of greater than 85% and specificity of more than 90% for the diagnosis of pulmonary embolism. An additional benefit is that where the CTPA is negative, additional and alternative diagnoses may become apparent.

CT thorax

CT thorax frequently yields more information (Table 4.2) than portable AP CXR in the critically ill but requires the patient to be moved from the ICU to the scanner. Any transfer of a critically ill patient carries an increased risk of patient harm. In addition, the overall radiation dose is much greater than portable CXR and studies of the aorta and pulmonary vasculature require potentially harmful radiocontrast administration. Contrast should not be administered through a multi-lumen CVC using an automated injection device because of the risk of lumen rupture secondary to high pressure. In the diagnosis of acute haemodynamic instability CT chest is useful in patients with chest trauma, aortic dissection, suspected pulmonary embolism (see 'Lung ultrasound' in section 4.5) and occult pneumothorax. In addition, perdicardial effusions may be diagnosed with CT scanning.

4.7 Invasive catheterisation procedures

The ready availability of senior and experienced operators in both diagnostic and interventional cardiac catheterisation is essential for investigation and management of critically ill cardiac patients. Although non-invasive investigation of coronary artery disease is a rapidly developing field, the cardiac catheter laboratory is uniquely positioned by being able to offer not only diagnosis but also the potential for immediate therapy. In the critically ill, this has obvious advantages. In addition to right and left heart catheterisation, angiography may be required in a number of circumstances, including performance of renal and mesenteric angiography, and in patients with congenital heart disease to delineate venous access. The more common indications for catheter laboratory investigations in the critically ill are described below.

Right and left heart catheterisation
Left heart catheterisation

The indications for coronary angiography in the critically ill are shown in Table 4.3. In any patient where cardiac surgery has involved re-implantation or manipulation of the coronary arteries, there should be a high index of suspicion for coronary obstruction. Here, prompt liaison

Table 4.2 The potential abnormalities detectable using CT thorax in various conditions affecting critically ill patients. Where relevant, comments are shown regarding the use of CT for guided invasive procedures, and the planning of a surgical strategy.

Clinical problem	Findings and notes	
Chest trauma	Aorta	Aortic tear, intimal flap
		Blood in mediastinum
	Lung	Consolidation
		Pneumothorax, haematomas, pneumatoceles
	Chest wall	Vertebral, rib and sternal fractures
		1st rib fracture – associated with vascular injuries
		9th, 10th and 11th rib fractures – associated with hepatic and splenic injury
	Pleura	Haemothorax, pneumothorax, chylothorax
		Pleural effusions
	Trachea/bronchi	Pneumothorax, pneumomediastinum
	Oesophagus	Pneumothorax, pneumomediatinum
		Pleural effusions
Pneumothorax	Particularly useful in diagnosis of anterior and loculated pneumothoraces – CT guided drainage may reduce risk of complications	
Pulmonary embolus	Spiral contrast CT pulmonary angiography has high sensitivity and specificity and will provide information about other potential diagnoses	
Occult infection	Diagnosis of sternal wound and mediastinal infection, empyema and lung abscess	
Acute respiratory distress syndrome	Assessment and diagnosis of coexisting problems, e.g. pleural effusions, anterior penumothorax, lung abscess	
Pleural effusions	Useful in differentiating effusion, empyema and lung abscess and for guiding percutaneous drainage	
Pre-cardiac or aortic surgery	Assessment of aortic aneurysm and dissection	
	Planning of re-sternotomy	
Diagnosis of pulmonary disease	Pneumonia, interstitial lung disease, neoplasms, COPD	

ARDS, acute respiratory distress syndrome.

with the surgical team is essential, and early surgical re-exploration should be considered, particularly if catheter laboratory investigation may lead to a delay in diagnosis.

Right heart catheterisation

Although measurement of right-heart pressures is routinely performed on the ICU, there are certain occasions where formal right heart catheterisation may be necessary (see Table 4.4). This is particularly relevant in patients with complex congenital heart disease.

Table 4.3 Indications for coronary angiography in the critically ill, differential diagnoses, potential causes and other, complementary investigations.

Clinical features	Potential diagnosis	Potential causes	Other investigations
Haemodynamic instability	Myocardial ischaemia	Coronary obstruction Graft malfunction Pericardial disease	ECG Echo (RWMA) Positive troponin
Ventricular arrhythmias	Myocardial ischaemia	Coronary obstruction Graft malfunction	ECG Echo (RWMA)
Failure to wean from ventilator	Myocardial ischaemia	Coronary obstruction Ischaemic MR	Positive troponin Stress echo
Failure to wean from ventilator Haemodynamic instability	Dynamic MR	Ventricular dilatation	Pulmonary oedema Stress echo RHC
Clinical history Unequal pulses Haemodynamic instability	Aortic disruption	Dissection Trauma	Echo CXR CT/CMR Aortography Coronary angiography

ECG, electrocardiogram; RWMA, regional wall motion abnormality; MR, mitral regurgitation; RHC, right heart catheterisation; CXR, chest X-ray; CT, computerised tomography; CMR, cardiac magnetic resonance.

4.8 Cardiac magnetic resonance scanning and nuclear medicine

The superior image quality of cardiac magnetic resonance scanning (CMR) makes it an attractive imaging modality in the investigation of patients with cardiac disease; however, there are particular considerations where imaging of the critically ill is concerned. These relate to interaction of the magnetic field with ferro-magnetic items, which may result in injury from projectiles and from movement of, or induction of current within implanted devices (pacemakers, cerebral clips, etc.). Although scanning the critically ill patient may be performed quickly, and reveal a diagnosis that may have a major impact on intervention and outcome, specific precautions must be taken into consideration. All anaesthetic and trolley equipment must be fully MR compatible, piped oxygen only should be used and all machines should remain in the control room, connected to the patient with long lines passed through a waveguide [21].

Nuclear medicine may be used in the investigation of the cardiovascularly critically ill on occasion as an adjunct to echocardiography

Table 4.4 Indications for right heart catheterisation in the critically ill, differential diagnoses, potential causes and other, complementary investigations.

Clinical features	Potential diagnosis	Potential causes	Other investigations
Unexplained hypoxia	Intracardiac shunt Intrapulmonary shunt	ASD, VSD Collaterals	Echo CXR ECG CT CMR
Pulmonary hypertension	Primary PHT Secondary PHT	Idiopathic Congenital heart disease Structural acquired heart disease Pulmonary disease	ECG Echo CXR CTPA V/Q LHC Reversibility studies Pulmonary angiography
Massive haemoptysis	PHT Bronchial bleeding Pulmonary bleeding	Pulmonary thrombo-embolic disease Aspergillosis Malignancy	CXR CTPA Pulmonary angiography
SVC/IVC obstruction	Internal obstruction External obstruction	Tumour Venous thrombosis Multiple instrumentation	Ultrasound CT CMR TOE

ASD, atrial septal defect; VSD, ventricular septal defect; PHT, pulmonary hypertension; CXR, chest X-ray; ECG, electrocardiograph; CT, computerised tomography; CMR, cardiac magnetic resonance; CTPA, computerised tomographic pulmonary angiography; V/Q, ventilation/perfusion scan; LHC, left heart catheterisation.

in the diagnosis of endocarditis, and in determining the extent of ischaemia and infarction. Although TOE is considered the gold standard in the investigation of potential endocarditis, radiolabelled white blood cell scintigraphy may be used in conjunction where cases are complicated by extra-cardiac infection (aortic cannulation sites, previous shunts in congenital heart disease) and where it is uncertain whether a lesion seen on echocardiography remains actively infected. The more widespread use of nuclear medicine in cardiology relates to determining regions of ischaemia, viable myocardium, infarction and ejection fraction. Although there are few circumstances in which the diagnosis cannot be made using alternative imaging modalities which can be performed by the bedside (echocardiography) or allow the potential for intervention (angiography), on occasion nuclear scanning may be useful in patient management (see case study).

4.9 Biochemistry

Markers of cardiac ischaemia, infarction and function
Troponins
Elevated concentrations of the proteins troponin I and T in blood are
sensitive markers of myocardial cell damage. Elevated creatinine kinase
isoenzyme MB (muscle brain) concentrations are a less sensitive marker
of myocardial cell necrosis than troponins. Skeletal muscle necrosis
secondary to ischaemia will cause elevated CK concentrations. Studies in
critically ill patients, particularly with severe sepsis, septic shock and renal
dysfunction, have shown that up to 70% of patients can have elevated
troponin I and T concentrations without other evidence of myocardial
ischaemia. Following cardiac surgery, an elevated troponin concentration
is associated with increased myocardial infarction rates and mortality [22].
Some studies have shown worse myocardial function and outcomes
associated with elevated troponin levels in patients with non-cardiac
reasons for admission. These markers are therefore not specific enough to
be used as daily screening tests for myocardial ischaemia or used as sole
criteria for the diagnosis of acute myocardial infarction. Furthermore
where there is a high index of suspicion of cardiac ischaemia other
investigations may be more appropriate to facilitate early intervention
(section 4.2).

Natriuretic peptides
Increased concentrations of natriuretic peptides have been correlated with
poor myocardial function and worse prognosis in patients with
decompensated heart failure and acute coronary syndromes. In ICU
patients, brain natriuretic peptide (BNP) and its inactive fragment N-
terminal Pro B-type natriuretic peptide (NTproBNP) concentrations
correlated with myocardial contractility [23], but one-off measurements do
not correlate well with pulmonary artery occlusion pressure (PAOP).
NTproBNP concentrations taken on admission in unselected patients
predicted ICU mortality as effectively as the APACHE II score [24]. There
thus may be a role for natriuretic peptide concentrations to be used for
outcome prediction.

Endocrine abnormalities
Thyroid function
Thyroid function is altered in critically ill patients even without pre-existing
thyroid disease. In the acute phase of severe illness total T3 concentrations
are decreased initially because of lower peripheral conversion from T4.
Later total T4 concentration is decreased and reverse T3 concentrations are
increased. Free T4 concentrations usually remain normal in acute illness.
The magnitude of alterations in total T3 and T4 have been correlated with
mortality. TSH concentration is low or normal despite the decreased T3
concentration, probably because of decreased hypothalamic TRH
production. Patients with hyperthyroidism usually have a larger

suppression of TSH. Administration of T4 did not improve outcomes in critically ill patients without thyroid disease and decreased T3 and T4 concentrations.

Thyroid function should be measured regularly in patients receiving amiodarone in whom interpretation may be challenging. Thyroid function abnormalities may occur rapidly in the acutely ill.

Adrenal function

The hypothalamic-pituitary-adrenal (HPA) axis is stimulated in critically ill patients and the magnitude is related to the severity of illness. HPA axis activation results in increased secretion of corticotrophin-releasing hormone (CRH), adrenocorticotropic hormone (ACTH) and cortisol. Severe adrenal insufficiency can present as a number of clinical scenarios, including haemodynamic compromise despite fluid resuscitation, variably associated with hypoglycaemia, hypokalaemia or hyponatraemia. An impaired response of the adrenal cortex to stimulation with adrenocorticotropic hormone (ACTH) (so-called relative adrenal insufficiency) has been reported in up to 60% of critically ill patients, depending on the criteria that are used, with a high incidence in patients with severe sepsis and septic shock.

Diagnosing adrenal insufficiency is not straightforward. Approximately 90% of plasma cortisol is protein-bound and most studies have measured total cortisol rather than the active free concentration, making interpretation difficult. Poor patient outcomes have been associated with both low, indicating a poor adrenal response, and high (more severe illness) baseline cortisol concentrations [25]. Patients with severe adrenal insufficiency have a low total cortisol concentration, but there is no widely accepted normal cortisol concentration range in critically ill patients.

Recent interest in investigating patients with potential 'relative' adrenal insufficiency was increased by a study in patients with septic shock. In a randomised controlled trial increased survival was reported in patients with an impaired response (increase in total cortisol < 248 nmol/l) to a short Synacthen test (250 µg) and who subsequently received hydrocortisone and fludrocortisone treatment [26]. However, in the larger CORTICUS study of 499 patients, hydrocortisone treatment had no effect on mortality in responders and non-responders to a short Synacthen test [27]. The 2008 update of the Surviving Sepsis guidelines suggests that the ACTH stimulation test should not be used to identify the subset of adults with septic shock who should receive hydrocortisone, and that intravenous hydrocortisone be given only to adult septic shock patients after blood pressure has been identified to be poorly responsive to fluid resuscitation and vasopressor therapy [28]. However, it is important to note that Addisonian crisis due to severe adrenal insufficiency can have a clinical presentation similar to that of septic shock. If a short Synacthen test is to be carried out, this should be done before hydrocortisone is administered.

Chromaffin tumours

Phaeochromocytomas are rare tumours arising from the chromaffin cells of the adrenal medulla. The screening test of choice is measurement of plasma-free and urinary fractionated metanephrine concentrations, which is more sensitive than plasma and urinary catecholamine concentrations in the diagnosis of secretory chromaffin tumours [29]. CT and MRI scanning are used for tumour imaging.

Carcinoid tumours

Screening for carcinoid tumours involves measurement of serotonin or its metabolite 5-hydroxyindoleacetic acid (5-HIAA) in blood or 24-hour urine collection. Metastatic carcinoid tumours are associated with right-sided valvular heart disease.

4.10 Summary

There is a tendency in critical care to accept diagnoses, for example the acute respiratory distress syndrome, without uncovering the underlying causes with sufficient rigour. Conversely, patients may be harmed and resources wasted through the unthinking application of unnecessary 'routine' investigations. Basic investigations are still valuable in the management of critically ill patients, when deployed appropriately, but many investigations have not been well-validated in the critically ill. The risk:benefit ratio should be considered for each investigation in the context of the patient's current state. Despite the use of invasive investigations which themselves may cause harm, and the risks inherent in transporting patients out of the critical care unit for tests in other departments, the greatest risk to the patient is misinterpretation of investigations, and expert opinion is often warranted.

Case study

A 66-year-old man was admitted as an emergency to the ICU because of severe acute pulmonary oedema that occurred at the start of diagnostic coronary angiography. He had known coronary artery disease and had undergone coronary revascularisation several years before, involving saphenous vein grafts to the left anterior descending, circumflex and right coronary arteries. In addition he had type II diabetes mellitus, peripheral vascular disease and chronic renal impairment. He was treated with oxygen, vasodilators and diuretics but deteriorated rapidly, requiring endotracheal intubation and mechanical ventilation. TTE demonstrated new RV and LV ischaemic changes associated with severe biventricular dysfunction. He underwent urgent coronary angiography that revealed an occluded graft to the Cx, and tight stenosis of the vein grafts to the RCA (Figure 4.3) and LAD. He underwent stenting to the

Continued

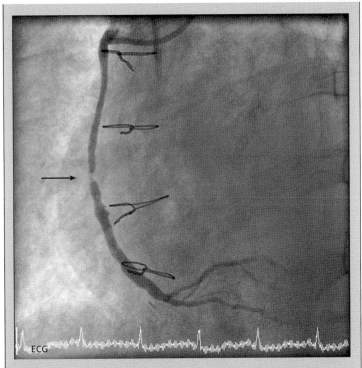

Figure 4.3 Coronary angiography with selective intubation of the vein graft to the right coronary artery, demonstrating a tight stenosis (arrowed) in the mid-portion of the graft. ECG Electrocardiogram.

RCA and LAD grafts. After initial improvement he developed cardiogenic shock, requiring inotropic support. ECG excluded new ischaemia and echocardiography demonstrated high left atrial pressure, severe LV dysfunction and no evidence of ongoing ischaemia. As echo features of ischaemia may be masked by high left atrial pressure, coronary angiography was performed to confirm stent patency. He was treated for severe left ventricular dysfunction and despite echocardiographic improvement in LV systolic function, he continued to develop pulmonary oedema on ventilatory weaning. At this stage nuclear imaging was performed to determine whether the circumflex territory was in fact viable and could be potentially revascularised. This confirmed infarction of the Cx territory and further revascularisation was not indicated.

As the patient was unable to progress owing to a low CO state and pulmonary oedema on ventilatory weaning, he underwent echocardiography to determine whether he might benefit from biventricular pacing. Following echocardiographic confirmation of ventricular dyssynchrony (Figures 4.4a and 4.4b) a biventricular pacemaker was implanted and the patient was eventually successfully weaned and discharged. *Continued*

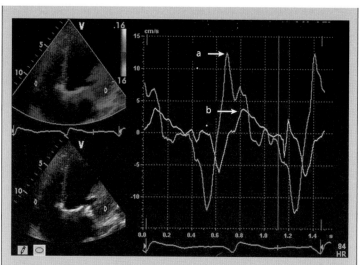

Figure 4.4a Tissue velocity mapping demonstrating inter-ventricular dyssynchrony (trans-thoracic echocardiography). Left of the image shows the 2D representation of the heart (lower) and TVI mapping (upper) with sample volumes placed at the annulus of the right ventricle (green) and free wall of the left ventricle (yellow). Right of the image, the corresponding tissue velocities sampled are shown (x axis time in seconds, y axis velocity in centimetres per second) for the right ventricle (arrowed, a) and the left ventricle (arrowed, b). (See also colour plate 4.1a).

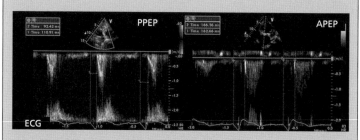

Figure 4.4b Corresponding ejection from the right and left heart resulting from the dyssynchrony shown in Figure 4.4a. Here, a difference in pre-ejection period between the right heart (pulmonary pre-ejection period, PPEP) and left heart (aortic pre-ejection period, APEP) of > 40 msec is shown, resulting from inter-ventricular dyssynchrony. ECG Electrocardiogram. (See also colour plate 4.1b).

References

1. Landesberg G, Vesselov Y, Einav S, et al. Myocardial ischemia, cardiac troponin, and long-term survival of high-cardiac risk critically ill intensive care unit patients. *Crit Care Med* 2005; 33(6):1281–7.
2. Kress JP, Vinayak AGMD, Levitt JMD, et al. Daily sedative interruption in mechanically ventilated patients at risk for coronary artery disease. *Crit Care Med* 2007; 35(2): 365–71.

3. Maisel WH, Rawn JD, Stevenson WG. Atrial fibrillation after cardiac surgery. *Ann Intern Med* 2001; 135: 1061–73.

4. Sukhija R, Aronow WS, Ahan C, et al. Electrocardiographic abnormalities in patients with right ventricular dilation due to acute pulmonary embolism. *Cardiology* 2006; 105(1): 57–60.

5. Fijewski TR, Pollack ML, Chan TC, et al. Electrocardiographic manifestations: right ventricular infarction. *J Emerg Med*. 2002; 22: 189–94.

6. Oliva PB, Hammill SC, Edwards WD. Electrocardiographic diagnosis of postinfarction regional pericarditis. Ancillary observations regarding the effect of reperfusion on the rapidity and amplitude of T wave inversion after acute myocardial infarction. *Circulation* 1993; 88: 896–904.

7. Krainin FM, Flessas AP, Spodick DH. Infarction-associated pericarditis. Rarity of diagnostic electrocardiogram. *N Engl J Med* 1984; 311: 1211–14.

8. Rivers E, Nguyen B, Havstad S, et al. Early goal-directed therapy in the treatment of severe sepsis and septic shock. *N Engl J Med* 2001; 345(19):1368–77.

9. Linton RA, Linton NW, Kelly F. Is clinical assessment of the circulation reliable in postoperative cardiac surgical patients? *J Cardiothorac Vasc Anesth* 2002; 16(1): 4–7.

10. Price S, Prout J, Jaggar SI, et al. 'Tamponade' following cardiac surgery: terminology and echocardiography may both mislead. *Eur J Cardiothorac Surg* 2004; 26(6): 1156–60.

11. Sutton J, Gibson DG. Measurement of postoperative pericardial pressure in man. *Br Heart J* 1977; 39(1): 1–6.

12. Sturgess DJ, Joyce C, Marwick TH, et al. A clinician's guide to predicting fluid responsiveness in critical illness: applied physiology and research methodology. *Anaes Int Care* 2007; 35(5): 669–78.

13. Lichtenstein D. *General Ultrasound in the Critically Ill*. Springer-Berlin, 2007, 2nd edn.

14. Graat ME, Stoker J, Vroom MB, et al. Can we abandon daily routine chest radiography in intensive care patients? *J Inten Care Med* 1995; 20(4): 238–46.

15. Breitkreutz R, Walcher F, Seeger FH. Focused echocardiographic evaluation in resuscitation management: concept of an advanced life support-conformed algorithm. *Crit Care Med* 2007; 35(5 Suppl): S150–61.

16. Charron C, Caille V, Jardin F, et al. Echocardiographic measurement of fluid responsiveness. *Curr Opin Crit Care* 2006; 12(3): 249–54.

17. Cholley BP, Payen D. Noninvasive techniques for measurements of cardiac output. *Curr Opin Crit Care* 2005; 11(5): 424–9.

18. Price S, Nicol E, Gibson DG, et al. Echocardiography in the critically ill: current and potential roles. *Int Care Med* 2006; 32(1): 48–59.

19. Miller RR, Ely EW. Radiographic measures of intravascular volume status: the role of vascular pedicle width. *Curr Opin Crit Care* 2006; 12(3): 255–62.

20. British Thoracic Society. Suspected acute pulmonary embolism – a practical approach. *Thorax* 1997; 52(Suppl 3): S2–24.

21. Prasad SK, Pennell DJ. Safety of cardiovascular magnetic resonance in patients with cardiovascular implants and devices. *Heart* 2004; 90(11): 1241–4.

22. Nesher N, Alghamdi AA, Singh SK, et al. Troponin after cardiac surgery: a predictor or a phenomenon? *Ann Thorac Surg* 2008; 85(4): 1348–54.

23. Jefic D, Lee JW, Jefic D, et al. Utility of B-type natriuretic peptide and N-terminal pro B-type natriuretic peptide in evaluation of respiratory failure in critically ill patients. *Chest* 2005; 128(1): 288–95.

24. Meyer B, Huelsmann M, Wexberg P, et al. N-terminal pro-B-type natriuretic peptide is an independent predictor of outcome in an unselected cohort of critically ill patients. *Crit Care Med* 2007; 35(10): 2268–73.

25. Arafah BM. Hypothalamic pituitary adrenal function during critical illness: limitations of current assessment methods. *J Clin End Metab* 2006; 91(10): 3725–45.

26. Annane D, Sébille V, Charpentier C, et al. Effect of treatment with low doses of hydrocortisone and fludrocortisone on mortality in patients with septic shock. *JAMA* 2002;288:862–71.

27. Sprung CL, Annane D, Keh D, et al. Hydrocortisone therapy for patients with septic shock. *NEJM* 2008; 358: 111–24.

28. Dellinger RP, Levy MM, Carlet JM, et al. Surviving Sepsis Campaign: international guidelines for management of severe sepsis and septic shock. *Int Care Med* 2008; 34: 17–60.

29. Chrisoulidou A, Kaltsas G, Ilias I, et al. The diagnosis and management of malignant phaeochromocytoma and paraganglioma. *Endocr Rel Cancer* 2007; 14: 569–85.

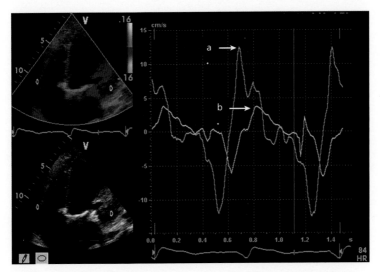

Plate 4.1a Tissue velocity mapping demonstrating inter-ventricular dyssynchrony (transthoracic echocardiography). Left of the image shows the 2D representation of the heart (lower) and TVI mapping (upper) with sample volumes placed at the annulus of the right ventricle (green) and free wall of the left ventricle (yellow). Right of the image, the corresponding tissue velocities sampled are shown (x axis time in seconds, y axis velocity in centimetres per second) for the right ventricle (arrowed, a) and the left ventricle (arrowed, b).

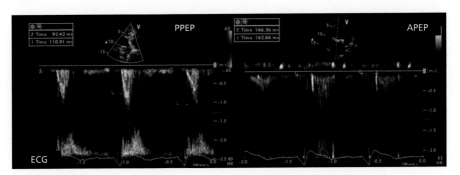

Plate 4.1b Corresponding ejection from the right and left heart resulting from the dyssynchrony shown in Figure 4.4a. Here, a difference in pre-ejection period between the right heart (pulmonary pre-ejection period, PPEP) and left heart (aortic pre-ejection period, APEP) of > 40 msec is shown, resulting from inter-ventricular dyssynchrony. ECG Electrocardiogram.

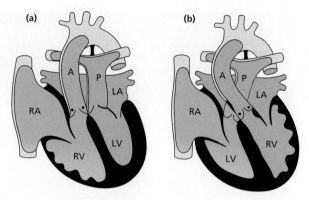

Plate 10.1 Variants of transposition. (**a**) Transposition of the great arteries, with normal atrio-ventricular connections but discordant ventriculo-atrial connections. (**b**) Congenitally corrected transposition of the great arteries, with discordant atrio-ventricular and ventriculo-atrial connections. RA, right atrium; RV, right ventricle; LA, left atrium; LV, left ventricle; A, aorta; P, pulmonary artery.

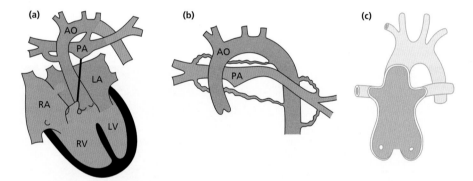

Plate 10.2 Examples of systemic-pulmonary shunts. (**a**) Pulmonary atresia plus VSD – here, pulmonary blood flow is via a patent ductus arteriosus. (**b**) Pulmonary atresia with blood supply to confluent pulmonary arteries from sytemic-pulmonary collaterals. (**c**) Common arterial trunk, where there is a common valve and arterial trunk from the ventricles, giving rise to the left and right pulmonary arteries from the ascending aorta. RA, right atrium; RV, right ventricle; LA, left atrium; LV, left ventricle; PA, pulmonary artery; AO, aorta.

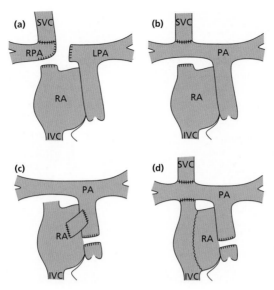

Plate 10.3 Different types of venous anastamosis used in patients with absent or deficient right-sided connections. (**a**) Classical Glenn. (**b**) Bidirectional Glenn. (**c**) Atrio-pulmonary Fontan. (**d**) Total cavo-pulmonary connection (TCPC) – lateral tunnel. RA, right atrium; IVC, inferior vena cava; RPA, right pulmonary artery; LPA, left pulmonary artery; SVC, superior vena cava.

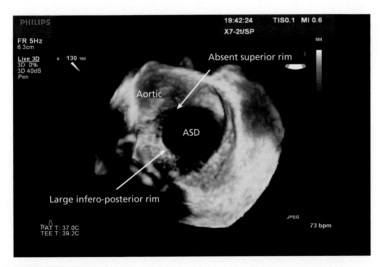

Plate 10.4 Three-dimensional TOE of a large secundum atrial septal defect (ASD) in a patient prior to surgical closure. The image is taken from the left atrium, looking through the ASD into the right atrium.

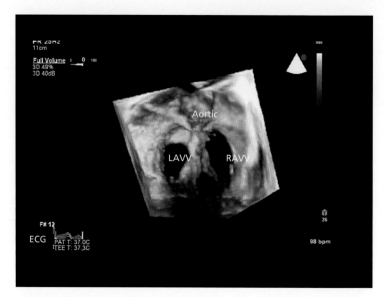

Plate 10.5 Three-dimensional TOE of a patient with an unoperated incomplete atrio-ventricular septal defect (AVSD). The image is shown from the roof of the atria, looking down on the two separate orifices of the atrio-ventricular valves during diastole. Note the absence of inter-atrial septum and abnormal anatomical arrangement of the aortic valve with respect to the atrio-ventricular valves. LAVV left atrio-ventricular valve, RAVV right atrio-ventricular valve, Aortic aortic valve, ECG electrocardiogram.

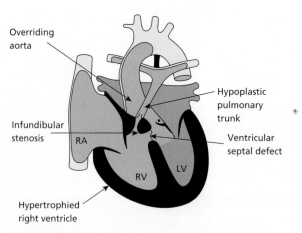

Plate 10.6 Unoperated tetralogy of Fallot, with the various components marked. In addition to the classical four components, there are frequently abnormalities of the pulmonary valve and/or pulmonary trunk (as shown). RA, right atrium; RV, right ventricle; LV, left ventricle.

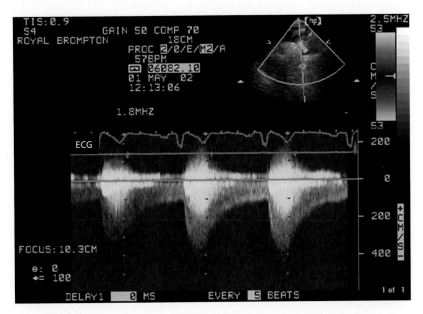

Plate 16.1 Doppler continuous wave (CW) sample in the area of coarctation, showing a peak velocity at the excess of 4 m/sec (pressure gradient more than 64 mmHg) and increased velocity throughout systole and diastole (diastolic tail), both indicative of significant, severe coarctation.

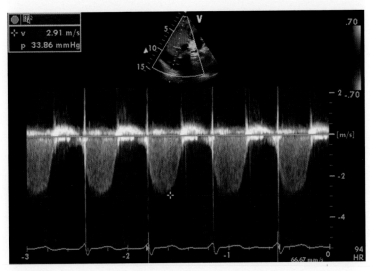

Plate 18.1 Continuous wave Doppler of tricuspid regurgitation demonstrating a peak velocity of 2.9 m/sec (pressure drop 34 mmHg).

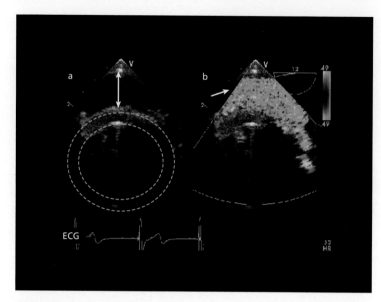

Plate 18.2 TOE demonstrating severe paraprosthetic regurgitation. In the left side of the figure (**a**) outline of the valve leaflets (inner circle) and sewing ring (outer circle) are highlighted. Arrow indicates the space between the sewing ring and annulus. In the right side of the figure (**b**) colour Doppler demonstrates flow between the sewing ring and annulus in systole (arrowed).

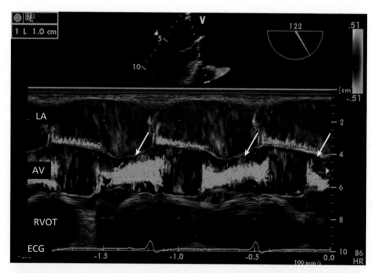

Plate 19.1 M-mode trans-oesophageal echocardiography (mid-oesophageal, left ventricular outflow tract view) in a patient with severe aortic valve endocarditis. Here, the colour jet represents blood flow back into the left ventricle during diastole (arrowed), and is 10 mm in depth, representing severe aortic regurgitation. For reference, a two-dimensional picture is shown at the top of the image. LA left atrium, AV aortic valve, RVOT right ventricular outflow tract, ECG electrocardiogram.

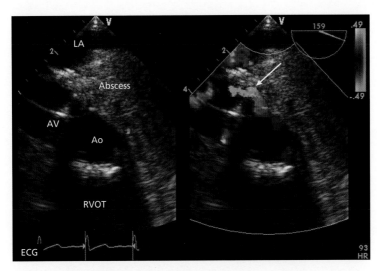

Plate 19.2 Two-dimensional trans-oesophageal echocardiography (mid-oesophageal, left ventricular outflow tract view) in a patient with previous St Jude aortic valve replacement and an aortic root abscess. Note the small paraprosthetic jet (arrowed in the figure on the right) and the absence of vegetations on the valve. At operation the abscess was found to extend to the level of the pulmonary artery bifurcation, providing the only continuity between the ascending aorta above this level and the aortic root. LA left atrium, AV aortic valve, Ao ascending aorta, RVOT right ventricular outflow tract, ECG electrocardiogram.

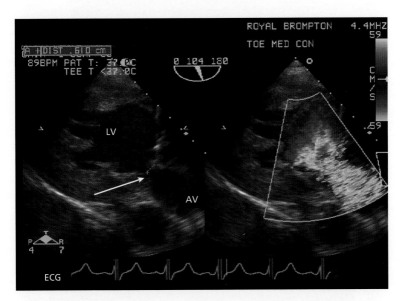

Plate 19.3 Two-dimensional trans-oesophageal echocardiography (trans-gastric left ventricular outflow tract view) in a patient with bicuspid aortic valve and sub-aortic stenosis (arrowed). In the figure on the right, colour Doppler reveals flow acceleration and aliasing of the colour jet, indicating high velocity blood flow due to the sub-aortic membrane. LV left ventricle, AV aortic valve, ECG electrocardiogram.

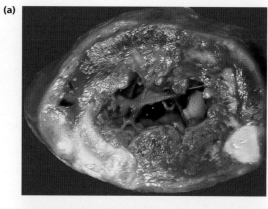

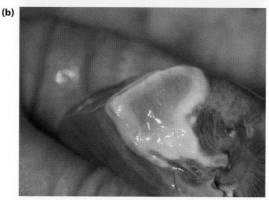

Plate 20.1 Post-mortem findings in a patient with *Staph. aureus* endocarditis with multiple abscesses. (**a**) Myocardial abscess. (**b**) Renal abscess.

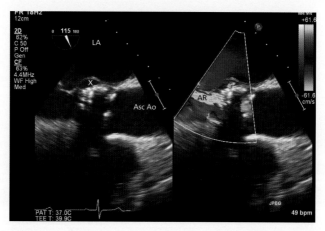

Plate 20.2 TOE of same patient as Figure 20.2a, but after 3 months ICU care with MRSA-infected bed-sores. Note the development of aortic root abscess (X) in the left panel. Note flow in and out of the abscess on colour flow Doppler in the right panel, together with a jet of aortic regurgitation (AR).

5 Haematological Aspects of Cardiovascular Critical Care

Kanchan Rege[1] and Mark J.D. Griffiths[2]
[1]Papworth Hospital, Cambridge, UK
[2]Royal Brompton & Harefield NHS Foundation Trust, London, UK

Take Home Messages

- There are very few data to guide the management of coagulation and transfusion issues in cardiac ICU.
- The main risk of blood transfusion is receiving the wrong blood component. Checking procedures are therefore the single most important aspect of care in this field.
- After cardiac surgery, correcting the clotting with blood products of patients who are not bleeding is almost never justified.
- Heparin-induced thrombocytopenia syndrome is a potentially devastating haematological complication whose management requires close co-operation between haematologists and intensivists.
- Developments in near patient testing may change the traditional relationship between the laboratory and ICU.

5.1 Introduction

The patient returning from cardiac surgery to the Intensive Care Unit (ICU) presents unique haematological challenges. Unfortunately, there is very little evidence from randomised controlled trials to guide management and the clinician often has no alternative to reliance on 'custom and practice'.

5.2 Management of bleeding

Bleeding is a common complication of cardiac surgery owing to complex interactions between an acquired platelet function defect, fibrinolysis and heparin usage [1]. This discipline consumes a significant proportion of the

---

Cardiovascular Critical Care. Edited by M. Griffiths, J. Cordingley and S. Price.
© 2010 Blackwell Publishing Ltd.

blood supply, but, as is frequent in transfusion medicine, there are no randomised controlled trials to direct best practice. Whilst withholding blood products was previously thought to be unethical, unnecessary exposure is now considered to be equally unjustifiable. Transfusion rates per procedure vary widely amongst centres and clinical teams [2]. The likelihood of transfusion depends as much on the preferences of the surgical team as on any other variable.

Nowadays, the majority of patients undergoing cardiac surgery should not need blood transfusion. Clinicians must distinguish between those in whom blood product transfusion is indicated and those who need surgical re-exploration. This may be done by regular measurement of the amount of blood loss and comparison with 'expected' values. One method of separating these three scenarios is to produce a centile chart (Figure 5.1). This has been derived from the data on blood loss from patients undergoing the same surgical procedure but not requiring blood transfusion. A gradual departure from the centile line suggests the need for blood products, whilst a more dramatic deviation suggests that surgical intervention may be required. Re-sternotomy is associated with a an increased incidence of complications and a longer ICU stay, but the outlook is significantly worse in cases where re-exploration is delayed [3]. In a series of almost 3000 patients, 3.1% underwent re-exploration for bleeding; risk factors included smaller body mass index, increased age, emergency surgery, five or more distal anastomoses and pre-operative use of aspirin and heparin. Bleeding vessels were found in 67% of cases of re-exploration [4] and in these cases transfusion of blood products is unlikely to stop bleeding.

The greatest risk of blood transfusion is 'incorrect blood component transfused', that is a patient receives a blood component that was either not allocated to them or did not fulfil their requirements, which accounts for approximately 66% of all reported errors [5]. Correct labelling and checking procedures, therefore, remain the cornerstone of safe transfusion practice.

Red cells

Since the Transfusion Requirements in Critical Care (TRICC) study in 1999 [6], there has been growing confidence in allowing critically ill patients to remain anaemic. Most cardiac centres accept a transfusion trigger of a haemoglobin concentration of 8 g/dl, but there are no specific data to substantiate a precise trigger, nor information pertaining to patients with coronary disease. The literature is also conflicting as to whether blood transfusion causes immunosuppression in the era of universal leukocyte depletion, which was introduced in the UK in 1999.

Platelets

Platelets suffer functional damage during and immediately after cardiopulmonary bypass (CPB). The contributory factors associated with CPB include the huge doses of unfractionated heparin (UFH) to which they are exposed, and contact with surface-absorbed fibrinogen leading to alpha granule release and damage to surface Glycoprotein Ib (the von Willebrand factor receptor) and Glycoprotein IIb/IIIa (the fibrinogen receptor) [7].

Papworth Hospital NHS Trust

Cumulative post-operative blood loss

Patient Name _____

Date of surgery:_____

Hospital Number _____

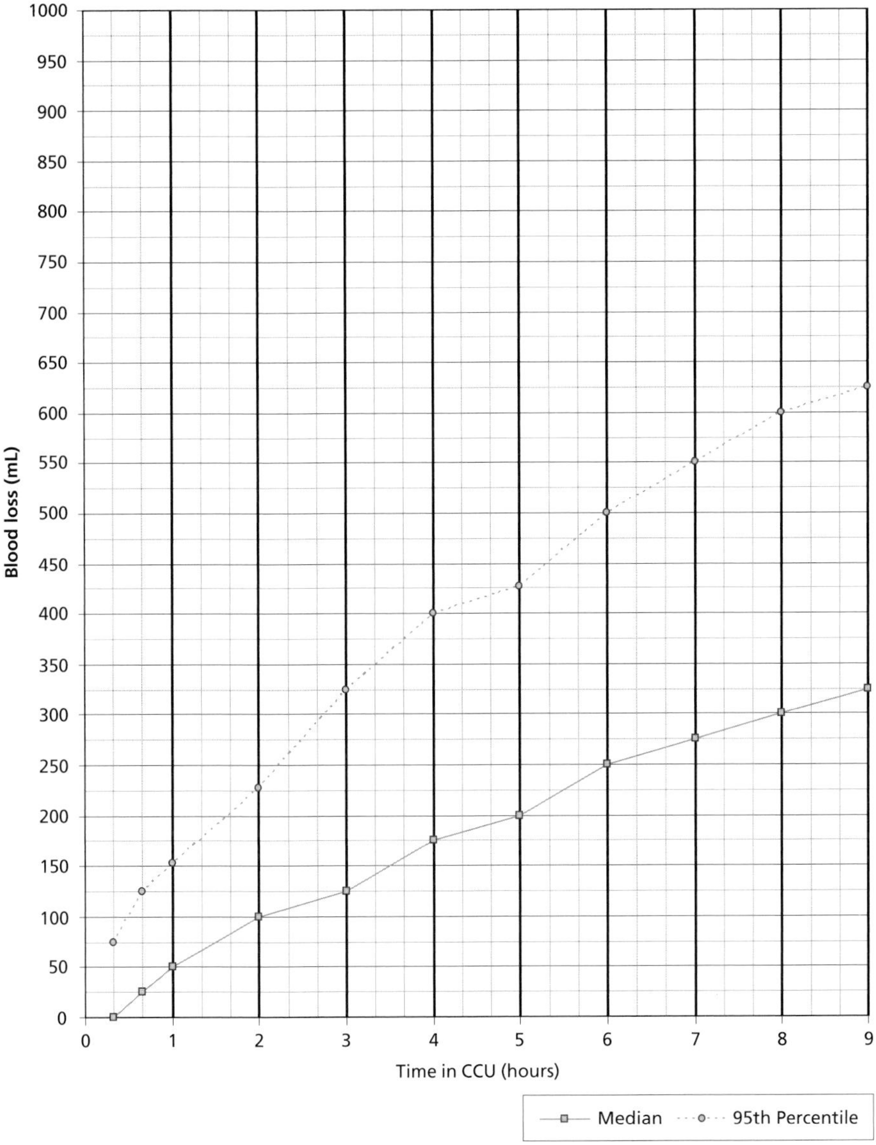

Figure 5.1 Centile chart of expected bleeding based on 700 patients undergoing first-time coronary artery bypass grafting and not requiring transfusion. (Reproduced with permission from Papworth Hospital, Cambridge, UK.)

Platelet aggregometry studies show normal aggregation on the day following surgery, prior to administration of aspirin or other antiplatelet agents [8]. This indicates that the platelet damage sustained may be reversible or more probably that the damaged platelets have been destroyed and replaced by healthy ones. In practice, therefore, platelet transfusion may be of benefit, in the *immediate* post-operative period, at levels higher than the 50×10^9/l trigger normally employed in massive transfusion policies [9], but thereafter the trigger should return to 50×10^9/l. This difficult decision may, in principle, be guided by the use of near patient testing devices (see below).

Fresh frozen plasma (FFP)

Shortly after starting CPB, predictable reductions in the plasma concentrations of coagulation factors occur, although, typically, they remain above the level considered to be adequate for haemostasis even in heavy bleeding. Generally all coagulation factors except fibrinogen normalise within 12 hours after CPB [10]. There is no role for prophylactic FFP given prior to cardiac surgery in reducing post-operative blood loss [11]. There are no reported studies examining its therapeutic efficacy in cardiac surgery. Despite this, appreciable quantities of FFP are used in this setting [12]. This practice exposes patients to unnecessary risks, including transfusion-transmitted infections, anaphylaxis, haemolysis, fluid overload and transfusion-related acute lung injury (TRALI) [5].

In an effort to control and rationalise the use of blood products, the use of FFP is commonly restricted to a dose of 12–15 ml/kg in actively bleeding patients with an activated partial thromboplastin time (APTT) or prothrombin time (PT) ratio of greater than 1.5. An isolated prolonged APTT should always be confirmed by an antiXa assay where available or thrombin and ideally reptilase times to check for the presence of heparin prior to the issue of FFP. Where indicated the effect of heparin should be reversed by protamine and the relevant test repeated (Figure 5.2).

Cryoprecipitate

Clinically significant fibrinogen deficiency develops after a loss of about 150% of blood volume – earlier than any other haemostatic abnormality when packed red cell concentrates are used in replacing major blood loss [10]. Fibrinogen levels should be maintained above 1.5 g/dl by the use of an adult pooled unit of cryoprecipitate [13].

Recombinant Factor VIIa

This product was originally introduced in 1996 as a haemostatic agent for haemophilia patients with inhibitory antibodies to Factors VIII and IX. It is able to bypass the defective parts of the coagulation cascade in these patients by its mechanism of action on the surface of platelets activated at the site of vascular injury [14]. Several small case series have supported its use in reducing rather than preventing bleeding in a variety of clinical settings. Although it is unlicenced in cardiac surgery its off-label use is increasing and being incorporated into local policies for management of

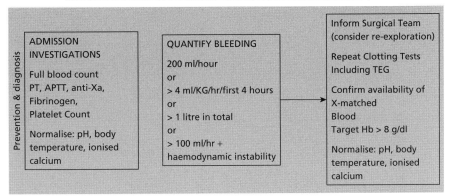

Remember the 'rule' no bleeding, no products   Remember the 'rule' no bleeding, no products

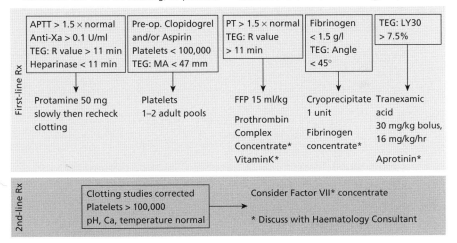

Figure 5.2 An example of an algorithm using laboratory parameters to guide the management of bleeding after cardiac surgery. Asterisks denote second-line agents to be used after consultation with a senior haematologist. PT, prothrombin time; APTT, activated partial thromboplastin time; PCC, prothrombin complex concentrate; TEG, thromboelastography: 'R' time to initial thrombin formation, an index of intrinsic, extrinsic and common pathways; 'α' angle, an index of the rate of fibrin formation; MA, maximum amplitude, reflecting clot strength and the interaction between platelets (number and function) and fibrin; LY30 the rate of amplitude reduction 30 minutes after MA, an indication of the stability of the clot and thrombolysis (see also Figure 5.4).

life-threatening bleeding. Anecdotal reports suggest that it is more efficacious with a platelet count above $50 \times 10^9/l$ in a normothermic, non-acidotic patient.

Antifibrinolytic drugs
Fibrinolysis contributes to bleeding after cardiac surgery. There is, however, insufficient evidence to suggest the use of drugs such as tranexamic acid in a

therapeutic rather than prophylactic role in reducing post-operative blood loss. These agents are contra-indicated in disseminated intravascular coagulation as there is a risk of fortifying thrombi in the small vasculature of the brain or renal bed.

5.3 Thromboprophylaxis in the ICU

Despite being exposed to large doses of UFH during CPB, patients undergoing cardiac surgery have a similar risk of post-operative venous thromboembolism (VTE) to patients undergoing major general or gynaecological surgery [15–16].

As in other arenas, thromboprophylaxis using subcutaneous UFH has largely been superseded by the use of once daily subcutaneous low molecular weight heparin (LMWH). Low molecular weight heparin (LMWH) has predictable pharmacokinetics and a long half-life. Unlike UFH, it is not necessary to monitor levels routinely, although this may be done by measuring anti-Xa activity. There is no definitive evidence to correlate anti-Xa levels with risk of VTE. LMWH is not fully reversible by protamine and caution must be employed in the immediate post-operative period when a risk of bleeding persists, as LMWH is exclusively renally excreted and renal dysfunction is common after cardiac surgery [17]. Twice daily dosing regimens may offer more uniform anticoagulation [18] and allow the drug to be withheld more promptly in the event of bleeding. The effect of LMWH should not be treated with FFP as this is likely to intensify anticoagulation by the provision of additional antithrombin.

Atrial fibrillation is a common occurrence early after cardiac surgery. The accepted long-term benefits of anticoagulation in preventing atrial thrombus formation and stroke must be weighed against the risk of bleeding and pericardial collection formation in the post-operative period. In the absence of definitive evidence for critically ill patients, the authors' practice is not to anticoagulate patients who develop atrial fibrillation, beyond the standard prophylaxis against VTE, in the absence of additional risk factors for atrial clot formation, such as massive left atrial enlargement, pre-existing intra-cardiac thrombus and a Fontan circulation. The American College of Chest Physicians Guidelines recommend that high risk patients (aged over 75 years, hypertensive, left ventricular dysfunction) benefit most from heparin therapy in the ICU while oral vitamin K antagonist (VKA) therapy is being established, but emphasise that the balance between risk and benefit should be assessed on an individual patient basis [19].

5.4 Anticoagulation of patients with prosthetic heart valves

There is wide agreement on the need to use VKA for long-term anticoagulation after mechanical heart valve replacement. In the immediate post-operative period, whilst the patient is unstable it can be difficult to achieve therapeutic levels of VKA. LMWH offers a safe effective bridging anticoagulation until therapeutic VKA levels can be achieved [20]. It is not necessary for these levels to be within the target range prior to the patient's discharge from hospital providing LMWH therapy is maintained.

The anticoagulation of bioprosthetic valves poses a more contentious question. Several retrospective non-randomised studies have shown that there is an increased risk of thromboembolism prior to the formation of endothelium over the sutures and valve in the first 3 months following bioprosthetic valve replacement. These studies suggest that VKA reduce the risk of thromboembolism at the cost of a slightly increased risk of bleeding [21]. Others argue that aspirin alone is sufficient to reduce thromboembolism without incurring the additional risk of bleeding [22]. There are at present no data from randomised trials to settle the argument.

5.5 Heparin-induced thrombocytopenia (HIT)

Heparin-induced thrombocytopenia is a potentially fatal haematological complication [23]. Two processes need to be distinguished from the outset. HIT type I is a benign non-immune self-limiting asymptomatic mild fall in platelet count which occurs soon after commencement of heparin therapy. It has no clinical significance. HIT type II, however, is a syndrome with an immune basis leading to thrombocytopenia and possible venous and arterial thrombosis. The following remarks pertain only to HIT type II.

Pathophysiology
HIT is caused by an IgG antibody that recognises both heparin and Platelet Factor 4 (PF4). Heparin induces a conformational change in PF4, causing presentation of a neo-antigen which stimulates development of the HIT antibody. The heparin/PF4 complex binds to the platelet surface attracting the HIT antibody. It is thought that the IgG Fc regions bind and cross-link the platelets. Clearing of this complex accounts for the thrombocytopenia. The cause of the thrombosis has not been fully elucidated, but it has been speculated that the binding of the IgG to the heparin/PF4 complex is effective in activating platelets. Moreover, the IgG may also promote vessel injury when binding to PF4 complexed with glycosaminoglycans on endothelial cells [24]. An iceberg model has been proposed to represent the relationship between the different phases of the process (Figure 5.3).

Laboratory testing
Thrombocytopenia is not uncommon on cardiac ICU (see Table 5.1), although diagnoses other than HIT are more likely. The correct diagnosis can be difficult to reach in this setting. Both false negative and false positive diagnoses can have far-reaching consequences. A missed diagnosis can subject the patient to potentially avoidable fatal thrombosis. A false positive diagnosis may result in prolonged therapy with expensive drugs, which in the worst case can cause irreversible bleeding. Unfortunately, laboratory

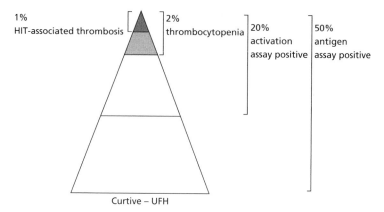

Figure 5.3 The 'iceberg' schema to show the relationship between the phases of heparin-induced thrombocytopenia (HIT).

Table 5.1 Causes of thrombocytopenia in the ICU.

Anti-thymocyte globulin*
Post cardiopulmonary bypass*
Heparin-induced thrombocytopenia (type 1)*
Haemofiltration
Sepsis
Disseminated intravascular coagulation
Intra-aortic balloon pump
Massive transfusion
Liver dysfunction
Drug-induced immune thrombocytopenia
Heparin-induced thrombocytopenia thrombosis (type 2)

* Platelet count not usually lower than 75–125 × 10⁹/l.

testing for HIT in cardiac patients is also not straightforward. It is essential that it is used only in conjunction with the pre-test probability (PTP) as there are wide variations in the sensitivities and specificity of the available tests.

There are two main types of tests for HIT. Platelet activation assays are technically demanding tests that have a good specificity and sensitivity when washed platelets are used. The rigours of the procedure, however, preclude its use in non-expert laboratories. Antigen assays are easier to perform and offer a high sensitivity. Specificity, however, is poor, with a false positive rate approaching 50% in patients following cardiac surgery [25].

Management

The frequency of HIT in cardiac surgical patients is about 2% and about 50% of these will suffer thrombosis [23]. HIT is seen more commonly in cardiac surgical patients than other patients because CPB is associated with high fluctuating levels of UFH and PF4 [24]. LMWH is much less likely to cause HIT than the longer molecules of UFH. Classically, 5–10 days after the first exposure to heparin, the platelet count begins to fall. The platelet count usually falls by more than 50% to a mean nadir of $55 \times 10^9/l$ (severe thrombocytopenia is unusual); if the patient has been exposed to heparin in the previous 3 months a more rapid fall may occur. At this point the PTP of HIT should be considered (see Table 5.2). Half of the patients developing HIT develop thrombosis; the other half (isolated HIT) are at high risk of thrombosis if heparin continues to be given and alternative anticoagulation with agents such as danaparoid, hirudins or argatroban (available in the USA) is not immediately instituted. LMWH is unsuitable as cross-reactivity with the HIT antibody occurs in up to 50% of cases [26].

If the thrombocytopenia is caused by HIT, the platelet count should improve promptly and anticoagulation should continue until the platelet count has been fully restored. Warfarin alone should not be used in the acute setting as this may precipitate warfarin-induced skin necrosis. It may be introduced once the platelet count has normalised and with an overlap with the alternative anticoagulant. Bleeding is uncommon in HIT. Platelet transfusions are relatively contraindicated as they may heighten the thrombotic risk.

The HIT antibody usually resolves after approximately 100 days providing heparin is *completely* withdrawn. The few molecules present in heparin/saline flushes may be sufficient to cause catastrophic thrombosis during this period. In cardiac patients requiring cardiopulmonary bypass, anticoagulation with UFH may be contemplated once the platelet count has normalised and the HIT antibody has become completely undetectable. If the clinical urgency does not allow the luxury of time, anticoagulation may proceed with alternative agents [27]. There are reported case series of anticoagulation with lepirudin and danaparoid, but serious post-operative bleeding is a well-documented risk.

5.6 Near patient testing

The perceived lengthy delay between sending specimens to and receiving results from the laboratory is a potential source of tension between the cardiac ICU and the Haematology/Transfusion service. The tests are often used as a 'gate-keeping' aide to ensure rational prescription of blood products. This has led to the growth of interest in near patient testing. There is already the well-established precedent of the activated clotting times (ACT) used to measure the adequacy of heparin levels for CPB in the operating theatre.

The standard laboratory repertoire gives no information on platelet function or rates of fibrinolysis. Furthermore, the results of routine clotting tests are frequently abnormal after cardiac surgery. They are associated with reduced levels of clotting factors, but it is not clear whether they are clinically useful. Some studies have shown that the PT and APTT do not discriminate between bleeders and non-bleeders [28], whilst other authors describe a clear correlation [29]. Whilst certain point of care devices measuring PT and APTT have enjoyed success in the field of self-testing of

Table 5.2 Estimating the pretest probability of HIT: the 'four Ts'.

	Points (0, 1 or 2 for each of four categories: maximum possible score = 8)		
	2	1	0
Thrombocytopenia	> 50% fall or platelet nadir 20–100 × 10⁹/l	30–50% fall or platelet nadir 10–19 × 10⁹/l	Fall < 30% or platelet nadir < 10 × 10⁹/l
Timing* of platelet count fall or other sequelae	Clear onset between days 5 and 10; or less than 1 day (if heparin exposure within past 100 days)	Consistent with immunisation but not clear (e.g. missing platelet counts or onset of thrombocytopenia after day 10)	Platelet count fall too early (without recent heparin exposure)
Thrombosis or other sequelae (e.g. skin lesions)	New thrombosis; skin necrosis; post heparin bolus acute systemic reaction	Progressive or recurrent thrombosis; erythematous skin lesions; suspected thrombosis not yet proven	None
Other causes for thrombocytopenia not evident	No other cause for platelet count fall evident	Possible other cause is evident	Definite other cause is present

Pretest probability score: 6 – 8 = high; 4 – 5 = intermediate; 0 – 3 = low.

* First day of immunising heparin exposure is considered day 0; the day the platelet count begins to fall is considered the day of onset of thrombocytopenia (it generally takes 1–3 days more until an arbitrary threshold that defines thrombocytopenia is passed.

Reprinted from Warkentin and Heddle (2003) Laboratory diagnosis of immune heparin-induced thrombocytopenia. *Current Haematology Reports*, 2, 148–57. Copyright *Current Medicine*, used with permission.

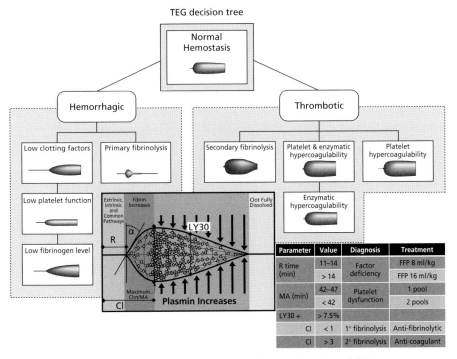

TEG decision tree

Figure 5.4 A guide to the interpretation of thromboelastography. 'R' time to initial thrombin formation, an index of intrinsic, extrinsic and common pathways; 'α' angle, an index of the rate of fibrin formation; MA, maximum amplitude, reflecting clot strength and the interaction between platelets (number and function) and fibrin; LY30 the rate of amplitude reduction 30 minutes after MA, an indication of the stability of the clot and thrombolysis. FFP, fresh frozen plasma.

the International Normalised Ratio (INR), they have not flourished in the ICU setting owing to poor reliability [30].

Thromboelastography (TEG: Figure 5.4) is enjoying a revival of interest since it was first introduced in the 1950s. This is a whole blood test which offers a global assessment of haemostasis to include the coagulation cascade, red cells, platelets and fibrinolytic pathways. The TEG examines the visco-elastic properties of blood using two mechanical parts: a cuvette that is oscillated at 4.5 Hz and a suspended pin connected to a computer. Its renaissance is partly due to its computerisation that has enabled speedier results to be produced [30]. Refinements of the technique include heparinase cups which eliminate the effect of heparin and increasingly sophisticated platelet function cups. There is a body of literature pointing to decreases in blood product usage when TEG is employed [31], yet other authors remain to be convinced [30]. It is agreed that TEG still has to be fully validated to achieve the standards of quality control demanded from traditional laboratory tests.

Exciting developments in point of care assessment of platelet function have been made to ascertain the efficacy of platelet function antagonists such as aspirin and clopidogrel. These devices are particularly useful in the cardiology setting for determining drug absorption after coronary artery stenting and monitoring compliance with drug therapy in stable out-patients. As yet there is insufficient familiarity and experience with their use in evaluating the complex platelet defect in the setting of the ICU following cardiopulmonary bypass.

5.7 Blood sparing techniques for surgery

These techniques are aimed at optimising haemoglobin prior to surgery, reducing bleeding and re-using shed blood to keep the patient's haemoglobin above the transfusion trigger. These interventions are only appropriate for patients who are likely to need blood transfusion. A blanket application of techniques is likely to add cost and risk to patients' management.

Preoperative interventions
Haematinic therapy
The pre-operative assessment should include a Full Blood Count. Abnormalities of red cell indices should prompt further investigation, such as iron studies, serum vitamin B_{12} and red cell folate levels, as appropriate. Oral iron replacement therapy can increase the haemoglobin by 0.2 g/dl/day in uncomplicated iron deficiency. A more rapid response can be achieved using the intravenous route. The cause of iron deficiency must always be established and cannot merely be attributed to aspirin use.

Drug management
Anticoagulants and antiplatelet agents should be withheld prior to surgery according to local protocols. For urgent cases, the INR may be safely reduced by small doses (0.5–3 mg) of intravenous or oral vitamin K; larger doses may cause resistance to VKA post-operatively. In an emergency, the INR may be normalised by the use of prothrombin complex concentrates (PCC). These are freeze dried, virally inactivated products with quality controlled levels of Factors II, VII, IX and X and as such are preferable to FFP for this indication. If surgery on a patient who has been taking clopidogrel in the 7 days prior to the operation is unavoidable, platelet transfusion may be necessary.

Recombinant human erythropoietin (rHuEPO) has been used for years to increase haemoglobin in chronic renal insufficiency and chemotherapy-induced anaemia. In the context of cardiac surgery it may be employed in two ways: pre-operatively as a blood sparing technique or post-operatively to lessen transfusion in chronically anaemic unwell patients in the ICU. Several studies have shown that a higher preoperative haemoglobin is related to a lower transfusion rate. This technique may also be employed for Jehovah's Witnesses and others who refuse blood transfusion. RhuEPO does, however, offer a risk of hypertension and thromboembolism that should be monitored. In the latter group, chronic illness and surgery itself may blunt endogenous erythropoietin (EPO) production [32]. There are no baseline predictive factors of response to rHuEPO in this setting, in contrast to that of haematological malignancies where a low serum EPO level predicts for a good response [33]. The addition of intravenous iron gives a superior response compared to oral iron. The optimal dosage regimen has not been established.

Pre-operative autologous donation (PAD)

This technique involves venesecting patients' units of their own blood prior to surgery (with or without rHuEPO support) and storing them for up to 5 weeks. This allows the haemoglobin to be supported peri- and post-operatively by homologous rather than allogeneic blood. The concept was originally popular when the main risks of transfusion were thought to be viral transmission rather than receipt of the incorrect blood component. PAD does not lessen this risk nor does it alter the risk of transfusion-transmitted bacterial infection. Owing to theoretical concerns about myocardial ischaemia caused by venesection and governance issues about local storage of blood, this technique is rarely used.

Peri-operative techniques
Antifibrinolytic agents

Aprotinin is a serine protease inhibitor and an antifibrinolytic drug that has been in clinical use for several years as a prophylactic agent which aimed to decrease the risk of bleeding in high-risk cardiac surgery. Tranexamic acid and ε aminocaproic acid are lysine analogue antifibrinolytic drugs which have been used for the same indication, but the literature is not so extensive. Aprotinin significantly reduces the need for peri-operative red cell transfusion and rate of return to theatre for bleeding compared to controls [34]. Recently, however, controversy has emerged over the safety profile of aprotinin, particularly its propensity to cause renal impairment, myocardial infarction and stroke [35]. The Blood Conservation using Antifibrinolytics in a Randomized Trial (BART) study compared aprotinin with the lysine analogues in patients undergoing high-risk cardiac surgery, demonstrating that aprotinin was marginally more effective at preventing bleeding [36]. However, at 30 days, patients who received aprotinin had an increased risk of death of more than 50%. It is not clear from these data whether aprotinin causes harm through its intended procoagulant action or through a different effect of inhibiting unrelated serine proteases. It seems likely that the use of aprotinin will be completely replaced by other agents, for example tranexamic acid.

Acute normovolaemic haemodilution (ANH)

This procedure involves venesecting a unit of whole blood from a patient just prior to the operation and *leaving it attached to the patient*, so that any operative blood loss will be of a lower haematocrit. On completion of the operation, the fresh whole blood (including platelets unexposed to UFH or cardiopulmonary bypass) can be safely reinfused to restore the haematocrit and support haemostasis. Whilst ANH reduces exposure to allogeneic blood, its place in a rigorous panoply of blood sparing techniques has not been substantiated [37].

Cell salvage

This technique has loyal proponents in cardiothoracic surgery. It is the process in which blood shed in the surgical field is retrieved by an anticoagulated suction apparatus and collected within a reservoir, from where it is centrifuged, washed and pumped into an infusion bag, whence it can be returned to the patient. This process is effective in reducing the need for allogeneic red cell transfusion and has been widely used in adult orthopaedic and cardiac surgery without complication [38]. Again, its contribution to the overall management of blood avoidance remains to be established. Systematic reviews in cardiothoracic surgery may have shown less impressive results than in orthopaedic surgery due to the inclusion of early trials using unprocessed blood which is known to cause coagulopathy and is likely to contain significant concentration of potentially damaging free haemoglobin.

Post-operative techniques

Placement of wound drains to collect blood for later reinfusion has become a standard blood sparing technique in some types of orthopaedic surgery. It has not, however, been developed for post-cardiotomy drainage.

5.8 Conclusion

The use of high doses of antiplatelet agents, heparin and extra-corporeal circuits in patients undergoing procedures leading to cardiac intensive care requires close co-operation between haematologists, operators and intensivists to optimise patient safety.

Case study

A 55-year-old woman was admitted to ICU for management of refractory heart failure. She had undergone septomymectomy and mitral valve replacement several years earlier without complication. In the 12 months prior to admission she had been admitted on several occasions for treatment of heart failure. At the time of admission she was taking warfarin. During her stay in the ICU, she required constant inotropic support and an intra-aortic balloon pump was inserted, necessitating an infusion of UFH to keep the APTT ratio twice normal. Five days after commencing the UFH infusion, the platelet count fell from $359 \times 10^9/l$ to $26 \times 10^9/l$ (see Figure 5.5). The UFH was switched to danaparoid and a particle gel immunoassay test was done which was strongly positive. Over the next 5 days the platelet count returned to $178 \times 10^9/l$. The clinical condition failed to improve so the patient was listed for an urgent cardiac transplant. Seven days later a suitable organ became available. As there was prior familiarity with this protocol,

Continued

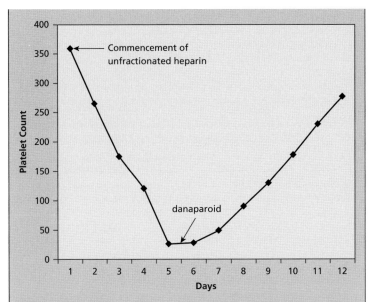

Figure 5.5 Daily platelet count of the patient in the case study. The commencement of heparin and time of diagnosis of HIT are indicated.

anticoagulation was provided with lepirudin. Levels were monitored using the Ecarin clotting test [26]. Post-operatively the patient suffered torrential bleeding into her drains with concurrent high lepirudin levels. These were then brought down by the use of continuous veno-venous haemofiltration. This markedly reduced the bleeding and the patient continued on an uneventful post-operative course.

References

1. Bevan DH. Cardiac bypass haemostasis: putting blood through the mill. *Br J Haematol* 1999; 104: 208–19.
2. Hutton B, Fergusson D, Tinmouth A, et al. Transfusion rates vary significantly amongst Canadian medical centres. *Can J Anaes* 2005; 52(6): 581–90.
3. Karthik S, Grayson AD, McCarron EE, et al. Reexploration for bleeding after coronary artery bypass surgery: risk factors, outcomes, and the effect of time delay. *Ann Thorac Surg* 2004; 78: 527–34; discussion 534.
4. Unsworth-White MJ, Herriot A, Valencia O, et al. Resternotomy for bleeding after cardiac operation: a marker for increased morbidity and mortality. *Annals Thor Surg* 1995; 59: 664–7.
5. Stainsby D, Davison K. *Serious Hazards of Transfusion (SHOT) – Annual Report 2004.* Royal College of Pathologists.
6. Hebert PC, Wells G, Blajchman MA, et al. A multicenter, randomised, controlled clinical trial of transfusion requirements in critical care. *New Engl J Med* 1999; 340: 409–17.

7. Woodman RC, Harker LA. Bleeding complications associated with cardiopulmonary bypass. *Blood* 1990;76:1680–97.

8. Zimmerman N, Kienzle P, Weber A-A, et al. Aspirin resistance after coronary artery bypass grafting. *J Thor Cardiovasc Surg* 2001; 121: 982–4.

9. Hippala S. Replacement of massive blood loss. *Vox Sanguinis* 1998; 74: 399–407.

10. Gans H, Siegel DL, Lillehai CW, et al. Problems in haemostasis during open heart surgery. II. On the hypercoagulability of blood during cardiac bypass. *Annals Surg* 1962; 156: 19–23.

11. Casbard AC, Williamson LM, Murphy MF, et al. the role of prophylactic fresh frozen plasma in decreasing blood loss and correcting coagulopathy in cardiac surgery. A systematic review. *Anaesthesia* 2004; 59(6): 550–8.

12. Stainsby D, Burrowes-King V. Audit of the appropriate use of fresh frozen plasma. *Blood Matters* 2002; 10: 8–10.

13. Stainsby D, Maclennan S, Hamilton PJ. Commentary. Management of massive blood loss: a template guideline. *Br J Anaes* 2000; 85: 487–91.

14. Hoffman M, Munroe DM. The action of high-dose factor VIIa (FVIIa) in a cell-based model of haemostasis. *Seminars Haematol* 2001; 38 (4 Suppl 12): 6–9.

15. Ramos R, Salem BI, De Pawlikowski MP, et al. The efficacy of pneumatic compression stockings in the prevention of pulmonary embolism after cardiac surgery. *Chest* 1996; 109: 82–5.

16. Ambrosetti M, Salerno M, Zambelli M, et al. Deep vein thrombosis among patients entering cardiac rehabilitation after coronary artery bypass surgery. *Chest* 2004; 125(1): 191–6.

17. Jones HU, Muhlestein JB, Jones KW, et al. early postoperative use of unfractionated heparin or enoxaparin is associated with increased surgical re-exploration for bleeding. *Annals Thor Surg* 2005; 80(2): 518–22.

18. Rutherford EJ, Schooler WG, Sredzienski E, et al. Optimal dose of enoxiparin in critically ill trauma and surgical patients. *J Trauma* 2005; 58(6): 1167–70.

19. Epstein AE, Alexander JC, Gutterman DD, et al. Anticoagulation. American College of Chest Physicians guidelines for the prevention and management of postoperative atrial fibrillation after cardiac surgery. *Chest* 2005; 128(2): 24–7.

20. Spyropoulos AC, Turpie AG, Dunn AS, et al. Clinical outcomes with unfractionated heparin or low-molecular-weight heparin as bridging therapy in patients on long-term oral anticoagulants: the REGIMEN registry. *J Thrombosis Haemostasis* 2006; 4(6): 1246–52.

21. Heras M, Chesebro JH, Fuster V, et al. High risk of thromboemboli early after bioprosthetic cardiac valve replacement. *J Am Coll Cardiol* 1995; 25(5): 214–19.

22. Moinuddeen K, Quin J, Shaw R, et al. Anticoagulation is unnecessary after biological aortic valve replacement. *Circulation* 1998; (19S): 496–500.

23. Warkentin TE, Greinacher AG, eds. *Heparin-Induced Thrombocytopenia*, 2nd edn. Marcel Dekker, New York, 2001.

24. Keeling D, Davidson S, Watson H. The management of heparin-induced thrombocytopenia. *Br J Haematol* 2006; 133: 259–69.

25. Warkentin TE, Sheppard JI, Horsewood P, et al. Impact of the patient population on the risk of heparin-induced thrombocytopenia. *Blood* 2000; 96: 1703–8.

26. Keeling DM, Richards EM, Baglin TP. Platelet aggregation in response to four low molecular weight heparins and the heparinoid ORG 10172 in patients with heparin-induced thrombocytopenia. *Br J Haematol* 1994; 86: 425–6.

27. Pötzsch B, Madlener K, Seeling C, et al. The whole blood ecarin clotting time assay allows rapid and accurate monitoring of the anticoagulant response of r-hirudin during cardiopulmonary bypass. *Thrombosis Haemostasis* 1997; 77: 920–5.

28. Gravlee GP, Arora S, Lavender SW, et al. Predictive value of blood clotting tests in cardiac surgical patients. *Annals Thorac Surg* 1994; 58: 216–21.

29. Blome M, Isgro F, Kiessling AH, et al. Relationship between Factor XIII activity, fibrinogen, haemostasis screening tests and postoperative bleeding in cardiopulmonary bypass surgery. *Thrombosis Haemostasis* 2005; 93(6): 1101–7.

30. Samama CM, Ozier Y. Near-patient testing of haemostasis in the operating theatre: an approach to appropriate use of blood in surgery. *Vox Sanguinis* 2003; 84: 251–5.

31. Shore-Lesserson L, Manspeizer HE, Deperio M, et al. Thromboelastography-guided transfusion algorithm reduces transfusions in complex cardiac surgery. *Anaes Anal* 1999; 88: 312–19.

32. Clemens J, Spivak JL. Serum immunoreactive erythropoietin during the perioperative period. *Surgery* 1994; 115: 510–5.

33. Bokemeyer C, Aapro MS, Courdi A, et al. EORTC guidelines for the use of erythropoietic proteins in anaemic patients with cancer: 2006 update. *Eur J Cancer* 2007; 43: 258–70.

34. Henry DA, Carless PA, Moxey AJ, et al. Anti-fibrinolytic use for minimising perioperative allogeneic blood transfusion. *Cochrane Database of Systematic Reviews* 2007, Issue 3. Art. No.: CD001886. DOI: 10.1002/14651858.CD001886.pub2.

35. Ray WA, Stein CM. The aprotinin story – is BART the final chapter? *N Engl J Med* 2008; 358: 2398–400.

36. Fergusson DA, Hébert PC, Mazer CD, et al. A comparison of aprotinin and lysine analogues in high-risk cardiac surgery. *N Engl J Med* 2008; 358: 2319–31.

37. Carless P, Moxey A, O'Connell D, Henry D. Autologous transfusion techniques: a systematic review of their efficacy. *Transfus Med* 2004; 14: 123–44.

38. Carless PA, Henry DA, Moxey AJ, et al. Cell salvage for minimising perioperative allogeneic blood transfusion. *Cochrane Database of Systematic Reviews* 2006, Issue 2. Art. No.: CD001888. DOI:10.1002/14651858.CD001888.pub2.

6 Cardiovascular Support: Pharmacological

Joseph E. Arrowsmith and Florian Falter
Papworth Hospital, Cambridge, UK

Take Home Messages

- The purpose of pharmacological haemodynamic intervention is the restoration and maintenance of adequate oxygen delivery to vital organs through the manipulation of circulating volume, cardiac output and perfusion pressure.
- Knowledge of the range of normal physiological responses, an understanding of the dynamics of the pathological processes and familiarity with vasoactive drugs permit targeted pharmacological intervention.
- Effective pharmacological cardiovascular support requires consideration of the underlying cause(s) of circulatory insufficiency, adequate monitoring, the selection of therapeutic goals and an empirical approach that permits alterations in therapy when interventions are deemed to have failed.

6.1 Introduction

Normal cardiovascular function relies on a multitude of neural, hormonal and local homeostatic mechanisms that maintain organ perfusion by controlling intra-vascular volume, vascular tone, heart rate and myocardial contractility. Pathological conditions such as sepsis interfere with these mechanisms on different levels, leading to impaired end-organ perfusion. As early as 1969, Joly and Weil [1] described a direct correlation between toe skin temperature, cardiac output and survival. Since then numerous studies have evaluated strategies to increase cardiac output, arterial blood pressure and organ perfusion in conditions frequently met in the intensive care environment. Only when we have knowledge of the range of normal physiological responses and understand the dynamics of the pathological

---

Cardiovascular Critical Care. Edited by M. Griffiths, J. Cordingley and S. Price.
© 2010 Blackwell Publishing Ltd.

processes will we be able to provide therapy by targeted pharmacological intervention.

6.2 Cardiovascular physiology

The components of cardiovascular homeostasis act in concert. However, it is more convenient to consider them separately:

- Mean Arterial Pressure (MAP) is the time-weighted average of arterial pressures during a pulse cycle.
- Blood pressure is the product of two components – cardiac output (CO) and systemic vascular resistance (SVR).
- Cardiac output is defined as the volume of blood pumped by the heart during a given time period, usually over 1 minute. It is the product of stroke volume (SV) and heart rate (HR).
- While SVR corresponds to the arterial impedance to ejection and is mainly determined by arteriolar tone, stroke volume is determined by preload, myocardial contractility and afterload (Figure 6.1).

Haemodynamic parameters
Preload

Preload is the end-diastolic ventricular volume, which exerts a passive force that stretches the resting muscle. The Frank–Starling law governs the relationship between end-diastolic filling and cardiac output, where the initial fibre length determines the force of the cardiac muscle contraction. Assuming a constant heart rate, cardiac output is directly proportional to

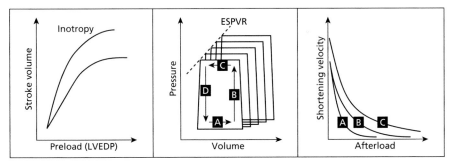

Figure 6.1 The determinants of stroke volume (SV). *Left* The Frank–Starling relationship. Preload is represented by left ventricular end-diastolic pressure (LVEDP). *Centre* The left ventricular pressure/volume relationship. A ventricular filling; B isovolumic contraction; C ventricular ejection; D isovolumic relaxation. Dotted lines represent the pressure/volume relationship at increasing levels of preload. The end-systolic pressure/volume relationship (ESPVR) describes contractility independent of load. *Right* The effect of afterload on the velocity of muscle fibre shortening (arbitrary units). Increasing preload (curve B) increases shortening velocity for a given afterload but has no impact on maximum shortening velocity. Inotropic action (curve C) increases the maximum shortening velocity for a given preload and afterload.

preload until excessive end-diastolic volumes are reached, i.e. until the maximum isometric force is achieved. A further increase in preload beyond this point produces a fall in cardiac output. Preload is influenced by intravascular volume, gravity, respiratory pattern, atrial compliance and contractility, ventricular compliance (i.e. dP/dV – change in pressure with respect to volume), heart rate and afterload.

Intravascular volume is largely regulated by hormonal and neuronal homeostatic mechanisms under the influence of the hypothalamus. Activation of osmoreceptors in the preoptic area in response to very small changes in the osmolality of extracellular fluid (ECF) induces thirst. Neurones in the supraoptic and paraventricular area shrink with increasing osmolality, inducing the release of antidiuretic hormone (ADH) from the posterior pituitary which decreases urine output.

Myocardial contractility

This intrinsic ability of the myocardium essentially describes the extent and rate of cardiac muscle shortening, which is dependent on the cytosolic calcium concentration. The ability to alter contractility in a variety of conditions is a unique property of cardiac muscle. Contractility is best described by the slope of the end-systolic pressure/volume relationship (ESPVR) – also known as the end-systolic elastance (E_{ES}) [2].

Heart rate

Heart rate is predominantly under the control of the sympathetic nervous system (SNS) acting via the so-called *cardiac plexus* (T_1–T_4) and catecholamines from the adrenal medulla. SNS activity increases the rate of slow diastolic (phase IV) depolarisation in the sinoatrial (SA) node (i.e. chronotropy) and increases action potential conduction velocity in the atrioventricular node (i.e. dromotropy). This is mainly achieved by adrenergic β_1-receptors and to a lesser extent by β_2-receptors. Circulating catecholamines increase the rate of slow diastolic depolarisation in *all* cardiomyocytes. In contrast, the parasympathetic nervous system (PNS) – acting via the vagi and muscarinic (M_2) receptors to increase potassium conductance in the SA node – reduces both conduction velocity and the rate of spontaneous diastolic depolarisation.

Afterload

Afterload – often described as 'vascular impedance' – can be thought of as the pressure that must be overcome by the ventricle to decrease its size during systole. The *force–velocity relationship* describes the inverse relationship between afterload and the extent and rate of cardiomyocyte fibre shortening. Systolic ventricular pressure is largely determined by the force necessary to achieve ventricular contraction, the viscoelastic properties of the aorta and proximal vessels, blood viscosity and density, and the systemic vascular resistance (SVR).

Arteriolar muscle tone – the key determinant of SVR – is controlled by the SNS acting via the sympathetic chain and vascular α_1 (vasoconstriction) and β_1 (vasodilatation) receptors, and a wide variety of compounds that are 'delivered' to vascular smooth muscle by the circulation, autonomic neurones and endothelial cells. Most regional circulations possess the ability to regulate blood flow autonomously (i.e. autoregulation). Periods of increased tissue oxygen demand or low perfusion pressure induce vasodilatation, whereas low tissue oxygen demand or high perfusion pressure induce vasoconstriction. Over a physiological range of MAP (60–150 mmHg) the cardiac, renal and cerebral circulations are capable of autoregulation, maintaining near-constant blood flow by local mechanisms which vary the diameter of precapillary resistance vessels. This phenomenon has been explained on the basis of an active arteriolar smooth muscle response to tension (myogenic theory) and the influence of local vasodilatory metabolites such as O_2, CO_2, NO, K^+, H^+, eicosanoids, kinins and adenosine (metabolic theory).

Vascular endothelium produces or modifies numerous substances that are directly involved in blood pressure control and local perfusion. Shearing forces created by blood flow over the endothelium and circulating substances (e.g. insulin, bradykinin, acetylcholine, substance P) acting via endothelial membrane receptors lead to variations in endothelial metabolic activity. Prominent amongst endothelium-derived factors are vasoconstrictors such as endothelins and thromboxane A, vasodilators such as nitric oxide (NO) and prostacyclin, anticoagulants and fibrinolytics. The release of endothelin-derived vasoconstrictors is triggered by adrenaline and thrombin (Figure 6.2).

Regulation of cardiovascular physiology

Blood flow in the great arteries is pulsatile; however, in the capillary system flow becomes laminar. MAP drops from a normal value of 90–100 mmHg in the arterial system to nearly 0 in the large veins as it returns to the heart. The most dramatic pressure drop of 50% occurs in the arteriolar bed.

Short-term regulation
Baroreceptors
The short-term regulation of arterial pressure is principally achieved by stretch receptors (baroreceptors) located both centrally in the brain stem and hypothalamus and peripherally in the aortic arch, carotid sinuses, ventricles, atria and vena cavae. A rise in MAP and arterial pulsatility increases the firing rate of high-pressure (aortic and carotid) baroreceptors, which produces vasomotor inhibition and a reduction in heart rate, SV and SVR (Figure 6.3).

Chemoreceptors
Receptors sensitive to small changes in pH, PaO_2 and $PaCO_2$ are located in the medulla oblongata and in the carotid bodies. Although the principal function of these receptors is the regulation of respiration, they play a minor but important role in cardiovascular homeostasis. Hypercarbia, acidosis and hypoxia produce SNS stimulation leading to a rise in heart rate and SVR.

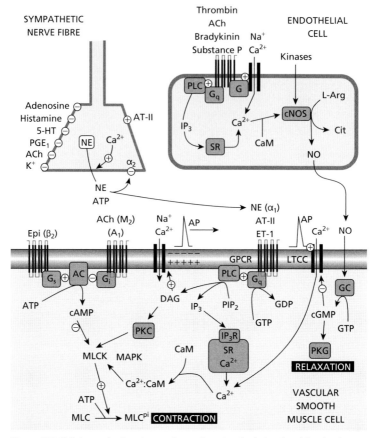

Figure 6.2 Cellular mechanisms in smooth muscle contraction/relaxation. AC, adenylate cyclase; AT-II, angiotensin II; ATP, adenosine triphosphate; CaM, calmodulin; cAMP, cyclic adenosine monophosphate; cGMP, cyclic guanosine monophosphate; DAG, diacylglycerate; ET-1, endothelin 1; GC, guanylate cyclase; GDP, guanosine diphosphate; GPCR, G-protein coupled receptor; G_q, G_i and G_s, G-proteins; GTP, guanosine triphosphate; IP_3, inositol triphosphate; IP_3R, inositol triphosphate receptor; LTCC, L-type calcium channel; MLC, myosin light chain; MLCK, myosin light chain kinase; NE, norepinephrine; NO, nitric oxide; PIP_2, phosphatidyl inositol biphosphate; PKC, protein kinase C; PLC, phospholipase C.

Intermediate regulation

A sustained decrease in arterial pressure will, within minutes, activate a series of compensatory mechanisms, which serve to preserve organ perfusion and restore the circulation. The renin–angiotensin–aldosterone system mediates vasoconstriction via angiotensin II (AT_1 receptors) and renal sodium and water retention. Release of ADH in response to baroreceptors, osmoreceptors and the central action of aldosterone produces vasoconstriction (V_1 receptors) and an anti-diuresis (V_2 receptors). Alteration in the balance of hydrostatic and oncotic pressures in capillaries results in the net transfer of fluid from the interstitial space into the vascular compartment (Figure 6.4).

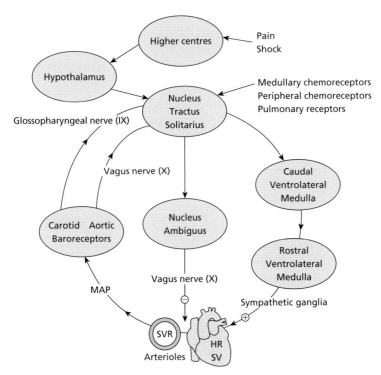

Figure 6.3 Baroreceptor reflexes. HR, heart rate; MAP, mean arterial pressure; SV, stroke volume; SVR, systemic vascular resistance.

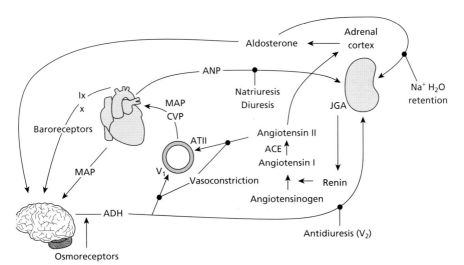

Figure 6.4 Control of intravascular volume. ACE, angiotensin converting enzyme; ADH, antidiuretic hormone (vasopressin); ANP, atrial natriuretic peptide; ATII, angiotensin II; CVP, central venous pressure; IX, glossopharyngeal nerve; JGA, juxtaglomerular apparatus; MAP, mean aterial pressure; X, vagus nerve.

Long-term regulation

Sustained hypotension leads to increased renal water and sodium reabsorption through the kidneys. However, these renal mechanisms to restore normal blood pressure only become effective after several hours of sustained low blood pressure.

6.3 Therapeutic pharmacological intervention

A thorough knowledge of the mechanisms of action of drugs and the pathophysiology of underlying diseases permits targeted pharmacologic intervention. Drugs acting on the cardiovascular system can be considered under the following categories:

- Inotropes – increasing the rate and force of myocardial contraction.
- Lucitropes – increasing the rate of myocardial relaxation.
- Chronotropes – increasing heart rate.
- Antidysrhythmics – restoring normal cardiac rate and rhythm.
- Vasoactive drugs – acting on systemic and pulmonary vascular smooth muscle.
- Diuretics – reducing circulating volume.

Antidysrhythmic drugs are considered by Montgomery and Sivaraman in Chapter 7 and will not be discussed further.

Positive inotropes

Commonly used inotropic agents include catecholamines and their synthetic derivatives, phosphodiesterase (PDE) inhibitors, digitalis glycosides, calcium sensitisers and a number of uncategorised agents. Inotropes have been classified [3, 4] according to their mode of action:

Class I   Drugs that increase intracellular levels of cyclic adenosine monophosphate (cAMP) via G_s protein receptor complex-mediated activation of adenylate cyclase (β agonists) and inhibition of cAMP metabolism by phosphodiesterase.

Class II   Drugs that increase intracellular levels of Ca^{2+} via non-cAMP-dependent mechanisms mediated by G_q protein receptor complex activation of phospholipase C (α_1 agonists).

Class III   Drugs that affect ion channel conductance or ion exchange mechanisms such as the N^+/K^+ ATPase.

Class III   Drugs that modulate intracellular calcium regulation.

Class IV   Drugs that augment contractility through multiple pathways.

Catecholamines

Naturally occurring catecholamines are derived from the tyrosine metabolite 3,4-dihydroxy-L-phenylalanine (L-DOPA). Through a number of enzyme-catalysed reactions L-DOPA is transformed into dopamine, noradrenaline and adrenaline. Synthetic substitution of the aminoethyl

Table 6.1 Compounds produced as a result of modification of the catecholamine nucleus.

	R_1	R_2		R_3	R_4	R_5
L-DOPA	OH	OH		H	COOH	H
Dopamine	OH	OH		H	H	H
Noradrenaline	OH	OH		OH	H	H
Adrenaline	OH	OH		OH	H	CH_3
Dobutamine	OH	OH		H	H	$CH(CH_3).CH_2.CH_2.(C_6H_4).OH$
Dopexamine	OH	OH		H	H	$(CH_2)_6.NH.CH_2.CH_2.(C_6H_5)$
Isoproterenol	OH	OH		OH	H	$CH(CH_3)_2$
Salbutamol	OH	CH_2OH		OH	H	$C(CH_3)_3$
Metaraminol	OH	H		OH	CH_3	H
Ephedrine	H	H		OH	CH_3	CH_3
Phenylephrine	OH	H		OH	H	CH_3
Atenolol	H	$O.CH(OH).CH_2.NH.CH(CH_3)_2$		H	O	H

chain of the catecholamine nucleus (Table 6.1) yields a series of compounds with β_1 (dobutamine, dopexamine), α_1 (metaraminol, phenylephrine), non-selective β (isoproterol) and selective β_2 (salbutamol) agonist properties, whereas modification of the benzene ring yields compounds with β antagonist properties (atenolol).

Properties shared by most catecholamines include: mild central nervous system stimulation, bronchodilatation, hyperglycaemia (secondary to inhibition of insulin secretion, and stimulation of glucagon release and glycogenolysis), an increase in circulating free fatty acids, lactic acidosis and hypokalaemia.

Adrenaline

Adrenaline is a positive inotrope and chronotrope, with predominantly β-adrenergic effects (α_1 ++, α_2 ++, β_1 +++, β_2 +++). At low doses (0.01–0.04 μg/kg/min) it produces a transient tachycardia (β_1), a rise in systolic pressure and a fall in SVR and diastolic pressure (β_2). At higher doses (0.1–0.5 μg/kg/min) it produces a tachycardia (β_1) and rise in SVR, PVR and MAP (α_1). It is a potent bronchodilator and a mild stimulant effect induces an increase in both respiratory rate and tidal volume (β_2). Increased platelet adhesiveness and factor V activity induces a mild thrombophilic state.

Dopamine

Dopamine is a positive inotrope and chronotrope with selective vasodilator properties which acts on both adrenergic (α_1 ++, α_2 +, β_1 ++, β_2 +++) and dopaminergic (D_1 +++, D_2 +++) receptors. Vasoconstriction is mediated via α_1-adrenoceptors, whilst splanchnic vasodilatation is mediated via D_1 receptors. At low doses (< 3 μg/kg/min) dopamine produces a modest increase in cardiac output (β_1) and renal/splanchnic blood flow (D_1). The notion that a low-dose infusion confers protection against renal failure (so-called renal dopamine dose) should be abandoned, because multiple clinical trials have demonstrated that dopamine is ineffective in this role [5, 6]. At intermediate doses (3–6 μg/kg/min) dopamine increases cardiac output and renal/splanchnic blood flow (β_1), with a modest increase in heart rate (β_2) and SVR (α_1). At higher doses (> 6 μg/kg/min) it increases heart rate (β_2) and SVR (α_1). Dopamine inhibits the release of aldosterone and prolactin (D_2) and, rarely, may cause nausea via a central serotoninergic action.

Dobutamine

Dobutamine is a synthetic positive inotrope and chronotrope with predominantly β_1-adrenergic effects (α_1 +, α_2 +, β_1 +++, β_2 +). It produces a dose-dependent increase in cardiac output with β_1 effects predominating at doses < 10 μg/kg/min. At doses > 15 μg/kg/min therapy is often limited by tachycardia secondary to reflex response to vasodilatation rather than direct β_1 effect [7]. Undoubtedly the use of the drug in Shoemaker's early work on goal-directed therapy [8] served to popularise the use of dobutamine in critical care, although there is little evidence that it is superior to any other inotrope [9].

Dopexamine

Dopexamine is a synthetic positive inotrope and chronotrope devoid of any significant α-adrenergic effects (β_1 +++, β_2 ++, D_1 +, D_2 +). Its relatively weak inotropic action is thought to be mediated by both a direct action via β_2-receptors and an indirect action via β_1-mediated inhibition of catecholamine reuptake. In addition, it produces vasodilatation via β_2, D_1 and prejunctional D_2 receptors and β_2-mediated bronchodilatation. Early studies suggested that dopexamine (0.5–6 μg/kg/min) increased splanchnic blood flow in critically ill patients [10, 11]. In contrast, more recent studies suggest that dopexamine has no selective effect on splanchnic vasculature and that changes in splanchnic blood flow were proportional to changes in cardiac output [12].

Isoproterenol

Isoproterenol (isoprenaline) is a synthetic positive inotrope and chronotrope (β_1 +++, β_2 ++). Vasodilatation and bronchodilatation is mediated via β_2 receptors. Although the drug can be administered orally (90–840 mg/day) it undergoes extensive first-pass metabolism. Parenteral administration (bolus 1–2 μg, infusion 0.5–10 μg/min) is more usual. Isoproterenol is particularly useful in the treatment of complete heart block, atropine-resistant bradycardia, torsade de pointes and following cardiac transplantation.

Phosphodiesterase (PDE-III) inhibitors

PDE-III inhibitors currently available for clinical use include enoximone, milrinone and inamrinone (formerly known as amrinone). Milrinone is by far the most potent of the three agents. Inhibition of PDE-III leads to an increase in cAMP in myocytes and vascular smooth muscle, which prolongs protein kinase-mediated inotropy, lusitropy, chronotropy and vasodilatation [13]. PDE-III inhibitors are typically used in combination with other inotropes with or without a vasoconstrictor in advanced heart failure and pulmonary hypertension [14], following cardiac surgery [15] and as a pharmacological bridge to cardiac transplantation.

Digitalis glycosides

Digoxin possesses both positive inotropic and negative chronotropic and dromotrophic properties. Inhibition of sarcolemmal $Na^+K^+ATPase$ mediates a rise in the intracellular sodium and calcium concentration and a fall in potassium concentration. This in turn mediates inotropy, reduced atrioventricular conduction velocity and reduced sinus node discharge. An indirect vagotonic effect enhances cardiac slowing and may explain the gastrointestinal side effects of the drug. While slowing of ventricular response rate in atrial fibrillation remains the most common indication for digoxin therapy, it is increasingly used in patients with impaired left ventricular function in sinus rhythm [16–18].

Calcium sensitisers

Drugs such as levosimendan are thought to mediate their positive inotropic effects by (i) increasing the affinity of troponin C for Ca^{2+}, (ii) stabilising the conformational change in troponin C mediated by Ca^{2+}, (iii) activating protein kinases that mediate muscle contraction and (iv) inhibition of phosphodiesterase-III. Because there is believed to be no net increase in intracellular calcium concentration, inotropy is said to be achieved without an increase in either myocardial oxygen consumption or arrhythmogenesis. In addition to its inotropic effects, levosimendan causes vasodilatation via activation of ATP-dependent potassium channels in smooth muscle cells. Most clinical experience has been gained in patients with acute decompensated left ventricular failure after acute coronary syndromes [19]. Two recently published studies of patients hospitalised with worsening cardiac failure demonstrated that while levosimendan improved symptoms, it conferred no survival advantage [20, 21]. Although the drug is currently only licensed for administration over 24 hours (5–10 µg/kg followed by 0.5–0.20 µg/kg/min) the clinical effects may last for 3–4 days, particularly in patients with renal dysfunction owing to the presence of a long-lived active acetylated metabolite.

Miscellaneous agents

Glucose, insulin and potassium: the infusion of glucose, insulin and potassium (GIK) has been used to ameliorate ischaemic myocardial dysfunction for over four decades [22]. It is only recently, however, that large-scale clinical trials have demonstrated significant benefit in the settings of myocardial infarction and cardiac surgery. Typically a solution containing glucose 500 mg/ml and soluble insulin 1 iu/ml is infused at 10–50 ml/hour and KCl administered to maintain a serum potassium concentration of 4.5–5.5 mmol/l. It is recommended that serum glucose and potassium be measured every 30 minutes.

Calcium salts: the intravenous administration of calcium (chloride or gluconate) typically produces a short-lived rise in cardiac output and MAP. In the setting of low cardiac output, calcium salts may be of use as an intermediate or 'rescue' therapy, while other inotropic drugs are prepared. Parenteral calcium is particularly useful in the management of calcium channel blocker toxicity and hyperkalaemic dysrhythmias. Care should be taken when administering calcium to patients with arterial coronary artery bypass grafts owing to the risk of inducing spasm.

Glucagon: in addition to its use in the treatment of hypoglycaemia, glucagon may be used in cardiogenic shock [23]. Its positive inotropic, chronotropic and lusitropic actions are mediated via adenylate cyclase and a rise in intracellular cAMP. It acts synergistically with β_2 agonists and has the advantage that it does not increase myocardial irritability. Because of its short elimination half-life (~ 5 minutes) glucagon must be administered every 30 minutes (1–5 mg) or by infusion (5–20 mg/hour).

Vasoconstrictors
Alpha agonists
Noradrenaline
Noradrenaline is a positive inotrope and chronotrope, and a potent vasoconstrictor (α_1 +++, α_2 +++, β_1 ++, β_2 ++). At low doses (< 0.005 µg/kg/min) it produces a transient tachycardia (β_1), a rise in systolic pressure and a fall in both SVR and diastolic pressure (β_2). At higher doses (0.01–0.4 µg/kg/min) it produces a tachycardia (β_1) and rise in SVR, PVR and MAP (α_1). In patients with impaired right heart function, a rise in PVR coupled with a rise in venous return secondary to venoconstriction may lead to a paradoxical fall in cardiac output.

Metaraminol and phenylephrine
Regarded as 'pure' α_1 agonists, metaraminol (Aramine®) and phenylephrine (Neosynephrin®) are commonly used to treat transient hypotension. Severe reflex bradycardia may accompany the administration of a large dose. Phenylephrine hydrochloride is typically 8–10 times more expensive than metaraminol. Furthermore, it is metabolised by monoamine oxidase (MAO) and should be used with great caution or avoided in patients taking type-A MAO-inhibitor antidepressants.

Ephedrine
Ephedrine is a synthetic sympathomimetic amine chemically related to amphetamine. While it possesses weak direct α and β adrenergic activity, ephedrine's principal mode of action is indirect via the release of presynaptic noradrenaline stores. In addition to vasoconstriction, ephedrine may induce tachycardia and dysrhythmias. Its principal role

appears to be the treatment of acute hypotension during anaesthesia. Because of its use as a recreational drug, ephedrine is regarded as a controlled substance in the USA.

Other vasoconstrictors
Vasopressin
Arginine vasopressin (argipressin; antidiuretic hormone; ADH) is a nonapeptide released from the posterior pituitary gland in response to a variety of stimuli. It acts on at least three receptor types to produce: vasoconstriction, hepatic gluconeogenesis, platelet aggregation (V_{1a}); corticotropin release (V_{1b}); and increased free water reabsorption in the renal collecting ducts (V_2). Vasopressin may be used in the presence of pathological vasodilatation unresponsive to α_1 agonists such as noradrenaline [24]. Its minimal effects on the pulmonary vasculature make vasopressin a useful alternative to α_1 agonists in patients with right ventricular dysfunction or established pulmonary hypertension [25]. Vasopressin is frequently administered as part of hormone replacement therapy in brainstem-dead multi-organ donors.

Vasodilators
Centrally acting agents
Alpha methyldopa
This oral antihypertensive agent is metabolised to α-methylnorepinephrine which acts on central α receptors to induce peripheral vasodilatation. The wide range of side effects (rebound hypertension, haemolytic anaemia, lupus-like syndrome, etc.) and the introduction of newer agents have relegated α-methyldopa to the history books.

Clonidine
Clonidine is a centrally acting α_2 agonist, which induces vasodilatation via a reduction in the sympathetic activation of the adrenal medulla. In common with other drugs in this class (e.g. dexmedetomidine) clonidine produces dose-dependent sedation and reduces the minimal alveolar concentration (MAC or ED_{50}) of anaesthetic agents.

Ganglion blockers
Blockade of postganglionic nicotinic acetylcholine receptors in sympathetic ganglia results in hypotension and a reflex tachycardia. Historically, drugs such as trimetaphan (1–5 mg/min) were used in combination with halothane and D-tubocurarine to induce deliberate hypotension during anaesthesia. The unpredictable nature of ganglion blockers, their direct actions on vascular smooth muscle and associated histamine release make them unsuitable for use in critical care.

Peripherally acting agents
Angiotensin converting enzyme (ACE) inhibitors
The ACE inhibitors (e.g. captopril, enalapril, lisinopril) have become a mainstay of treatment for systemic hypertension and chronic cardiac

failure. Their principal mode of action is prevention of the conversion of angiotensin I to angiotensin II. This typically results in a 20–40% fall in SVR and a rise in cardiac output. Reliance on enteral administration and renin-induced aldosterone release (which may cause deterioration in renal function and hyperkalaemia) limits the usefulness of ACE inhibitors in acute circulatory compromise with worsening renal function.

Peripheral dopamine (D_1) agonists

Fenoldopam (Corlopam®), a benzazepine derivative, is the first selective D_1 agonist that has been approved for clinical use. Although it possesses some α_2 activity, its principal actions include arteriolar vasodilatation and diuresis. It is indicated for the short-term management of severe hypertension. It may cause hypokalaemia and raised intraocular pressure, and at doses > 0.1 µg/kg/min may induce tachycardia.

In critically ill patients with early renal dysfunction, the use of fenoldopam may improve renal function [26]. Fenoldopam has recently been investigated as prophylaxis against contrast-associated nephropathy and renal dysfunction following cardiac surgery [27]. Despite initial promising case studies the first randomised controlled trials failed to demonstrate any advantage for patients treated with fenoldopam for either indication.

Nitric oxide donors

Sodium nitroprusside (SNP): the nitroprusside anion – $[Fe(CN)_5 NO]^{2-}$ – is an iron-nitrosyl complex which produces profound, short-lived dilatation of both resistance and capacitance vessels. This produces a dose-dependent (0.5–5 µg/kg/min) fall in systemic blood pressure and a reflex tachycardia. SNP has no direct chronotropic or inotropic action. Cardiac output is usually unchanged in normal individuals, but typically increases in patients with cardiac failure. Inhibition of hypoxic pulmonary vasoconstriction increases intrapulmonary shunt, leading to a reversible fall in PaO_2. The major disadvantage of SNP is cyanide-induced lactic acidosis, which is more likely in malnourished patients and those with renal and hepatic dysfunction. The likelihood of cyanide intoxication increases with the duration of the infusion, but there have been reports of cyanide poisoning after short periods of infusion.

Glyceryl trinitrate (GTN): as well as being widely used for the treatment of chronic stable angina and acute coronary syndromes, GTN ($CH_2NO_3.CHNO_3.CH_2NO_3$) is frequently used to control blood pressure in the perioperative period. While GTN acts on both resistance and capacitance vessels, venodilatation predominates at low doses (10–200 µg/min) [2]. GTN induces a fall in arterial pressure (systolic > diastolic), CVP, LVEDP and myocardial oxygen consumption. There is often a mild reflex increase in heart rate, and cardiac output typically remains unchanged or decreases slightly. The precise mechanism of action of GTN remains unknown, although denitration (to yield NO) and activation of smooth muscle guanylate cyclase seems likely. In addition to acute side effects such as headache, the major drawback of long-term GTN therapy is tolerance.

Hydralazine

Hydralazine is a hydrazine derivative that acts directly on arteriolar smooth muscle to produce vasodilatation. It is frequently used in the treatment of acute severe hypertension in the settings of pre-eclampsia, acute aortic dissection and acute heart failure. Cardiac output and heart rate (if not already elevated) tend to rise. Stimulation of the renin-aldosterone system leads to fluid retention and peripheral oedema in long-term use. Prolonged use (> 6 months) is associated with an increased likelihood of blood dyscrasias, a lupus-like syndrome and peripheral neuropathy.

Diazoxide

This benzothiadiazine analogue is a directly acting arteriolar vasodilator that may be used to treat hypertensive emergencies (5 mg/kg) and intractable hypoglycaemia. Its mechanisms of action are thought to include inhibition of phosphodiesterase and calcium entry. Inhibition of insulin release leads to elevation of blood glucose. Activation of the renin-aldosterone system leads to fluid retention.

Angiotensin II receptor antagonists (ARA)

These agents are indicated for the treatment of hypertension and cardiac failure. Emerging evidence suggests that ARAs may also delay the progression of nephropathy in diabetic patients. Unlike ACE inhibitors, which inhibit the breakdown of bradykinin and other kinins, the ARAs do not generally cause the persistent dry cough characteristic of ACE inhibitor therapy. The unavailability of parenteral preparations of ARAs restricts their use in the acute setting.

α-Adrenoceptor blockers

An infusion of labetalol (α_1 β_1 β_2; 0.5–2.5 mg/min) or, less frequently, intermittent intravenous doses of phentolamine (α_1 α_2; 25–100 μg) are used to provide acute control of MAP in patients with acute hypertension or acute proximal aortic dissection. Prazosin (α_1) may be a suitable alternative in patients able to take oral medication. The long duration of action of phenoxybenzamine (α_1) makes it unsuitable in unstable patients and those likely to undergo surgery with cardiopulmonary bypass. α_1 antagonists are frequently used to control symptoms and reverse severe vasoconstriction as seen in the presence of a phaeochromocytoma. Their action results in a drop in systemic blood pressure, leading to an increase in circulating blood volume.

β-Adrenoceptor blockers

β-Adrenoceptor blockers possess negative inotropic, chronotropic and dromotropic (β_1) properties as well as causing vasoconstriction and bronchoconstriction (β_2). In contrast to non-selective β-blockers (e.g. propranolol), the so-called cardio-selective β_1-blockers (e.g. atenolol, metoprolol, bisoprolol) are associated with fewer pulmonary and peripheral vascular side effects. Although short-acting β-blockers, such as esmolol (50–200 μg/kg/min) and labetalol (see above) may be used to treat systemic hypertension, they should be used with extreme caution in patients with impaired myocardial function.

In general, β-blockers have no place in the management of acute circulatory failure unless the principal cause is supraventricular tachyarrhythmia or dynamic left ventricular outflow tract obstruction. In chronic, severe cardiac failure, however, the non-specific agent carvedilol, which possesses α_1-antagonist properties, reduces morbidity and mortality [28]. In addition to its action on β-adrenoceptors, sotalol inhibits inward K^+ channels, thereby prolonging repolarisation, lengthening the QT interval and reducing automaticity. In addition it slows conduction through the AV node. This Vaughan-Williams class III action is used to treat both ventricular and atrial tachyarrhythmias.

Pulmonary vasodilators

In patients with pulmonary hypertension (defined as a mean pulmonary artery pressure > 25 mmHg or pulmonary vascular resistance > 2.5 Wood units/200 dynes/s/cm^5) pharmacological pulmonary vasodilatation may improve right ventricular function and, by improving left ventricular filling, increase cardiac output. The resulting redistribution of pulmonary blood flow has the potential to improve or worsen hypoxia.

Pulmonary vasodilators can be classified according to their selectivity, pharmacological class and route(s) of administration. Parenteral administration of GTN, SNP and prostaglandins produces both systemic and pulmonary vasodilatation, and increases intrapulmonary shunt. The administration of a wide range of vasodilators by inhaled aerosol has been shown to be highly effective and largely avoids adverse systemic side effects.

Nitric oxide

Inhaled NO (1–20 ppm) causes selective pulmonary vasodilation, bronchodilatation, inhibition of the function, adhesion and activation of inflammatory cells and platelets, inhibition of cell proliferation, and reduction in intrapulmonary shunt. NO is rapidly deactivated by binding to haemoglobin. Metabolism of NO to nitrogen dioxide (NO_2 – a pulmonary toxin), nitric acid (HNO_3) and nitrous acid (HNO_2) limits the dose of NO that can be safely administered for prolonged periods. NO can only be delivered through a dedicated delivery system and requires endotracheal intubation for reliable application.

Prostacyclins

Prostacyclin or prostaglandin I_2 (PGI_2) is a naturally occurring derivative of ω-6 arachidonic acid produced in endothelial cells by the action of prostacyclin synthetase on PGH_2. When used therapeutically it is referred to as epoprostenol. The short half-life of less than 6 minutes necessitates epoprostenol to be given by continuous infusion. Systemic administration produces marked hypotension and tachycardia, and interferes with coagulation. Synthetic analogues of PGI_2, such as iloprost and cisaprost, are more stable than epoprostenol and have longer half-lives.

Inhaled aerosolised prostacyclin (IAP) was first described in the late 1970s. While clear benefit has been demonstrated in patients with primary pulmonary hypertension, the usefulness of IAP in cardiac failure (measured by mortality) remains unproven. In acute haemodynamic decompensation secondary to pulmonary hypertensive crisis following heart and lung transplantation, IAP may obviate the need for mechanical ventricular assist or extracorporeal oxygenation. Iloprost (Ventavis®) is the only form of inhaled prostacyclin currently licenced for use in Europe and the USA.

Phosphodiesterase (PDE-V) inhibitors

Originally developed for the treatment of erectile dysfunction, the orally active drugs sildenafil (Viagra®, Revatio®), tadalafil (Cialis®) and vardenafil (Levitas®) all act on pulmonary vascular cyclic nucleotide phosphodiesterase type-V (PDE-V) to produce pulmonary vasodilatation. Sildenafil was licenced for use in pulmonary hypertension in 2005.

Endothelin receptor antagonists

Bosentan (Tracleer®) is an orally active, non-peptide, competitive antagonist of endothelin ($ET_A > ET_B$) receptors. It has been successfully used in patients with idiopathic pulmonary hypertension and in patients with pulmonary hypertension associated with congenital heart disease and connective tissue disease. Despite its potential for hepatotoxicity, bosentan has been used and administered continuously for periods exceeding 12 months. Selective ET_A antagonists are currently under development.

6.4 A rational approach to managing haemodynamic impairment?

The purpose of pharmacological haemodynamic intervention is the restoration and maintenance of adequate oxygen delivery to vital organs through the manipulation of circulating volume, cardiac output and perfusion pressure. Several principles are key to this process:

1. Monitoring sufficient to allow accurate assessment and diagnosis, and sufficient to permit an assessment of the response to therapeutic interventions. In the majority of cases this entails advanced cardiovascular monitoring (Table 6.2).
2. A working diagnosis or, at the very least, a differential diagnosis. Treatment of associated or causative conditions (e.g. sepsis) is an essential component of managing acute circulatory failure. When drug therapy produces unexpected results (e.g. when inotropic therapy causes a *fall* in cardiac output and a *rise* in pulmonary artery wedge pressure) an alternative diagnosis should be considered (e.g. left ventricular outflow tract obstruction) as well as additional monitoring, such as echocardiography.
3. Selection of *end-points* at which treatment is deemed to have been successful. These end-points or 'therapeutic goals' will typically

Table 6.2 Advanced haemodynamic monitoring.

Invasive pressure	Systemic arterial
	Central venous
	Pulmonary arterial
Cardiac output	Thermodilution
	Lithium dilution
	Oesophageal Doppler
	Pulse contour analysis
Tissue oxygenation	Mixed venous oxygen saturation
	Intestinal tonometry
Imaging	Echocardiography
Organ function	Urine output
	Arterial blood gases (pH, base deficit)
	Conscious level

incorporate indices of both cardiovascular function (i.e. heart rate, CVP, MAP, PAP, cardiac output) and end organ function (i.e. urine output, metabolic state, conscious level).

4. Empirical approach: adoption of a mind-set that permits the acceptance of defeat. Careful consideration should be given to the withdrawal of any drug therapy that has failed to achieve the desired clinical response either within a predetermined time interval or within a predetermined dose range.

In selecting drugs for therapeutic intervention it is important to bear in mind that:

● Few, if any, drugs are 'clean' – acting solely on heart rate, contractility or vascular tone.
● Cardiovascular function is affected by metabolic derangement (e.g. acidosis, hypokalaemia, hypocalcaemia), posture, mechanical ventilation and interaction between the ventricles.
● Whenever possible, stabilisation of cardiac rhythm, institution of cardiac pacing and optimisation of circulating volume should precede pharmacological cardiovascular support.
● Patients react to drugs in different ways – cell surface receptors and intracellular signal transduction mechanisms are subject to genetic variability.
● Drug potency and efficacy (i.e. the dose-response curve) is frequently altered by disease states (e.g. sepsis, renal impairment and hepatic impairment) and chronic drug therapy (e.g. β_1 antagonists).
● The response to a particular drug may change over time.
● The combination of several agents at low to medium doses may be more beneficial than the use of a single agent in escalating doses.
● Drugs should be selected on the basis of clinical experience rather than putative benefits.
● Effective treatment of the underlying cause of haemodynamic disturbance (e.g. myocardial ischaemia, valvular dysfunction, sepsis) is essential.

Case study 1

Following surgical repair of an incompetent mitral valve, a patient could not be weaned from cardiopulmonary bypass (CPB). Preoperative transthoracic echocardiography had suggested significant pulmonary hypertension, and on this basis an infusion of dopamine (~ 6 µg/kg/min) had been started following removal of the aorta cross-clamp. Following the failed attempt to wean from CPB, calcium chloride (10 mmol slow bolus) and enoximone (0.4 mg/kg bolus, then 5 µg/kg/min) were administered. Noradrenaline (0.075 µg/kg/min) was used to offset the enoximone-induced hypotension and maintain an aortic root pressure > 60 mmHg. Over the course of the next 30 minutes the patient was gradually weaned from CPB. Transoesophageal echocardiography (TOE) was used to monitor ventricular function and the rate of noradrenaline infusion adjusted to maintain a mean arterial pressure (MAP) > 60 mmHg.

Case study 2

During the course of a laparoscopic adrenalectomy for phaechromocytoma, an elderly patient became hypotensive and tachycardic, with elevation of central venous pressure (CVP). Intravenous boluses of phenylephrine (100–200 µg) produced only short-lived improvements in mean arterial pressure (MAP). Dopamine (5 µg/kg/min) was commenced on the basis that the problem was likely to be primary myocardial failure. Within minutes the heart rate had risen from 105 to 130 beats/min without improvement in MAP. At this stage a pulmonary artery flotation catheter was inserted, revealing low cardiac index (1.2 l/min/m^2) and marked elevation of the pulmonary capillary wedge pressure (PCWP; 24 mmHg). Prominent *cv*-waves in the PCWP trace suggested significant mitral valve incompetence. Increasing the rate of dopamine administration to 10 µg/kg/min produced a further increase in heart rate but no improvement in cardiac output. Transoesophageal echocardiography (TOE) revealed gross left ventricular (LV) hypertrophy, virtual obliteration of the LV cavity at end-systole and systolic anterior motion of the anterior mitral leaflet with associated LV outflow tract obstruction (LVOTO; peak gradient ~ 81 mmHg) and severe mitral regurgitation. On the basis of these findings, the dopamine infusion was discontinued; colloid was administered in 100 ml aliquots (whilst monitoring LV end-diastolic area with TOE) and repeated esmolol boluses (10–20 mg) used to control heart rate. Over the course of the next 15 minutes the LVOTO and mitral regurgitation resolved with restoration of cardiac index > 2.0 l/min/m^2.

References

1. Joly HR, Weil MH. Temperature of the great toe as an indication of the severity of shock. *Circulation* 1969;39(1):131–8.
2. White P, Arrowsmith J. Ventricular performance. In: Mackay J, Arrowsmith J (Eds). *Core Topics in Cardiac Anaesthesia*. Cambridge: University Press; 2004. pp. 17–21.
3. Elliott P. Rational use of inotropes. *Anaesth Intensive Care* 2006;7(9):326–30.
4. Feldman AM. Classification of positive inotropic agents. *J Am Coll Cardiol* 1993;22(4):1223–7.
5. Bellomo R, Chapman M, Finfer S, et al. Low-dose dopamine in patients with early renal dysfunction: a placebo-controlled randomised trial. Australian and New Zealand Intensive Care Society (ANZICS) Clinical Trials Group. *Lancet* 2000;356(9248):2139–43.
6. Kellum JA, M Decker J. Use of dopamine in acute renal failure: a meta-analysis. *Crit Care Med* 2001;29(8):1526–31.
7. Sasada M, Smith S. *Drugs in Anaesthesia & Intensive Care*. Oxford: University Press; 1997.
8. Shoemaker WC, Appel PL, Kram HB, et al. Prospective trial of supranormal values of survivors as therapeutic goals in high-risk surgical patients. *Chest* 1988;94(6):1176–86.
9. El Mokhtari N, Arlt A, Meissner A, et al. Inotropic therapy for cardiac low output syndrome: comparison of hemodynamic effects of dopamine/dobutamine versus dopamine/dopexamine. *Eur J Med Res* 2007;12(11):563–7.
10. Meier-Hellmann A, Bredle D, Specht M, Hannemann L, et al. Dopexamine increases splanchnic blood flow but decreases gastric mucosal pH in severe septic patients treated with dobutamine. *Crit Care Med* 1999;27(10): 2166–71.
11. Smithies M, Yee T, Jackson L, et al. Protecting the gut and the liver in the critically ill: effects of dopexamine. *Crit Care Med* 1994;22(5): 789–95.
12. Lisbon A. Dopexamine, dobutamine, and dopamine increase splanchnic blood flow: what is the evidence? *Chest* 2003;123(5 Suppl):460S–3S.
13. Zausig Y, Stowe D, Zink W, et al. A comparison of three phosphodiesterase type III inhibitors on mechanical and metabolic function in guinea pig isolated hearts. *Anesth Analg* 2006;102(6):1646–52.
14. Patel M, Katz S. Phosphodiesterase 5 inhibition in chronic heart failure and pulmonary hypertension. *Am J Cardiol* 2005;96(12B):47M–51M.
15. Rathmell J, Prielipp R, Butterworth J, et al. A multicenter, randomized, blind comparison of amrinone with milrinone after elective cardiac surgery. *Anesth Analg* 1998;86(4):683–90.
16. White H. Heart failure: to digitalise or not? The view against. *Aust N Z J Med* 1992;22(5 Suppl):626–30.
17. Belz G, Breithaupt-Grögler K, Osowsk U. Treatment of congestive heart failure – current status of use of digitoxin. *Eur J Clin Invest* 2001;31(Suppl 2):10–7.
18. Dec G. Digoxin remains useful in the management of chronic heart failure. *Med Clin North Am* 2003;87(2):317–37.
19. Follath F, Cleland J, Just H, et al. Efficacy and safety of intravenous levosimendan compared with dobutamine in severe low-output heart failure (the LIDO study): a randomised double-blind trial. *Lancet* 2002;360(9328):196–202.

20. Moiseyev V, Põder P, Andrejevs N, et al. Safety and efficacy of a novel calcium sensitizer, levosimendan, in patients with left ventricular failure due to an acute myocardial infarction. A randomized, placebo-controlled, double-blind study (RUSSLAN). *Eur Heart J* 2002;23(18):1422–32.

21. Lehtonen L, Põder P. The utility of levosimendan in the treatment of heart failure. *Ann Med* 2007;39(1):2–17.

22. Broomhead C, Wright S, Colvin M. The inotropic action of glucose-insulin-potassium infusions. In: Arrowsmith J, Simpson J (Eds). *Problems in Anesthesia: Cardiothoracic Surgery.* London: Martin Dunitz; 2002. pp 127–32.

23. White C. A review of potential cardiovascular uses of intravenous glucagon administration. *J Clin Pharmacol* 1999;39(5):442–7.

24. Russell J. Vasopressin in septic shock. *Crit Care Med* 2007;35(9 Suppl):S609–15.

25. Jeon Y, Ryu J, Lim Y, et al. Comparative hemodynamic effects of vasopressin and norepinephrine after milrinone-induced hypotension in off-pump coronary artery bypass surgical patients. *Eur J Cardiothorac Surg* 2006;29(6): 952–6.

26. Brienza N, Malcangi V, Dalfino L, et al. A comparison between fenoldopam and low-dose dopamine in early renal dysfunction of critically ill patients. *Crit Care Med* 2006;34(3):707–14.

27. Garwood S, Swamidoss C, Davis E, et al. A case series of low-dose fenoldopam in seventy cardiac surgical patients at increased risk of renal dysfunction. *J Cardiothorac Vasc Anesth* 2003;17(1):17–21.

28. Krum H, Roecker E, Mohacsi P, et al. Effects of initiating carvedilol in patients with severe chronic heart failure: results from the COPERNICUS Study. *JAMA* 2003;289(6):712–8.

7 Arrhythmias

Hugh Montgomery[1] and Vivek Sivaraman[2]

[1]Institute for Human Health and Performance, University College London, London, UK
[2]Anaesthetics and Critical Care, Central London School of Anaesthesia, London, UK

Take Home Messages

Epidemiology
- Arrhythmias in critically ill patients occur most frequently after cardiac or thoracic surgery.
- Atrial fibrillation is the commonest arrhythmia.
- The onset of arrhythmias in critically ill patients adversely affects morbidity and mortality.
- A variety of non-modifiable and potentially modifiable factors are associated with arrhythmias, but evidence of causation is generally weak.

Treatment
- In all cases treat the underlying cause.
- Pharmacological treatment may be avoided if the patient is not suffering haemodynamic compromise. If drug use is unavoidable, use familiar drugs and avoid polypharmacy.
- Amiodarone is associated with acute lung injury in the critically ill and its incidence appears to be higher in post-operative cardiothoracic patients.

7.1 Introduction

Arrhythmias commonly complicate critical illness, occurring most frequently in the intensive care unit (ICU) after cardiothoracic surgery. The commonest documented arrhythmia in this setting is atrial fibrillation. However, the nature and duration of arrhythmias vary greatly: indeed, the full spectrum of abnormal rhythm and conduction is seen, from simple ectopic beats to intractable and terminal ventricular fibrillation. Whilst the clinical gravity of pulseless rhythms is self-evident, the significance of rhythms that would elsewhere be considered more benign is less clear – as is the need (and urgency) for treatment. Confusion also surrounds the causal

Cardiovascular Critical Care. Edited by M. Griffiths, J. Cordingley and S. Price.
© 2010 Blackwell Publishing Ltd.

and potentially remediable factors that drive arrhythmia pathogenesis in intensive care. Indeed, association has often been taken to infer causation, whilst scrutiny of the available literature reveals a paucity of evidence supporting the latter. Indeed, many of our established 'therapeutic responses' are underpinned by a poor evidence base. Such issues are of substantial clinical relevance: arrhythmias can be associated with high morbidity and mortality, but so, too, is inappropriate pharmacotherapy. Analysis of the risk:benefit ratio of such therapy is also confounded by the fact that anti-arrhythmic agents have generally not been trialled extensively in the critically ill, amongst whom pharmacokinetics, pharmacodynamics and tissue end-effector mechanisms (such as receptor populations) may be far from normal.

This chapter reviews the nature and prevalence of the common ICU arrhythmias, and discusses those factors associated with their presence. It also critically appraises evidence of causation, where this exists.

7.2 Incidence of arrhythmias

Atrial arrhythmias

Atrial dysrhythmias are common amongst the critically ill, occurring in around 11% of patients (Table 7.1). The incidence is similar for mixed non-cardiothoracic post-operative surgical patients admitted to ICU (10.2%), with approximately two thirds of these developing atrial fibrillation (AF) and one third paroxysmal supraventricular tachycardia (PSVT) [1]. Comparison across studies should be done with caution, as patient populations, location, case identification/diagnostic criteria vary substantially between studies, and different arrhythmias are often grouped and reported together. Nonetheless, the available data suggest that 4–5% of intensive care patients will develop an episode of AF.

When compared with other cardiac surgical cases, however, the incidence of AF after coronary artery bypass surgery is significantly higher [2], literature review suggesting that perhaps one in three of such individuals suffers an episode of AF. Similarly, after thoracic surgery, the incidence of arrhythmias is higher than that seen amongst general surgical patients, but lower than that following cardiac surgery. Most of these arrhythmias are also supraventricular in origin (Figures 7.1A and B).

Incidence of ventricular arrhythmias

Atrial arrhythmias are the most common abnormal rhythms in general surgical ICU, and ventricular arrhythmias occur rarely [2]. Ventricular arrhythmias seen more frequently in mixed ICUs, the commonest being monomorphic ventricular tachycardia (VT), occurring in up to 41% of patients [3]. This may relate to the relatively high proportion of medical patients with primary cardiac pathology (including myocardial infarction, heart failure, myocarditis or cardiogenic shock). Indeed, it would seem that ventricular arrhythmias in critically ill patients occur mainly in the setting of ischaemic heart disease or poor ventricular function.

Table 7.1 Incidence of arrhythmias in intensive care units.

Author	Sample size	Rhythm	Site	Definition of arrhythmia	Incidence
Reinelt [3]	756	Atrial fibrillation	ICU	Sustained clinically significant arrhythmias. Sustained if > 30 s, clinically significant if sustained and/or intervention/termination was required	8.3%
		Ventricular tachycardia			7.1%
Seguin [74]	460	Atrial fibrillation	ICU	Ventricular response rate of < 110/min or < 110/min with irregular R-R interval confirmed on ECG	5.3%
Christians [75]	13,780	Atrial fibrillation	ICU + Ward	ICD-9 coding used to retrospectively identify patients, with subsequent review of notes	0.37%
Batra [76]	226	Supraventricular and ventricular arrhythmias	HDU	On ECG monitoring	13%
Bender [77]	206	Supraventricular tachycardias	ICU	NA	13.6%
Kahn [78]	583	Atrial arrhythmias	Ward	Obtained on a 12-lead ECG	4.8%
Goldman [79]	916	Supraventricular tachyarrhythmia	ICU + Ward	NA	4%

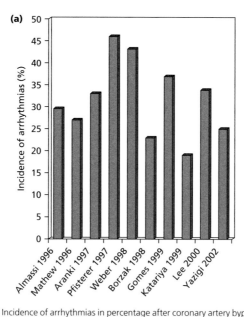

Figure 7.1a Incidence of arrhythmias in percentage after coronary artery bypass surgery [4–6, 10, 64–69].

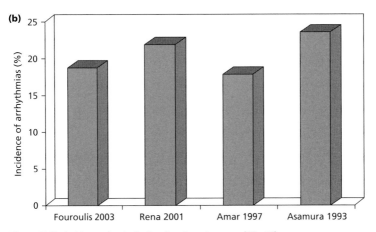

(b)

Figure 7.1b Incidence of arrhythmias after thoracic surgery [70 – 73].

7.3 Arrhythmias and morbidity

Atrial arrhythmias

New-onset post-operative atrial arrhythmia is associated with substantially increased mortality (23% vs. 4% for sufferers vs. non-sufferers), ICU stay (8.5 vs. 2 days) and hospital length of stay (23.3 vs. 13.3 days) after general surgery [1]. Similar associations are seen after cardiothoracic surgery, where post-operative AF is associated with increased rates of ICU readmission, myocardial infarction, congestive cardiac failure, re-intubation and stroke, as well as a higher mortality 6 months after surgery (4.16% vs. 9.36%) [4]. However, such association does not prove causation. Indeed, the cause of death in the majority of patients with new onset atrial fibrillation is non-cardiac. In fact, sepsis is the most common cause of death [1, 4–6], and development of the systemic inflammatory response syndrome (SIRS) increases arrhythmic risk 36-fold [2], possibly as a result of associated myocardial dysfunction [7, 8]. Interestingly, the 174G/C interleukin-6 genetic polymorphism that modulates interleukin-6 levels is also associated with the development of post-operative atrial fibrillation in patients [9].

Thus, AF-impaired cardiac function might impair gut perfusion, promoting endotoxaemia and thus sepsis/SIRS-related morbidity. Alternatively, sepsis and systemic inflammation may drive post-operative morbidity, with AF merely representing a 'bystander' effect. It might also exhibit confounding association with other non-modifiable risk factors for poor outcome, including possibly increasing age, male gender, pre-existing hypertension and African-American race [5, 10 –13]. Further, a variety of potentially modifiable factors including central venous pressure, serum potassium and magnesium concentrations, arterial oxygen and carbon dioxide tensions, and concurrent drug administration may also be associated with development of AF, and may also independently influence outcome.

Despite the potential for such confounding associations, however, AF may yet carry an independent burden of morbidity: multivariate logistic regression analysis ascribes nearly three full days of excess hospital stay to episodes of AF after coronary grafting [4]. Perhaps more compellingly, a recent Cochrane systematic review found evidence of benefit for pharmacoprophylaxis of post cardiac-surgical AF, with therapy being associated with a reduced hospital length of stay for three different classes of agent [5]. A similar systematic review also suggested that post-operative magnesium supplementation might also reduce both AF risk and morbidity and mortality [6].

Ventricular arrhythmias

Ventricular arrhythmias commonly complicate primary cardiac disease which can itself precipitate intensive care admission, including ischaemic heart disease, myocarditis, congestive cardiac failure and cardiogenic shock. Whilst data relating specifically to the critical care environment are sparse, survival rates following in-hospital VT/VF cardiac arrest are much better than non-VF/VT arrests [14]. Amongst elderly patients, length of intensive care and hospital stay are associated with the nature of the underlying arrhythmia. Hospital stay following ventricular fibrillation was 7.8 days (2.7 days in intensive care) and 7 days (1.7 days in intensive care) after ventricular tachycardia, but only 4.7 days in atrial fibrillation (0.9 ITU days), 4.5 days in atrial flutter (1 ITU day) and 5.6 days in complete heart block (1.5 ITU days). However, such data cannot confirm that the arrhythmia caused the longer stay rather than the underlying disease state which precipitated the arrhythmia.

7.4 Modifiable risk factors for arrhythmia

Substantial efforts are devoted to the prevention and treatment of peri-operative atrial fibrillation. However, data supporting the efficacy of such interventions (whether prophylactic or therapeutic) are sparse, and many interventions are themselves not without risk.

Central venous cannulae

Whilst the position of the central venous catheter (CVC) tip is anecdotally reported to be associated with an increased risk of AF, the only published supporting data relate to pulmonary artery (rather than central venous) catheter use [15–17]. Nonetheless, many clinicians will consider adjusting CVC position if episodes of AF are recurrent. In addition, many modulate central venous pressure (CVP) in an effort to treat AF. In support, experiments in both animal models and humans demonstrate a direct relationship between right atrial pressure, sympathetic activity and cycle length in atrial arrhythmias. A decrease in right atrial pressure causes an increase in sympathetic activity and a cycle-length prolongation in human atrial flutter [18], whilst higher sympathetic activity is itself associated with the onset of tachyarrhythmia [19]. More directly, the occurrence of AF is associated with a higher antecedent CVP, suggesting that volume overload post operatively could instigate the onset of an arrhythmia. Indeed, the relative risk of AF attributable to a rise in CVP of 1 mmHg has been suggested to be 1.26 [2, 12]. However, it is possible that factors associated with a higher CVP (e.g. lower cardiac or central venous compliance, or higher volume loading) may independently have caused the excess AF risk.

Arterial oxygen and carbon dioxide tensions

Arterial hypoxaemia or hypercarbia have traditionally been associated with AF, but evidence supporting causation is generally lacking. Although it is well established that progressive hypoxia may be causally associated with a rise in heart rate, the effects of hypercapnia are more unpredictable, being associated with either a rise or a fall in the heart rate [20]. Hypoxia in patients with chronic lung disease causes a higher QTc dispersion on the electrocardiogram, which is significantly reduced with even a partial correction of hypoxia with oxygen therapy [21]. Hypercapnic patients with chronic obstructive pulmonary disease (COPD) have a higher incidence of arrhythmias [22, 23] and, postoperatively, these are associated with significant morbidity and mortality [2, 24]. However, proof of causality is lacking, and a variety of confounding factors (such as beta-agonist use, cor pulmonale, smoking-related vascular disease and changes in pH) have been implicated.

Magnesium

Magnesium is frequently used for the prophylaxis and treatment of AF. However, whilst ICU mortality is inversely associated with serum magnesium, such data derive from small studies [25] and do not demonstrate causality. Furthermore, hypomagnesaemia is often associated with hypocalcaemia or hypokalaemia, through which any associations may, in reality, be mediated. Thus Passakiotou's study of 95 patients showed hypomagnesaemia at the time of ICU admission to be associated with greater ICU length of stay and poorer outcome, but this was unaffected by magnesium supplementation [26]. Further better-powered studies are required.

Cardiopulmonary bypass is thought to be associated with depletion of electrolytes including magnesium, and this is offered as one possible explanation for the increased risk of arrhythmias in these patients [27]. Anecdotal reports suggest the widespread use of intravenous magnesium in both the prevention and treatment of post-cardiac surgical AF. However, of the large number of reported trials, many were underpowered or poorly designed, and the benefits of routine use of magnesium in either context remains unproven [28–34]. A systematic review suggests that routine magnesium supplementation after CABG surgery reduces the incidence of post-operative atrial fibrillation with an attendant reduction in morbidity and mortality [35]. However, there is no evidence to support the routine use of magnesium after off-pump coronary artery surgery [36].

The use of magnesium in patients with ST elevation myocardial infarction (STEMI) has been examined in two large randomised control trials [37, 38]. Given the lack of conclusive proof of benefit, and the potential for significant hypotension (an increase in incidence of hypotension of 11 per 1000 was noted in the ISIS-4 study, considered severe enough to terminate the trial [37]), the American Association of Chest Physicians (Box 7.1) still recommends against the routine use of magnesium in the prevention of atrial fibrillation and flutter.

> **Box 7.1 Causes of atrial fibrillation /flutter.**
>
> AV valve disease
> Restictive cardiomyopathy
> Pulmonary embolism
> Congestive heart failure
> Atrial septal defects
> Myocardial infarction/ischaemia
> Sino atrial disease
> Wolff–Parkinson–White (WPW) syndrome
> Infiltrative tumours
> Constrictive pericarditis
> Myopericarditis
> Cardiac and thoracic surgery
> Pneumonia
> Thyrotoxicosis
> Alcohol
> Idiopathic – lone atrial fibrillation

Potassium

Potassium is an intracellular ion that increases trans-membrane resting potential, hastens depolarisation, delays repolarisation (and lengthens QT interval) and increases cell excitability. Profound hypokalaemia is thus associated with (potentially fatal) ventricular tachyarrhythmias, and with atrial ectopic activity/tachyarrhythmia. The rationale for a causal association of more modest hypokalaemia is thus strong. Further, hypokalaemia increases the risk of drug-induced torsades, which is benefited by potassium replacement. In the general intensive care setting, however, there is only one report that falling serum potassium levels correlate with a higher incidence of ventricular tachycardia [39].

In the context of myocardial infarction (MI), the ischaemic myocardium is thought to extrude potassium, increasing the risk of developing arrhythmias. Furthermore, the catecholamine response to MI causes a redistribution of potassium to the intracellular compartment, resulting in hypokalaemia and thus an excitable myocardium [40]. In the case of MI, therefore, ventricular fibrillation /tachycardia are strongly associated with lower potassium levels [41–45], and maintaining serum K^+ above 4.6 mmol/l is an effective prophylactic measure, even abolishing VF risk in one study. Similarly in heart failure, hypokalaemia is an independent predictor of mortality [46], and victims of sudden cardiac death generally have lower myocardial potassium than controls [47]. The relation of hypokalaemia to ventricular arrhythmias in the ICU setting for such patients is, however, unclear.

Before cardiac surgery, serum potassium levels of < 3.5 mmol/l predict not only post-operative atrial fibrillation /flutter (OR 1.7) but also serious peri-operative and intra-operative arrhythmias such as ventricular tachycardia or those leading to the need for cardiopulmonary resuscitation [39, 48]. However, one study reported the incidence of post-operative AF to have fallen from 21% to 11% between 1990 and 1993 – a time-frame during which the use of potassium chloride supplements increased from 0 to 96%, and the use of intravenous frusemide decreased from 12 to 3% [49]. Other studies, however, have failed to demonstrate a correlation between hypokalaemia and tachyarrhythmia after cardiac surgery [2]. Thus, the case for potassium supplementation for prophylaxis or treatment of AF after cardiac surgery remains unproven. A randomised control trial of targeted potassium replacement with monitoring of potassium levels is thus needed to elucidate the role of potassium in patients undergoing cardiac surgery. Meanwhile, avoidance of levels < 3.5 mmol/l seems sensible on the grounds of avoiding potentially fatal ventricular arrhythmias.

7.5 Management of arrhythmias

General principles

There are some general rules that can be followed in managing arrhythmias in critically ill patients:

Principle	Notes
In all cases treat the underlying cause	See Box 7.1
Treatment may be avoided if the patient is not suffering haemodynamic compromise, or if this is not incipient	High-risk patients with congenital heart disease should be regarded differently (Chapter 10)
Reduce an unnecessarily high CVP to reduce risk of (recurrent) atrial fibrillation	Conclusive proof of benefit is lacking
Correct hypokalaemia	Particularly in ischaemic heart disease
Correct hypomagnesaemia	Note recommendations [50] in atrial arrhythmias
Avoid hypoxia/hypercapnia	May not be possible in certain cardiothoracic patients
Ensure central venous access is correctly positioned	Avoid Swan–Ganz catheters if possible
If ischaemic, consider revascularisation	Additional measures: IABP, beta blockade
DC cardioversion/pacing is generally safer than pharmacotherapy	Patients with congenital heart disease should be regarded differently (Chapter 10)
Use familiar drugs where possible	
Avoid polypharmacy	All anti-arrhythmic drugs have pro-arrhythmic potential

Atrial fibrillation – rhythm or rate control?

The management of atrial fibrillation (outside the context of critical care) has been specifically examined in two complete trials – AFFIRM and PIAF [51, 52] – and are summarised in a Cochrane review [53]. It is concluded that rhythm control was in no way superior to rate control but was, in fact, associated with a higher risk of adverse complications and increased hospitalisation. However, the recommendations for non-critically ill patients may not be relevant to the ICU setting. Specifically, in cardiac surgical patients, there may be a higher rate of conversion to sinus rhythm a few days after starting treatment with an anti-arrhythmic agent. This might, in part, be driven by the heightened adrenergic state in the post-operative period. However, if atrial fibrillation is recurrent and/or persistent, then rate-control may be the only alternative.

In general, digoxin offers poor rate control, in the context of heightened adrenergic states such as occur in ICU, and it has no role in preventing episodes of paroxysmal atrial fibrillation (PAF). The necessity to measure digoxin levels, their vulnerability to changes in (for instance) renal function, the amplification of toxicity by changes in potassium, and the associated dangers of administering other agents such as calcium further complicate its use. Beta-blockade is generally more effective at rate control (and at preventing PAF), but may be inappropriate in many patients, such as those with asthma, or who are requiring administration of beta-1 adrenoceptor agonists such as adrenaline. Diltiazem may reduce ventricular rate in AF. Meanwhile, amiodarone is effective at PAF prevention and also at rate control. Extensive experience, anecdotally reported, suggests that the use of such agents is relatively safe. It must be emphasised once again, however, that there have been no formal trials of anti-arrhythmics in general ICU patients, and that all drugs must be used with caution. This applies especially to other classes of agent (and especially to other class I agents, such as flecainide). If rate control is sought, and atrial fibrillation is likely to be longstanding, then consideration must be given to the risk of left atrial thrombus formation and thus to thrombo-embolic prophylaxis.

Guidelines for anticoagulation in sustained atrial fibrillation have been drawn up by, amongst others, the National Institute for Clinical Excellence [54]. However, these are not generally applicable to the ICU environment, for a number of reasons. First, many ICU patients experience a degree of auto-anticoagulation, whilst others are anticoagulated for other reasons (such as haemofiltration). Second, the risk of unexpected spontaneous hemorrhage (for instance, from the GI tract) is greater that that in the general population. Third, the use of aspirin in ICU is associated, in some, with an increased risk of gastric ulceration. Meanwhile, there is the ever-present likelihood that ongoing vascular (placement of arterial and central venous catheters) or surgical interventions will be required, often rendering the use of long-acting anticoagulant agents inappropriate. Finally, the instability of factors affecting warfarin action (vitamin K absorption, albumin levels, antibiotic use) make warfarin use more awkward to manage. Thus, thromboembolic risk must be assessed. This is perhaps best judged in ICU based on left atrial size, presence of mitral valve disease (and especially mitral stenosis) and impaired left ventricular function. This must then be weighed against the actuarial risk of a thromboembolic event during the timescale of ICU admission. In non-ICU populations, those suffering sustained non-rheumatic AF have a 5% chance of a systemic embolus [55], making the risk over a short ICU admission comparatively low. However, growing evidence supports the use of thromboprophlaxis where AF after cardiothoracic surgery persists for > 2 days [56].

Electrical or chemical cardioversion is warranted if AF causes clinically relevant haemodynamic compromise. Thromboembolic risk associated with cardioversion is low when AF has been present for < 2 days. If sustained for a longer period, then transoesophageal echocardiography is generally suggested, with 3 weeks of formal anticoagulation instigated prior to cardioversion if left atrial thrombus is detected [54]. However, in critical care, 'elective' cardioversion of this nature is rarely warranted, and where haemodynamic compromise is present, concerns over the need for transoesophageal echocardiography to exclude left atrial thrombus, or the need for anticoagulation, are here balanced against the need for urgent action. In life-threatening cases, external electrical cardioversion should be performed. Chemical cardioversion may be preferred: intravenous amiodarone (300 mg bolus or 5 mg/kg over 3–5 minutes through a central venous catheter) offers rapid rate-control and high likelihood of cardioversion [54, 57]. After cardiac surgery, atrial overdrive pacing may be possible using atrial wires, if present. However, UK 'NICE' guidelines recommend that (a) rhythm control should be the primary intervention for AF after cardiac surgery, and (b) AF after any other surgery should be managed as for any new-onset AF [54].

In all cases, the presence of recurrent or unresponsive AF should warrant a more detailed search for underlying drivers. Thereafter, polypharmacy should be avoided, and expert help sought (for instance, guidance as to a role for single or biatrial pacing, or electrophysiological intervention).

Pharmacotherapy/pharmacoprophylaxis for cardiac surgery

Whilst there have been few trials of pharmacotherapy for dysrhythmias in general intensive care, many studies have examined drug prophylaxis before, during and after cardiac surgery. Most have addressed the role of amiodarone, cardio-selective beta adrenoceptor antagonists, or sotalol. A Cochrane systematic review (2004) supported use of all three drugs [58]. However, whilst intervention benefited length of stay, the trend for benefit in terms of cost of hospitalisation did not reach statistical significance. In the light of such data, the American Association of Chest Physicians issued guidelines in 2006 for the prevention and management of atrial fibrillation after cardiac surgery (Box 7.2) [50]. These are similar to those issued by the

> **Box 7.2 Summary of recommendations by the American College of Chest Physicians for the post-operative prophylaxis of atrial fibrillation [50].**
>
> 1. In patients in whom prophylaxis against post-cardiac surgery AF is indicated, including those patients receiving long-term therapy with beta-blockers prior to surgery for whom therapy should be reinstated, the use of Vaughan-Williams class II beta-blockers is recommended (strength of recommendation, A; evidence grade, fair; net benefit, substantial).
> 2. Sotalol (Vaughan-Williams class III agent) therapy may be considered for postoperative AF prophylaxis, but is associated with increased toxicity (strength of recommendation, B; evidence grade, good; net benefit, intermediate).
> 3. In individual patients for whom therapy with class II beta-blockers is contraindicated, therapy with amiodarone should be considered (strength of recommendation, B; evidence grade, good; net benefit, intermediate).
> 4. To prevent AF/flutter in patients following cardiac surgery, we recommend against the use of calcium channel antagonists (i.e. verapamil and diltiazem) (strength of recommendation, D; evidence grade, low; net benefit, none).
> 5. For the prevention of AF/flutter in patients following cardiac surgery, we recommend against routine treatment with magnesium (strength of recommendation, D; evidence grade, low; net benefit, none).
> 6. For reducing the incidence of post surgical AF, we do not recommend digitalis for use as monotherapy (strength of recommendation, I; evidence grade, low; net benefit, none).

National Institute for Clinical Excellence in the UK, which supports the continuation of beta-blockade or amiodarone therapy, or initiation of either in the perioperative period as a matter of routine [54].

Amiodarone

Amiodarone has a wide spectrum of action, including inhibition of potassium and calcium channels, and blockade of both α and β adrenergic receptors. It carries a low proarrhythmic risk, and can therefore be used with caution in patients with structural heart disease (Chapter 17). Almost all tachyarrhythmias, whether atrial or ventricular in origin, respond to amiodarone, whatever the context (from ischaemia to heart failure to post-resuscitation scenarios) [59]. The clear exception is ventricular torsade, in which underlying QT prolongation may be worsened by amiodarone therapy.

There have been several reports and small studies of amiodarone causing acute pulmonary toxicity or a picture similar to Acute Respiratory Distress

Syndrome (ARDS), especially when given to postoperative cardiothoracic patients in ICU. A retrospective study of patients receiving amiodarone treatment after cardiac surgery [60] demonstrated a 50% prevalence of ARDS amongst surgical survivors. None of the patients who had received no amiodarone fulfilled the ARDS criteria. A later prospective trial of amiodarone in the prophylaxis of supraventricular tachycardias in patients undergoing lung surgery demonstrated that the incidence of ARDS in the amiodarone group was 11% and in the untreated group was 1.8%. This further strengthened the notion that amiodarone was a critical factor in the development of ARDS after lung surgery [61].

The mechanism of such pulmonary toxicity remains unclear. However, amiodarone and its metabolite, desethylamiodrone (DEA), accumulate in the pulmonary parenchyma at levels that exceed that of the heart [62]. It has been suggested that such loading increases lung oxidative stress, and that this contributes to the pathogenesis of ARDS [63]. The use of high partial pressures of inhaled oxygen are thus implicated in ARDS causation in such patients.

Beta receptor antagonists

Multiple trials have addressed the use of beta blockers (class II anti-arrhythmic agents) to prevent atrial fibrillation after cardiac surgery, with the drugs being administered at various times in the peri-operative period [50]. It is proposed that beta blockade counters the heightened adrenergic state associated with cardiothoracic surgery, thus reducing the incidence of arrhythmias. A Cochrane meta-analysis suggests that prophylaxis with beta blockers reduces the incidence of atrial fibrillation following cardiac surgery, although many of the studies supporting their use excluded the elderly, or patients with congestive cardiac failure, pulmonary disease or diabetes [58].

In addition to its beta-blocking properties, sotalol blocks potassium channels (class III anti-arrhythmic agent). Although there is some evidence supporting its use in the postoperative period [58], the major limitation relates to its propensity to prolong the QT interval – and its use should be avoided in those with the long QT syndrome. The American Association of Chest Physicians thus recommends the use of beta blockers over sotalol.

7.6 Conclusion

Atrial tachyarrhythmias (especially AF) are common in intensive care, especially after cardiac surgery, and are associated with excess hospital morbidity, length of stay and mortality. Such an association may be causal and, if so, the costs attributable to AF episodes may be very substantial: the adjusted length of hospital stay attributable to AF has been estimated as 4.9 days, corresponding to > $10,055 in hospital charges per patient [5].

A host of associated – and possibly causal – factors have been identified. However, there has yet to be an appropriately powered large-scale randomised controlled trial for interventions addressing these factors, including the use of magnesium, potassium, adjustment in CVP or arterial blood gas tensions, or even the use of many drugs. Large-scale trials are needed. In the meantime, substantial efforts continue to be made to prevent or treat such episodes using a range of interventions, generally based on data from retrospective association studies, with causality merely inferred.

Case study

A 74-year-old male has severe smoking-related lung disease, with an exercise tolerance measured in yards. He has a past history of anterior myocardial infarction, and his notes document 'left ventricular ejection fraction 28%'. He has had a gastric ulcer treated in the past. Until recently, he drank 60–70 units of alcohol each week. He has suffered 3 months of progressive anorexia, abdominal bloating, diarrhoea and fatigue. When seen in clinic, he is cachexic and frail, with a serum albumin concentration of 18 g/l. He has clinical large bowel obstruction.

After 3 days of intravenous fluids and nasogastric drainage, an anterior resection for colonic villous adenocarcinoma was performed under epidural anaesthesia, after which he was admitted to the intensive care unit. Twelve hours later he developed new onset atrial fibrillation at a rate of 163 bpm which persisted beyond 30 minutes. His blood pressure is sustained.

Action: This man is unlikely to tolerate fast atrial fibrillation for long: rates of > 150 bpm (especially in the elderly) confer risk of haemodynamic compromise. All underlying predisposing factors should be treated at once. His total body potassium is likely to be low as he has had diarrhoea from a villous adenocarcinoma and poor nutrition for months. Diarrhoea and alcohol use are both associated with hypomagnesemia. He may still be intravascularly volume deplete, his colloid osmotic pressure being low due to a low albumin concentration. He should be given potassium to raise his serum K^+ to > 4.5 mmol/l, and 20–40 mmol magnesium chloride over 30 minutes. He should receive cautious colloid challenges against his CVP. Attention should be made to his oxygenation.

His ventricular rate fell to 128 bpm; however, ST segment depression was noted across the anterior leads.

Action: Urgent treatment is now required. The choice lies between rate control and cardioversion. With regards to the latter, electrical cardioversion is to be avoided because tracheal intubation and muscle relaxation would here be hazardous, given his parlous pulmonary state. He was thus given amiodarone 300 mg over 5 minutes through his central venous catheter, and sinus rhythm was restored.

Continued

Two hours later, AF returned (118 bpm), again with associated ST segment depression.

Action: The same management plan should be followed. Another dose of amiodarone was given.

On this occasion, the ventricular rate fell to 98 bpm and ST segment changes resolved. However, AF was sustained despite an infusion of 900 mg over the next 24 hours. Amiodarone therapy continued for 3 days without converting AF to sinus rhythm.

Action: Urgent action is not warranted. Attention should be paid to possible drivers which are sustaining the AF. Are the electrolyte concentrations and fluid balance normal?

In fact, this patient had received a furosemide infusion for severe oedema, and his arterial catheter has been removed.

The serum K^+ on a venous sample fell to 3.4 mmol/l. This was corrected, but AF continued. Electrical cardioversion is best avoided for reasons given above, and chemical cardioversion failed. Rate control was achieved, but this patient is at high risk of thromboembolism (sustained AF for > 48 hours, very poor left ventricular function).

Action: The patient would seem to need anticoagulation. However, consideration must be given to timing. Nothing can be done while his epidural catheter remains *in situ*. Once removed, is he likely to go back to theatre? Consideration must also be given to the choice of anticoagulant. He now has an albumin of 11 g/l, and enteral feeding is not fully established. Vitamin K levels may be low, and establishing warfarinisation is going to be very hard, and risk of mechanical fall not inconsiderable. Aspirin would seem a risk, given the past gastric ulcer and poor enteral nutrition. Subcutaneous unfractionated heparin might be considered, but his massive subcutaneous oedema makes assessment of his true underlying lean weight unreliable, and absorption similarly so. He is started on an infusion of unfractionated heparin, sustained until discharge to the ward.

References

1. Brathwaite D, Weissman C. The new onset of atrial arrhythmias following major noncardiothoracic surgery is associated with increased mortality. *Chest* 1998;114(2):462–8.
2. Knotzer H, Mayr A, Ulmer H, et al. Tachyarrhythmias in a surgical intensive care unit: a case-controlled epidemiologic study. *Intensive Care Med* 2000;26(7):908–14.
3. Reinelt P, Karth GD, Geppert A, et al. Incidence and type of cardiac arrhythmias in critically ill patients: a single center experience in a medical-cardiological ICU. *Intensive Care Med* 2001;27(9):1466–73.
4. Almassi GH, Schowalter T, Nicolosi AC, et al. Atrial fibrillation after cardiac surgery: a major morbid event? *Ann Surg* 1997;226(4):501–11; discussion 11–13.

5. Aranki SF, Shaw DP, Adams DH, et al. Predictors of atrial fibrillation after coronary artery surgery. Current trends and impact on hospital resources. *Circulation* 1996;94(3):390–7.

6. Mathew JP, Parks R, Savino JS, et al. Atrial fibrillation following coronary artery bypass graft surgery: predictors, outcomes, and resource utilization. MultiCenter Study of Perioperative Ischemia Research Group. *JAMA* 1996;276(4):300–6.

7. Jardin F, Brun-Ney D, Auvert B, et al. Sepsis-related cardiogenic shock. *Crit Care Med* 1990;8(10):1055–60.

8. Schremmer B, Dhainaut JF. Heart failure in septic shock: effects of inotropic support. *Crit Care Med* 1990;18(1 Pt 2):S49–55.

9. Gaudino M, Andreotti F, Zamparelli R, et al. The –174G/C interleukin-6 polymorphism influences postoperative interleukin-6 levels and postoperative atrial fibrillation. Is atrial fibrillation an inflammatory complication? *Circulation* 2003;108 Suppl 1:II195–9.

10. Borzak S, Tisdale JE, Amin NB, et al. Atrial fibrillation after bypass surgery: does the arrhythmia or the characteristics of the patients prolong hospital stay? *Chest* 1998;113(6):1489–91.

11. Creswell LL, Schuessler RB, Rosenbloom M, et al. Hazards of postoperative atrial arrhythmias. *Ann Thorac Surg* 1993;56(3):539–49.

12. Frost L, Jacobsen CJ, Christiansen EH, et al. Hemodynamic predictors of atrial fibrillation or flutter after coronary artery bypass grafting. *Acta Anaesthesiol Scand* 1995;39(5):690–7.

13. Leitch JW, Thomson D, Baird DK, et al. The importance of age as a predictor of atrial fibrillation and flutter after coronary artery bypass grafting. *J Thorac Cardiovasc Surg* 1990;100(3):338–42.

14. Gwinnutt CL, Columb M, Harris R. Outcome after cardiac arrest in adults in UK hospitals: effect of the 1997 guidelines. *Resuscitation* 2000;47(2): 125–35.

15. Elliott CG, Zimmerman GA, Clemmer TP. Complications of pulmonary artery catheterization in the care of critically ill patients. A prospective study. *Chest* 1979;76(6):647–52.

16. Iberti TJ, Benjamin E, Gruppi L, et al. Ventricular arrhythmias during pulmonary artery catheterization in the intensive care unit. Prospective study. *Am J Med* 1985;78(3):451–4.

17. Patel C, Laboy V, Venus B, et al. Acute complications of pulmonary artery catheter insertion in critically ill patients. *Crit Care Med* 1986;14(3): 195–7.

18. Vulliemin P, Del Bufalo A, Schlaepfer J, et al. Relation between cycle length, volume, and pressure in type I atrial flutter. *Pacing Clin Electrophysiol* 1994;17(8):1391–8.

19. Mayr A, Knotzer H, Pajk W, et al. Risk factors associated with new onset tachyarrhythmias after cardiac surgery – a retrospective analysis. *Acta Anaesthesiol Scand* 2001;45(5):543–9.

20. Sanders MH, Keller FA. Chronotropic effects of progressive hypoxia and hypercapnia. *Respiration* 1989;55(1):1–10.

21. Sarubbi FA, Vasquez JE. Spinal epidural abscess associated with the use of temporary epidural catheters: report of two cases and review. *Clin Infect Dis* 1997;25(5):1155–8.

22. Shih HT, Webb CR, Conway WA, et al. Frequency and significance of cardiac arrhythmias in chronic obstructive lung disease. *Chest* 1988;94(1):44–8.

23. Levine PA, Klein MD. Mechanisms of arrhythmias in chronic obstructive lung disease. *Geriatrics* 1976;31(11):47–56.
24. Cohen A, Katz M, Katz R, et al. Chronic obstructive pulmonary disease in patients undergoing coronary artery bypass grafting. *J Thorac Cardiovasc Surg* 1995;109(3):574–81.
25. Rubeiz GJ, Thill-Baharozian M, Hardie D, et al. Association of hypomagnesemia and mortality in acutely ill medical patients. *Crit Care Med* 1993;21(2):203–9.
26. Passakiotou MLC, Kopatzidis E, Sounidakis N, et al. Magnesium at admission: is it an outcome marker in the critically ill patient? *Crit Care* 2005; 9(Suppl 1):P416.
27. Polderman KH, Girbes AR. Severe electrolyte disorders following cardiac surgery: a prospective controlled observational study. *Crit Care* 2004;8(6): R459–66.
28. Fanning WJ, Thomas CS, Jr, Roach A, et al. Prophylaxis of atrial fibrillation with magnesium sulfate after coronary artery bypass grafting. *Ann Thorac Surg* 1991;52(3):529–33.
29. England MR, Gordon G, Salem M, et al. Magnesium administration and dysrhythmias after cardiac surgery. A placebo-controlled, double-blind, randomized trial. *JAMA* 1992;268(17):2395–402.
30. Karmy-Jones R, Hamilton A, Dzavik V, et al. Magnesium sulfate prophylaxis after cardiac operations. *Ann Thorac Surg* 1995;59(2):502–7.
31. Jensen BM, Alstrup P, Klitgard NA. Magnesium substitution and postoperative arrhythmias in patients undergoing coronary artery bypass grafting. *Scand Cardiovasc J* 1997;31(5):265–9.
32. Treggiari-Venzi MM, Waeber JL, Perneger TV, et al. Intravenous amiodarone or magnesium sulphate is not cost-beneficial prophylaxis for atrial fibrillation after coronary artery bypass surgery. *Br J Anaesth* 2000;85(5):690–5.
33. Toraman F, Karabulut EH, Alhan HC, et al. Magnesium infusion dramatically decreases the incidence of atrial fibrillation after coronary artery bypass grafting. *Ann Thorac Surg* 2001;72(4):1256–61; discussion 61–2.
34. Yeatman M, Caputo M, Narayan P, et al. Magnesium-supplemented warm blood cardioplegia in patients undergoing coronary artery revascularization. *Ann Thorac Surg* 2002;73(1):112–8.
35. Alghamdi AA, Al-Radi OO, Latter DA. Intravenous magnesium for prevention of atrial fibrillation after coronary artery bypass surgery: a systematic review and meta-analysis. *J Card Surg* 2005;20(3):293–9.
36. Zangrillo A, Landoni G, Sparicio D, et al. Perioperative magnesium supplementation to prevent atrial fibrillation after off-pump coronary artery surgery: a randomized controlled study. *J Cardiothorac Vasc Anesth* 2005;19(6):723–8.
37. ISIS-4: a randomised factorial trial assessing early oral captopril, oral mononitrate, and intravenous magnesium sulphate in 58,050 patients with suspected acute myocardial infarction. ISIS-4 (Fourth International Study of Infarct Survival) Collaborative Group. *Lancet* 1995;345(8951):669–85.
38. Early administration of intravenous magnesium to high-risk patients with acute myocardial infarction in the Magnesium in Coronaries (MAGIC) Trial: a randomised controlled trial. *Lancet* 2002;360(9341):1189–96.
39. Johnson RG, Shafique T, Sirois C, et al. Potassium concentrations and ventricular ectopy: a prospective, observational study in post-cardiac surgery patients. *Crit Care Med* 1999;27(11):2430–4.

40. Macdonald JE, Struthers AD. What is the optimal serum potassium level in cardiovascular patients? *J Am Coll Cardiol* 2004;43(2):155–61.

41. Solomon RJ, Cole AG. Importance of potassium in patients with acute myocardial infarction. *Acta Med Scand Suppl* 1981;647:87–93.

42. Madias JE, Shah B, Chintalapally G, et al. Admission serum potassium in patients with acute myocardial infarction: its correlates and value as a determinant of in-hospital outcome. *Chest* 2000;118(4):904–13.

43. Nordrehaug JE, Johannessen KA, von der Lippe G. Serum potassium concentration as a risk factor of ventricular arrhythmias early in acute myocardial infarction. *Circulation* 1985;71(4):645–9.

44. Nordrehaug JE, von der Lippe G. Serum potassium concentrations are inversely related to ventricular, but not to atrial, arrhythmias in acute myocardial infarction. *Eur Heart J* 1986;7(3):204–9.

45. Hulting J. In-hospital ventricular fibrillation and its relation to serum potassium. *Acta Med Scand* Suppl. 1981;647:109–16.

46. Cleland JG, Dargie HJ, Ford I. Mortality in heart failure: clinical variables of prognostic value. *Br Heart J* 1987;58(6):572–82.

47. Johnson CJ, Peterson DR, Smith EK. Myocardial tissue concentrations of magnesium and potassium in men dying suddenly from ischemic heart disease. *Am J Clin Nutr* 1979;32(5):967–70.

48. Wahr JA, Parks R, Boisvert D, et al. Preoperative serum potassium levels and perioperative outcomes in cardiac surgery patients. Multicenter Study of Perioperative Ischemia Research Group. *JAMA* 1999;281(23):2203–10.

49. Gaylard E. Changing incidence of atrial fibrillation following coronary artery bypass grafting: a retrospective analysis. *Br J Clin Pract* 1996;50(3): 164–5.

50. Bradley D, Creswell LL, Hogue CW, Jr, et al. Pharmacologic prophylaxis: American College of Chest Physicians guidelines for the prevention and management of postoperative atrial fibrillation after cardiac surgery. *Chest* 2005;128(2 Suppl):39S–47S.

51. Wyse DG, Waldo AL, DiMarco JP, et al. A comparison of rate control and rhythm control in patients with atrial fibrillation. *N Engl J Med* 2002;347(23):1825–33.

52. Hohnloser SH, Kuck KH, Lilienthal J. Rhythm or rate control in atrial fibrillation – Pharmacological Intervention in Atrial Fibrillation (PIAF): a randomised trial. *Lancet* 2000;356(9244):1789–94.

53. Cordina J, Mead G. Pharmacological cardioversion for atrial fibrillation and flutter. *Cochrane Database Syst Rev* 2005;(2):CD003713.

54. *CG36 Atrial Fibrillation – Full Guideline. 2006* (cited 28 June 2006). Available from http://guidance.nice.org.uk/CG36/guidance/pdf/English.

55. Tonkin A. Non-rheumatic atrial fibrillation and stroke. *Aust N Z J Med* 1999;29(3):467–72.

56. Maisel WH, Rawn JD, Stevenson WG. Atrial fibrillation after cardiac surgery. *Ann Intern Med* 2001;135(12):1061–73.

57. Kumar A. Intravenous amiodarone for therapy of atrial fibrillation and flutter in critically ill patients with severely depressed left ventricular function. *South Med J* 1996;89(8):779–85.

58. Crystal E, Garfinkle MS, Connolly SS, et al. Interventions for preventing post-operative atrial fibrillation in patients undergoing heart surgery. *Cochrane Database Syst Rev* 2004;(4):CD003611.

59. Naccarelli GV, Wolbrette DL, Patel HM, et al. Amiodarone: clinical trials. *Curr Opin Cardiol* 2000;15(1):64–72.

60. Greenspon AJ, Kidwell GA, Hurley W, et al. Amiodarone-related postoperative adult respiratory distress syndrome. *Circulation* 1991;84(5 Suppl):III407–15.

61. Van Mieghem W, Coolen L, Malysse I, et al. Amiodarone and the development of ARDS after lung surgery. *Chest* 1994;105(6):1642–5.

62. Brien JF, Jimmo S, Brennan FJ, et al. Distribution of amiodarone and its metabolite, desethylamiodarone, in human tissues. *Can J Physiol Pharmacol* 1987;65(3):360–4.

63. Ashrafian H, Davey P. Is amiodarone an underrecognized cause of acute respiratory failure in the ICU? *Chest* 2001;120(1):275–82.

64. Pfisterer ME, Kloter-Weber UC, Huber M, et al. Prevention of supraventricular tachyarrhythmias after open heart operation by low-dose sotalol: a prospective, double-blind, randomized, placebo-controlled study. *Ann Thorac Surg* 1997;64(4):1113–9.

65. Weber UK, Osswald S, Buser P, et al. Significance of supraventricular tachyarrhythmias after coronary artery bypass graft surgery and their prevention by low-dose sotalol: a prospective double-blind randomized placebo-controlled study. *J Cardiovasc Pharmacol Ther* 1998;3(3):209–16.

66. Gomes JA, Ip J, Santoni-Rugiu F, et al. Oral *d,l* sotalol reduces the incidence of postoperative atrial fibrillation in coronary artery bypass surgery patients: a randomized, double-blind, placebo-controlled study. *J Am Coll Cardiol* 1999;34(2):334–9.

67. Katariya K, DeMarchena E, Bolooki H. Oral amiodarone reduces incidence of postoperative atrial fibrillation. *Ann Thorac Surg* 1999;68(5):1599–603; discussion 603–4.

68. Lee JH, Abdelhady K, Capdeville M. Clinical outcomes and resource usage in 100 consecutive patients after off-pump coronary bypass procedures. *Surgery* 2000; 128(4):548–55.

69. Yazigi A, Rahbani P, Zeid HA, et al. Postoperative oral amiodarone as prophylaxis against atrial fibrillation after coronary artery surgery. *J Cardiothorac Vasc Anesth* 2002;16(5):603–6.

70. Foroulis CN, Kotoulas C, Lachanas H, et al. Factors associated with cardiac rhythm disturbances in the early post-pneumonectomy period: a study on 259 pneumonectomies. *Eur J Cardiothorac Surg* 2003;23(3):384–9.

71. Rena O, Papalia E, Oliaro A, et al. Supraventricular arrhythmias after resection surgery of the lung. *Eur J Cardiothorac Surg* 2001;20(4):688–93.

72. Amar D. Prevention and management of dysrhythmias following thoracic surgery. *Chest Surg Clin N Am* 1997;7(4):817–29.

73. Asamura H, Naruke T, Tsuchiya R, et al. What are the risk factors for arrhythmias after thoracic operations? A retrospective multivariate analysis of 267 consecutive thoracic operations. *J Thorac Cardiovasc Surg* 1993;106(6):1104–10.

74. Seguin P, Signouret T, Laviolle B, et al. Incidence and risk factors of atrial fibrillation in a surgical intensive care unit. *Crit Care Med* 2004;32(3): 722–6.

75. Christians KK, Wu B, Quebbeman EJ, et al. Postoperative atrial fibrillation in noncardiothoracic surgical patients. *Am J Surg* 2001;182(6):713–5.

76. Batra GS, Molyneux J, Scott NA. Colorectal patients and cardiac arrhythmias detected on the surgical high dependency unit. *Ann R Coll Surg Engl* 2001;83(3):174–6.

77. Bender JS. Supraventricular tachyarrhythmias in the surgical intensive care unit: an under-recognized event. *Am Surg* 1996;62(1):73–5.

78. Kahn RL, Hargett MJ, Urquhart B, et al. Supraventricular tachyarrhythmias during total joint arthroplasty. Incidence and risk. *Clin Orthop Relat Res* 1993;(296):265–9.

79. Goldman L. Supraventricular tachyarrhythmias in hospitalized adults after surgery. Clinical correlates in patients over 40 years of age after major noncardiac surgery. *Chest* 1978;73(4):450–4.

8 Mechanical Heart Failure Therapy

Richard Trimlett

Royal Brompton & Harefield NHS FoundationTrust, London, UK

> ## Take Home Messages
>
> - Mechanical assist devices have a role to play both in short-term support post-cardiotomy and longer-term support whilst awaiting transplantation or recovery.
> - Early identification of cardiac failure and prompt device implantation, before the onset of multi-organ dysfunction, improves outcome.
> - Meticulous haemostasis is essential to ensure improved outcomes in these high-risk patients as bleeding is a frequent and major complication.
> - Assess recovery regularly using multiple sources of data including clinical parameters and echocardiography to ensure correct timing for successful explantation.
> - Percutaneous mechanical assist devices may be a realistic option when an intra-aortic counter pulsation device is insufficient and a left ventricular assist device is not desirable.

8.1 Introduction

This chapter is concerned primarily with the indications and management of patients requiring advanced mechanical support for heart failure in the acute setting. Heart failure is defined as the inability of the cardiac output to meet the demands of the body. It is a common condition affecting over 14 million people across Europe [1] and approximately 710,000 people within the UK [2]. The annual incidence is 1.2–1.4 per 1000 of the population [3], increasing to 10–17 per 1000 in those over 85 years of age [4]. Heart failure severely impacts on a patient's quality of life, and the prognosis remains poor despite advances in medical and surgical therapies. Indeed, only 25% of patients live longer than 5 years after diagnosis [5] and survival rates are worse than those of most cancers [6].

Cardiovascular Critical Care. Edited by M. Griffiths, J. Cordingley and S. Price.
© 2010 Blackwell Publishing Ltd.

Table 8.1 Commonest indications for mechanical cardiac support.

Acute myocardial infarction resulting in cardiogenic shock
Decompensation of chronic heart failure
Cardiomyopathy (myocarditis, dilated cardiomyopathy)
Transplant rejection
Arrhythmia
Hypothermia
Drug-related cardiomyopathy
Post-cardiac surgery

The most common cause of heart failure in the western world is ischaemic cardiomyopathy. Over 2.1 million people in the UK have coronary artery disease which represents the greatest cause of mortality in the developed world [6]. In addition, hypertension is a common cause of heart failure, accounting for 10% of all deaths worldwide [7]. Additional causes include valvular heart disease, the rarer cardiomyopathies and myocarditis which principally affects younger patients (Table 8.1).

For many years, heart transplantation has been the gold standard of treatment for heart failure, with 10-year survival of approximately 50% [8]. However, only a minority of patients with end-stage cardiac failure are transplanted, as the demand is hugely outstripped by the supply. This is due in part to organ donation practice, but also due to improvements in road traffic safety reducing the number of incidents of isolated unrecoverable head injuries [9]. Thus, although medical therapy remains the mainstay of treatment for the majority of patients, in recent years mechanical support has been developed to provide an alternative.

8.2 The physics of mechanical assist

It is worth considering the physics of mechanical support devices in some detail as, although industrial engineers have made great advances in fluid mechanics, there are several reasons why these technologies are not directly translatable to human physiology.

Mechanical support of the heart became a realistic option with the introduction of cardiopulmonary bypass first being used successfully to repair an atrial septal defect [10]. At this time, the purpose of cardiopulmonary bypass was to provide short-term support of the circulation whilst the heart was operated on. It was apparent that the technology could potentially be extended to provide longer-term support; however, it took 13 years from the first successful cardiopulmonary bypass procedure for this potential to be realised [11]. In 1975 it was demonstrated that the duration of cardiopulmonary bypass was one of the three key determinants of outcome following cardiac surgery [12]. This was due in part to the surface area required for oxygenation. Early attempts to provide left ventricular mechanical support with a pump alone remained hazardous, with mixed outcomes eventually leading to the banning of the total artificial heart in the USA by 1990 [13]. Other potential avenues for mechanical support of the heart have continued to be explored.

The ideal artificial heart would be: safe (not thrombogenic or toxic), reliable, inexpensive, easily implantable and of appropriate size. No single pumping system satisfies all these criteria and consequently a choice must be made as to which system best suits the needs of each patient. All mechanical pumps can be divided, according to how they function, into either positive displacement pumps or centrifugal pumps.

Positive displacement pumps

A positive displacement pump moves a fixed amount of fluid with each stroke/cycle irrespective of the speed of operation. By having a fixed chamber capacity, the same amount of fluid is moved with each stroke and so the total pumping rate is a product of the rate and stroke volume. An unintended but useful consequence of this design is that when the pump is stopped, backflow cannot occur.

Centrifugal pumps

Centrifugal pumps use the viscosity of the fluid. The fluid enters the pump close to the centre of the impeller and due to the speed of rotation the fluid is thrown towards the outer edge of the impeller. Once beyond the tips of the spinning impeller, the fluid carries on tangentially where it passes into the pump outflow tract. The impeller does not make contact with the casing of the pump and at low speeds it is a relatively inefficient device. Efficiency and hence pumping capacity increase with rotational speed, giving rise to a non-linear relationship between rotational speed and pumping rate. Two major advantages of the non-contact design are (1) the reduction of trauma to cellular elements of blood, and (2) the very low viscosity of air which means that at physiologically relevant rotational speeds gases are not viscous enough to be pumped, and so entrainment of air into the system will prevent the pump from working. This makes the potential for accidental massive arterial air embolus very low. However, the non-occlusive design will allow reverse flow to occur when the impeller stops.

Pulsatile vs. non-pulsatile flow

Physiological delivery of blood to end organs is pulsatile. The velocity varies throughout the cardiac cycle, with flow close to zero at the end of the cardiac cycle (end diastole) and at its highest after iso-volumetric contraction during systole. The velocity therefore oscillates about the mean. There are several theoretical advantages to this mode of perfusion, with energy of the moving blood being proportional to the square of the velocity. During pulsatile flow, when the velocity is significantly greater than the mean, more energy is delivered to the end organs which may improve capillary flow and lead to improved tissue perfusion. This remains an area of controversy, with research supporting both pulsatility and non-pulsatility.

Achieving pulsatile flow presents a technical challenge as the flow of blood must be cyclically interrupted and then recommenced at a higher rate than for continuous flow to compensate for the period of reduced or no flow. These peak higher levels of flow may well cause turbulent flow in a system delivering the same flow but at a continuous rate. Turbulence wastes energy and can be harmful by exerting shear forces on the blood components, increasing the risk of cellular injury. Dimensions may need to be increased to avoid turbulence, which would be a disadvantage for implantable devices as well as at cannulation sites. In addition, stopping and starting devices that use very high pump speeds 4,000 plus times per hour may reduce their long-term durability. All of these obstacles can be overcome, and indeed several of the presently available pumps used in cardio-pulmonary bypass have a pulsatile operating mode, but at present there is no overwhelming evidence supporting pulsatility. Consequently most systems are non-pulsatile as they can be smaller and simpler.

8.3 Types of assist devices

Until all of the engineering challenges have been met there will continue to be a range of cardiac assist devices available for use (Table 8.2). These devices can be usefully considered in separate groups according to clinical indications for use. Whilst some traits are desirable for all types of device, the duration of intended implantation will have implications for design. For short-term support, ease of implantation is more important than size. As many recipients remain on the Intensive Care Unit, the device can be located outside the body. By contrast, for longer-term therapy, a fully implantable device is preferable.

Table 8.2 Types of assist devices.

Short-term	Long-term	Third generation
Biomedicus Biopump	Heartmate XVE	Incor/Berlin Heart
Terumo Capiox	Novacor LVAS	Ventrassist
Jostra Rotaflow	Thoractec	Worldheart
St Jude Lifestream		Novacor II
Heartmate	**Axial flow devices**	Heartmate III
Nikkiso	Micromed Debakey	Terumoheart
Cardiac Assist iVAD & pVAD	Jarvik 2000	Coraide blood pump
Medos Deltastream	Heartmate II	Levitronix centrimag
CorAide		
VentrAssist	**Totally implantable**	
Levitronix Centri-Mag	Arrow Lionheart LVD2000	
Sarns Centrifugal		
	Total artificial heart	
	Cardiowest TAH	
	Abiocor	

8.4 Indications for use

The principal aims of cardiac assist are to maintain cardiac output, whilst resting the heart and awaiting recovery of ventricular function. Heart failure is often defined according to the New York Heart Association Functional Classification of Physical Activity (NYHA class I–IV) [14]. This classification is useful in the management of patients with heart failure, and as an endpoint in clinical studies. In practice, it can, however, be difficult to differentiate objectively between mild and moderate or moderate and severe limitation of activities. Therefore, when considering the initiation of mechanical cardiac support, additional objective markers of cardiac output may be used, including acid-base status or cardiac index (Figure 8.1). Predicting the risk of use of a cardiac assist device is challenging, as with advances in technology and safer implantation techniques, both the mortality and morbidity of mechanical cardiac assist falls.

Acute myocardial infarction complicated by cardiogenic shock

Two hundred thousand people per year are admitted to hospital in the UK with the diagnosis of ischaemic heart disease and more than 64,000 with a myocardial infarction [15]. Cardiogenic shock is a complicating factor in 6.6% of patients presenting with an ST elevation infarction and 3% of those with non-ST elevation infarction [16]. In this context cardiogenic shock is usually defined as a systolic blood pressure below 90 mmHg for more that 30 minutes post-infarction, or evidence of inadequate end-organ perfusion, and is associated with an overall mortality of 70–80% [17].

Decompensated chronic cardiac failure

Heart failure affects more than 600,000 people in the UK and is responsible for 5% of all hospital admissions [18]. Mechanical assist devices are playing

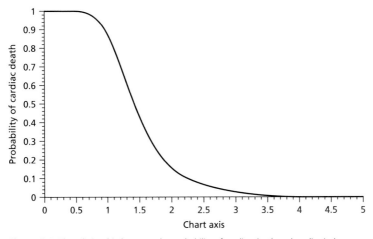

Figure 8.1 The relationship between the probability of cardiac death and cardiac index.

an increasing role not only in facilitating survival until a suitable donor is available but also potentially as a permanent replacement to a failed heart, also called 'destination therapy'.

Myocarditis and cardiomyopathy

These conditions occur in a younger age group and identifying those patients where recovery will occur is extremely difficult. As the risk of device implantation reduces, mechanical treatment can be instituted at an earlier stage, reducing the risk to the patient of sudden cardiac death from low cardiac output whilst waiting for either recovery or transplantation.

Post-cardiac surgery

Pre-operative cardiac function is one of the three most important predictors of outcome following cardiac surgery, along with age and length of cardiopulmonary bypass [12]. In many cases, post-operative cardiac failure can be anticipated and mechanical assist can be implemented before cessation of cardio-pulmonary bypass. However, in about 5% of cases cardiac failure after surgery is not anticipated [19]. Survival without mechanical support is related to cardiac function (Figure 8.1), whilst that following device implantation is greater than 50% [20]. In the New York registry data, of those requiring mechanical support post-cardiopulmonary bypass, 40% were successfully weaned from the device and 25% were discharged from hospital [21].

8.5 Short-term/long-term implantation

The choice of mechanical assist device used for support should be dependent on the duration of expected support. For acute conditions such as cardiogenic shock after cardiopulmonary bypass and myocardial infarction the expectation would be for recovery to occur in days to weeks. By contrast, in chronic heart failure, for example, support of the circulation in patients awaiting transplantation would be expected to be required for many months, and in some cases years.

Clearly, those patients not expected to recover intrinsic cardiac function and not suitable for transplantation will become dependent on the implanted device, and long-term durability is the key factor in the choice of device. In some cases where the duration of recovery does not easily fall into either category, a short-term device can be implanted and if recovery becomes prolonged then it is possible to switch to a long-term fully implantable device.

8.6 Methods of implantation

Artificial replacement of cardiac function necessitates delivery of several litres of blood to and from the pump every minute. This imposes some limitations on the way in which these devices can be connected to the circulation.

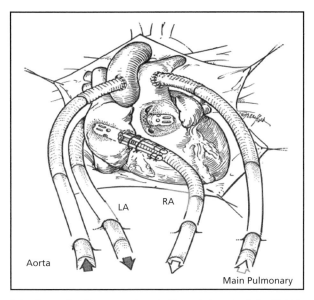

Figure 8.2 Inflow and outflow connections of a bi-ventricular assist device (BiVAD) circulation.

Surgical connection

For isolated assistance of the right or left ventricle, access is needed to the heart or at least the pulmonary circulation (Figure 8.2). For left heart support, blood must be taken from the left atrium or pulmonary veins. These techniques require access to the central vessels, where large-bore cannulae are sutured in place to ensure satisfactory haemostasis between the synthetic tubes leading to and from the device and the vessels (Figure 8.3). This process is very similar to cannulation for cardiopulmonary bypass. There is the additional option of locating the device within the thoracic or abdominal cavity or exteriorising the pipes to an external pump. Combined right and left support with extra-corporeal membrane oxygenation (ECMO) can be achieved via large-capacity veins and arteries more remote from the heart.

Connection tubing plays an important role in mechanical cardiac assist. Whilst long connecting lines may make transfer of the patient easier and facilitate turning of the patient, the length of the lines is directly proportional to the resistance to flow, as well as increasing the thrombogenic surface area, increasing the priming volume and providing a greater volume of extra-corporeal blood from which heat can be lost. The balance is in favour of the shortest line length compatible with safe management of the bedside pump. Insulated sheaths can be useful in combating heat loss.

Percutaneous devices

Many assist devices can be deployed percutaneously whilst the pump remains extra-corporeal. For long-term support, as in bridge to

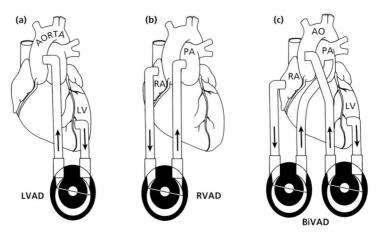

Figure 8.3 Inflow and outflow connections for a left ventricular assist device (LVAD), right-sided device (RVAD) and bi-ventricular assist device (BiVAD). (**a**) Surgical connection of an LVAD showing blood diverted from the left ventricular (LV) apex and returning to the body via the ascending aorta (AO), above the closed aortic valve. (**b**) RVAD diverting blood from the right atrium (RA) and returning it to the pulmonary trunk, above the pulmonary valve (PA). (**c**) Both pumps connected to provide total cardiac support.

transplantation or destination therapy, the device needs to be internal for the patient to achieve a satisfactory quality of life, and due to the size of the device required for full circulatory support. This is usually done through an open procedure with direct, central cannulation.

Advances in assist device design and the introduction of the high-speed impeller pump have enabled the manufacture of devices small enough to be delivered percutaneously. The device is fitted to the end of a long arterial catheter and is inserted retrogradely through percutaneous femoral access. For satisfactory function, the body of the device must site across the aortic valve. The device inlet sits within the left ventricular chamber of the heart, and blood is drawn into the device and passes through the screw-impeller. Blood is ejected above the aortic valve into the aorta.

Due to the constraints of size these devices are not capable of delivering the higher flows of conventional pumps, but can deliver 2.5 or 5.0 litres/min depending on the size [22]. There are several obvious advantages to a fully contained ventricular support device, including avoiding the need for an extra-corporeal circulation, removing the contact of blood with pump tubing, cooling, priming volume, safer transit and ease of insertion. With the choice of circulatory support there is a relatively large transition from the Intra-Aortic Counter-Pulsation Device (balloon pump) to full ventricular support, and percutaneous devices present the opportunity to provide further support beyond the balloon pump without the need for full left ventricular assist device (LVAD) support with all its attendant risks.

Acute management of mechanical cardiac assist
General principles

Whilst a high cardiac output may be considered more desirable there are several considerations relating to pump speed and cardiac output. There is close correlation between low cardiac index and mortality, but at the higher flows that are possible with a mechanical pump, trauma to the cellular components of the blood increases [23, 24]. Delivery of blood to the pump can also be problematic at high flows, causing high negative pressures and cavitation, once again affecting the cellular elements adversely. Furthermore, at high flow rates all cardiac return arriving in the relevant atrium may be directed entirely towards the pump, leaving no forward flow through the atrioventricular valve(s) into the ventricle, and with a competent aortic or pulmonary valve no blood will enter the ventricle. Thrombus can form on the ventricular surface of any valve where flow has ceased, and indeed can form within the valve sinuses if the return cannula from the pump is placed far enough away from the valve so that minimal flow occurs at valve level. The thrombus can be extremely difficult to access surgically, as manipulation of the heart or pump cannulae frequently reduces pump flow, which can allow blood to flow through the heart, pushing the thrombus into the circulation before it can be retrieved.

A combination of low-level ventricular ejection and appropriate anticoagulation can prevent thrombus formation within the circulation whilst on mechanical support, but in order for the ventricle to eject, this does increase the effort required by the ventricle to eject the blood.

Thromboembolism

All devices present an increased risk of thromboembolism, and anticoagulation is required for most devices to a recommended target International Normalised Ratio (INR) of 2.5–3.5 [25]. The risk varies enormously according to the reported series and the condition of the patient, but approximately 30% of patients with a cardiac assist device suffer this complication [26].

The increased risk is due to the presentation of a foreign surface to the blood during transit of the blood through the pump and also the reduced flow through the native cardiac chamber which is being assisted by the pump. Advances in manufacturing techniques have resulted in the development of internal coatings which are less thrombogenic, and scintered titanium is currently used without anticoagulation with a comparable rate of thromboembolism [27].

The most important principle in the prevention of this complication is rigorous control of anticoagulation along with antiplatelet therapy. Regular inspection of the device, if external, and the cardiac chambers by echocardiography is necessary to identify thrombus. If this occurs in an external device, the pump should be replaced immediately. If thrombus has developed within the heart, removal should be attempted as the treatment of choice, if the procedure is possible.

Bleeding

This is a common complication occurring in between 25% and 50% of cases [28]. The cause of the bleeding is multifactorial. The requirement for anticoagulation with most current devices increases the risk of post-implantation haemorrhage. In addition, patients requiring mechanical support frequently have deranged clotting and require significant transfusion. In addition, the devices require that cannulae be inserted into large vessels or chambers of the heart, and achieving a haemostatic seal between these and tissue can be challenging. Moreover, the return of high-pressure blood from the pump poses a further challenge for haemostasis, as not only must the interface between the cannulae and the vessels into which the blood is returning be haemostatic, but also the sutures must have sufficient purchase to ensure that the cannulae do not become displaced at any point during what might be a prolonged period of support.

Bleeding is either revealed (increased drainage through chest drains) or concealed (blood remains within the thoracic cavity). When tamponade occurs in the presence of mechanical assist, extrinsic pressure on the drainage chamber reduces the flow of blood to the pump is manifested by a reduction in measured flow through the pump. The classical features of tamponade [29] are not normally seen – either clinically or on echocardiography. The external manifestation of either tamponade or excessive blood loss on pump function is typical. With centrifugal pumps the flow will oscillate as the pump attempts to suck more blood than can be delivered. This causes a sudden drop in pressure in the line supplying the pump, revealed as a judder when the pipe is held (or a coarse vibration of the pipe if it is not firmly fixed). The sudden drop in flow allows blood to accumulate within the supplying chamber of the heart, which then allows the pump to recommence flow with a rapid increase in velocity again. It represents a simple supply versus demand problem and can be used as a useful test of circulatory filling. Here, if the pump is functioning satisfactorily at the required flow rate, momentarily increasing the flow until juddering of the lines occurs will allow assessment of the venous return to the heart. This is useful in determining the intravascular filling status of the patient, especially if a strategy of fluid removal is planned.

When flow is compromised by inadequate venous return, echocardiography (usually trans-oesophageal in the acute stage) is necessary to exclude tamponade and confirm optimal cannula placement and filling status. The former two may require immediate surgical exploration either to decompress the tamponade and deal with the cause or to reposition the drainage cannula(e).

Infection

Data from the Randomised Evaluation of Mechanical Assistance for the Treatment of Congestive Heart Failure (REMATCH) trial demonstrated that infection was the leading cause of mortality in patients with cardiac assist devices, accounting for almost 40% of deaths, with the highest risk being the first month following implantation [30]. Infections relating directly to the device most frequently occur at the sites of breaches of the epithelium, such as exit sites for drivelines or main blood send and return lines. In addition there may be either local collections occurring around the device, or sepsis related to the circulation such as bacteraemia or potentially endocarditis. Patients requiring cardiac assist have, by definition at least, single and frequently multi-organ dysfunction. Further, the presence of intravenous and intra-arterial cannulae and the catabolic state due to nutritional issues provide both potential sites for infection and a reduction in immune capacity, making infection more likely. Common pathogens include *Staphylococcus*, *Pseudomonas* and fungal species.

The cornerstones of treatment of infection relating to a foreign implant are the removal of foreign material, drainage of collections and appropriate antimicrobial therapy. If device infection is suspected and cardiac support is still required, this does not exclude the possibility of transplantation.

Mechanical failure

Mechanical failure is a significant cause of death in this group of patients, second only to infection, with a 12-month rate of just over 10% rising to over 30% at 2 years [30]. Failure of the device can occur at any point, with occlusion, obstruction or disconnection of the send or return cannulae. Valves within the inflow and outflow channels are subject to the same complications as conventional prosthetic heart valves, and the pumping mechanism may fail due to power loss or component failure.

These devices are highly complex with essential electronic, electromagnetic and hydraulic components. Here an important difference can again be seen between the positive displacement and the centrifugal pumps. The failure of a positive displacement pump effectively turns the pump into a two-way obstruction to blood flow through the device. Stasis occurs and the heart will begin to fill in the normal way as blood is no longer diverted out of the heart. If the intrinsic myocardial function is satisfactory then cardiac output will be maintained. By contrast, if a centrifugal device fails, it becomes a passive two-way conduit. Even when the heart contracts, cardiac output will be reduced by retrograde blood flow, in effect equivalent to massive aortic or pulmonary regurgitation, depending upon which ventricle is being supported. In this situation a clamp must be immediately applied to any external part of the circuit to prevent reverse flow whilst the underlying problem is identified and dealt with. In some of the newer systems, diagnostic information is displayed warning that there has been a failure but allowing the pump to continue whilst preparation is made to rectify the problem.

Multi-organ failure and immunocompromise

Cardiac assist devices are associated with a high mortality, and as a result are often considered a last line of treatment. In addition, patients with end-stage cardiac failure frequently have multi-organ dysfunction due to a combination of hypoperfusion and high filling pressures. Commencing cardiac mechanical assistance in any patient with multi-organ dysfunction cannot guarantee the reversal of non-cardiac organ failure, and as a result this is one of the commonest causes of death in these patients. The duration of organ failure is inversely proportional to the chance of recovery [31] and therefore early implantation of cardiac assist (or before the onset of established organ failure) is preferable. Multi-organ failure further complicates recovery as it is an independent marker of the severity of the insult, resulting in the need for cardiac support [32]. In addition it correlates with immune system function and therefore increases the likelihood of infection [33]. In those patients surviving to transplantation, a further complication relating to the immune system is the prolonged stimulation of the T-cells by the foreign surfaces within the pump and conduits [34]. This leads to a higher incidence of acute rejection following transplantation [34].

8.7 Weaning and device removal

The most desirable outcome for mechanical cardiac support is full recovery. The requirement for successful weaning of mechanical cardiac support is accurate assessment of the underlying ventricular performance. This can only be done by assessing the heart under different loading conditions and should be carried out using a combination of echocardiography with manipulation of pre- and after-load. The process of weaning is complicated by the reduction in inotropic support once the ventricular assist device is *in situ*. It is therefore necessary to recommence inotropic support when the weaning process is commenced and it will be frequently necessary to repeatedly evaluate whether the ventricle(s) will be capable of sustaining an adequate cardiac output. In the presence of appropriate anticoagulation, pump flow is slowly reduced in a stepwise manner, and the pre- and after-load values are observed together with detailed physiological echocardiography. When cardiac performance is judged to be adequate and sustainable (judged over a short time-frame), flows are returned to normal and device removal planned.

Device removal is usually undertaken surgically and requires a reversal of the steps for implantation. The process is potentially more hazardous if the device has been in situ for a long time, but once the cannulae have been removed the anticoagulation may be reversed if there is no contra-indication. Frequently, the change in lung compliance and the reduction of pericardial space with the apposition of the sternum together with filling of the heart may require the chest to be splinted open as an interim step towards definitive closure once further improvement has occurred.

8.8 Conclusion

The poor long-term outlook for patients with medically managed end-stage cardiac failure, coupled with a severe limitation in supply of organs for transplantation, has resulted in an increase in use of mechanical cardiac assist devices. The evidence now supports the role for these devices in both the acute and chronic heart failure setting, but there remain limitations in the technologies. Further work is required to improve our understanding of the increasing role of these devices in a potentially large population of heart failure patients, whilst reducing major complications such as infection, thromboembolism and device failure. With an increasing number of heart failure patients this technology offers a significant hope of better outcomes in the future, and the potential to overcome the current obstacles within transplantation.

Case study

A 56-year-old man presented with severe shortness of breath of 18 months duration. He had previously undergone three cardiac surgical procedures in the last 30 years, including two redo-aortic homograft replacements. He lived abroad and had failed to attend valve follow-up clinic for the last 2 years. He was admitted as an emergency and investigations revealed severe prosthetic aortic valve degeneration with severe aortic regurgitation, and a dilated left ventricle with biventriular failure.

He consented for a third time to redo-aortic root replacement. This was a high-risk procedure due to the complexity of the surgery and the poor pre-existing cardiac function. The procedure was difficult due to the level of calcification and the previous coronary ostial re-implantations; however, a porcine stentless root replacement was completed successfully. The ischaemic time was 165 minutes and expectation was that inotropic support and intra-aortic balloon counter pulsation would be required. He was able to separate from cardiopulmonary bypass successfully, but, despite significant support, the cardiac index remained low. Haemostasis presented a problem and as the operation progressed the requirement for inotropes increased. A decision was taken to support the left ventricle with a short-term extra-corporeal device, inserted through the previous aortic cannulation site and the right superior pulmonary vein vent site. Flow was steadily increased, but the poor function of the right ventricle limited the maximum flow of the left-sided assist device, despite reducing the right ventricular afterload with pulmonary vasodilators. A right-sided device was then inserted, again using one of the right atrial cannulation sites and the pulmonary trunk. Both devices were now able to achieve adequate flows and the inotropic requirements were reduced.

Following satisfactory haemostasis, the man was returned to Intensive Care where he made a good recovery. Daily assessments using trans-oesophageal echo and haemodynamic parameters allowed accurate indication of ventricular recovery, and 2 weeks later with sufficient improvement of biventriular function first the left and then the right devices were explanted, and some time later the man was discharged from the hospital having made a full recovery.

References

1. *SHAPE Survey Results to the General Public*. Annual Congress of the European Society of Cardiology, Vienna, September 2003.
2. Davies, Hobbs F, Davis R, et al. Heart of England Screening Study. *Lancet* 2001;358(9280):432–4.
3. Cowie MR, Wood DA, Coats AJ, et al. Survival of patients with a new diagnosis of heart failure: a population based study. *Heart* 2000;83(5): 505–10.
4. Cowie MR, Wood DA, Coats AJ, et al. Incidence and aetiology of heart failure; a population-based study. *Eur Heart J* 1999;20(6):421–8.
5. Stewart S, MacIntyre K, Hole DJ, et al. More 'malignant' than cancer? Five-year survival following a first admission for heart failure. *Eur J Heart Failure* 2001;3(3):315–22.
6. *Office for National Statistics (2000) Key Health Statistics from General Practice*. The Stationery Office, London.
7. World Health Organisation. *The World Health Report 2002: Risks to Health 2002*. WHO, Geneva.
8. Zuckermann A, Dunkler D, Deviatko E, et al. Long-term survival (> 10 years) of patients > 60 years with induction therapy after cardiac transplantation. *Eur J Cardiothorac Surg* 2003;24:283–91.
9. Thomas J. Road traffic accidents before and after seatbelt legislation – study in a district general hospital. *J R Soc Med* 1990;83(2):79–81.
10. Dennis C, Spreng DS, Nelson GE, et al. Development of a pump-oxygenator to replace the heart and lungs; an apparatus applicable to human patients, and application to one case. *Ann Surg* 1951;134(4):709–21.
11. Cohn LH. Fifty years of open-heart surgery. *Circulation* 2003;107:2168–70.
12. Järvinen A. Low-output syndrome as a complication of open-heart surgery in 85 patients. *Ann Clin Res* 1975;7(6):379–93.
13. *Food and Drugs Administration Import Alert #74-02*. 27 April 1990. FDA, Silverspring, Maryland.
14. The Criteria Committee of the New York Heart Association. *Nomenclature and Criteria for Diagnosis of Diseases of the Heart and Great Vessels*, 9th edn. Little, Brown & Co, Boston, 1994, pp 253–6.
15. Jarman B, Aylin P, Bottle A. Trends in admissions and deaths in English NHS hospitals. *BMJ* 2004;328:855, doi: 10.1136/bmj.328.7444.855.
16. Lindholm MG, Boesgaard S, et al. and DANAMI-2 investigators. Percutaneous coronary intervention for acute MI does not prevent in-hospital development of cardiogenic shock compared to fibrinolysis. *Eur J Heart Failure* 2008;10(7):668–74. See also *Rev Cardiovasc Med* 2003;4(3):131–5.
17. *AHA/ACC Guidelines for Stemi – 482–3, 772–3*. AHA, Dallas, Texas, and ACC, Washington, DC.
18. Department of Health. *Hospital Episode Statistics 2000–2001*. DH, London, 2002, http://www.doh.gov.uk/hes/.
19. Farkas B, Vánky MD, Håkanson E, et al. Long-term consequences of postoperative heart failure after surgery for aortic stenosis compared with coronary surgery. *Ann Thorac Surg* 2007;83:2036–43.
20. Nwaejike N, Bonde P, Campalani G. Complete mechanical circulatory support using ventricular assist devices for post-cardiotomy biventricular failure. *Ulster Med J* 2008;77(1):36–8.
21. Kimble Jett G. ABIOMED BVS 5000: experience and potential advantages. *Ann Thorac Surg* 1996;61:301–4.

22. Henriques J, Remmelink M, Baan J. Jr, et al. Safety and feasibility of elective high-risk percutaneous coronary intervention procedures with left ventricular support of the impella recover LP 2.5. *Am J Cardiol* 2006;97:990–2.

23. Chales G, Nevaril CG, Lynch EC, et al. Erythrocyte damage and destruction induced by shearing stress. *J Lab Clin Med* 1968;71:784–90.

24. Indeglia RA, Shea MA, Forstrom R, et al. Influence of mechanical factor on erythrocyte sublethal damge. *Trans Am Soc Artif Intern Organs* 1968;14:264–72.

25. *HeartMate II Registry*. Thoratec Corporation, Pleasonton, California, 2006.

26. Schmid C, Weyand M, Nabavi DG, et al. Cerebral and systemic embolization during left ventricular suport with the Novacor N100 device. *Ann Thorac Surg* 1998;65:1703–10.

27. Rafii Shahin MD, Oz MC, Seldomridge JA, et al. Characterization of hematopoietic cells arising on the textured surface of left ventricular assist devices. *Ann Thorac Surg* 1995;60:1627–32.

28. Goldstein DJ, Beauford B. Left ventricular assist devices and bleeding: adding insult to injury. *Ann Thorac Surg* 2003;75:S42–7.

29. Morgagni JB. De sedibus et causes morborum, lipsiae sumptibus Leopoldi Vossii, 1829. (Beck CS. Wounds of the heart. The technic of suture.) *Arch Surg* 1926;13:205–27.

30. Rose EEA, Gelijns AC, Moskowitz AJ, et al. The Randomized Evaluation of Mechanical Assistance for the Treatment of Congestive Heart Failure (REMATCH) Study Group.
Long-term use of a left ventricular assist device for end-stage heart failure. *N Engl J Med* 2001;345:1435–43.

31. Knaus WA, Draper EA, Wagner DP, et al. Prognosis in acute organ-system failure. *Ann Surg* 1985;202:685–93.

32. Morgan JA, John R, Rao V, et al. (2004) Bridging to transplant with the HeartMate left ventricular assist device: the Columbia Presbyterian 12-year experience. *J Thorac Cardiovasc Surg* 127:1309–16.

33. Deitch EA. Multiple organ failure. Pathophysiology and potential future therapy. *Ann Surg* 1992;216(2):117–34.

34. Itescu S, Burke E, Lietz K, et al. Intravenous pulse administration of cyclophosphamide is an effective and safe treatment for sensitized cardiac allograft recipients. *Circulation* 105:1214–19.

9 Care of the High Risk Patient Undergoing Surgery

Justin Woods and Andrew Rhodes
St George's Hospital, London, UK

9.1 Introduction

Complex high-risk surgery is associated with a substantial morbidity and mortality despite recent advances in medical and surgical techniques. It has been estimated that there are approximately 2.3 million operative procedures performed annually in the UK with a mortality of 1.4%. Similar complication rates have also been reported from around the world. Within this large group of patients undergoing surgery it is possible to identify a subset of patients that make up 12% of the overall population and have a mortality of 12% [1, 2]. The patients in this subgroup account for 83% of all deaths. This chapter discusses the methods that can be used to identify this group of 'high risk' patients and the techniques that have been tried to reduce their complications.

9.2 Identification of high-risk patients

In order to concentrate resources appropriately it is necessary to identify patients who are at high risk of peri-operative morbidity and mortality. Once identified, the risk should be discussed with patients and the clinician should plan interventions aimed at decreasing the potential risks, according to the type of surgery. It is important to remember that the risk should only be quantified after all treatable medical co-morbidities have been corrected. Multiple studies have looked at risk factors in an effort to classify patients into at-risk groups (Table 9.1) [3].

There are many different ways of identifying patients with an excessive risk of complications following major surgery. Traditionally, risk has been assessed using simple clinical criteria. Now, risk can also be assessed by a number of monitoring technologies that quantify the underlying physiological disturbance and reserve required to deal with stress.

Perhaps the simplest method of identifying high-risk patients is also the most commonly used in clinical research studies. The Shoemaker criteria (Table 9.2) consist of nine [4] clinical scenarios that describe patients'

Cardiovascular Critical Care. Edited by M. Griffiths, J. Cordingley and S. Price.
© 2010 Blackwell Publishing Ltd.

Table 9.1 Critical elements for risk stratification in patients undergoing non-cardiac surgery.

● Tool must be accurate:
  Predicts peri-operative events with a positive likelihood ratio > 1*
  Predicts absence of peri-operative events with a negative likelihood ratio < 0.2
● Influences outcome:
  Identifies subgroups in which surgery should be cancelled/postponed/modified
  Identifies subgroups that do or do not benefit from therapies that aim to decrease risk
● Favourable risk/benefit ratio

---

* The likelihood ratio is the chance of a given result occurring in a patient with the target disorder compared with the likelihood that the same result would be expected in a patient without the disorder.
Adapted from Grayburn et al. [3].

Table 9.2 Risk criteria for mortality following major surgery.

● Previous severe cardio-respiratory illness (acute MI, COPD, stroke, etc.)
● Extensive ablative surgery planned for carcinoma; e.g. oesophagectomy and total gastrectomy, prolonged surgery (> 8 hours)
● Age over 70 years and evidence of limited physiologic reserve of one or more vital organs
● Shock: MAP < 60 mmHg, CVP < 15 cm H_2O and urine output < 20 ml/hour
● Septicaemia, positive blood culture or septic focus, WBC > 13,000, spiking fever to 101°F for 48 hours, and haemodynamic instability
● Respiratory failure, e.g. PaO_2 60 mmHg on FiO_2 > 0.4, Q_{sp}/Q_t > 30%, mechanical ventilation needed > 48 hours
● Acute abdominal catastrophe with haemodynamic instability, e.g. pancreatitis, gangrenous bowel, peritonitis, perforated viscus, GI bleeding
● Acute renal failure
● Late-stage vascular disease involving aortic disease

MI, myocardial infarction; COPD, chronic obstructive pulmonary disease; MAP, mean arterial pressure; CVP, central venous pressure; WBC, white blood cell count; GI, gastrointestinal.
Adapted from Pearse et al. [4].

clinical condition. Use of these criteria allows identification of patients undergoing major surgery with a mortality that ranges from 10 to 50%. Probably the most significant of these criteria is a patient's cardiovascular and respiratory status. Any patient who has severe cardiac or respiratory disease is at high risk of peri-operative complications.

There are many scoring systems that have been designed to quantify cardiac or respiratory risk. Goldman [5] identified nine factors associated with increased risk of peri-operative cardiac events. Each factor has points assigned dependent on the associated risk. High risk was ascribed to those patients with a cumulative score of more than 12 (the maximum was 53). When the ASA (American Society of Anesthesiologists) chronic health status was combined with the Goldman risk index the predictive power was

Table 9.3 Risk factors used in the revised cardiac risk index (RCRI) and the associated cardiac event rates.

Insulin therapy for diabetes		
Ischaemic heart disease		
Serum creatinine > 2 mg/dl (168 μmol/l)		
Cardiovascular disease		
Cerebrovascular disease		
High-risk surgery		
Congestive cardiac failure (at any time)		
Major cardiac event rates with the RCRI [9]		
Class	Events/patients (*n/n*)	Event rate (95% CI) (%)
I (no risk factors)	2/488	0.4 (0.05–1.5)
II (1 risk factor)	5/567	0.9 (0.3–2.1)
III (2 risk factors)	17/258	6.6 (3.9–10.3)
IV (3 or more risk factors)	12/109	11.0 (5.8–18.4)

Adapted from Lee et al. [9].

increased, but the risk index alone was not as good at predicting post-operative mortality as ASA status [6]. Currently, only the Detsky [7] and Lee [8] scores have been evaluated prospectively in non-cardiac surgery. Of all the indices for non-cardiac surgery the Lee index is 'the best validated and most accurate' of the generic predictors in non-emergency, non-cardiac surgery (Table 9.3) [9].

The ACC/AHA (American College of Cardiology/American Heart Association) algorithm and risk groups are derived from multiple studies, have not been evaluated prospectively against other indices and are more complex [8]. The Detsky and Goldman scores, ASA status and the Canadian Cardiovascular Society Index (CCSI) were all better than chance at predicting myocardial events [10]. The most reasonable approach seems to be to use the RCRI but to be aware of its limitations in that it does not take account of obstructive cardiac lesions or define ventricular wall motion abnormalities on echocardiography. The presence of regional wall motion abnormality correlates with ischaemia and has been shown to be a better predictor than electrocardiogram (ECG) monitoring for adverse cardiac events outcomes post-operatively [11, 12].

Additional testing and investigation as an adjunct to risk stratification may improve the predictive power [13]. There has been a tendency to use a single test such as an exercise ECG or echocardiogram to risk stratify patients, but such undirected investigations are not useful unless they answer a specific question centred around the risk stratification process. Modalities available include: cardiopulmonary exercise testing, 24-hour Holter monitoring, exercise electrocardiography, echocardiography, dobutamine stress echocardiography and stress magnetic resonance imaging (MRI), contrast ventriculography, thallium scintigraphy and angiography. To date, cardiac MRI has not been widely used as a routine test but may become more established. The tests allow us to focus resources on at-risk groups to define the extent of the disease or its morbidity, which then may allow us to direct and modify therapy [13].

9.3 Intervention strategies

Major surgery is associated with a significant inflammatory response, which to a certain extent is necessary to facilitate healing. There is general consensus that variables associated with oxygen delivery (DO_2I) and consumption are important determinants of survival from major surgery. The main strategies recommended to facilitate good outcome from major surgery are based on ensuring adequate DO_2I during the peri-operative period without causing further complications.

Cardiovascular interventions

The concept of augmenting cardiac output peri-operatively to improve the outcome of surgical patients has been described by many authors as 'optimisation' (Figure 9.1). The main aim of all optimisation strategies for high-risk surgical patients has been to ensure that the circulatory status of the patients is adequate for their needs in the peri-operative period. This has been achieved with a number of differing protocols using different time periods, resuscitation endpoints and pharmacological agents. There are little to no data describing the relative efficacy of different protocols, as they have nearly all been compared against 'standard' care.

$$\text{Oxygen delivery (ml/min)} = \text{Cardiac output (l/min)} \times \text{Oxygen content (ml/100 ml)}$$

$$\text{Oxygen content} = ([1.34 \times Hb \times (SaO_2/100)] + (0.023 \times PaO_2))$$

The theory behind resuscitation strategies to enhance cardiovascular performance in the peri-operative period is based on the equation describing DO_2I. Thus there are three factors of primary importance when managing high-risk patients: the haemoglobin (Hb) concentration, the arterial saturation of Hb with oxygen (SaO_2) and cardiac output. The target Hb concentration is determined by the clinical situation as well as the underlying pathophysiological process, but many authors would aim to keep the Hb level above 9 g/dl in a stable peri-operative setting [14]. SaO_2 is usually targeted to at least 95% using increased FiO_2 and/or continuous positive airways pressure (CPAP). There is increasing evidence that atelectasis in the post-operative period is associated with a pro-inflammatory response that potentiates tissue injury [13]. Recent data suggest that patients with post-operative atelectasis have better outcomes if this is reversed by CPAP in the immediate post-operative period [15–18].

Traditionally most investigators have measured cardiac output with a pulmonary artery catheter or more recently using an oesophageal Doppler probe or pulse contour analysis technique. If cardiac output is too low, strategies to increase it include optimisation of heart rate (HR), preload,

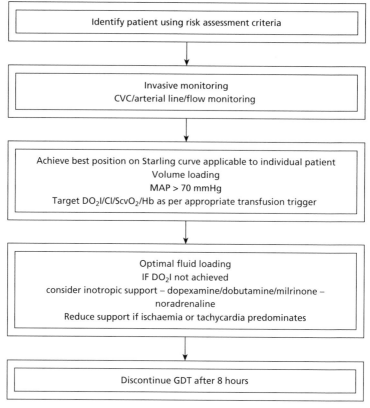

Figure 9.1 Generic flowchart for optimisation. CVC, central venous catheter; MAP, mean arterial pressure; DO_2I, oxygen delivery index; CI, cardiac index; $ScvO_2$, central mixed venous oxygen; Hb, haemoglobin; GDT, goal-directed therapy. (Modified from Tote and Grounds [19].)

afterload and use of inotropic drugs. The results of multiple studies support the use of peri-operative optimisation in elective surgical patients [20, 21].

The emphasis to date has been focused on oxygen supply and demand imbalance [22]. Sub-optimal values of cardiac index (CI), DO_2I and excessive oxygen consumption result in abnormal microcirculatory blood flow as a result of vasoconstriction in the capillary beds. Oxygen debt can exist in the presence of normal cardiac output, arterial blood gases and other indices of malperfusion [19, 22]. In addition, hypovolaemia may be present despite normal cardiac filling and systemic blood pressure [22].

Shoemaker utilised supra-physiological targets of CI, DO_2I and consumption [23] (4.5 l/min/m², $DO_2I > 600$ ml/min/m² and $VO_2 > 170$ ml/min/m²) and found that repayment of an incurred oxygen debt within 8 hours resulted in improved survival [20]. He derived these targets from previous work that had shown them to be the median levels of these variables in patients who survived from surgery. It was subsequently demonstrated, in elective major surgical patients, that if tissue oxygenation was inadequate ($DO_2I < 390$ l/min/m², the amount of oxygen delivered to the tissues related to the body surface area), the use of low-dose inotropes with fluid optimisation improved both mortality and morbidity [24]. It has been consistently shown that reductions in mortality and morbidity are obtained when supra-normal levels of DO_2I are achieved and that, in conjunction with decreased complications, there is a reduced length of hospital stay.

Despite this evidence there is continuing debate about which targets to pursue and how to achieve them. Not all patients will achieve the Shoemaker targets even with the techniques described above. For these patients an increase in DO_2I may still be beneficial, although it is unclear exactly how hard to drive them so that the complications do not outweigh any benefit accrued. Most successful trials have targeted an DO_2I of 600 ml/min/m². Other goals or targets include: maximal stroke volume (SV), central or mixed venous oxygen ($ScvO_2$) saturations and lactate concentration. Until other end-points of resuscitation have been proven to be better, it would be prudent to continue with targeting DO_2I. This contrasts with Hayes who suggests that in shocked patients, the ability to achieve these goals merely reflects their physiological reserve and that aggressive efforts to increase oxygen consumption may be deleterious [25].

Appropriate intravenous fluid administration is a cornerstone of post-operative optimisation (Figure 9.2). Excessive fluid administration is detrimental to critically ill and post-operative patients [22, 26–28]. Fluid administration and its effects must be monitored invasively where clinical signs of preload status are inadequate. Defining the point at which intravascular volume is optimal and the need for inotropic therapy begins is difficult. Plateauing of SV, maximising flow time as determined by oesophageal doppler, or minimising SV and blood pressure variation can all be used to optimise fluid loading. It seems intuitive and important that the endpoints of resuscitation are reached with minimal fluid and inotrope administration. Fluid response may be defined as those patients who raise their SV by 10% in response to a fluid challenge or, in the absence of invasive monitoring, sustain a rise in their central venous pressure of 2 mmHg for 20 minutes [4].

The timing of goal-directed therapy (GDT) may influence its efficacy. Most of the interventions that have had significant impacts on mortality have been started prior to surgery and continued throughout the peri-operative period. Due to resource constraints this has proved difficult to implement, so the effects of GDT administered either only during surgery or during the post-operative period have been studied. Although nearly all of these have also demonstrated benefit, the effects are not as dramatic as when intervention was started pre-operatively [29] (Figure 9.3; Rhodes, unpublished data). Whether this is a real effect or whether it is an artefact of study design is difficult to ascertain. It does seem sensible, however, to cover as much of the 'at risk' period as possible. In practice this means that GDT should be started as early as possible and continued until the patient is stable in the post-operative period. The duration, timing and setting of therapy will mandate the type of monitoring technology used, for

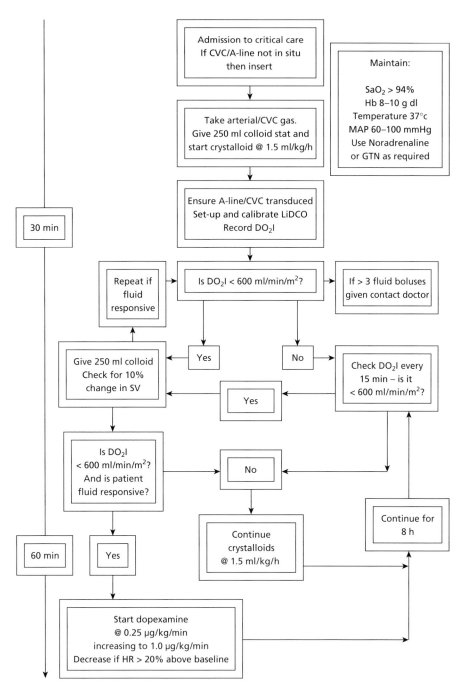

Figure 9.2 An example of a post-operative, goal-directed optimisation protocol from St George's Hospital, London. CVC, central venous catheter; MAP, mean arterial pressure; DO_2I, oxygen delivery index; SaO_2, saturation of Hb with oxygen; Hb, haemoglobin; A-line, arterial line; LiDCO, lithium dilution cardiac output monitoring; GTN, glyceryl trinitrate; SV, stroke volume; HR, heart rate. (Adapted from Tote and Grounds [19].)

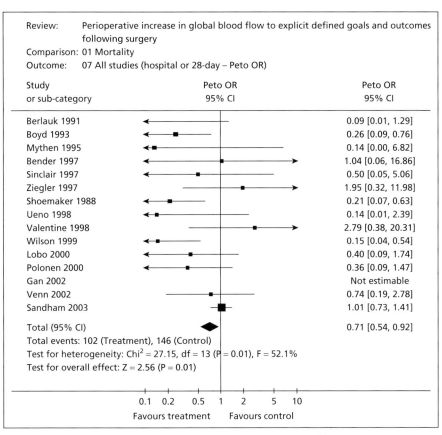

Review: Perioperative increase in global blood flow to explicit defined goals and outcomes
             following surgery
Comparison: 01 Mortality
Outcome: 07 All studies (hospital or 28-day – Peto OR)

Study or sub-category	Peto OR 95% CI	Peto OR 95% CI
Berlauk 1991		0.09 [0.01, 1.29]
Boyd 1993		0.26 [0.09, 0.76]
Mythen 1995		0.14 [0.00, 6.82]
Bender 1997		1.04 [0.06, 16.86]
Sinclair 1997		0.50 [0.05, 5.06]
Ziegler 1997		1.95 [0.32, 11.98]
Shoemaker 1988		0.21 [0.07, 0.63]
Ueno 1998		0.14 [0.01, 2.39]
Valentine 1998		2.79 [0.38, 20.31]
Wilson 1999		0.15 [0.04, 0.54]
Lobo 2000		0.40 [0.09, 1.74]
Polonen 2000		0.36 [0.09, 1.47]
Gan 2002		Not estimable
Venn 2002		0.74 [0.19, 2.78]
Sandham 2003		1.01 [0.73, 1.41]
Total (95% CI)		0.71 [0.54, 0.92]

Total events: 102 (Treatment), 146 (Control)
Test for heterogeneity: $Chi^2 = 27.15$, df = 13 (P = 0.01), $I^2 = 52.1\%$
Test for overall effect: Z = 2.56 (P = 0.01)

0.1   0.2   0.5   1   2   5   10
Favours treatment   Favours control

Figure 9.3 Meta-analysis of peri-operative optimisation. Peto OR Peto odds ratio.

instance awake patients do not readily tolerate the oesophageal Doppler probe. However, there is encouraging evidence that a softer nasal probe may be more bearable, thereby extending our monitoring capablitities [30].

Prevention of myocardial ischaemia

Patients should where possible have all co-morbidities, including ischaemic heart disease, treated prior to surgery. If a patient is at high risk of an ischaemic cardiac event peri-operatively, pre-operative treatment may include beta-blockade and in some instances coronary intervention [3]. There is little evidence to suggest a survival benefit with a revascularisation strategy. Godet demonstrated that in over 1,000 patients needing high-risk surgery, who underwent percutaneous coronary intervention (PCI), whilst the procedure could be performed safely, it conferred no benefit in terms of modifying risk [31]. The consensus opinion is that if revascularisation is required as part of the long-term management of angina, then it should be undertaken. However, there is no benefit in carrying out the procedure in order to facilitate non-cardiac surgery and may result in a poorer outcome, and stent placement should be avoided when possible [32–34].

The key issue, therefore, is the identification of the patients most likely to benefit. There are published clinical guidelines for investigation and treatment of this patient group [35]. A detailed examination is beyond the scope of this chapter, but in broad terms those individuals necessitating acute cardiological intervention, poor functional states – as defined by such tests as cardiopulmonary exercise testing or metabolic equivalents – coupled with clinical predictors of peri-operative risk mandate further investigation and stratification according to the classification of operative risk. The full description of clinical risk predictors is contained within the referenced AHA/ACC guidelines but include problems such as previous infarction, unstable angina, dysrhythmias, diabetes and renal failure [36, 37]. Several studies have demonstrated benefit from beta-blockade in highly selected patients considered to be most at risk of a peri-operative ischaemic event [38–40]. It is not appropriate to start beta-blocker therapy in all patients undergoing surgery; rather it should be reserved for the small subgroup of patients with active ischaemic heart disease who are the most likely to benefit [41, 42]. Even after patients have received beta-blockade therapy it is still vital to optimise fluid administration and monitor the cardiac output during and immediately after surgery. In cardiac patients it has recently been shown that chronic beta-blockade therapy has been associated with a decrease in 30-day mortality, although the precise benefit has yet to be elucidated [43] (a retrospective analysis of chronic beta-blockade in 1,586 patients undergoing coronary artery bypass surgery).

9.4 Conclusions

It is relatively easy to identify patients who are at high risk of significant complications following major surgery. There is good observational evidence linking poor tissue perfusion to these complications. There is also good evidence showing that augmentation of DO_2I in the peri-operative period can reduce both morbidity and mortality in these patients. This type of therapy mandates cardiac output monitoring and GDT, although there remains some controversy concerning the choice of appropriate goals.

In summary we should aim to achieve:

- Stratification of risk.
- Early aggressive GDT/optimisation/resuscitation (< 12 hours).
- Avoidance of tachycardia.
- Tailored goals according to individual physiological requirements/needs.
- Cardiac output/flow and biochemical marker monitoring.
- Care in a high-dependency area with sufficient numbers of adequately trained staff.

Case study

A 78-year-old man with a symptomatic 7-cm abdominal aortic aneurysm diagnosed on contrast enhanced computed tomography (CT) was admitted to ICU post-endovascular aortic aneurysm repair (EVAR) for optimisation. His co-morbidities included a non-ST elevation myocardial infarction 6 weeks previously, NHYA (New York Heart Association) III heart failure, limited exercise tolerance, chronic obstructive pulmonary disease (COPD) as evidenced by a protracted history of smoking and FEV1:FVC (forced expiratory volume in 1s:forced vital capacity) < 0.6, mild chronic renal failure (creatinine > 150 μmol/l), and mild anaemia. His medications included clopidogrel, aspirin, atenolol, perindopril and frusemide. He had significant right coronary disease (50% stenosis proximally and a distal 90% stenosis) with a dominant right coronary system. The cardiologist had elected for medical management of his disease symptoms and he was pain free at rest but had moderate exertion-induced angina.

Anaesthesia was induced uneventfully and he tolerated the stent placement with an estimated blood loss of 250–500 ml. He received 500 ml of gelofusine per-operatively. He was admitted to the ICU extubated, with saturations of 99% on 40% oxygen, but his central venous blood gas analysis showed a saturation of 55%, the base excess was −4 mmol/L, standard bicarbonate 22.3 mmol/L, lactate 2.2 mmol/L, pH 7.36, and Hb at this time was 8.7 g/dL. He was placed on lithium dilution cardiac ouput (LiDCO) monitoring in addition to standard monitoring and DO_2I was calculated to be 350 ml/min/m^2. Colloid (as blood and gelofusine) was titrated to central venous saturations > 70% and DO_2I 600 ml/min/m^2. His beta-blockade had been continued peri-operatively and chronotropic agents were avoided. His blood lactate, bicarbonate and base excess normalised within 4 hours. He received, in total, 1.25 L of colloid in 125- to 250-ml aliquots. He was discharged from a level 2 bed to a level 1 bed the following morning after 16 hours and subsequently was discharged uneventfully from the hospital.

References

1. *Quality and Performance in the NHS: NHS Performance Indicators.* London: NHS Executive; 2000.
2. Pearse R, Harrison D, James P, et al. Identification and characterisation of the high-risk surgical population in the United Kingdom. *Critical Care* 2006;10:R81.
3. Grayburn PA, Hillis LD. Cardiac events in patients undergoing noncardiac surgery: shifting the paradigm from noninvasive risk stratification to therapy. *Ann Intern Med* 2003;138:506–11.
4. Pearse R, Dawson D, Fawcett J, et al. Early goal-directed therapy after major surgery reduces complications and duration of hospital stay. A randomised, controlled trial (ISRCTN38797445). *Critical Care* 2005, 9:R687–93.

5. Goldman L, Caldera D, Nussbaum S, et al. Multifactorial index of cardiac risk in non-cardiac surgical procedures. *N Engl J Med* 1977;845–50.

6. Prause G, Ratzenhofer-Comenda B, Pierer G, et al. Can ASA grade or Goldman's cardiac risk index predict peri-operative mortality? A study of 16 227 patients. *Anaesthesia* 1997;52(3):203.

7. Detsky A, Abrams H, McLaughlin J, et al. Predicting cardiac complications in patients undergoing non-cardiac surgery. *J Gen Intern Med* 1986;1:211–9.

8. Lee T, Marcantonio E, Mangione C, et al. Derivation and prospective validation of a simple index for prediction of cardiac risk of major noncardiac surgery. *Circulation* 100:1043–9.

9. Devereaux P, Goldman L, Cook D, et al. Perioperative cardiac events in patients undergoing noncardiac surgery: a review of the magnitude of the problem, the pathophysiology of the events and methods to estimate and communicate risk. *CMAJ* 2005;173:627–34.

10. Gilbert K, Larocque B, Patrick L. Prospective evaluation of cardiac risk indices for patients undergoing noncardiac surgery. *Ann Intern Med* 2000;356–9.

11. Comunale M, Body S, Ley C, et al. The concordance of intraoperative left ventricular wall-motion abnormalities and electrocardiographic S-T segment changes: association with outcome after coronary revascularization. *Anesthesiology* 1998;88(4):945–54.

12. Leung J, O'Kelly B, Browner W, et al. Prognostic importance of postbypass regional wall-motion abnormalities in patients undergoing coronary artery bypass graft surgery. SPI Research Group. *Anesthesiology* 1989;71(1):16–25.

13. Davies SJ, Wilson RJT. Preoperative optimization of the high-risk surgical patient. *Br J Anaesth* 2004;93:121–8.

14. Hebert PC, Wells G, Blajchman MA, et al. A multicenter, randomized, controlled clinical trial of transfusion requirements in critical care. *N Engl J Med* 1999;340:409–17.

15. Duggan M, Kavanagh B. Atelectasis in the peri-operative patient. *Curr Opin Anaesthesiol* 2007;20(1):37–42.

16. Lellouche F. Noninvasive ventilation in patients with hypoxemic acute respiratory failure. *Curr Opin Crit Care* 2007;13(1):12–19.

17. Warner DO. Preventing postoperative pulmonary complications: the role of the anesthesiologist. *Anesthesiology* 2000;92:1467–72.

18. Squadrone V, Coha M, Cerutti E, et al. Continuous positive airway pressure for treatment of postoperative hypoxemia: a randomized controlled trial. *JAMA* 2005;293:589–95.

19. Tote S, Grounds M. Performing perioperative optimization of the high-risk surgical patient. *Br J Anaesth* 2006;97:4–11.

20. Goldhill D. Preventing surgical deaths: critical care and intensive care outreach services in the postoperative period. *Br J Anaesth* 2008;95:88–94.

21. Older P, Hall A, Grocott M, et al. Should perioperative management target oxygen delivery? *Br J Anaesth* 2004;92:597–8.

22. Grocott M, Mythen M, Michael G, et al. Perioperative fluid management and clinical outcomes in adults. *Anesth Analg* 2005;100:1093–106.

23. Shoemaker WC, Appel PL, Kram HB, et al. Prospective trial of supranormal values of survivors as therapeutic goals in high-risk surgical patients. *Chest* 1988;94:1176–86.

24. Wilson J, Woods I, Fawcett J. Reducing the risk of major elective surgery: randomised controlled trial of preoperative optimisation of oxygen delivery. *BMJ* 1999;318:1099–103.

25. Hayes M, Timmins AC, Yau EH, et al. Elevation of systemic oxygen delivery in the treatment of critically ill patients. *N Eng J Med* 1994;331(17):1160–1.

26. Joshi GP. Intraoperative fluid restriction improves outcome after major elective gastrointestinal surgery. *Anesth Analg* 2005;101:601–5.

27. The National Heart, Lung, and Blood Institute Acute Respiratory Distress Syndrome (ARDS) Clinical Trials Network. Pulmonary-artery versus central venous catheter to guide treatment of acute lung injury. *N Engl J Med* 2006;354:2213–24.

28. Lobo S, Lobo F, Polachini C, et al. Prospective, randomized trial comparing fluids and dobutamine optimization of oxygen delivery in high-risk surgical patients (ISRCTN42445141). *Crit Care* 2006;10:R72.

29. Kern JW, Shoemaker WC. Meta-analysis of hemodynamic optimisation in high-risk patients. *Crit Care Med* 2002;30:1686–92.

30. Walker D, Usher S, Hartin J, et al. Early experiences with the new awake oesophageal Doppler probe. *Br J Anaesth* 2004;93:471.

31. Godet G, Riou B, Bertrand M, et al. Does preoperative coronary angioplasty improve perioperative cardiac outcome? *Anesthesiology* 2005;102: 739–46.

32. Kaluza GL, Joseph J, Lee JR, et al. Catastrophic outcomes of noncardiac surgery soon after coronary stenting. *J Am Coll Cardiol* 2000;35:1288–94.

33. Wilson S, Fasseas P, Orford J, et al. Clinical outcome of patients undergoing non-cardiac surgery in the two months following coronary stenting. *J Am Coll Cardiol* 2003;42:234–40.

34. Howard-Alpe G, de Bono J, Hudsmith L, et al. Coronary artery stents and non-cardiac surgery. *Br J Anaesth* 2007;98:560–74.

35. Poidermans D, Bax JJ, Boersma E, et al. Guidelines for pre-operative cardiac risk assessment and perioperative cardiac management in non-cardiac surgery. *European Heart Journal* 2009;30:2769–2812.

36. Park K. Preoperative cardiology consultation. *Anesthesiology* 2003; 98(3):754–62.

37. Eagle K, Berger P, Calkins H, et al. ACC/AHA guideline update for perioperative cardiovascular evaluation for noncardiac surgery – executive summary: a report of the American College of Cardiology/American Heart Association Task Force on Practice Guidelines (Committee to Update the 1996 Guidelines on Perioperative Cardiovascular Evaluation for Noncardiac Surgery). *J Am Coll Cardiol* 2002;39:542–53.

38. Mangano D, Layug E, Wallace A, et al. Effect of atenolol on mortality and cardiovascular morbidity after noncardiac surgery. *N Engl J Med* 1996;335:1713–20.

39. Poldermans D, Boersma E, Bax JJ, et al. The effect of bisoprolol on perioperative mortality and myocardial infarction in high-risk patients undergoing vascular surgery. Dutch Echocardiographic Risk Evaluation Applying Stress Echocardiography Study Group. *N Engl J Med* 1999;341:1789–94.

40. Lindenauer PK, Pekow P, Wang K, et al. Perioperative beta-blocker therapy and mortality after major noncardiac surgery. *N Engl Med* 2005;353:349–61.

41. Palda V, Detsky A. Perioperative assesment and management of risk from coronary artery disease. *Ann Intern Med* 1997;313–28.

42. Fleisher L, Beckman J, Brown K, et al. ACC/AHA 2006 guideline update on perioperative cardiovascular evaluation for non-cardiac surgery: focused update on perioperative beta-blocker therapy. A report of the American College of Cardiology/American Heart Association Task Force on Practice

Guidelines (Writing Committee to Update the 2002 Guidelines on Perioperative Cardiovascular Evaluation for Noncardiac Surgery). *Circulation* 2006;113:2662–74.

43. ten Broecke PWC, de Hert SG, Mertens E, et al. Effect of preoperative ß-blockade on perioperative mortality in coronary surgery. *Br J Anaesth* 2003;90:27–31.

10 Adult Congenital Heart Disease: Principles of Management in Critical Care

Susanna Price and Brian Keogh

Royal Brompton & Harefield NHS Foundation Trust, London, UK

Take Home Messages

- Investigation and management of the critically ill adult congenital heart disease (ACHD) patient is complex and requires expertise from an appropriately trained multi-disciplinary team.
- The key to good management involves understanding the cardiopulmonary anatomy and physiology of each individual patient.
- Standard intensive care unit (ICU) parameters in the non-ACHD population may not be applicable in the ACHD patient.
- The response to standard ICU therapies may be unpredictable.

10.1 Introduction

Advances in surgical and interventional cardiological techniques have resulted in increasing numbers of patients with congenital heart disease surviving to adulthood [1]. It is estimated that in excess of 10 million people aged over 20 in the USA have congenital heart disease, and in the UK the number of adult patients with moderate–severe lesions is predicted to increase by around 1,600 per annum [2]. The majority of adult congenital heart disease (ACHD) patients that require ongoing specialist medical attention are at the more severe end of the disease spectrum, requiring repeated surgical interventions to replace prosthetic valves or conduits, and to address persistent or worsening abnormal haemodynamics. In addition, the high incidence of arrhythmias in those with complex congenital heart disease results in a large number of admissions for specialist electrophysiological interventions or repeated cardioversion. Many of these patients will require admission to the intensive care unit (ICU) for both cardiological and non-cardiological indications [3].

Cardiovascular Critical Care. Edited by M. Griffiths, J. Cordingley and S. Price.
© 2010 Blackwell Publishing Ltd.

Although many of the principles that underpin the investigation and management of patients in the general and cardiac ICU setting are equally applicable to the ACHD population, there are some important areas that require special consideration. For this reason, international recommendations suggest that specialist experience in specific aspects of cardiopulmonary physiology are crucial for those responsible for the care of critically ill AHCD patients [4]. In addition, whilst admitting that standard management principles apply to most patients with ACHD, these guidelines also suggest that certain trends in modern ICU management, particularly relating to fluid administration and systemic oxygen delivery, may not be well tolerated by this patient population. Consequently, some authorities suggest that certain ACHD patients should be managed in specialist cardiac centres, even when undergoing non-cardiac surgery [5]. However, with improved patient survival, and the small number of such specialist centres, it is inevitable that ACHD patients will present to their local hospitals for emergency care that will, on occasion, require ICU admission.

The aim of this chapter is to outline the general principles involved in the care of the critically ill ACHD patient, particularly where they differ from those of the general population. In addition, principles of the management of the more common medical indications for ICU admission will be discussed, together with those regarding the management of the ACHD patient following cardiac surgery.

10.2 Principles of management of the critically ill ACHD patient

General principles

Patients are generally classified as having simple, moderately complex and complex congenital heart disease (Table 10.1), according to the Canadian Consensus definitions [6]. ACHD patients are surviving longer, and the complexity of procedures undertaken is increasing [7]. In the critically ill ACHD patient, increasing complexity is associated with higher ICU morbidity and mortality [3]. The first principle of ACHD ICU management is to understand the cardiopulmonary anatomy. This involves knowledge of the primary lesion, any subsequent surgery or intervention and the presence of any residual haemodynamic lesions, either dynamic or fixed. Second, an understanding of the normal physiology of the patient is essential. This includes the "normal" haemoglobin, oxygen saturations, systemic and pulmonary blood pressure and surface electrocardiogram for that patient. Third, the ICU physician must consider how supportive and therapeutic interventions might affect the circulation. This is of particular importance in the univentricular heart, in the presence of systemic-pulmonary shunts and in the Fontan circulation. An example of the importance of understanding basic ACHD cardiopulmonary anatomy and physiology to enable correct patient management is given in the case study.

Table 10.1 Canadian Consensus Conference classification of disease complexity in ACHD.

Simple congenital heart disease

Native disease
Isolated congenital AV disease
Isolated congenital MV disease
Isolated PFO/ASD
Isolated small VSD
Mild pulmonic stenosis

Repaired conditions
Previously ligated/occluded PDA
Fully repaired secundum/SV ASD
Repaired VSD with residua

Moderately severe congenital heart disease
Aorto-left ventricular fistulae
Anomalous pulmonary venous drainage (partial or total)
Atrioventricular canal defects (partial or complete)
Ostium primum atrial septal defect
Pulmonary valve regurgitation (moderate to severe)
Patent ductus arteriosus (not closed)
Subvalvar or supravalvar aortic stenosis (except HOCM)
Ventricular septal defect with absent valve or valves
Sinus of Valsalva fistula/aneurysm
Infundibular right ventricular outflow obstruction of significance
RVOT obstruction
Coarctation of the aorta
Ebstein's anomaly
Tetralogy of Fallot
Aortic regurgitation
Mitral valve disease
Subaortic stenosis
Straddling TV/MV
Sinus venosus ASD

Complex congenital heart disease
Conduits, valved or non-valved
Cyanotic congenital heart (all forms)
Double-outlet ventricle
Eisenmenger's syndrome
Fontan procedure
Mitral atresia
Single ventricle (double inlet or outlet, common or primitive)
Pulmonary atresia (all forms)
Pulmonary vascular obstructive disease
Transposition of the great arteries
Tricuspid atresia
Truncus arteriosus/hemitruncus
Other abnormalities of atrioventricular or ventriculoarterial connection not included above

AV, aortic valve; MV, mitral valve; PFO, patent foramen ovale; ASD, atrial septal defect; VSD, ventricular septal defect; PDA, patent ductus arteriosus; SV ASD, sinus venosus ASD; HOCM, hypertrophic obstructive cardiomyopathy; RVOT, right ventricular outflow tract; TV, tricuspid valve.

In patients with ACHD (particularly where complex) performance of relatively simple investigations and interventions may differ from those in the non-ACHD population. In addition to the basic anatomy and physiology, there are further aspects relevant to ICU care that must be considered (Table 10.2). Close liaison between specialists in ACHD, heart failure, congenital cardiac surgeons and echocardiography is crucial as the management of such patients demands a multi-disciplinary approach [3]. As in the non-ACHD population, where no potentially reversible causes for deterioration exist, and there is no prospect of intervention or transplantation, the appropriateness of ICU admission should be considered.

Patients with cyanotic ACHD

Cyanotic ACHD is not a contra-indication to ICU admission as these patients may have a relatively good prognosis. Their mortality is usually related to the admission diagnosis, rather than the underlying diagnosis. The ICU physician should be aware of the normal physiological changes that occur in response to prolonged cyanosis and also the associated pathology.

The cyanotic ACHD patient will have developed adaptive mechanisms to increase oxygen delivery, including a rightward shift in the oxyhaemoglobin dissociation curve, an increase in cardiac output and an increased haematocrit [8]. The corresponding erythrocytosis may result in the hyperviscosity syndrome; however, routine venesection is not recommended and iron deficiency in these patients is common [8]. Haemostatic abnormalities are also common, and correlate with the level of erythrocytosis. Abnormalities in prothrombin time, partial thromboplastin time, factors V, VII, VIIII and IX, and thrombocytopaenia have been documented, but do not usually require treatment [8]. When assessing the cyanotic patient, citrate bottles adjusted for the haematocrit must be used. Bleeding is usually minor, but it may be life-threatening particularly if the patient is anticoagulated. In such circumstances, close liaison with haematological experts is essential.

Renal dysfunction is common ('blue kidneys') and occurs due to the combination of hyperviscosity with arteriolar vasoconstriction which results in renal hypoperfusion and progressive glomerulosclerosis. This may manifest as proteinuria, hyperuricaemia or varying degrees of renal failure. Any investigation of the cyanotic patient that requires intravenous contrast should be performed with the patient well hydrated, and using appropriate precautions to prevent further renal injury. In particular, those with renal failure are prone to developing marked hyperkalaemia following administration of contrast.

Finally, when a cyanotic patient is admitted with abnormal neurology, headache or post-ictal, a high index of suspicion should exist for cerebral abscess or haemorrhage.

The failing morphological right ventricle

The morphological right ventricle may be sub-pulmonary, sub-aortic or the only effective ventricle in the univentricular heart (see below). Causes of

Table 10.2 Common pathologies associated with congenital heart disease that may impact on ICU care. The more common associated pathology seen in the cardiovascular, pulmonary, gastro-intestinal, renal and endocrine systems are outlined, with potential implications for ICU investigation and management.

Cardiovascular	Pulmonary	Gastrointestinal/renal/endocrine
Absent or abnormal connections • Expected (Fontan/TCPC) • Unexpected (LSVC)	Intubation • Craniofacial abnormalities in associated syndromes may complicate	Associated anatomical defects • Asplenia • GI or renal malformation
Multiple previous cannulations • Challenging vascular access	Associated congenital pulmonary disease • Hypoplastic lung • Severe congenital V/Q mismatch	Cyanotic congenital heart disease • Associated renal impairment common
Potential/actual right–left shunting • Air filters required on all lines	Lung reperfusion injury post-operatively • ARDS/ALI-like picture • Unilateral/bilateral	Enteral feeding • Severe RHF may necessitate low feeding rates
Cardiac output measurement • Intracardiac shunt may complicate • No PA/R-sided connection • Small aorta may invalidate OD	Pulmonary hypertension • May not need treating per se • In presence of an inadequate CO, consider iNO, PC and sildenafil	Tolerance to fluid loading/restriction • Univentricular circulations require relatively full circulation • Acute RH dilatation may occur (i.e. Ebstein's anomaly)
Transvenous pacing • No access to R heart (i.e. Fontan/TCPC)	Tracheostomy • Presence of collateral blood vessels, abnormal neck anatomy	Liver function • Abnormal LFTs common post-operatively and associated with increased mortality
ECG interpretation • Atrial re-entry may mimic sinus tachycardia	Previous cardiac surgery • Phrenic nerve palsy	Thyroid function • Commonly abnormal in ACHD
Differential effects of vasoactive drugs on systemic/pulmonary vasculature • Unpredictable • May affect CO and saturations	Difficulty with ventilatory weaning • Associated congenital musculoskeletal deformities not uncommon	Haemoglobin • Cyanotic ACHD associated with erythrocytosis may necessitate more liberal transfusion policy

TCPC, total cavo-pulmonary connection; LSVC, persistent left-sided superior vena cava; GI, gastro-intestinal; V/Q, ventilation/perfusion; ARDS, adult respiratory distress syndrome; ALI, acute lung injury; RHF, right heart failure; PA, pulmonary artery; R-sided connection right-sided intracardiac connection; OD, oesophageal Doppler; CO, cardiac output; iNO, inhaled nitric oxide; PC, prostacyclin; RH, right heart; LFT, liver function test; ACHD, adult congenital heart disease.

right ventricular dysfunction include previous cardiac surgery, pulmonary hypertension, Ebstein's anomaly, a significant shunt, systemic right ventricle and volume overload. When in the sub-pulmonary position, the failing right ventricle may be supported using standard inotropic agents whilst avoiding pulmonary vasoconstrictors. Further, cardiac output may be maintained or improved by minimising right ventricular afterload optimising airway pressures in ventilated patients balanced against the development of basal collapse and hypoxaemia, aggressive drainage of pleural collections, bronchodilation, the use of pulmonary vasodilators and early extubation. In some centres, balloon counterpulsation in the pulmonary circulation is used [9]. Pulmonary hypertension, even if only moderate, should be treated if the cardiac output is inadequate in the context of right heart failure; inhaled nitric oxide, nebulised prostacyclin, and oral or intravenous sildenafil have been used with variable effect.

Where the morphological right ventricle is systemic (congenitally corrected transposition of the great arteries (ccTGA) and TGA after Mustard or Senning procedures) and failing, treatment is equally challenging (Figure 10.1). Reversible causes, including arrhythmia and volume overload, should be aggressively sought and treated. Although fibrosis of the systemic right ventricle in the adult is common, the coronary arteries are usually angiographically unobstructed. Standard management of the failing systemic ventricle should be used, including pharmacological and mechanical support, but these may be less effective than when used to treat the failing morphological left ventricle. Specifically, the use of intra-aortic balloon counter pulsation (particularly in younger patients) may be less useful, and the role of newer inodilators (e.g. Levosimendan) remains uncertain. In some centres the use of multi-site right ventricular pacing has been used with good effect. Management of the univentricular right ventricle that is failing is discussed in the next section.

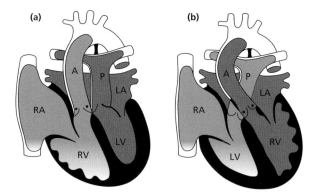

Figure 10.1 Variants of transposition. (**a**) Transposition of the great arteries, with normal atrio-ventricular connections but discordant ventriculo-atrial connections. (**b**) Congenitally corrected transposition of the great arteries, with discordant atrio-ventricular and ventriculo-atrial connections. RA, right atrium; RV, right ventricle; LA, left atrium; LV, left ventricle; A, aorta; P, pulmonary artery (See also colour plate 10.1).

The univentricular heart

Management of the failing univentricular heart presents many challenges, from prevention of air embolism, to the unpredictability of the effects of vasoactive agents and the adverse effects of positive pressure ventilation. All patients at risk of paradoxical embolism should have filters placed on lines, with scrupulous care to avoid entrainment of air when placing central and peripheral venous lines. It is important to know the current and most recently documented function of the single ventricle (morphologically right or left), as recent rapid deterioration is often caused by an arrhythmia. Assessment of function of the univentricular heart may be difficult, particularly in the presence of inotropic support. Expert echocardiography is indicated in this situation.

When considering the use of inotropic and vasoactive agents, the nature of the pulmonary connections must be considered. The unprotected pulmonary circulation with Eisenmenger physiology should be managed so as to minimise any further increase in pulmonary artery pressures. Where the pulmonary vasculature is protected by pulmonary artery banding, the relative effects of pulmonary versus systemic constriction or dilatation may be different when compared with cases where there is an absent pulmonary connection with systemic-pulmonary collaterals or shunts (Figure 10.2). In the patient with absent pulmonary connection and systemic-pulmonary collaterals/shunts, a small increase in pulmonary vascular resistance (PVR) may result in a significant reduction in pulmonary blood flow and dramatic desaturation. In contrast, an increase in systemic vascular resistance (SVR) or a fall in PVR may result in an increase in systemic-pulmonary shunting with fall in cardiac output. Attention should also be paid to oxygen administration; this may also alter the balance between pulmonary and systemic circulation. Thus, any vasoactive drug should be used with care as

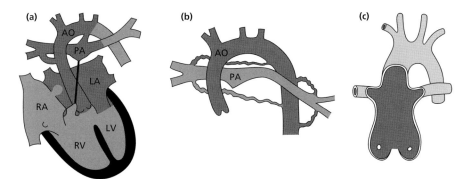

Figure 10.2 Examples of systemic-pulmonary shunts. (**a**) Pulmonary atresia plus VSD – here, pulmonary blood flow is via a patent ductus arteriosus. (**b**) Pulmonary atresia with blood supply to confluent pulmonary arteries from sytemic-pulmonary collaterals. (**c**) Common arterial trunk, where there is a common valve and arterial trunk from the ventricles, giving rise to the left and right pulmonary arteries from the ascending aorta. RA, right atrium; RV, right ventricle; LA, left atrium; LV, left ventricle; PA, pulmonary artery; AO, aorta (See also colour plate 10.2).

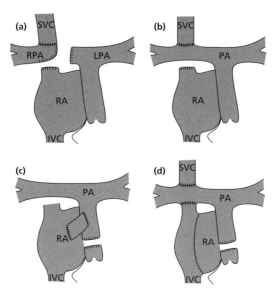

Figure 10.3 Different types of venous anastamosis used in patients with absent or deficient right-sided connections. (**a**) Classical Glenn. (**b**) Bidirectional Glenn. (**c**) Atrio-pulmonary Fontan. (**d**) Total cavo-pulmonary connection (TCPC) – lateral tunnel. RA, right atrium; IVC, inferior vena cava; RPA, right pulmonary artery; LPA, left pulmonary artery; SVC, superior vena cava (See also colour plate 10.3).

the results may be unpredictable. The univentricular heart with absent right-sided venous connections (including the Fontan and Fontan-type circulation; see Figure 10.3) presents a specific challenge to the intensivist, and is discussed in more detail below.

10.3 Anaesthesia in the critically ill ACHD patient

General principles

The 2003 report of the European Society of Cardiology Task Force on the Management of Grown-Up Congenital Heart Disease stated that there was little evidence-based information regarding the choice of anaesthetic technique in ACHD patients undergoing cardiac and non-cardiac procedures [10]. Despite subsequent publication of several reviews, evidence still remains limited [11, 12] and thus practice remains based largely on personal or institutional preference. A well-compensated, stable ACHD patient requiring anaesthesia for a non-cardiological and unrelated indication in ICU (e.g. limited trauma management) can usually be managed successfully without anaesthetic difficulty. Although many ACHD patients are young and appear to be well, despite profound circulatory abnormalities, there is in some patient groups great potential for profound destabilisation under anaesthesia. Thus anaesthetists undertaking such procedures should be experienced and familiar with the pathophysiology of the patient as well as the agents and techniques they elect to use.

Anaesthetic assistance and patient monitoring in critical care

Guidelines relevant to the conduct of 'minor' procedures in the ICU state that anaesthetists must have dedicated qualified assistance wherever anaesthesia is administered, whether in the operating department or any other area [13]. Minimum standards of patient monitoring for induction and maintenance of anaesthesia include the following [14]:

- Pulse oximeter
- Non-invasive blood pressure monitor
- Electrocardiograph
- Airway gas monitoring: oxygen, carbon dioxide and anaesthetic vapour
- Airway pressure

The following must also be available:

- A nerve stimulator whenever a muscle relaxant is used
- A means of measuring the patient's temperature

In the ACHD patient, invasive arterial pressure should also be considered in the emergency situation or in patients with limited reserve. Central venous access may also be indicated, particularly if transvenous pacing might be required.

Induction of anaesthesia

The choice of induction agent in ACHD patients is less important than the dose chosen and speed of administration. Slow injection, possibly over several minutes, taking into account delayed circulation time and both negative inotropic and systemic vasodilatory effects, is prudent. Although propofol is still most commonly used for induction, etomidate is perceived to have less hypotensive effects and is preferred by many experienced ACHD anaesthetists for induction, particularly in those with limited reserve. Ketamine, used more widely in paediatric congenital practice, may also be preferred in such patients due to its maintenance of sympathetic tone, although its use in adults is limited by dysphoria and post-procedural nightmares. Opiates are not normally administered as part of the induction process in ACHD patients until the haemodynamic effects of the induction agent have been fully assessed.

Regardless of the choice of induction agent, alpha-adrenergic agonists or another vasoconstrictor must be prepared in advance and used if necessary to modulate reductions in vascular resistance, either by small repeated bolus injections of metaraminol ($10-20$ µg) or phenylephrine ($2-5$ µg) or, more appropriately in the decompensating patient, by low-dose adrenaline infusion (usually $0.02-0.05$ µg/kg/min).

Maintenance of anaesthesia

Options for maintenance of anaesthesia in the ICU setting include propofol infusion alone or supplemented with short-acting opiates. Volatile agents, typically sevoflurane, may safely be employed if appropriate facilities for delivery are available.

Neuromuscular blockade
A procedure that mandates tracheal intubation may be facilitated by short-acting muscle relaxants. Vecuronium or similar agents that do not cause tachycardia or liberate histamine are usually preferred.

Analgesia
Adequate analgesia must be administered during any procedure and also for post-procedural comfort. Systemic analgesics should be employed according to local practice and include intravenous paracetamol. Systemic non-steroidal anti-inflammatory agents should be used with care in ACHD patients, who are often anticoagulated and at risk of adverse renal effects. Alternative anaesthesic modalities, including local nerve block, should always be considered.

Procedures on intubated and sedated patients
In patients already intubated and receiving ongoing sedation in the ICU, anaesthetic supplementation is likely to be required for minor diagnostic and interventional procedures. The options available include administration of an appropriately reduced bolus of an anaesthetic induction agent followed by its infusion and/or supplementation with potent short-acting narcotics. Alternatively, a short-term increase in benzodiazepine administration may be used, although there is an incidence of recall if these agents are used alone. Short-term vasoconstrictors may also be required. The principles of post-procedure analgesia techniques also apply in these patients.

Elective cardioversion in the ACHD population
Anaesthesia for cardioversion represents the most frequent call for anaesthesia services in ACHD patients in the ICU. The anaesthetic principles are generally applicable to other minor or short procedures. In general, the following recommendations apply to any patient undergoing cardioversion [15]:
- Resuscitation equipment must be checked within the previous 24 hours – or since any other resuscitation event.
- External pacing equipment must be available.
- Anticoagulated patients must have a current therapeutic coagulation result.
- All patients should have current electrolyte results.
- Cardioversion devices with biphasic waveforms should be used.

Four additional considerations apply to the ACHD population:
- Patients with poorly tolerated arrhythmias or degrees of heart failure represent a considerable anaesthetic challenge.
- Profound haemodynamic collapse following induction of anaesthesia may occur, in particular in those with a univentricular circulation.
- ACHD patients with cyanotic heart disease or effectively univentricular circulation tolerate hypovolaemia poorly, and intravenous fluids should normally be started at the time the patient is required to be nil by mouth.

● Some patients may have no means of transvenous access to the heart (i.e. Fontan, total cavo-pulmonary connection (TCPC)). Here, it is crucial that external pacing is available and functioning, and the operator performing cardioversion is fully trained in its use.

Recently the use of trans-oesophageal echocardiography (TOE) in conjunction with cardioversion has greatly increased, and is now almost universal in the ACHD population. The anaesthetic duration may thus be prolonged and ongoing maintenance of anaesthesia required. Anaesthetic options include tracheal intubation with muscle relaxant, a laryngeal mask airway (removed and re-sited after TOE insertion) and remifentanil infusion with or without tracheal intubation. The choice of technique will be largely dictated by the individual anaesthetist's assessment of the patient. Where 3D TOE is required, tracheal intubation provides a superior technique, facilitating breath-holding for image acquisition. Intravenous paracetamol should be administered to patients undergoing cardioversion and topical ibuprofen 5% cream applied prophylactically [16].

Emergency electrophysiological interventions

A more challenging scenario is the ACHD patient admitted emergently to the ICU with poorly tolerated arrhythmia and associated haemodynamic collapse. These patients require immediate stabilisation including anti-arrhythmic therapy with attention to electrolyte and fluid balance disturbances, and usually (if no automated internal cardioverter defibrillator (AICD) in situ) early external cardioversion.

The anaesthetic issues associated with such a presentation are challenging and complicated. Inotropic support may be indicated, but may also drive the arrhythmia. Induction of anaesthesia is usually accompanied by significant hypotension, but in the presence of significant systemic atrio-ventricular valve regurgitation, both vasoconstriction and further fluid administration may be deleterious. TOE should be used to direct ongoing management, but a degree of systemic vasodilatation and resultant hypotension may need to be tolerated in these patients. Specifically, the benefits of further fluid administration to patients with signs of cardiac failure must be carefully considered before administration. Intra-aortic balloon counter pulsation may be indicated, especially in refractory ventricular arrhythmia; however, in patients with chronically low cardiac output states, insertion may be challenging due to the small dimensions of the systemic vessels, and the benefit limited by tachycardia.

Thus, the degree of achievable stabilisation may be less than desired and anti-arrhythmic therapy poorly effective or limited by adverse haemodynamic effects. In practice, such arrhythmias are poorly tolerated and the therapeutic window may be short; in such a situation, there may be little option other than to resuscitate the patient as feasible and then transfer him or her to the catheter laboratory.

Elective electrophysiogical interventions

Complicated electrophysiological interventions are increasingly undertaken in ACHD patients for a variety of arrhythmias. The often-complex anaesthetic management of these patients in the catheter laboratory is outside the scope of this chapter, but of relevance is that patients with complex ACHD undergoing such elective interventions are ideally recovered in the ICU. Despite their apparently stable pre-intervention condition, such patients may suffer recurrent periods of poorly tolerated arrhythmia and low cardiac output during the electrical mapping or treatment phases, superimposed on already limited cardiac reserve. A minority may require ongoing high level ICU support. It is vital that appropriate level post-operative care facilities are organisationally integrated and predictably available.

Specific ACHD conditions and anaesthesia in the ICU

The ACHD anaesthetist encounters a wide variety of conditions. Several more common or challenging issues deserve specific consideration.

Systemic-pulmonary shunts.

Induction of anaesthesia and the resultant hypotension may result in reduced pulmonary blood flow and desaturation requiring systemic vasoconstriction with volume resuscitation.

Pulmonary hypertension.

Patients with moderate and certainly severe pulmonary hypertension represent an anaesthetic challenge. A further rise in pulmonary vascular resistance must be avoided; thus ventilation with high inspired oxygen to at least normocapnia, maintaining alveolar stability while avoiding high airway pressures and preventing metabolic acidosis are the sometimes difficult-to-apply principles. Severe pulmonary hypertension is often fixed and in this scenario further ventilatory manipulation will have little favourable effect. The combination of the negative inotropic effect of anaesthesia and systemic vasodilatation, which may create a mismatch of oxygen supply and demand across the right ventricle (with an already fixed high afterload), may be catastrophic. If anaesthesia is required in such patients, systemic vasodilatation must be counteracted by administration of systemic vasoconstrictors. Invasive arterial monitoring is nearly always mandatory in patients with severe pulmonary hypertension.

The same principles apply in the anaesthetic management of patients with Eisenmenger's syndrome. Such patients will exhibit some degree of baseline cyanosis but may become profoundly desaturated with systemic vasodilatation due to increased right to left shunting. Pulse oximetry must be secure and reliable in such patients and can be used to titrate administration of vasoconstrictors in very short procedures. Arterial access is desirable for anything other than minor procedures.

Fontan circulation

This circulation (Figure 10.3) is considered in detail in Chapter 16. Patients with Fontan circulations may present for several reasons, and often with arrhythmia requiring urgent cardioversion if decompensation and intra-cardiac thrombus formation are to be avoided. If the systemic ventricle is failing and the systemic atrio-ventricular valve is regurgitant, further fluid administration and vasoconstriction in response to anaesthesia-induced systemic vasodilatation will probably prove disastrous. In contrast, if the Fontan circulation is obstructed or PVR is high and the systemic atrial pressure is low, systemic vasoconstriction may be appropriate along with pulmonary vasodilators. Fluid administration may also be appropriate, and the presence of a fenestration between left and right heart circulation may facilitate anaesthetic management in this context. Ventilatory strategies should aim to reduce PVR (high FiO_2, low $paCO_2$ and low mean airway pressures), and extra-pulmonary collections, which are common in the failing Fontan, should be aggressively sought and drained.

10.4 Medical indications for ICU admission

Mortality in ACHD patients requiring admission to the ICU for medical indications (excluding arrhythmia) is high (36%) and accurately predicted by the APACHE II score [3]. In contrast, although arrhythmia is a common indication for acute deterioration of the ACHD patient, even when ICU admission is indicated, the mortality is generally low. Where the indication for admission is non-cardiological, the principles of management of the admission diagnosis do not differ from the non-ACHD population. The attending intensivist must always consider the underlying cardiopulmonary pathophysiology, and the principles of management as described above should be applied in parallel.

Arrhythmia

The commonest indication for medical admission in the ACHD population is arrhythmia, and on occasion this will require ICU admission, or input from the critical care team. The management of arrhythmia in the ACHD ICU population is covered in Chapter 17 in detail; however, some principles warrant particular mention. The diagnosis of an arrhythmia may be challenging; for example, atrial tachycardia may mimic sinus tachycardia. Comparison with previous 12-lead ECGs and interrogation of implanted pacemakers may be critical in making the diagnosis. Given the high incidence of thyroid dysfunction and amiodarone prescription, thyroid function tests should be performed upon diagnosis of a tachycardia or bradycardia. Although patients with a univentricular circulation in atrial tachycardia may tolerate a tachyarrhythmia well initially, decompensation may be rapid, and cardioversion should be considered at the earliest opportunity. Cardioversion to a malignant arrhythmia is not uncommon, and as there may be no venous access to the heart, transvenous pacing may be impossible and transcutaneous pacing should always be available.

Heart failure

The causes of heart failure in the ACHD population that require ICU admission include one or more of the following: impaired ventricular function, volume overload, arrhythmia, stenotic lesions or an excessive shunt. The principles of management of heart failure in these patients are in essence those that underpin the management of non-congenital patients with heart failure: primarily circulatory support to maintain cardiac output and exclusion of treatable causes. Once an arrhythmia has been excluded, echocardiography is required to make or confirm the precise anatomical diagnosis and determine the cause of inadequate cardiac output.

Where indicated, urgent surgical or catheter intervention may be required. Pre-optimisation of cardiac output prior to surgical intervention has not been shown to improve patient survival, but as with non-ACHD patients, pulmonary oedema and sepsis should be treated prior to surgery. Once surgically or catheter-directed correctable causes have been excluded, management is directed to treating ventricular dysfunction. The principles of treatment of sub-systemic morphological left ventricular failure are as for the non-ACHD population, including the use of inodilators, and device therapy. As mentioned previously, younger patients may not benefit from intra-aortic balloon pump (IABP) counter pulsation, and where the aorta is small due to a chronically low cardiac output, insertion may be challenging. The management of right and univentricular failure is described above.

Haemoptysis

Haemoptysis in this population, particularly those with pulmonary hypertension, should always be considered a serious event and early transfer to high-level care should be considered. A minor haemoptysis may herald a major bleed, and patients with major haemoptysis usually die from airway obstruction rather than blood loss. Haemoptysis in the ACHD population has been attributed to bronchitis, bleeding diathesis, pulmonary arterial rupture, pulmonary embolism, tracheo-arterial fistula (in prolonged intubation or tracheostomy) and rupture of aorto-pulmonary collaterals. In patients with Eisenmenger physiology, haemoptysis accounts for 11–15% of deaths [17]. Investigation will depend upon the skills available locally, but would normally include plain chest radiography, bronchoscopy, computed tomography (CT) angiography and embolisation, which may be life-saving.

Endocarditis

Endocarditis as a primary indication for ICU admission indicates a high level of valve destruction leading to significant haemodynamic abnormalities. The diagnosis of endocarditis requires physicians to have a high index of suspicion, the performance of multiple blood cultures and expert echocardiography. Echocardiography to exclude endocarditis in this patient population is particularly challenging as it may not be confined to intra-cardiac structures. Infection has been reported on conduits, shunts, sites of previous coarctation repair, aortic cannulation sites, pacemaker wires and ventricular surgical vent sites. It is unusual to see vegetations on mechanical valves; often the only echocardiographic evidence of endocarditis is a new paraprosthetic leak. On occasion, nuclear medicine (white cell scanning) or cardiac magnetic resonance scanning may give further indication as to the site of infection. Management of endocarditis is as in the non-ACHD population; however, discussion with congenital surgeons should be undertaken at an early stage following diagnosis.

10.5 Post-operative admissions

The majority of ACHD patients who are admitted to the ICU will be post-operative, and the complexity of both the cases undertaken and of the underlying cardiac disease is increasing [7]. In post-operative patients, the mortality relates to the complexity of the underlying disease; however, unlike in medical ACHD admissions, standard scoring systems do not reflect the severity of illness of the patients, as they tend to overestimate mortality in those with more simple disease, and underestimate predicted mortality in those with more complex disease (Figure 10.4) [3].

In specialist centres peri-operative mortality and morbidity is low, but increases significantly with increasing disease complexity, and in the presence of pre-operative abnormalities in renal, liver or thyroid function [3]. As in the paediatric population, haemodynamically significant residual lesions post-operatively are associated with a significantly increased ICU morbidity. Mortality and morbidity for the more complex or numerous groups of ACHD patients undergoing surgery in a cardiac centre are shown in Table 10.3. As with all cardiac surgical patients, good post-operative management relies on a clear understanding of not only the underlying

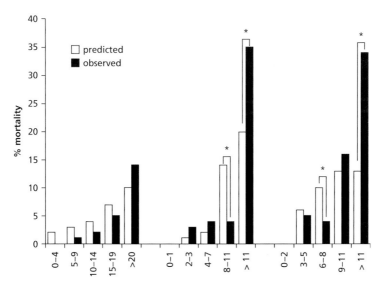

Figure 10.4 Graphs comparing observed outcomes of surgery in ACHD patients shown as a function of pre-operative risk assessment using the Parsonnet, Logistic EuroSCORE and Ontario systems. Scores are divided into low/fair/moderate/high/extremely high risk categories. Asterisks denote $p < 0.05$ [3].

Table 10.3 Underlying cardiac diagnosis and outcome in patients with ACHD requiring ICU admission. Number of patients, duration of ICU/hospital admission and mortality are shown by disease category [3].

Diagnosis	Number of admissions	ICU admission (days)	Ward admission (days)	Hospital mortality n (%)	Two-year mortality n (%)
Aortic valve (AV)	56	†1.4 + 0.2	*10.0 + 1.4	0 (0%)	0 (0%)
AV + other disease	27	†1.6 + 0.2	10.0 + 1.1	0 (0%)	0 (0%)
Sub-aortic stenosis	12	†1.1 + 0.3	6.8 + 2.7	0 (0%)	0 (0%)
Coarctation of aorta	19	3.2 + 1.2	10.2 + 1.2	0 (0%)	0 (0%)
Secundum ASD	53	†1.5 + 0.3	8.6 + 0.5	0 (0%)	0 (0%)
VSD	14	†1.4 + 0.1	6.3 + 0.8	0 (0%)	0 (0%)
Sinus venosus ASD	9	1.8 + 0.6	6.6 + 1.2	0 (0%)	0 (0%)
AVSD	24	6.3 + 3.5	10.2 + 0.8	1 (4.2%)	1 (4.2%)
Tetralogy of Fallot	35	5.0 + 1.1	9.5 + 0.9	2 (5.6%)	3 (8.3%)
Ebstein's anomaly	8	3.4 + 0.7	*13.7 + 2.6	1 (12.5%)	1 (12.5%)
Pulmonary stenosis	6	†1.0 + 0.2	8.8 + 2.6	1 (17%)	1 (17%)
PA + VSD	21	4.5 + 0.3	*20.5 + 3.2	2 (10%)	4 (20%)
Fontan circulation	14	6.9 + 4.0	*21.2 + 2.3	3 (21.4%)	5 (35.7%)
TGA	11	4.2 + 1.2	12.1 + 3.1	1 (9.1%)	2 (18.1%)
CcTGA	11	9.0 + 5.2	*22.0 + 1.7	2 (20%)	2 (20%)
Eisenmenger	6	1.5 + 0.4	7.3 + 1.8	1 (16.7%)	1 (16.7%)
Left atrial isomerism	4	3.4 + 0.5	*15.5 + 4.0	0 (0%)	0 (0%)
Other ACHD	12	3.1 + 2.5	*16.0 + 3.2	1 (8.3%)	1 (8.3%)
Non-ACHD	6315	5.7 + 0.1	7.4 + 0.1	215 (4.0%)	not available

Data are shown as mean ± SEM.
* Significant increase. † Significant reduction when compared with non-ACHD patients, $p < 0.05$.
AV, aortic valve disease; ASD, atrial septal defect; VSD, ventricular septal defect; AVSD, atrio-ventricular septal defect; PA + VSD, pulmonary atresia and ventricular septal defect; TGA, transposition of the great arteries; ccTGA, congenitally corrected transposition of the great arteries/double discordance, Eisenmenger Eisenmenger physiology; Other ACHD, other adult congenital heart disease; Non-ACHD, acquired heart disease.

disease, but also the precise surgical procedure and outcome, and also the haemodynamic responses of the patient in the operating theatre. Close liaison with and detailed handover from the operating surgeon and cardiac anaesthetist are essential.

Simple congenital heart disease
Aortic valve and root disease
Abnormalities of the left heart constitute the majority of post-operative cardiac surgical admissions and have an extremely low ICU mortality and morbidity, even with the high percentage of multiple re-operations seen in this patient group (Table 10.3). Although ACHD patients undergoing aortic surgery have a relatively high requirement for re-exploration for bleeding or tamponade and permanent pacemaker insertion, the requirement for prolonged or sophisticated ICU support is relatively low (Figure 10.5a and b) [3].

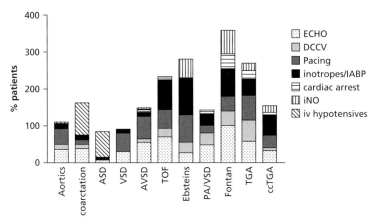

Figure 10.5a Graph denoting cardiovascular investigations/interventions in post-operative patients. Data are shown by diagnostic category and expressed as a cumulative percentage of total surgical ACHD patients admitted to ICU. Aortics, aortic valve disease; ASD, atrial septal defect; VSD, ventricular septal defect; AVSD, atrio-ventricular septal defect; TOF, tetralogy of Fallot, Ebsteins Ebstein's anomaly of the tricuspid valve; PA/VSD, pulmonary atresia with ventricular septal defect, Fontan previous or current Fontan circulation; TGA, transposition of the great arteries; ccTGA, congenitally corrected transposition of the great arteries/double discordance; INO, inhaled nitric oxide; DCCV, cardioversion; ECHO, echocardiography.

Aortic coarctation

Adult patients undergoing surgical coarctation repair have a low ICU mortality and morbidity, whether as primary or repeat operation. The main indication for remaining in the ICU is the requirement for close control of rebound arterial hypertension that may require intravenous hypotensive agents (Figure 10.5b). Mesenteric arteritis possibly due to the institution of pulsatile flow has been reported [18]. In some centres, enteric feeding is witheld for 24 hours post-procedure to avoid gastro-intestinal ischaemia. An additional rare but serious complication is spinal neurological damage. The use of cerebrospinal fluid drainage following thoracoabdominal aortic surgery has reduced the incidence of neurological injury [19] and there are numerous anecdotal reports of the use of this strategy following less extensive surgery [20]. The role of cerebrospinal fluid drainage following either open repair or endovascular stenting of coarctation in the ACHD population is unknown. Where a patient is suspected of having spinal cord damage after surgery it may be worth considering this intervention, although its mechanism of potential benefit differs and it is as yet unproven [21].

Atrial septal defect

The treatment of choice for closure of a simple atrial septal defect (ASD) (Figure 10.6) is percutaneous device closure; however, some large or complex defects will require surgical closure. Although in the younger ACHD patient population the procedure (either percutaneous or open surgical) is well tolerated, there is a high incidence of post-operative arrhythmia (tachy- and bradycardia). Pulmonary hypertension recorded

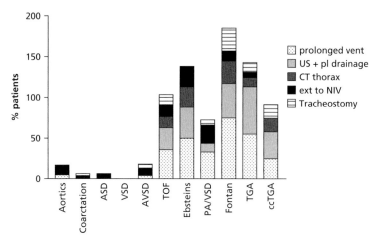

Figure 10.5b Graph denoting respiratory investigations/interventions in post-operative patients. Data are shown by diagnostic category and expressed as a cumulative percentage of total surgical ACHD patients admitted to ICU. Aortics, aortic valve disease; ASD, atrial septal defect; VSD, ventricular septal defect; AVSD, atrio-ventricular septal defect; TOF, tetralogy of Fallot, Ebsteins Ebstein's anomaly of the tricuspid valve; PA/VSD, pulmonary atresia with ventricular septal defect, Fontan previous or current Fontan circulation; TGA, transposition of the great arteries; ccTGA, congenitally corrected transposition of the great arteries/ double discordance.

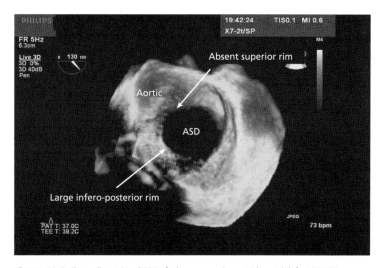

Figure 10.6 Three-dimensional TOE of a large secundum atrial septal defect (ASD) in a patient prior to surgical closure. The image is taken from the left atrium, looking through the ASD into the right atrium. (See also colour plate 10.4)

pre-operatively may not resolve immediately and in the presence of an adequate cardiac output will not require treatment. The more elderly patient may have restrictive ventricular disease (right and/or left) which limits cardiac output. Where this is diagnosed, pacing should be optimised

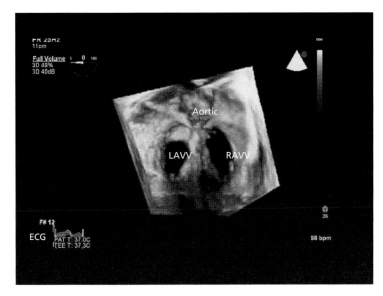

Figure 10.7 Three-dimensional TOE of a patient with an unoperated partial atrio-ventricular septal defect (AVSD). The image is shown from the roof of the atria, looking down on the two separate orifices of the atrio-ventricular valves during diastole. Note the absence of inter-atrial septum and abnormal anatomical arrangement of the aortic valve with respect to the atrio-ventricular valves. LAVV, left atrio-ventricular valve; RAVV, right atrio-ventricular valve; Aortic, aortic valve; ECG, electrocardiogram. (See also colour plate 10.5).

using echocardiography and continuous cardiac output monitoring to optimise the cardiac output. This may require heart rates of up to 130 beats per minute.

Moderately complex congenital heart disease
Atrio-ventricular septal defect
Complete atrio-ventricular septal defect (AVSD) (Figure 10.7) repair is usually performed in childhood; however, some adults may present with partial defects requiring surgical repair. In such patients, the most important determinant of outcome is a successful surgical repair – in particular ensuring the absence of left ventricular outflow tract obstruction (LVOTO). Where a patient has inadequate cardiac output post-operatively, in addition to exclusion of the usual post-operative complications, LVOTO should specifically be excluded using echocardiography, particularly where the fall in cardiac output is associated with increasing inotropic support. Although these patients do not usually have prolonged ICU admission, their requirement for specialist investigation and intervention post-operatively is relatively high (Figure 10.5a and b).

Tetralogy of Fallot
Patients admitted post-operatively with a diagnosis of tetralogy of Fallot (TOF) (Figure 10.8) will either have undergone redo-surgery (usually

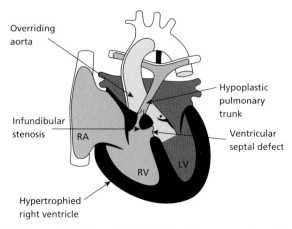

Figure 10.8 Unoperated tetralogy of Fallot, with the various components marked. In addition to the classical four components, there are frequently abnormalities of the pulmonary valve and/or pulmonary trunk (as shown). RA, right atrium; RV, right ventricle; LV, left ventricle. (See also colour plate 10.6).

pulmonary valve replacement) or, less frequently, primary repair. Although primary repair in the adult population is associated with significant ICU morbidity, even redo-surgery for pulmonary valve replacement should not be regarded as 'routine' (Figure 10.2). Complications and morbidity are usually associated with right ventricular dysfunction (redo-surgery); however, significant left ventricular dysfunction may co-exist, particularly in the presence of significant coronary artery disease. In patients undergoing primary repair the increased pulmonary blood flow may result in pulmonary capillary hyperpermeability, presenting with an ARDS-like picture, and managed as is standard for acute lung injury post-bypass (Chapter 11).

Ebstein's anomaly

The post-operative course of these patients is determined by the function of the post-operative right ventricle, meticulous intra-operative management (surgical and anaesthetic) and the technical expertise of the surgeon. Where there is significant right ventricular dysfunction, this should be managed in the standard way. Significant post-operative right ventricular dysfunction is associated with a high incidence of renal, gastrointestinal and hepatic dysfunction, and a significant requirement for prolonged respiratory support (Figure 10.5b). If the cardiac output is inadequate despite all measures and an intra-atrial communication does not exist, atrial fenestration may be considered if left ventricular function is thought to be adequate. The post-operative Ebstein's patient has a high incidence of atrial arrhythmias and these should be managed in collaboration with an electrophysiologist (see Chapter 17).

Complex congenital heart disease
Congenitally corrected transposition of the great arteries (ccTGA, Figure 10.1b)

Tricuspid valve replacement (the systemic atrio-ventricular valve) due to regurgitation is the most commonly performed operation in adult patients with ccTGA. In such cases, the added burden of significant volume overload on the systemic, morphologically right ventricle may result in significant ventricular dysfunction post-operatively. This should be managed as described in Section 2, 'The failing morphological right ventricle', and its relevance to post-operative management is seen in the high requirement for post-operative cardiorespiratory investigations and support (Figure 10.5a and b). Where required in the post-operative period, ventricular assist may be considered whilst the right ventricle recovers from the surgical insult. Where associated with a small left (sub-pulmonary) ventricle, either with or without an LV-PA (left ventricular-pulmonary artery) conduit, care must be taken to avoid LVOTO as a result of inotropic support required for the right ventricle. Here, IABP counter pulsation may be useful by providing systemic ventricular support and minimising the need for inotrope administration.

Transposition of the great arteries

Patients admitted to the ICU following surgery for transposition of the great arteries (TGA) (Figure 10.1a) will have undergone either a Rastelli procedure (physiologically normal communications), Mustard/Senning (systemic right ventricle, sub-pulmonary left ventricle) or arterial switch (normal connections). The post-operative management of these patients illustrates the importance of understanding the underlying anatomy, surgery and physiology of the ACHD patient.

In a Rastelli procedure, the normal ventriculo-arterial connections are restored, and adult patients are generally admitted following redo-surgery for conduit replacement. In an arterial switch procedure, the ventriculo-arterial connections are anatomically normal; however, late complications in adulthood include the requirement for aortic or pulmonary valve replacement, and ventricular dysfunction due to coronary disruption. In these patients, post-operative recovery is generally uneventful and does not significantly differ from standard post-cardiac surgical care. In patients with previous Mustard/Senning procedures the systemic ventricle remains morphologically a right ventricle and so these patients have a high incidence of post-operative ventricular dysfunction (Figure 10.5a). Where patients undergo surgery for systemic baffle obstruction, chronic venous hypertension results in hepatic and renal dysfunction, which does not resolve immediately and is associated with significant post-operative morbidity in some cases.

Systemic-pulmonary shunt

Patients with either central or Blalock–Taussig type aorto-pulmonary shunts rely on systemic arterial pressure to maintain pulmonary blood flow via the shunt (Figure 10.2). In such patients, pulmonary blood flow may be reduced by aggressive ventilatory manoeuvres, but the major determinant of pulmonary blood flow remains systemic aortic pressure; so that the appropriate response to desaturation may be systemic vasoconstriction.

ACHD patients previously palliated with either classical or modified Blalock–Taussig shunts and who have then proceeded to definitive repair will exhibit reduced arterial pressure in the ipsilateral arm. This may range from slight under-reading compared to aortic pressure to almost impalpable arm pulses. Arterial lines and non-invasive blood pressure cuffs placed on the ipsilateral arm will provide false low readings. Patients not infrequently present having undergone bilateral shunt procedures, in which case both upper limb pressures will under-reflect true aortic pressure.

Fontan and Fontan-type circulation

The Fontan and Fontan-type circulations (Figure 10.3) are described in Chapter 16. Surgery undertaken in this patient population is usually elective, comprising conversion from atrio-pulmonary Fontan to TCPC. The physiological effects of a univentricular circulation together with systemic venous hypertension over years in these adult patients present challenges to the intensivist in their post-operative management.

The presence of prolonged univentricular circulation results in ventricular dysfunction that should be managed using standard supportive measures (inodilators, pacing, mechanical support). Arrhythmias are common and may be difficult to diagnose (Chapter 17), particularly when temporary epicardial pacing is undertaken post-operatively. Where there is any haemodynamic disturbance and there is uncertainty regarding the underlying rhythm, an atrial ECG should be performed. Prevention of atrial arrhythmias is important, as they will significantly reduce cardiac output, with close attention to electrolytes, early administration of amiodarone and cardioversion where indicated.

The passive flow of blood from the systemic venous circulation to the pulmonary circulation depends upon adequate preload and avoidance of pulmonary hypertension. In the spontaneously breathing patient, negative intra-thoracic pressure generated on inspiration also increases pulmonary flow. In contrast, when the patient is mechanically ventilated, the positive pressure will significantly reduce cardiac output. Thus, in order to maximise cardiac output, PVR and intra-thoracic pressure should be kept as low as possible, with aggressive drainage of pleural collections, avoidance of pulmonary vasoconstrictors, treatment of bronchoconstriction, pulmonary vasodilators, optimising ventilator settings and extubation as early as the patient allows. Where the patient needs respiratory support and is intubated, ventilator settings and fluid balance may be titrated against venous return using echocardiography. In patients with a fenestrated circulation, the presence of hypoxia may represent V/Q mismatch or excessive right–left shunting through the fenestration. Differentiating between the two is important, as hypoxia resulting in pulmonary vasoconstriction will limit cardiac output.

The post-operative recovery of these patients is unpredictable, ranging from immediate extubation and ICU discharge to prolonged ICU admission with multisystem dysfunction. There is a high incidence of coagulopathy, renal dysfunction, hepatic dysfunction and requirement for ventilatory support after surgery undertaken in the presence of a significantly obstructed Fontan circulation associated with a low cardiac output (Figure 10.5b).

10.6 Conclusions

Management of the critically ill ACHD patient requires a highly trained multi-disciplinary team approach, and although it is best carried out in specialist centres, with improving patient survival patients will inevitably increasingly present to their local hospitals. Where possible, however, current recommendations are that the more complex ACHD population are cared for in specialist centres, even when undergoing non-cardiac surgery [5]. These issues have implications for future training, planning and funding of the critical care management of patients with ACHD.

Case study

A 47-year-old woman with previously unoperated congenitally corrected transposition of the great arteries (Figure 10.1) with ventricular septal defect and pulmonary stenosis was admitted to the ICU after total correction (closure of VSD and placement of LV-PA valved conduit). In the immediate post-operative period she was haemodynamically stable, requiring modest circulatory support (noradrenaline 0.08 mcg/kg/min and milrinone 0.3 mcg/Kg/min). On day 3 post-operatively, whilst weaning from invasive mechanical ventilation, she developed a catastrophic deterioration in her gas exchange (saturations 76%, FiO_2 1.0), followed rapidly by cardiac arrest. Clinically and radiographically there was florid pulmonary oedema.

The patient was successfully resuscitated, and echocardiography revealed moderate–severe systemic AV-valve regurgitation (TR) and significant systemic (RV) failure. She was treated with increased inodilatory support (milrinone 0.7 mcg/Kg/min); however, despite resolution of the pulmonary oedema and normalisation of arterial blood gases, her haemodynamics continued to deteriorate (BP 60/40 mmHg; milrinone 0.7 mcg/Kg/min, adrenaline 0.14 µg/kg/min). Repeat echocardiography demonstrated dynamic outflow tract obstruction from the LV to the PA conduit (Figure 10.9a), due to the increased inotropic support. An IABP was inserted which allowed rapid reduction of inotropic support and resolution of the LVOTO, whilst avoiding systemic AV valve regurgitation, maintaining arterial gas exchange and restoring haemodynamics to baseline (Figure 10.9b).

Continued

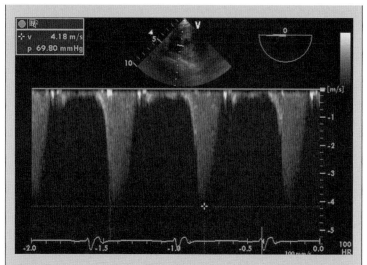

Figure 10.9a Continuous wave Doppler across the left ventricle-pulmonary conduit anastamosis (TOE) revealing a velocity of > 4 m/second consistent with significant outflow tract obstruction.

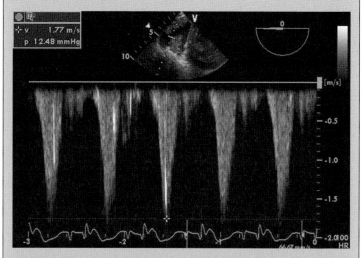

Figure 10.9b Continuous wave Doppler across the left ventricle-pulmonary conduit anastamosis (TOE) revealing a velocity of < 2 m/second, as a result of reduction in inotropic support and increasing circulatory volume (for full explanation, see text).

Subsequently, due to repeated failure to wean (resulting in systemic AV valve regurgitation) the patient underwent tricuspid valve replacement and was successfully discharged.

Comment
Knowledge of the complex haemodynamics and post-operative pitfalls in these patients allows intensivists to manage their post-operative

Continued

complications. Primary repair of complex congential heart disease in more elderly patients often results in haemodynamic changes that may be more easily tolerated in the younger patient, particularly where there is a significant change in ventricular–ventricular interaction. In congenitally corrected transposition, systemic ventricular failure and secondary tricuspid regurgitation are relatively common; however, in this patient, this only became apparent in the post-operative period. Although macroscopic coronary artery disease is unusual in this patient population, coronary arteriography should still be considered to exclude an ischaemic cause for deterioration in ventricular function. The use of IABP is controversial in the younger patient, as aortic compliance limits its usefulness; however, in the adult population it should be used where necessary. It is important to remember that many of these patients will have small descending aortas (due to a chronically low cardiac output state) and the size of balloon should be chosen with care. Close liaison with experts in congenital cardiology, surgery and echocardiography is essential.

References

1. Report of the British Cardiac Society Working Party. Grown-up congenital heart (GUCH) disease: current needs and provision of service for adolescents and adults with congenital heart disease in the UK. *Heart* 2002;88(Suppl 1):i1–14.
2. O'Sullivan JJ, Wren C. Survival with congenital heart disease and need for follow-up into adult life. *Heart* 2001;85:438–43.
3. Price S, Jaggar SI, Jordan S, et al. Adult congenital heart disease: intensive care management and outcome prediction. *Intensive Care Med* 2007;33(4):652–9.
4. Child JS, Collins-Nakai RL, Alpert JS, et al. Bethesda Conference Report – Task Force 3: Workforce description and education requirements for the care of adults with congenital heart disease. *J Am Coll Cardiol* 2001;37:1183–7.
5. Ammash NM, Connolly HM, Abel MD, Warnes CA. Noncardiac surgery in Eisenmenger syndrome. *J Am Coll Cardiol* 1999;33:227–9.
6. Warnes CA, Liberthson R, Danielson GK, et al. Bethesda Conference Report – Task Force 1: The changing profile of congenital heart disease in adult life. *J Am Coll Cardiol* 2001;37:1170–5.
7. Srinathan SK, Bonser RS, Sethia B, et al. Changing practice of cardiac surgery in adult patients with congenital heart disease. *Heart* 2005;91:207–12.
8. Thorne S. Management of polycythaemia in adults with cyanotic congenital heart disease. *Heart* 1998;79:315–16.
9. Karagöz HY, Babacan KM, Zorlutuna YI, et al. Postcardiotomy right ventricular failure: experience with pulmonary arterial balloon counterpulsation and pulmonary arterial venting. *Tex Heart Inst J* 1987;14(2):154–9.
10. Deanfield J, Thurlow E, Warnes C, et al. Management of grown up congenital heart disease. *Eur Heart J* 2003;24:1035–84.
11. Lovell AT. Anaesthetic implications of grown-up congenital heart disease. *Br J Anaes* 2004;93:129–39.

12. Chassot PG, Bettex DA. Anesthesia and adult congenital heart disease. *J Cardiothorac Vasc Anesth* 2006;20:414–37.
13. Association of Anaesthetists. www.aagbi.org/publications/guidelines/docs/anaesthesiateam05.pdf.
14. Association of Anaesthetists. www.aagbi.org/publications/guidelines/docs/standardsofmonitoring07.pdf.
15. Royal College of Anaesthetists. www.rcoa.ac.uk/docs/ARB-section6.pdf.
16. Ambler JJ, Zideman DA, Deakin CD. The effect of topical non-steroidal anti-inflammatory cream on the incidence and severity of cutaneous burns following external DC cardioversion. *Resuscitation* 2005;65:173–8.
17. Daliento L, Somerville J, Presbitero P, et al. Eisenmenger syndrome. Factors relating to deterioration and death. *Eur Heart J* 1998;19(12):1845–55.
18. Ho ECK, Moss AJ. The syndrome of 'mesenteric arteritis' following surgical repair of aortic coarctation. *Pediatrics* 1972;49(1):40–5.
19. Khan SN, Stansby G. Cerebrospinal fluid drainage for thoracic and thoracoabdominal aortic aneurysm surgery. *Cochrane Database of Systematic Reviews* 2004; Issue 1, Art. no. CD003635, DOI: 10.1002/14651858.CD003635.pub2.
20. Coselli JS, Lemaire SA, Köksoy C, et al. Cerebrospinal fluid drainage reduces paraplegia after thoracoabdominal aortic aneurysm repair: results of a randomized clinical trial. *J Vasc Surg* 2002:35;631–9.
21. Cheung AT, Pochettino A, McGarvey ML et al. Strategies to manage paraplegia risk after endovascular stent repair of descending thoracic aortic aneurysms. *Ann Thorac Surg* 2005;80(4):1280–8.

11 Common Complications of Cardiovascular Critical Illness

Simon J. Finney and Mark J.D. Griffiths
Royal Brompton & Harefield NHS Foundation Trust, London, UK

> ## Take Home Messages
>
> - Complications are common and often iatrogenic.
> - Acute pericardial collections may be localised following cardiac surgery and not present with classical clinical or echocardiographic signs of tamponade.
> - Systemic inflammation is common and may present as vasopressor dependence and multi-organ dysfunction syndrome. Management is supportive.
> - Renal failure is common and the management supportive. To date, no drugs have been demonstrated to accelerate renal recovery.
> - Pleural effusions are common following cardiac surgery. They are most often exudative but empyema is a very rare complication. Drainage of large effusions may improve oxygenation and aide weaning from mechanical ventilation.
> - Compartment syndromes may only be detected by clinical examination. Fasciotomy can be limb saving.

11.1 Introduction

Critically ill patients experience complications related to the underlying disease process and the therapies that they receive. The incidence is high and relates in part to the degree and complexity of disease and intervention. Some complications are encountered in all groups of critically ill patients; these include catheter-related bloodstream infections, ventilator-associated pneumonias and upper intestinal bleeding. These may be particularly problematic in patients with cardiovascular illness. For example, line sepsis is concerning in patients with prosthetic valves, and intestinal bleeding may be difficult to manage in patients who need anticoagulation. However, these general problems are not considered further in this chapter, which

Cardiovascular Critical Care. Edited by M. Griffiths, J. Cordingley and S. Price.
© 2010 Blackwell Publishing Ltd.

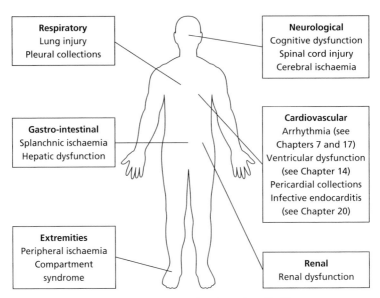

Figure 11.1 Sites of common complications of cardiovascular critical illness.

focuses on complications that are more specific to patients with cardiovascular disease or who have undergone cardiovascular interventions. Furthermore, certain complications such as cardiac arrhythmias, low cardiac output and coagulopathies are discussed in specific chapters and will not be further considered here.

11.2 Systemic disorders

Systemic inflammation

Systemic inflammation is common after any surgical insult and probably particularly so following cardiac surgery. The clinical manifestations are protean, ranging from systemic vasodilatation and a requirement for vasopressors to acute lung injury, acute renal failure, liver dysfunction and neurological disturbance. Indeed the systemic inflammatory component of acute confusional states is underappreciated and can persist [1]. Inflammation occurs following exposure of patients' blood to the components of the cardiopulmonary bypass (CPB) circuit and the activation of coagulation, complement and immune cells. However, there is biochemical and leukocyte evidence for inflammation in operations that do not require CPB, albeit of a lesser magnitude [2]. This reflects the other inflammatory stimuli that are present, such as surgical trauma and periods of low cardiac output followed by reperfusion.

Despite evidence that inflammation is common and associated with organ dysfunction and a worse outcome, there are no data to support the routine use of anti-inflammatory strategies such as corticosteroids, aprotinin and leukocyte-depleting filters during cardiac surgery. Thus, whilst intra-operative methylprednisolone leads to reduced plasma levels of cytokines and troponins this is not reflected in any reduction in length of stay or mortality [3, 4]. Moreover, it is well documented to affect adversely glycaemic control (*vide infra*) and has been associated with prolonged mechanical ventilation [5]. Aprotinin inhibits serine proteases such as the neutrophil-derived elastase and cathespin G, both of which have been implicated in organ dysfunction during systemic inflammation. Nevertheless, aprotinin has been implicated in increased renal dysfunction [6] and possibly increased mortality [7], such that its routine use could not be advocated. Finally, various studies of leukocyte-depleting filters used pre-, intra- or post-operatively have failed to demonstrate a beneficial effect on mortality or duration of mechanical ventilation following cardiac surgery [8].

Whilst there is no evidence for the routine application of anti-inflammatory therapy in cardiac surgery, it is possible that it may be appropriate in those patients who show signs of systemic inflammation. No studies have addressed this question specifically. To date, the only therapy demonstrated to reduce mortality due to severe sepsis in a randomised controlled trial is drotrecogin alfa (activated). This has been used following cardiac surgery despite concerns about haemorrhagic complications [9]. However, its role in patients with systemic inflammation due to tissue factor up-regulation for a reason other than sepsis is not known. Moreover, in surgical patients with sepsis and only one (in contrast to multiple) organ dysfunction, drotrecogin alfa use was associated with increased mortality [10].

Critical illness-related corticosteroid insufficiency

Critical illness-related corticosteroid insufficiency (CIRCI) is often implicated in shock states that are characterised by inflammation and systemic vasodilatation [11]. Previously termed relative adrenal insufficiency, it can be a consequence of dysfunction of the hypothalamic-pituitary-adrenal (HPA) axis or glucocorticoid receptor signalling pathway. Inflammatory cytokines, ischaemia, or 'endocrine exhaustion' may be causal. The incidence following cardiac surgery is uncertain due to variable diagnostic criteria and the variations in cortisol binding globulin that obscure the relationship between total and free cortisol [12]. Some data suggest that cardiac surgery *per se* may not be a risk for developing CIRCI [13]. However, the use of etomidate, an anaesthetic induction agent commonly employed in cardiovascularly unstable patients, can suppress HPA function after a single dose [14].

Recent studies in patients with systemic vasodilatation due to sepsis suggest that corticosteroid replacement accelerates shock reversal without any beneficial mortality effect and a possible increased incidence of nosocomial pneumonia [15]. It is not possible to determine which patients will benefit from steroid replacement with a corticotrophin stimulation test and this should not be undertaken [11]. The above observations are often extrapolated to patients with non-septic inflammation such as may occur following cardiac surgery. Indeed, many administer corticosteroids in this group of patients despite the lack of evidence. Nevertheless, some patients with concomitant myocardial dysfunction tolerate profound systemic vasodilatation poorly, with its consequences for perfusion of the heart and other organs. In these patients accelerated shock reversal may be advantageous if standard vasopressors are ineffective.

Hyperglycaemia

Hyperglycaemia is common in critically ill patients with cardiovascular disease and is related to the inflammatory response, administration of catecholamines and a high prevalence of diabetes mellitus in this population. Control of hyperglycaemia and/or the administration of insulin has been extensively investigated. To date, a single randomised controlled study demonstrated reduced mortality in critically ill patients given insulin aiming for a blood glucose target of 4.1–6.0 mM rather than a target of 10.0 –11.1 mM [16]. One of the several unique characteristics of this study was that most patients had undergone cardiac surgery, and the findings were corroborated with observational data [17]. However, other studies in different patient populations have shown that a target blood sugar of 4.1–6.0 mM has less clear cut benefits and risks inadvertent hypoglycaemia [18–20]. Furthermore, utilising this target during (rather than after) cardiac surgery may have an adverse effect [21]. A retrospective study predominantly of cardiothoracic patients suggested that most of the advantage of glucose control was accrued by maintaining blood glucose at a level below 8.0 mmol/l and proposed that this target may be safer [22].

11.3 Cardiovascular dysfunction

Myocardial dysfunction

Myocardial dysfunction is common following cardiac surgery and presents as a low cardiac output state, increased ventricular filling pressures or a requirement for inotropes to wean from cardiopulmonary bypass. It is related to underlying myocardial disease, peri-operative ischaemia, an alteration in the interaction between the two ventricles and the systemic inflammation that occurs following surgery. Pre-existing myocardial failure may be caused by previous infarction, long-standing valvular disease and intrinsic myocardial disease. Such pre-operative dysfunction increases pero-operative mortality and is reflected in risk evaluations such as the Parsonnet and Euroscore instruments.

Peri-operative ischaemia may occur in patients with coronary artery disease if oxygen demand is increased by hypertension or tachycardia, or supply is lowered by hypotension. Futhermore, intra-operative ischaemia is inevitable if a cross clamp is applied to the aorta in order to allow the left atrium, left ventricle or aorta to be opened or to allow the administration of cardioplegia to provide a non-moving heart for surgical intervention. Whilst the cross clamp is applied to the ascending aorta, coronary arterial perfusion does not occur. Ischaemia is mitigated by cooling the heart and the administration of a cardioplegia solution into the coronary circulation. Ischaemia may be exacerbated by poor distribution of cardioplegia due to coronary artery disease or ventricular hypertrophy and a prolonged ischaemic period. Finally, ischaemia and infarction in the territories of specific coronary arteries may occur if coronary artery bypass grafts fail, coronary ostia are distorted following reimplantation during aortic root surgery, or rarely if the circumflex coronary artery is damaged during mitral valve surgery.

Myocardial dysfunction may recover over a period of hours to months if the original insult is not ongoing. Management strategies include temporary cardiac support with inotropes (Chapter 6), intra-aortic balloon counterpulsation (Chapter 14) or even mechanical assist devices (Chapter 8).

Pericardial collections and tamponade
Aetiology
Acute pericardial collections of fluid, blood and clot are common following cardiac surgery. Indeed, small volumes of fluid are present in most patients; one study demonstrated fluid in 103 out of 122 patients that was visible on the second post-operative day, peaked on the tenth and tended to resolve within 30 days [23]. More significantly sized collections may occur in up to 64% of patients and tend to be more common in females, those on anticoagulants preoperatively and following valvular surgery. The pericardial collection is sufficient to compress the heart (cardiac tamponade) and compromise cardiac function in 0.8–6.0% of cases (Figure 11.2). Pericardial collections may also occur following cardiac catheterisation if coronary arteries are ruptured or if there is cardiac perforation, for example following trans-septal puncture or catheter ablation. The incidence of coronary rupture is estimated at 0.12% of cases and is more common if atheroablative techniques are used [24]. The deployment of covered stents may bridge the rupture and prevent significant tamponade.

Chronic pericardial effusions may occur in association with viral myocarditis, systemic inflammatory disorders such as systemic lupus erythematosus, neighbouring malignancies, uraemia, Dressler's syndrome and transplant rejection. They tend to be much larger since their slow development allows time for the pericardium to stretch so that pericardial pressure increases slowly.

Pathophysiology and diagnosis
The compliance of the fibrous pericardial sac is very low and small increases in volume result in marked rises in pressure. This rapid pressure rise is reduced if the pericardium and pleura are left open at the end of surgery. As pericardial pressure rises, transmural pressure falls and thus preload is reduced and cardiac output falls. The thinner walled right ventricle is particularly susceptible as its wall tension is lower. Elevated pericardial pressures may also compromise blood flow in epicardial coronary arteries and result in regional ischaemia. If the pressure rise occurs slowly, larger

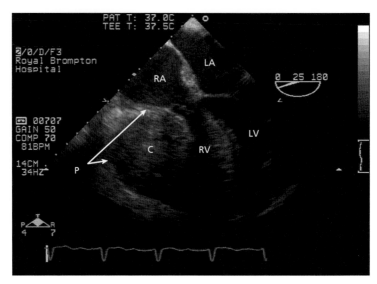

Figure 11.2 Trans-oesophageal echocardiogram (mid-oesophagus, four-chamber view) in a patient with a localised pericardial collection resulting in profound haemodynamic compromise. Here, although measured filling pressures were normal, there was a significant haematoma within the pericardial space, compressing the right ventricle and atrio-ventricular groove, resulting in tamponade. LA, left atrium; LV, left ventricle; RV, right ventricle; RA, right atrium; P, pericardium; C, collection.

volumes may accumulate within the pericardial space; however, with rapid collections, tamponade may occur with as little as 50 ml of fluid (Figure 11.3).

The classic syndrome of tamponade includes evidence of a low cardiac output state with an elevated right atrial pressure, although this is often normal. Low cardiac output states may manifest as low systemic blood pressure, tachycardia, oliguria, mental confusion, an elevated serum lactate, worsening metabolic acidosis and cool peripheries. In addition to an elevation in right atrial pressures the venous waveform changes. Thus increased pericardial pressure reduces atrial filling during atrial diastole and attenuates the v-wave. This attenuation of the v-wave leads to a diminished y-descent which represents passive ventricular filling when both chambers are in diastole. Ventricular filling becomes progressively dependent upon atrial systole and thus there is preservation of the a-wave. The x-descent is often marked as pericardial pressures fall rapidly during ventricular systole as the ventricles eject. It is often commented that the normal inspiratory fall in systemic blood pressure (pulsus paradoxicus) is exaggerated during cardiac tamponade, although this may not occur in patients with concomitant ventricular or pulmonary disease [25].

It is usually possible to visualise a collection using echocardiography, although it can be difficult to determine the haemodynamic significance of the collection. Classical echocardiographic signs of tamponade (Figure 11.2)

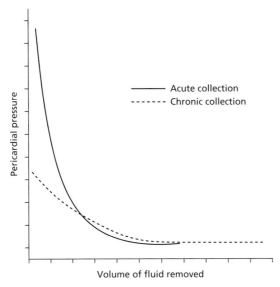

Figure 11.3 Schematic demonstrating the effects of rate of accumulation of a pericardial collection on intrapericardial pressure. In curve A (solid line) an acutely accumulating collection results in a rapid rise in intrapericardial pressure, rapidly resulting in critical tamponade. In curve B (dashed line) where a chronic collection is accumulating the curve is less steep, and tamponade results at a smaller volume of collection (*New England Journal of Medicine* 2003:347:7 (Figure 1).

include diastolic collapse of the right heart due to the negative transmural pressure. This can be visualised as abnormal inward movement of the right ventricular free wall during diastole, but occurs less often with hypertophic ventricles. Right atrial collapse is more common but less specific unless it is prolonged for over one third of the cardiac cycle. Left atrial collapse is very specific. It may also be possible to demonstrate pulsus paradoxicus in the absence of significant cardiac disease by the reciprocal variation in transtricuspid and transmitral flows with respiration.

As highlighted above, co-existing pathologies can influence the echocardiographic signs of tamponade. Furthermore localised collections can significantly compromise ventricular filling and have few other signs. The utility of echocardiography was investigated in a retrospective study of 148 consecutive patients who had returned to theatre for drainage of a collection [26]. In the acute setting only 21% of cases had the classical echocardiographic features and typically had small collections that were more likely to be detected using trans-oesophageal echocardiography. By contrast, collections presenting over 72 hours postoperatively were more likely to have classical echocardiographic features (70%) and were larger but had less classical clinical features. The key point is that in the acute setting if there is clinical suspicion of pericardial tamponade then echocardiography can reveal the collection but will not always reveal the haemodynamic significance. Increased cardiothoracic ratio on a plain chest X-ray is an insensitive and non-specific sign.

Management

Drainage of pericardial collections occurring after cardiac surgery is the treatment of choice. Options include re-sternotomy, drainage through a sub-xiphisternal incision and percutaneous drainage. The optimal method depends on the chronicity of the collection, the presence of clot or fibrinous strands, and the likelihood of ongoing bleeding that may require surgical repair. Drainage is typically associated with an immediate elevation in systemic blood pressure; however, the fall in right atrial pressure may be delayed. Paradoxically some patients subsequently require more vasoconstrictor for a period of time to maintain their systemic pressure. Whether this is due to a reduction in the sympathetic stimulation that was sustaining the blood pressure pre-drainage or a reperfusion-type inflammatory response is not clear.

The 'tight' pericardium

In a small number of patients there may be features of tamponade in the absence of a demonstrable pericardial collection (tight pericardium) as a consequence of opening the pericardium during surgery. This is a well-known entity in paediatric cardiothoracic surgery, but less well recognised in adult practice. The cause is thought to be insufficient space within the pericardium to allow normal cardiac function, and is most common in patients with significant chamber enlargement together with post-operative oedema. When a patient has elevated filling pressures and a low cardiac output state, together with marked respiratory variation in cardiac filling, this syndrome should be considered. Differential diagnoses include, for example, significant airway obstruction. Once differential diagnoses have been excluded and the patient has been resuscitated, re-sternotomy should be considered, with the chest stented open until the oedema resolves, aided where possible by encouraging a negative fluid balance.

Compartment syndrome

Compartment syndromes may develop in the limbs, typically the legs, following cardiac surgery. Inflammation and oedema of muscles within the confines of the anterior and posterior fascial compartments of the lower leg can be sufficient to compromise blood flow into the compartment and result in neural damage and muscle necrosis. This is particularly likely to occur in the setting of atherosclerotic disease or the presence of an intra-aortic balloon pump in the ipsilateral femoral artery resulting in poor flow. Up to 86% of post-operative compartment syndromes are associated with balloon pumps [27]. The origins of the inflammation are typically related to episodes of low cardiac output and ischaemia reperfusion, harvesting of saphenous vein for coronary artery bypass grafts or profound systemic inflammation.

Pain, parasthesiae and paralysis are cardinal signs in patients who are awake. However, the development of compartment syndromes is occult in ventilated patients. Thus poor peripheral pulses and biochemical markers of increased lactate, worsening acidosis and an elevated creatinine kinase, associated with low cardiac output states, should prompt clinical examination for a compartment syndrome. Surgical fasciotomies relieve the pressure and restore blood flow. They are essential in preventing debilitating damage to the limb.

Peripheral ischaemia

Critical limb ischaemia occurs in cardiac critical care units not only because many patients have concomitant peripheral vascular disease but also because patients frequently undergo interventions such as cardiac catheterisation or intra-aortic balloon pumping via their arterial systems. The insertion of devices via the femoral arteries may physically limit flow down atherosclerotic vessels or result in inadvertent dissection of the vessel. Alternatively, embolism of clot, originating from the heart or more commonly from intra-aortic balloon pumps, may occur. Signs include absent peripheral pulses, pallor or peripheral cyanosis, and poor capillary refill. Often advice from vascular surgeons is required.

Microvascular thrombosis and tissue ischaemia sometimes complicate profound systemic inflammation or sepsis and heparin-induced thrombocytopenia. The skin often appears mottled. Microvascular dysfunction is often exacerbated by the use of high-dose vasoconstrictors to sustain the systemic arterial pressure.

11.4 Renal dysfunction

Acute kidney injury (AKI) is common following cardiac intervention. It is associated with considerable morbidity, and in some studies is an independent risk factor for death on the intensive care unit (ICU). The aetiology is multifactorial, relating to pre-existing renal dysfunction, the use of radiographic contrast media, nephrotoxic drugs, episodes of hypotension and low cardiac output, renovascular disease, systemic inflammation and haemolysis during cardiopulmonary bypass. The incidence varies according to the definition employed. Moreover, a reduced urine output may reflect the rise in plasma anti-diuretic hormone that occurs following cardiac surgery [28], rather than any loss in renal function. A retrospective study of 29,623 patients illustrated that the incidences of 'Risk of renal failure', 'renal Injury' and 'renal Failure' as defined by the RIFLE criteria (Risk-Injury-Failure-Loss-End-stage: Table 11.1) are 9%, 5% and 2% respectively [29]. In the entire cohort,

Table 11.1 RIFLE classification of acute kidney injury [31].

RIFLE category	Creatinine	GFR	Urine output
Risk	1.5 × elevated	< 75%	< 0.5 ml/kg/h over 6 h
Injury	2 × elevated	< 50%	< 0.5 ml/kg/h over 12 h
Failure	3 × elevated	< 25%	< 0.3 ml/kg/h over 24 h or anuria for 12 h
Loss	Renal replacement therapy for over 4 weeks		
End-stage	Renal replacement therapy for over 3 months		

GFR, Glomerular filtration rate.

4.5% of patients required renal replacement therapy. Risk factors that have been associated with post-operative renal failure include female gender, diabetes mellitus, emergency surgery, left ventricular dysfunction and pre-existing renal dysfunction [30]. The incidence of pre-existing renal dysfunction is increasing in cardiothoracic ICUs, in part since it is a cardiovascular risk factor *per se*, but also as the demographics and co-morbidities of the patients change.

Contrast-induced nephropathy

Many therapies have been proposed to accelerate renal recovery, although none has proven efficacy in trials (see Table 11.2). The mainstay of management of renal dysfunction is maintenance of renal perfusion, relief of any obstruction and avoidance of nephrotoxic agents such as radiographic contrast, non-steroidal inflammatory agents and angiotensin converting enzyme inhibitors. Renal perfusion is maintained by restoring cardiac output through adequate fluid resuscitation, inotropes, and pacing and maintenance of an adequate blood pressure through the use of vasoconstrictors.

The failure of many pharmacological therapies in acute renal failure relates in part to late administration in the natural history of the condition, since substantial injury has occurred already when the serum creatinine and urine output start to change. By distinction, contrast induced nephropathy (CIN) provides an opportunity for pre-emptive therapy. Radiographic contrast induces renal dysfunction by triggering the release of vasoconstrictors, such as endothelin, which cause local renal ischaemia [56]. Since contrast is concentrated by the nephron the effects are amplified. Patients with chronic kidney disease stage II or more (i.e. with an estimated glomerular filtration rate of less than 60 ml/min/1.73 m^2) are particularly prone to CIN. Less toxic iso-osmolar agents should be used in this group [56].

Hypovolaemia exacerbates CIN and should be avoided by adequate rehydration and probably volume expansion. Proposed mechanisms of benefit include the dilution of contrast by higher urine flows and the inhibition of the renin angiotensin system (thereby countering renal vasoconstriction) by the increased sodium load. No specific regimen is clearly superior, although oral replacement and 0.45% sodium chloride solution appear less effective [57, 58]. Typical recommendations are that isotonic crystalloid (1.0–1.5 ml/kg/hour) is administered for 3–12 hours prior to the procedure and continued for 6–24 hours afterwards in patients with stage II or more chronic kidney disease [59]. Some data suggest that using 1.26% bicarbonate solutions as the hydration fluid may be more beneficial [60, 61]. It is hypothesised that alkalinisation of the urine may reduce the damaging local effects of reactive oxygen species.

N-acetylcysteine has been extensively investigated as an antioxidant that may mitigate CIN. Regimens typically are 600 mg administered twice daily commencing prior to administration of contrast. The results from studies are variable. Meta-analyses suggest only possible benefit, highlighting the

Table 11.2 Therapies investigated for the treatment of renal dysfunction.

Agent	Rationale	Evidence	References
Urodilatin	Atrial natriuretic peptide prohormone that causes vasodilation, natriuresis, diuresis and inhibition of aldosterone release	No reduction in need for renal replacement therapy or mortality in several studies. Bradycardiac and hypotension can be problematic	[32–34]
Fenoldopam	Selective dopamine receptor 1 (DA-1) agonist increasing renal blood flow	Metanalysis of 13 studies with variable dosing and limited quality suggested a possible beneficial effect. Fenoldopam causes significant vasodilatation which may limit its use	[35]
Minocycline	Anti-apoptotic and anti-inflammatory effects due to reduced free radical and cytokine production, interference with protein synthesis or modulation of matrix metalloproteinase activity	Reduced renal failure if administered pre-ischaemia in animal models. Clinical trial ongoing in patients following cardiac surgery	[36, 37]
Nesiritide	Recombinant human B-type natriuretic peptide licenced as a treatment in acute decompensated heart failure. It promotes natriuresis, dieresis and vasodilation	Varied effects on renal function and may increase renal injury if infused for over 24 hours	[38, 39]
AP214	Anti-inflammatory α-melanocyte-stimulating hormone analogue	Efficacious in murine model of sepsis-induced renal dysfunction. Currently in phase II human studies of patients undergoing cardiac surgery	[40–42]
Mannitol	Increased urine flow and scavenges free radicals	Several randomised studies showed no benefit, with one demonstrating the possibility of increased renal damage	[43–45]
Frusemide	Increased urine flow may prevent tubular obstruction and reduce tubular oxygen consumption	No evidence for reduced renal failure; possible increase in mortality in one study	[46–49]
Dopamine	Stimulation of DA-1 and DA-2 receptors, increasing renal blood flow and inhibiting proximal tubular sodium reabsorption	Increases urine output due to natriuresis. No evidence for reduced incidence of renal dysfunction or mortality. Inotropic effect may increase renal perfusion	[49–52]
Aminophylline	Non-selective adenosine antagonist that may prevent adenosine-1 (A1) receptor-induced vasoconstriction	Randomised controlled pilot study of 56 patients undergoing coronary artery surgery. No benefit demonstrated for a 96 hour infusion	[53]
Insulin	Post hoc observation made in a trial of intensive insulin therapy in a surgical ICU. No proposed mechanism	Single centre study of 1,573 patients randomised to receive insulin targeting their blood glucose to 4.4–5.1 mM in contrast to 10.0–11.1 mM	[16]
ISNP	Short ribonucleic acid interference molecule of p53, a transcription factor regulating cell cycle and apoptosis that has been implicated in ischaemic kidney injury	Currently in phase I human studies	[54, 55]

heterogeneity of the studies and the need for more data [59, 62, 63]. The interpretation of positive studies is complicated by the enhanced tubular excretion of creatinine caused by N-acetylcysteine. Another anti-oxidant, ascorbic acid, reduced the incidence of renal dysfunction (25% increase in serum creatinine) in patients undergoing cardiac catheterisation [64]. Further studies are merited.

Finally, contrast can be removed from the circulation by haemofiltration and dialysis. It has been demonstrated to be efficacious in preventing renal impairment, although it appeared to be necessary to start haemofiltration prior to the administration of contrast [65, 66], suggesting an effect other than removal of contrast from the circulation.

11.5 Respiratory dysfunction

Respiratory dysfunction is common following cardiovascular interventions. Aside from pulmonary oedema associated with cardiac pathology, patients may develop intrinsic pulmonary disease.

Acute lung injury

Acute lung injury (ALI) and the acute respiratory distress syndrome (ARDS) refer to the acute onset of refractory hypoxaemia in association with bilateral pulmonary infiltrates (Figure 11.3) with no evidence of elevated left atrial pressure. They differ only in the degree of hypoxaemia and represent the pulmonary manifestation of systemic inflammation. Transfusion of allogeneic blood products can trigger the syndrome – termed transfusion related ALI (TRALI). ARDS complicated 1.3% of cases undergoing cardiopulmonary bypass in one series and may be more common in the elderly and those undergoing prolonged cardiopulmonary bypass [67].

The management of ALI and ARDS is similar irrespective of the aetiology. General management includes nutrition, measures to reduce ventilator-associated pneumonia and fluid management. Whilst the pulmonary infiltrates are caused primarily by increased permeability of the alveolar-capillary membrane rather than fluid overload, the severity of pulmonary oedema will depend on the pulmonary capillary pressure and hence left ventricular function and volume status. In a recent study of liberal versus conservative fluid management, the conservative regimen was associated with a reduced length of mechanical ventilation without an increase in non-pulmonary organ failures [68]. Currently there are no data that support the routine application of corticosteroids or other pharmacotherapies either late or early in the natural history of the disease [69]. Most patients require mechanical ventilatory support. There is good evidence that aggressive (high tidal volume and airway pressure) ventilation contributes to the inflammatory process within the lung [70, 71]. The ARDS Network ARMA study demonstrated that ventilation with a tidal volume of 6 ml/kg predicted body weight was associated with approximately 10% less mortality than a 'conventional' tidal volume

(11 ml/kg) [71]. Lower tidal volumes may require the acceptance of a respiratory acidosis or the application of a higher respiratory frequency to maintain normocapnia [72]. Vigilance for complications such as ventilator-associated pneumonia and pneumothoraces should be maintained and managed appropriately.

Pulmonary atelectasis

Basal atelectasis and lobar collapse are common following cardiac procedures [73]. Left lower lobe collapse is to be expected in patients who are supine and mechanically ventilated, owing at least in part to the weight of the heart. Up to 3% of patients develop a pneumonia following cardiac surgery [74]. In elderly patients and those with concomitant lung disease, their functional residual capacity will fall below their closing volume, resulting in cyclical collapse of airways during tidal ventilation. This may be exacerbated by sputum retention, incomplete reinflation of the lungs following cardiopulmonary bypass and pain related to surgical incisions. Techniques that have been proposed to combat atelectasis include incentive spirometry, intermittent positive pressure breathing, physiotherapy and continuous positive airways pressure. None has been clearly demonstrated to be efficacious [75]. The available data support the practice of early mobilisation, which is beneficial also for the prevention of venous thrombosis.

Pleural effusions

Pleural effusions, particularly left sided, are common following cardiac surgery, being detectable on plain radiology in around 40% of patients [76]. Effusions may consist of serous fluid, blood, chyle or pus in the pleural cavity. Radiographic appearances depend on the positioning of the patient but include blunting of the costophrenic angle, loss of the distinction of the diaphragm and opacification of the hemithorax without air bronchograms.

Effusions result when pleural fluid accumulates faster than it is removed in the lymphatics of the pleura; lymphatic drainage may be impaired after cardiac surgery by surgical disruption and atelectasis. The lymphatics drain from the parietal surface to nodes in the chest wall and from the visceral surface to mediastinal nodes. The fluid may be further categorised as a transudate or exudate based on the fluid to plasma protein and lactate dehydrogenase ratios, which are less than 0.5 and 0.6 respectively (Light's criteria). Transudates are often bilateral and occur when capillary osmotic pressure exceeds oncotic pressure such as when the pleural venous pressure is high. The parietal pleural veins drain into the pulmonary veins and thus reflect the pressure in the left atrium. By contrast, exudates occur when vascular permeability is high and tend to be unilateral and associated with local inflammation in neighbouring structures. Indeed pericardial inflammation is thought to be the cause of post-operative left-sided effusions following cardiac surgery, the incidence of which does not appear to be affected by harvesting of the internal thoracic artery at surgery [76].

Bleeding may occur into the pleural cavity from the operative site following cardiac surgery. The usual manifestations are excessive losses from intercostal drains or cardiovascular and respiratory compromise. When blood loss is substantial and ongoing, patients should undergo surgical exploration to isolate the source (Chapter 5). In general, significant clots that occur following bleeding that has subsequently stopped should be evacuated since there is risk they may become an empyema or fibrothorax. Whilst instillation of urokinase and streptokinase may help up to 60% of clotted traumatic haemothoraces [77], it rarely has a place on the cardiothoracic ICU.

Chyle may accumulate if there is disruption of the lymphatic circulation, such as occurs with thoracic duct injuries. It can be damaged during cardiothoracic surgery anywhere along its course in the posterior mediastinum. Chyle has a milky appearance. Its nature can be confirmed biochemically in enterally fed patients by the presence of chylomicrons. Management includes parenteral nutrition or a fat-restricted oral diet supplemented with medium-chain triglycerides to reduce chylous flow, pleural drainage and surgical correction, which is required in approximately 50% of cases that fail conservative management.

Pleural effusions are often confirmed using ultrasound, which enables the differentiation from lung collapse or consolidation which often co-exist in the critically ill and can be difficult to differentiate with plain radiology. The effusion appears as a hypoechoic layer between the chest wall and lung which moves with respiration, and the volume of pleural fluid may be estimated. Ultrasound allows also the identification of a safe site for drainage [78], thereby reducing the complications of misplacement or inadvertent damage of neighbouring structures. The relationships between fluid and other structures can change dramatically with small changes in patient position and therefore it is the authors' belief that drainage should be undertaken immediately following ultrasonography or in real-time, rather than a site being marked for subsequent drainage. Samples of fluid should be sent for microbiological culture and biochemical evaluation of protein and lactate dehydrogenase.

Drainage of pleural effusions has variable effects on oxygenation in both ventilated and spontaneously breathing patients [79–82]. This variation is probably a consequence of the relative perfusion of any compressed lung. Thus if hypoxic pulmonary vasoconstriction is effective in collapsed segments, drainage is unlikely to have any great effect on V/Q matching and any oxygenation gradient. Similarly, in a small study of spontaneously ventilating patients, drainage had little effect on the physiological dead space (as predicted by the Bohr equation) and thus carbon dioxide clearance [82]. Thus the greatest effect of pleural drainage seems to be on respiratory mechanics and the work of breathing. One study demonstrated that pleural pressure decreased from a mean value of 10 to −7 cmH$_2$0 following drainage, thereby increasing the transpulmonary pressure gradient at similar airway pressures [82]. Furthermore, the reduction in thoracic volume reduces the mechanical disadvantage that occurs when intercostals are overstretched and the diaphragm is flattened.

The British Thoracic Society recommends that no more than 1.5 litres of fluid are drained in a single instance for fear of developing re-expansion pulmonary oedema [83]. This phenomenon probably represents an ischaemia-reperfusion injury to the previous collapsed lung and appears more likely if very large volumes are removed in patients who have had prolonged pulmonary collapse [84].

Phrenic nerve dysfunction

Phrenic nerve injury and the resultant diaphragmatic paralysis is common following cardiac surgery. It may result in delayed extubation and occasionally the need for non-invasive ventilatory support post-operatively, particularly if it is bilateral. The left phrenic nerve passes though the thorax over the left ventricle and a neuropraxia can result from the use of iced slush for topical myocardial protection [85]. Up to 30% may persist for over 6 months [86]. The right phrenic nerve passes through the thorax over the brachiocephalic artery and across the root of the right lung. It may be inadvertently damaged during harvesting of the right internal thoracic artery for coronary artery bypass grafting. The efficacy of diaphragmatic plication in persistent lesions associated with reduced respiratory function is not known.

11.6 Gastrointestinal dysfunction

Gastrointestinal complications have a reported incidence of 1–2% after cardiac surgery [87, 88]. Upper intestinal bleeding is the most common event and is particularly troublesome in patients who require anticoagulation and patients who have a persistently low cardiac output.

Liver dysfunction

Ischaemic hepatitis may complicate low cardiac output states particularly if there is systemic venous hypertension, as often occurs in right heart failure. It is associated with elevated transaminases that peak on the second day after injury [89, 90]. Hypoglycaemia and hyperlactataemia often occur early. By contrast, acute changes in serum bilirubin, alkaline phosphatase and gamma glutaryl transpeptidase are less striking except during recovery if the liver effectively becomes 'small-for-size' whilst it regenerates. Similarly, acute changes in prothrombin time, while common, are usually modest [90].

Management is supportive, including the administration of glucose and using high-flux haemofiltration with low lactate buffers to control the acid-base balance. Available data do not support the routine use of albumin dialysis (e.g. Molecular Adsorbent Recirculation System (MARS) or Prometheus) or N-acetylcysteine infusion.

Splanchnic ischaemia

Splanchnic ischaemia is a devastating complication of cardiovascular illness. It often relates to episodes of low cardiac output with or without concomitant atherosclerotic disease and the use of high-dose vasoconstrictors. In a retrospective study of 4,819 patients who underwent cardiac surgery, 30 (0.63%) suffered from intestinal ischaemia, with a roughly equal distribution between ischaemia of the large and small bowel [91]. Mortality was 47%. Common presentations include abdominal distension, metabolic acidosis, hyperlactataemia and haemodynamic instability. The diagnosis is generally confirmed by computed tomography of the abdomen. Ongoing management includes the restoration of cardiac output and consultation with gastrointestinal surgeons. Many patients decline rapidly and become too unwell for surgical resection and some have such extensive infarction that there is no surgical option. In the aforementioned case series, four patients considered too unwell for surgery subsequently survived [91].

Pancreatititis
Hyperamylasaemia may occur in up to 60% of patients following cardiac surgery. It may not always indicate pancreatic damage owing to a substantial contribution from the salivary isoenzyme [92]. Triggers for pancreatic injury include periods of low cardiac output, induced intra-operative hypothermia and the administration of calcium supplements. Hyperamylasaemia is often self-limiting. There is radiological evidence of pancreatic inflammation in about 3% of patients [93, 94]. There are no specific interventions, and the management of severe necrotising pancreatitis is as for other pancreatitis due to other aetiologies [95].

11.7 Neurological dysfunction

Spinal cord injury
Paraplegia due to spinal cord ischaemia may complicate surgical or endovascular repair of the thoracoabdominal aorta. The spinal cord is supplied by the anterior spinal artery and two posterior spinal arteries, supplemented by branches from the deep cervical, intercostal and lumbar arteries. The additional supply from the intercostals may be temporarily compromised during cross-clamping of the descending aorta or may be permanently lost if the vessels are occluded by a stent or tied off and not re-anastamosed to the surgical graft. The blood supply to the spinal cord may be further compromised by the rise in spinal cerebrospinal fluid (CSF) pressure that occurs during aortic cross-clamping. The peri-operative drainage of CSF through a spinal drain aiming for a pressure of 10 mmHg (13 cm CSF) reduces the incidence of paraplegia following extensive surgical repairs of thoracoabdominal aortic aneurysm [96]. Spinal drains have also been used for paraplegia that develops later, with dramatic improvements occurring [97–99]. Whilst the late insertion of drains has not been subjected to formal study and it is clear that some neurological deficits improve spontaneously, it is common practice to insert one in the presence of paraplegia in the hope of alleviating this devastating complication. This may be difficult in the setting of a coagulopathy or therapeutic anticoagulation.

Central nervous system dysfunction

Central neurological dysfunction is common following cardiac surgery [100] and cardiological intervention. It can range from subtle neurocognitive changes to an overt stroke. The aetiology is multifactorial.

Cerebral ischaemia is characterised by localisation. It may occur by several mechanisms. Atherosclerotic plaque, platelet clumps, clot and air may embolise into the cerebral circulation during cardiac catheterisation or surgical manipulation of the aorta. Haemorrhagic strokes may occur following the administration of thrombolytics for coronary thromboses or less commonly as a consequence of anticoagulation for cardiopulmonary bypass or a mechanical prosthetic valve. Cerebral ischaemia can occur also in the watershed regions between the territories of cerebral arteries if there are prolonged periods of hypotension or low cardiac output.

Aside from the administration of 100% oxygen to denitrogenate known air emboli, there are few specific interventions. Thus the management strategy is to prevent secondary brain injury in the ischaemic penumbra of an infarct through temperature control, avoidance of hyperglycaemia and maintenance of cerebral perfusion. Fever increases the cerebral oxygen demand and should be avoided. Lowering the body temperature reduces oxygen consumption further [101] and lessens the release of toxic reactive oxygen, nitrogen species and excitatory neurotransmitters [102]. This translates to an improved functional outcome in patients who have been successfully resuscitated from a cardiac arrest [103, 104]. These two randomised studies aimed to lower core temperature to 32–34°C; they differed in terms of the duration of hypothermia (18 vs. 24 hours), the timing at which hypothermia was commenced (pre-hosiptal vs. hospital) and the method of rewarming (passive vs. active). These differences did not appear to lessen the beneficial effect. More profound hypothermia has increasingly adverse effects on coagulation, the immune system and cardiac rhythm, and is not recommended. Cerebral perfusion is a consequence of the difference between systemic arterial pressure and intracranial pressure. It is thus maintained by the use of vasopressors, moderate head elevation, avoiding ties that may impair jugular venous drainage, manipulation of the arterial pCO_2 to a low to normal value, and the neurosurgical drainage of haematomas and hydrocephalus.

More generalised and less severe neurological dysfunction is usually manifest as agitation or delirium. Common causes include an inflammatory encephalopathy as part of more widespread systemic inflammation, alcohol withdrawal, sleep deprivation, the use of sedatives and psychological illness. Delirium is associated with increased mortality and length of stay on the ICU [105, 106]. It is not clear how to reduce the risks of delirium or whether drug therapy can improve the prognosis. Typically benzodiazepines are used for alcohol withdrawal and neuroleptics, such as haloperidol, are used for agitation. Most neuroleptic agents prolong the QT interval and are pro-arrhythmic. Other approaches include the avoidance of exacerbating drug therapy, facilitating a sleep–wake cycle through environmental changes, and improving sensory inputs and communication with spectacles, hearing aids, speech and writing aids.

11.8 Sternal wound complications

Sternal wound infection and dehiscence, whilst uncommon, can be devastating following cardiac surgery. Severity ranges from local skin infections to more extensive infection of the sternum and mediastinum associated with instability and ultimately wound dehiscence. These complications result in prolonged hospitalisation, significant morbidity and mortality [107]. Risk factors for these complications include the need for surgical re-exploration, the harvesting of both internal thoracic arteries for coronary arterial revascularisation, diabetes mellitus, female sex, obesity and smoking [108, 109].

Management strategies include antibiotic therapy, debridement of infected and devitalised tissues, repeat sternal closure or transpositions of musculocutaneous flaps after removal of the sternum. Complex vacuum-assisted dressings may help to keep a deep open wound relatively dry and clean.

11.9 Conclusion

The high frequency of impaired cardiac function in critically ill patients is inevitably accompanied by multiple organ dysfunction and a high risk of iatrogenic injury. Knowing the common patterns of complications associated with the various procedures associated with admission to cardiothoracic intensive care helps intensivists to detect and diagnose complications at the earliest opportunity.

Case study 1

A 76-year-old patient, who had previously undergone coronary artery bypass grafting, was admitted to the high dependency unit after balloon angioplasty of a stenosed vein graft. He had recently presented with recurrence of his anginal symptoms. The procedure was complicated by rupture of the vein graft and a visible leak into the pericardial cavity. This was managed by deployment of a covered stent across the rupture. Angiography at the end of the procedure demonstrated no ongoing leak.

During the following 12 hours he became more tachycardic (107 bpm) in contrast to his admission beta-blocked rate (44 bpm), more hypotensive (102 mmHg systolic) in contrast to admission systolic pressure (183 mmHg) and oliguric. His jugular venous pressure was elevated, his peripheries cool and the residual weakness from an old stroke appeared worse. The significant pericardial collection was not appreciated until the following day, when a transthoracic echocardiogram demonstrated a large localised clot that significantly compromised the right ventricular cavity. The patient underwent emergency right thoracotomy and drainage of a tense right pericardial

Continued

effusion. He had little haemodynamic benefit from the procedure and severe right ventricular dysfunction was demonstrated on transoesophageal echocardiography. Over the following 48 hours he developed multi-organ failure and profound vasodilation. Despite maximal support and re-sternotomy he died.

Learning points:

- A high index of suspicion should be maintained for clinical tamponade.
- Observations of vital signs should be considered relative to baseline values.
- Indicators of low cardiac output should prompt a search for the aetiology. Blood pressure is often maintained within the normal range despite profound cardiac dysfunction.

Case study 2

A 24-year-old man was admitted to the ICU following conversion of his atriopulmonary connection (Fontan) to a total cavopulmonary connection (TCPC), removal of intra-atrial clot and radiofrequency ablation of his right atrium. He was born with classic tricuspid atresia and acquired pulmonary atresia. This was managed initially with right and then left Blalock–Taussig shunts and conversion to a Fontan circulation at the age of 6 years. The indications for TCPC conversion were chronic atrial fibrillation and a massive intra-atrial clot despite systemic anticoagulation that could occlude his Fontan circuit imminently.

His intra-operative course was complicated by a prolonged period of haemostasis, coagulopathy and poor ventricular function. He was weaned from cardiopulmonary bypass on infusions of milrinone, adrenaline and noradrenaline. An intra-aortic balloon pump was inserted via his left femoral artery but removed after several hours since augmentation was poor and it was considered to be providing little support. During his early post-operative course he developed a lactic acidosis due to his low cardiac output state that resolved with large volumes of intravascular fluid replacement, inhaled nitric oxide as a pulmonary vasodilator and increased inotropic support. He developed acute renal failure which was managed using continuous veno-venous haemodiafiltration. On the second post-operative day his arterial blood lactate and base deficit started to rise once more despite continuous renal replacement therapy (against a lactate-free buffer), warmer peripheries and good capillary refill. Administration of adrenaline may have contributed to the lactic acidosis [110] but had been infused continuously since the operation. Closer examination revealed a tense

Continued

left calf and he underwent surgical fasciotomy and oedematous dusky muscle bulged from the incision. His lactate resolved over the subsequent hours. The appearance of his calf muscles improved and it was possible to perform a spilt skin draft to the fasciotomy site at day 59. His ICU course was complicated by ARDS and multiple episodes of pulmonary sepsis. He was discharged from the ICU on day 66. He was fully mobile on discharge home with no neurological deficit in his left limb.

Learning point:

• Elevated blood lactate may have causes other than a low cardiac output and should prompt a clinical examination for a compartment syndrome since surgical fasciotomy can be limb saving.

References

1. Wheeler, A.P. and Bernard, G.R. Treating patients with severe sepsis. *N Engl J Med*, 1999. 340(3): 207–14.

2. Raja, S.G. and Berg, G.A. Impact of off-pump coronary artery bypass surgery on systemic inflammation: current best available evidence. *J Card Surg*, 2007. 22(5): 445–55.

3. Liakopoulos, O.J., et al. Cardiopulmonary and systemic effects of methylprednisolone in patients undergoing cardiac surgery. *Ann Thorac Surg*, 2007. 84(1): 110–8; discussion 118–9.

4. Bourbon, A., et al. The effect of methylprednisolone treatment on the cardiopulmonary bypass-induced systemic inflammatory response. *Eur J Cardiothorac Surg*, 2004. 26(5): 932–8.

5. Chaney, M.A., et al. Methylprednisolone does not benefit patients undergoing coronary artery bypass grafting and early tracheal extubation. *J Thorac Cardiovasc Surg*, 2001. 121(3): 561–9.

6. Mangano, D.T., et al. Mortality associated with aprotinin during 5 years following coronary artery bypass graft surgery. *JAMA*, 2007. 297(5): 471–9.

7. Fergusson, D.A., et al. A comparison of aprotinin and lysine analogues in high-risk cardiac surgery. *N Engl J Med*, 2008. 358(22): 2319–31.

8. Warren, O., et al. The effects of various leukocyte filtration strategies in cardiac surgery. *Eur J Cardiothorac Surg*, 2007. 31(4): 665–76.

9. Pappalardo, F., et al. Drotrecogin alpha and anticoagulants in septic patients after cardiac surgery. *Eur J Anaesthesiol*, 2007. 24(3): 294–5.

10. Abraham, E., et al. Drotrecogin alfa (activated) for adults with severe sepsis and a low risk of death. *N Engl J Med*, 2005. 353(13): 1332–41.

11. Marik, E., et al. Recommendations for the diagnosis and management of corticosteroid insufficiency in critically ill adult patients: consensus statements from an international task force by the American College of Critical Care Medicine. *Crit Care Med*, 2008. 36(6): 1937–49.

12. Vogeser, M., et al. Corticosteroid-binding globulin and free cortisol in the early postoperative period after cardiac surgery. *Clin Biochem*, 1999. 32(3): 213–6.

13. Malerba, G., et al. Risk factors of relative adrenocortical deficiency in intensive care patients needing mechanical ventilation. *Intensive Care Med*, 2005. 31(3): 388–92.

14. Absalom, A., Pledger, D. and Kong, A. Adrenocortical function in critically ill patients 24 h after a single dose of etomidate. *Anaesthesia*, 1999. 54(9): 861–7.

15. Sprung, C.L., et al. Hydrocortisone therapy for patients with septic shock. *N Engl J Med*, 2008. 358(2): 111–24.

16. van den Berghe, G., et al. Intensive insulin therapy in the critically ill patients. *N Engl J Med*, 2001. 345(19): 1359–67.

17. Krinsley, J.S. Effect of an intensive glucose management protocol on the mortality of critically ill adult patients. *Mayo Clin Proc*, 2004. 79(8): 992–1000.

18. Devos, P., Presier, J. and Melot, C. Impact of tight glucose control by intensive insulin therapy on ICU mortality and the rate of hypoglycaemia., in European Society of Intensive Care Medicine. *Intensive Care Med*. 2007. S189.

19. Van den Berghe, G., et al. Intensive insulin therapy in the medical ICU. *N Engl J Med*, 2006. 354(5): 449–61.

20. Brunkhorst, F.M., et al. Intensive insulin therapy and pentastarch resuscitation in severe sepsis. *N Engl J Med*, 2008. 358(2): 125–39.

21. Gandhi, G.Y., et al. Intensive intraoperative insulin therapy versus conventional glucose management during cardiac surgery: a randomized trial. *Ann Intern Med*, 2007. 146(4): 233–43.

22. Finney, S.J., et al. Glucose control and mortality in critically ill patients. *JAMA*, 2003. 290(15): 2041–7.

23. Weitzman, L.B., et al. The incidence and natural history of pericardial effusion after cardiac surgery – an echocardiographic study. *Circulation*, 1984. 69(3): 506–11.

24. Fejka, M., et al. Diagnosis, management, and clinical outcome of cardiac tamponade complicating percutaneous coronary intervention. *Am J Cardiol*, 2002. 90(11): 1183–6.

25. Hoit, B.D. and Shaw, D. The paradoxical pulse in tamponade: mechanisms and echocardiographic correlates. *Echocardiography*, 1994. 11(5): 477–87.

26. Price, S., et al. 'Tamponade' following cardiac surgery: terminology and echocardiography may both mislead. *Eur J Cardiothorac Surg*, 2004. 26(6): 1156–60.

27. Allen, R.C., et al. Acute lower extremity ischemia after cardiac surgery. *Am J Surg*, 1993. 166(2): 124–9; discussion 129.

28. Kuitunen, A., et al. Anaesthesia affects plasma concentrations of vasopressin, von Willebrand factor and coagulation factor VIII in cardiac surgical patients. *Br J Anaesth*, 1993. 70(2): 173–80.

29. Heringlake, M., et al. Renal dysfunction according to the ADQI-RIFLE system and clinical practice patterns after cardiac surgery in Germany. *Minerva Anestesiol*, 2006. 72(7–8): 645–54.

30. Rosner, M.H. and Okusa, M.D. Acute kidney injury associated with cardiac surgery. *Clin J Am Soc Nephrol*, 2006. 1(1): 19–32.

31. Bellomo, R., et al. Acute renal failure – definition, outcome measures, animal models, fluid therapy and information technology needs: the Second International Consensus Conference of the Acute Dialysis Quality Initiative (ADQI) Group. *Crit Care*, 2004. 8(4): R204–12.

32. Allgren, R.L., et al. Anaritide in acute tubular necrosis. Auriculin Anaritide Acute Renal Failure Study Group. *N Engl J Med*, 1997. 336(12): 828–34.

33. Meyer, M., et al. Therapeutic use of the natriuretic peptide ularitide in acute renal failure. *Ren Fail*, 1999. 21(1): 85–100.

34. Brenner, R.M. and Chertow, G.M. The rise and fall of atrial natriuretic peptide for acute renal failure. *Curr Opin Nephrol Hypertens*, 1997. 6(5): 474–6.

35. Landoni, G., Biondi-Zoccai, G., Marino, T. et al. Fenoldopam reduces the need for renal replacement therapy and in-hospital death in cardiovascular surgery: a meta-analysis. *J Cardiothorac Vasc Anesth*, 2008. 22(1): 27–33.

36. Jo, S.K., Rosner, M.H. and Okusa, M.D. Pharmacologic treatment of acute kidney injury: why drugs haven't worked and what is on the horizon. *Clin J Am Soc Nephrol*, 2007. 2(2): 356–65.

37. ClinicalTrials.gov. *Minocycline to Prevent Acute Kidney Injury After Cardiac Surgery* (NCT00556491). St Louis University.

38. Chow, S.L., et al. Effect of nesiritide infusion duration on renal function in acutely decompensated heart failure patients. *Ann Pharmacother*, 2007. 41(4): 556–61.

39. Yancy, C.W. and Singh, A. Potential applications of outpatient nesiritide infusions in patients with advanced heart failure and concomitant renal insufficiency (from the Follow-Up Serial Infusions of Nesiritide (FUSION I) trial). *Am J Cardiol*, 2006. 98(2): 226–9.

40. Chiao, H., et al. Alpha-melanocyte-stimulating hormone protects against renal injury after ischemia in mice and rats. *J Clin Invest*, 1997. 99(6): 1165–72.

41. Doi, K., et al. AP214, an analogue of alpha-melanocyte-stimulating hormone, ameliorates sepsis-induced acute kidney injury and mortality. *Kidney Int*, 2008. 73(11): 1266–74.

42. ClinicalTrials.gov. *Safety Tolerability and Pharmacodynamics of AP214 Acetate in Patients Undergoing Cardiac Surgery* (NCT00628624). St Louis University.

43. Ip-Yam, C., et al. Renal function and proteinuria after cardiopulmonary bypass: the effects of temperature and mannitol. *Anesth Analg*, 1994. 78(5): 842–7.

44. Carcoana, O.V., et al. Mannitol and dopamine in patients undergoing cardiopulmonary bypass: a randomized clinical trial. *Anesth Analg*, 2003. 97(5): 1222–9.

45. Smith, M.N., et al. The effect of mannitol on renal function after cardiopulmonary bypass in patients with established renal dysfunction. *Anaesthesia*, 2008. 63(7): 701–4.

46. Lassnigg, A., et al. Lack of renoprotective effects of dopamine and furosemide during cardiac surgery. *J Am Soc Nephrol*, 2000. 11(1): 97–104.

47. Mehta, R.L., et al. Diuretics, mortality, and nonrecovery of renal function in acute renal failure. *JAMA*, 2002. 288(20): 2547–53.

48. Ho, K.M. and Sheridan, D.J. Meta-analysis of frusemide to prevent or treat acute renal failure. *BMJ*, 2006. 333(7565): 420.

49. Kellum, J.A. The use of diuretics and dopamine in acute renal failure: a systematic review of the evidence. *Crit Care*, 1997. 1(2): 53–9.

50. Woo, E.B., et al. Dopamine therapy for patients at risk of renal dysfunction following cardiac surgery: science or fiction? *Eur J Cardiothorac Surg*, 2002. 22(1): 106–11.

51. Bellomo, R., et al. Low-dose dopamine in patients with early renal dysfunction: a placebo-controlled randomised trial. Australian and New Zealand Intensive Care Society (ANZICS) Clinical Trials Group. *Lancet*, 2000. 356(9248): 2139–43.

52. Friedrich, J.O., et al. Meta-analysis: low-dose dopamine increases urine output but does not prevent renal dysfunction or death. *Ann Intern Med*, 2005. 142(7): 510–24.

53. Kramer, B.K., Preuner, J., Ebenberger, A., et al. Lack of renoprotective effect of theophylline during aortocoronary bypass surgery. *Nephrol Dial Transplant*, 2002. 17(5): 910−5.

54. Dagher, C. Apoptosis in ischemic renal injury: roles of GTP depletion and p53. *Kidney Int*, 2004. 66(2): 506−9.

55. ClinicalTrials.gov. *A Dose Escalation and Safety Study of I5NP to Prevent Acute Kidney Injury (AKI) in Patients at High Risk of AKI Undergoing Major Cardiovascular Surgery (QRK.004)* (NCT00683553). St Louis University.

56. McCullough, A. Contrast-induced acute kidney injury. *J Am Coll Cardiol*, 2008. 51(15): 1419−28.

57. Mueller, C., et al. Prevention of contrast media-associated nephropathy: randomized comparison of 2 hydration regimens in 1620 patients undergoing coronary angioplasty. *Arch Intern Med*, 2002. 162(3): 329−36.

58. Trivedi, H.S., et al. A randomized prospective trial to assess the role of saline hydration on the development of contrast nephrotoxicity. *Nephron Clin Pract*, 2003. 93(1): C29−34.

59. Stacul, F., et al. Strategies to reduce the risk of contrast-induced nephropathy. *Am J Cardiol*, 2006. 98(6A): 59K−77K.

60. Merten, G.J., et al. Prevention of contrast-induced nephropathy with sodium bicarbonate: a randomized controlled trial. *JAMA*, 2004. 291(19): 2328−34.

61. Briguori, C., et al. Renal Insufficiency Following Contrast Media Administration Trial (REMEDIAL): a randomized comparison of 3 preventive strategies. *Circulation*, 2007. 115(10): 1211−7.

62. Pannu, N., et al. Systematic review of the impact of N-acetylcysteine on contrast nephropathy. *Kidney Int*, 2004. 65(4): 1366−74.

63. Zagler, A., et al. N-acetylcysteine and contrast-induced nephropathy: a meta-analysis of 13 randomized trials. *Am Heart J*, 2006. 151(1): 140−5.

64. Spargias, K., et al. Ascorbic acid prevents contrast-mediated nephropathy in patients with renal dysfunction undergoing coronary angiography or intervention. *Circulation*, 2004. 110(18): 2837−42.

65. Marenzi, G., et al. Comparison of two hemofiltration protocols for prevention of contrast-induced nephropathy in high-risk patients. *Am J Med*, 2006. 119(2): 155−62.

66. Marenzi, G., et al. The prevention of radiocontrast-agent-induced nephropathy by hemofiltration. *N Engl J Med*, 2003. 349(14): 1333−40.

67. Messent, M., et al. Adult respiratory distress syndrome following cardiopulmonary bypass: incidence and prediction. *Anaesthesia*, 1992. 47(3): 267−8.

68. Wiedemann, H., et al. Comparison of two fluid-management strategies in acute lung injury. *N Engl J Med*, 2006. 354(24): 2564−75.

69. Cranshaw, J., Griffiths, M.J. and Evans, T.W. The pulmonary physician in critical care − part 9: non-ventilatory strategies in ARDS. *Thorax*, 2002. 57(9): 823−9.

70. Pinhu, L., et al. Ventilator-associated lung injury. *Lancet*, 2003. 361(9354): 332−40.

71. The Acute Respiratory Distress Syndrome Network. Ventilation with lower tidal volumes as compared with traditional tidal volumes for acute lung injury and the acute respiratory distress syndrome. *N Engl J Med*, 2000. 342(18): 1301−8.

72. Finney, S.J. and Evans, T.W. Mechanical ventilation in acute respiratory distress syndrome. *Curr Opin Anaesthesiol*, 2001. 14(2): 165−71.

73. Jain, U., et al. Radiographic pulmonary abnormalities after different types of cardiac surgery. *J Cardiothorac Vasc Anesth*, 1991. 5(6): 592−5.

74. Carrel, T., Eisinger, E., Vogt, M., et al. Pneumonia after cardiac surgery is predictable by tracheal aspirates but cannot be prevented by prolonged antibiotic prophylaxis. *Ann Thorac Surg*, 2001. 72(1): 143–8.

75. Pasquina, P., Tramer, M.R. and Walder, B. Prophylactic respiratory physiotherapy after cardiac surgery: systematic review. *BMJ*, 2003. 327(7428): 1379.

76. Peng, M.J., et al. Postoperative pleural changes after coronary revascularization. Comparison between saphenous vein and internal mammary artery grafting. *Chest*, 1992. 101(2): 327–30.

77. Inci, I., et al. Intrapleural fibrinolytic treatment of traumatic clotted hemothorax. *Chest*, 1998. 114(1): 160–5.

78. Lichtenstein, D., et al. Feasibility and safety of ultrasound-aided thoracentesis in mechanically ventilated patients. *Intensive Care Med*, 1999. 25(9): 955–8.

79. Wang, J.S. and Tseng, C.H. Changes in pulmonary mechanics and gas exchange after thoracentesis on patients with inversion of a hemidiaphragm secondary to large pleural effusion. *Chest*, 1995. 107(6): 1610–4.

80. Agusti, A.G., et al. Ventilation-perfusion mismatch in patients with pleural effusion: effects of thoracentesis. *Am J Respir Crit Care Med*, 1997. 156(4 Pt 1): 1205–9.

81. Talmor, M., et al. Beneficial effects of chest tube drainage of pleural effusion in acute respiratory failure refractory to positive end-expiratory pressure ventilation. *Surgery*, 1998. 123(2): 137–43.

82. Doelken, et al. Effect of thoracentesis on respiratory mechanics and gas exchange in the patient receiving mechanical ventilation. *Chest*, 2006. 130(5): 1354–61.

83. Laws, D., Neville, E. and Duffy, J. BTS guidelines for the insertion of a chest drain. *Thorax*, 2003. 58(Suppl 2): ii53–9.

84. Echevarria, C., et al. Does re-expansion pulmonary oedema exist? *Interact Cardiovasc Thorac Surg*, 2008. 7(3): 485–9.

85. Rousou, J.A., et al. Phrenic nerve paresis associated with the use of iced slush and the cooling jacket for topical hypothermia. *J Thorac Cardiovasc Surg*, 1985. 89(6): 921–5.

86. Cassese, M., et al. Topical cooling for myocardial protection: the results of a prospective randomized study of the 'shallow technique'. *J Card Surg*, 2006. 21(4): 357–62.

87. Yilmaz, A.T., et al. Gastrointestinal complications after cardiac surgery. *Eur J Cardiothorac Surg*, 1996. 10(9): 763–7.

88. Krasna, M.J., et al. Gastrointestinal complications after cardiac surgery. *Surgery*, 1988. 104(4): 773–80.

89. Birrer, R., Takuda, Y. and Takara, T. Hypoxic hepatopathy: pathophysiology and prognosis. *Intern Med*, 2007. 46(14): 1063–70.

90. Seeto, R.K., Fenn, B. and Rockey, D.C. Ischemic hepatitis: clinical presentation and pathogenesis. *Am J Med*, 2000. 109(2): 109–13.

91. Filsoufi, F., et al. Predictors and outcome of gastrointestinal complications in patients undergoing cardiac surgery. *Ann Surg*, 2007. 246(2): 323–9.

92. Ihaya, A., et al. Hyperamylasemia and subclinical pancreatitis after cardiac surgery. *World J Surg*, 2001. 25(7): 862–4.

93. Fernandez-del Castillo, C., et al. Risk factors for pancreatic cellular injury after cardiopulmonary bypass. *N Engl J Med*, 1991. 325(6): 382–7.

94. Rattner, D.W., et al. Hyperamylasemia after cardiac surgery. Incidence, significance, and management. *Ann Surg*, 1989. 209(3): 279–83.

95. Wyncoll, D.L. The management of severe acute necrotising pancreatitis: an evidence-based review of the literature. *Intensive Care Med*, 1999. 25(2): 146–56.

96. Coselli, J.S., et al. Cerebrospinal fluid drainage reduces paraplegia after thoracoabdominal aortic aneurysm repair: results of a randomized clinical trial. *J Vasc Surg*, 2002. 35(4): 631–9.

97. Widmann, M.D., et al. Reversal of renal failure and paraplegia after thoracoabdominal aneurysm repair. *Ann Thorac Surg*, 1998. 65(4): 1153–5.

98. Azizzadeh, A., et al. Reversal of twice-delayed neurologic deficits with cerebrospinal fluid drainage after thoracoabdominal aneurysm repair: a case report and plea for a national database collection. *J Vasc Surg*, 2000. 31(3): 592–8.

99. Hill, A.B., et al. Reversal of delayed-onset paraplegia after thoracic aortic surgery with cerebrospinal fluid drainage. *J Vasc Surg*, 1994. 20(2): 315–7.

100. Stroobant, N., et al. Neuropsychological functioning 3–5 years after coronary artery bypass grafting: does the pump make a difference? *Eur J Cardiothorac Surg*, 2008. 34(2): 396–401.

101. Hegnauer, A.H. and D'Amato, H.E. Oxygen consumption and cardiac output in the hypothermic dog. *Am J Physiol*, 1954. 178(1): 138–42.

102. Busto, R., et al. Effect of mild hypothermia on ischemia-induced release of neurotransmitters and free fatty acids in rat brain. *Stroke*, 1989. 20(7): 904–10.

103. Bernard, S.A., et al. Treatment of comatose survivors of out-of-hospital cardiac arrest with induced hypothermia. *N Engl J Med*, 2002. 346(8): 557–63.

104. Hypothermia after Cardiac Arrest Study Group. Mild therapeutic hypothermia to improve the neurologic outcome after cardiac arrest. *N Engl J Med*, 2002. 346(8): 549–56.

105. Ely, E.W., et al. Delirium as a predictor of mortality in mechanically ventilated patients in the intensive care unit. *JAMA*, 2004. 291(14): 1753–62.

106. Ely, E.W., et al. The impact of delirium in the intensive care unit on hospital length of stay. *Intensive Care Med*, 2001. 27(12): 1892–900.

107. Ivert, T., et al. Management of deep sternal wound infection after cardiac surgery–Hanuman syndrome. *Scand J Thorac Cardiovasc Surg*, 1991. 25(2): 111–7.

108. Stahle, E., et al. Sternal wound complications – incidence, microbiology and risk factors. *Eur J Cardiothorac Surg*, 1997. 11(6): 1146–53.

109. McDonald, W.S., et al. Risk factors for median sternotomy dehiscence in cardiac surgery. *South Med J*, 1989. 82(11): 1361–4.

110. Salak, N., et al. Effects of epinephrine on intestinal oxygen supply and mucosal tissue oxygen tension in pigs. *Crit Care Med*, 2001. 29(2): 367–73.

12 Haemodynamic Management of Severe Sepsis

Jean-Louis Vincent

Erasme University Hospital, University of Brussels, Brussels, Belgium

---

Take Home Messages

- Septic shock is associated with a hyperdynamic circulation, typically with a normal or high cardiac output.
- Early and rapid resuscitation of patients with septic shock can result in improved outcomes, and should be aimed at achieving a central venous oxygen saturation ($ScvO_2$) > 70% or a mixed venous oxygen saturation (SvO_2) > 65%.
- Colloids or crystalloids can be used for fluid resuscitation and repeated fluid challenges should be used to ensure adequate fluid administration with limited oedema formation.
- Vasopressor agents may be required to restore tissue perfusion and either dopamine or noradrenaline can be used as a first-line agent. Addition of low-dose vasopressin may be useful.
- Myocardial depression associated with septic shock may necessitate the use of inotropes to improve myocardial contractility and ensure adequate cardiac output. Pulmonary artery catheterisation may be useful for combined monitoring of cardiac output, SvO_2 and cardiac filling pressures in patients who fail to improve rapidly.
- Haemodynamic support should be titrated to the individual patient according to clinical status and global haemodynamic and oxygenation parameters.

12.1 Introduction

Sepsis is defined by the presence of both infection and a systemic inflammatory response [1]. Unfortunately, infection is often difficult to identify, particularly in the critically ill, and the 'systemic inflammatory response' is also difficult to define and characterise. The diagnosis of sepsis, therefore, currently relies on good clinical and laboratory detective work, in which the combined presence of various signs and symptoms make

---

Cardiovascular Critical Care. Edited by M. Griffiths, J. Cordingley and S. Price.
© 2010 Blackwell Publishing Ltd.

Table 12.1 Diagnostic criteria for sepsis [1]. Infection plus some of the following.

General variables
Fever (core temperature > 38.3°C) or hypothermia (core temperature < 36°C)
Unexplained tachycardia (> 90 beats/min or > 2 SD above the normal for age)
Unexplained tachypnoea/respiratory alkalosis
Unexplained disorientation or confusion
Significant oedema or positive fluid balance (> 20 ml/kg over 24 hours)
Unexplained hyperglycaemia (plasma glucose > 120 mg/dl)
Inflammatory variables
Altered white blood cell count
Increased C-reactive protein levels
Increased plasma procalcitonin levels
Haemodynamic and oxygenation variables
Increased cardiac output/low systemic vascular resistance
Unexplained arterial hypoxaemia (PaO_2/FiO_2 < 300)
Increased oxygen consumption
Unexplained lactic acidosis
Organ dysfunction variables
Thrombocytopenia/disseminated intravascular coagulation
Unexplained alteration in liver function tests
Unexplained alteration in renal function
Ileus

sepsis the most likely diagnosis (Table 12.1) [1]. Once sepsis has been diagnosed, the categories severe sepsis (sepsis complicated by organ dysfunction) and septic shock (severe sepsis plus persistent arterial hypotension unexplained by other causes) are relatively easy to identify [1]. Severe sepsis and septic shock are among the most important causes of morbidity and mortality in patients admitted to the intensive care unit (ICU). Severe sepsis affects 30% of ICU admissions and is associated with mortality rates of about 30%, while septic shock is present in about 15% of ICU admissions and is associated with mortality rates of more than 50% [2].

Severe sepsis is associated with a range of haemodynamic alterations that can lead to the development of tissue hypoperfusion and hypoxia, believed to be important in the development and maintenance of multiple organ failure, a common and frequently fatal sequel of severe sepsis and septic shock. Early correction of haemodynamic status is, therefore, an essential part of the management of patients with severe sepsis and septic shock, and this chapter focuses on this aspect, although other facets of treatment, including antimicrobial administration and source control, must, of course, also form part of the global care package for patients with severe sepsis.

12.2 Haemodynamic alterations in severe sepsis and septic shock

Septic shock is typically classified as a distributive form of shock, characterised by an increase in the vascular capacitance, although it may

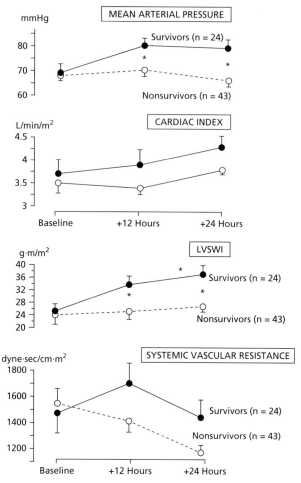

Figure 12.1 Changes in mean arterial pressure, cardiac index, left ventricular stroke work index (LVSWI) and systemic vascular resistance during the first 24 hours of septic shock in survivors and non-survivors. * $p < 0.05$ from previous measurements or between the two subgroups of patients. Data are expressed as mean ± SD. (Reproduced from Metrangolo et al. [3], with permission.)

also comprise components of hypovolaemic and cardiogenic shock. The typical haemodynamic pattern, following fluid resuscitation, is hyperdynamic with a normal or raised cardiac output and reduced vascular tone and, hence, systemic vascular resistance (Figure 12.1) [3]. Imbalance between vasodilating (e.g. nitric oxide (NO) and prostacyclin) and vasoconstricting (e.g. thromboxane and endothelin) mediators influences the degree of altered vascular tone, and is correlated with severity of sepsis and outcome [4].

Cardiac output may not be elevated in the initial phase of septic shock. Hypovolaemia may result from external (e.g. increased insensible losses and vomiting) and internal (e.g. oedema resulting from capillary leak) sources. Venous pooling can contribute to a reduction in venous return and cardiac output. Cytokines, including tumour necrosis factor (TNF-α) and interleukin (IL)-1, and other mediators released as part of the immune response to sepsis (e.g. NO) also cause myocardial depression, contributing to the haemodynamic alterations seen during severe sepsis [5]. Myocardial depression occurs early during the course of septic shock and manifests as reversible biventricular dilatation, decreased ejection fraction and decreased response to catecholamine stimulation. Interestingly, the left and right ventricles may respond differently in severe sepsis [5]. For example, decreased systemic vascular resistance results in reduced left ventricular afterload, which maintains a normal or high cardiac output despite the presence of depressed left ventricular contractility. However, increased pulmonary vascular resistance, related to the development of acute lung injury or adult respiratory distress syndrome (ARDS), often results in increased right ventricular afterload. Nevertheless, the development of right ventricular dysfunction in septic shock closely parallels the development of left ventricular dysfunction, and the presence of myocardial depression is correlated with a worse outcome [6, 7].

12.3 Haemodynamic management of severe sepsis

The approach to the haemodynamic management of the patient with severe sepsis should follow the VIP (ventilation, infusion, pump) schema initially proposed by Weil and Shubin [8] almost 40 years ago.

V for ventilation
Oxygen should be started immediately to treat hypoxia and thereby minimise pulmonary vasoconstriction which may limit cardiac output and oxygen delivery. There should be a lower threshold for tracheal intubation and invasive mechanical ventilation than in patients who are not septic. Not only will this ensure adequate ventilation and protect the airway in obtunded patients, but also it will reduce oxygen requirement by resting the respiratory muscles. The aim of oxygen administration should be to maintain arterial oxygen saturation (SaO_2) above 90%. The different modes of mechanical ventilation available are beyond the scope of this chapter, but non-invasive ventilation has little place in the acute management of critically ill patients with septic shock.

I for infusion
Fluid therapy is an essential part of the treatment of septic shock, to restore intravascular volume and, hence, cardiac output and arterial blood pressure. However, while too little fluid is clearly detrimental, too much fluid also carries risks, principally of pulmonary oedema. Fluid resuscitation must be initiated early. Patients admitted to the emergency department with severe sepsis and randomised to an early goal-directed therapy protocol for the first 6 hours had improved outcomes compared to patients who received standard care; this protocol involved the use of fluids,

vasopressors and blood transfusions to achieve a target central venous oxygen saturation (ScvO$_2$) of 70% [9]. Protocol-managed patients received 40% more intravenous fluids in those first 6 hours than did patients managed according to standard practice, supporting the role of adequate and early fluid resuscitation in patients with severe sepsis. However, while few would argue the need for fluid resuscitation in septic shock, there are several areas of controversy within this field, primarily related to the choice of fluid, and the choice of endpoint.

Type of fluid

Although the traditional debate has focused on the choice between crystalloid and colloid, within each of these two groups there are several fluid types to choose from.

The crystalloid solutions (e.g. normal saline, Ringer's lactate) are cheap and generally well tolerated, but they are less well retained in the intravascular space than colloid solutions, and more fluid is needed to achieve the same haemodynamic endpoints [10]. This in turn increases the risks of peripheral and pulmonary oedema developing, which can be associated with impaired oxygenation, wound healing and myocardial and gut function [11–13]. One approach to limiting the risks of oedema formation is to add colloids to crystalloids to decrease the total amount of fluid required to restore haemodynamic instability.

There are four main groups of colloid solutions: albumin, gelatins, dextrans and hydroxyethyl starch (HES) solutions. Gelatins are not very effective because they leave the circulation rapidly, and dextrans are now rarely used. It has been suggested that HES solutions may have beneficial properties in addition to their volume expansion effects, including reducing microvascular permeability [14] and anti-inflammatory properties [15]. However, their use has recently been challenged with the Efficacy of Volume Substitution and Insulin Therapy in Severe Sepsis (VISEP) study reporting an increased risk of renal failure in patients with severe sepsis who received 10% HES solution compared to those who received Ringer's lactate (35 versus 23%, $p = 0.002$) [16].

Albumin has been widely used in ICUs for years, but its use has generated considerable controversy over the last decade or so. A famous meta-analysis published in 1998 [17] suggested that resuscitation with albumin solutions was associated with a 6% increase in the absolute risk of death compared to crystalloids, and a recent propensity score analysis of 339 patients from a database of 3,147 patients admitted to 198 European ICUs showed that patients who received albumin had higher mortality rates than those who did not [18]. However, the Saline versus Albumin Fluid Evaluation (SAFE) study randomised 7,000 critically ill patients receiving either 4% albumin or 0.9% normal saline for their initial fluid resuscitation, and reported no significant differences between groups in mortality or ICU stay in the population as a whole [19]. In the subgroup of patients with sepsis, there was a trend to improved mortality in the patients who had received albumin. In addition, a meta-analysis of 71 randomised controlled trials suggested that albumin administration may reduce complications in critically ill patients [20], and a recently published pilot study investigating the effects of 20% albumin or placebo in patients with hypoalbuminaemia suggested that patients who received albumin had improved organ function compared to those who received placebo [21]. Albumin is an expensive solution, but its relative costs are decreasing as more expensive new therapies appear on the market. Clearly, it is not indicated in all patients, but further studies are needed to help define those patients in whom it may improve outcomes.

Overall, there are relatively few randomised controlled data comparing different fluids in patients with septic shock, and none that demonstrates a definite advantage of one fluid type over another, despite the potential apparent advantages of colloid solutions over crystalloids in terms of longer intravascular persistence. Until other evidence becomes available, fluid resuscitation should consist of natural or artificial colloids or crystalloids [22], and the choice will depend on patient factors, including the severity of the shock, renal function, risk of bleeding, physician preference and cost considerations.

Endpoints for fluid resuscitation

The main target of fluid resuscitation in septic shock is to restore an adequate cardiac output and perfusion pressure to ensure continued tissue blood flow. However, as sensitive tools for monitoring regional microcirculatory blood flow and oxygenation are not yet available, precise endpoints for fluid resuscitation are difficult to define. Although systemic variables are widely used to assess the adequacy of tissue oxygenation, these may appear to be normal even when regional tissue perfusion is still inadequate [23]. A fluid challenge technique, first suggested several decades ago [24], is the best method of determining a patient's ongoing need for fluids. This approach, reserved for patients in whom the response to fluids is uncertain, is thus very different to fluid loading or simple fluid administration. The fluid challenge technique is aimed at prompt correction of fluid deficits and quantification of the cardiovascular response to volume infusion, while minimising the risk of fluid overload [25]. The fluid challenge approach essentially incorporates four phases [25]:

- The type of fluid – either crystalloid or colloid can be used (see above).
- The rate of fluid administration – the amount of fluid to be administered over a specified interval must be defined. The Surviving Sepsis Campaign Guidelines for the management of severe sepsis and septic shock recommend $\geq$ 1000 ml of crystalloids or 300–500 ml of colloids over 30 min [22].
- The target for the fluid challenge should be identified, so that a target or goal of fluid administration can be set. This goal needs to be a variable that reacts sufficiently rapidly to indicate the acute effects of fluid administration and often an adequate mean arterial pressure is used. The recent update of the Surviving Sepsis Campaign Guidelines [22] suggests that the initial

target of fluid resuscitation should be a central venous pressure (CVP) of 8 mmHg (or 12 mmHg in mechanically ventilated patients).
- The safety limit(s) – clearly safety limits need to be set to avoid potential complications of fluid overload. Generally the pulmonary artery occlusion pressure (PAOP) or the CVP are used to define safety limits. It is important that, when assessing the result of *volume* loading by monitoring *pressure*, consideration is given to vascular compliance. It is possible for venous pressures to remain normal or even elevated in a hypovolaemic patient because of arteriolar and venous constriction. Similar considerations are important when resuscitating patients with known or suspected abnormalities of ventricular compliance.

Repeating the fluid challenge will allow the physician to continuously reassess a patient's ongoing fluid needs while limiting the risks of adverse effects.

P for pump
Vasopressor agents

In the majority of patients with septic shock, vasopressor agents will be required in addition to fluids in order to restore an adequate perfusion pressure, and in many patients vasopressors and fluid resuscitation will be started concomitantly. Vasopressors should then be tapered as soon as possible, once fluid resuscitation is complete. Several drugs are available for this purpose, the effects of each depending largely on the receptors on which they act: the two main agents are noradrenaline and dopamine.

Dopamine is a naturally occurring compound (the precursor of noradrenaline) that combines dopaminergic effects with α- and β-adrenergic properties. The dopaminergic effects predominate at very low doses (< 3 µg/kg/min) and may dilate the hepatosplanchnic and renal circulations [26, 27], thereby selectively increasing flow in these important regions. However, the clinical benefits of these dopaminergic effects have not been demonstrated [28] and the routine administration of low-dose dopamine to prevent renal failure is not recommended [22, 29]. At doses of $3-10$ µg/kg/min, β_1-adrenergic effects predominate, increasing cardiac contractility and heart rate, and at higher doses (> 10 µg/kg/min), α_1-adrenergic effects come to the fore, with arterial vasoconstriction and an increase in blood pressure. Importantly, these are not strict cut-off ranges and there is considerable overlap in dopaminergic, α and β effects and variation in response among patients.

Noradrenaline is another naturally occurring compound, secreted by the adrenal medulla and the post-ganglionic sympathetic nerves. Noradrenaline has predominantly α-adrenergic properties, increasing mean arterial pressure largely by its effects on vascular smooth muscle. The normal dose-range is $0.05-1$ µg/kg/min, although larger doses may be needed in septic shock, possibly due to α-receptor down-regulation. Although there have been concerns that excessive vasoconstriction with noradrenaline may have negative effects on blood flow, particularly in the hepatosplanchnic and renal circulations, studies have suggested that it can successfully increase blood pressure without causing any deterioration in

Table 12.2 Potential advantages and disadvantages of dopamine versus noradrenaline.

Dopamine	Noradrenaline
Advantages	
Greater increase in blood flow	Less arrhythmogenic
Increased renal blood flow (?)	
Increased splanchnic blood flow (?)	
Increased oedema clearance	
Improved muscle function	
Disadvantages	
Decreased gut mucosal blood flow (?)	Risk of excessive vasoconstriction (?)
Immunosuppression	
Arrhythmias	

organ function, particularly in the presence of decreased vascular tone, as in septic shock [30, 31].

Considerable effort has been put into trying to determine whether one agent may have specific beneficial effects on the regional (hepatosplanchnic) circulation, believed to be important in the development of multiple organ failure, a common sequel to severe sepsis, but again there is little evidence to demonstrate any clinically relevant differences between the two drugs in this respect [31] (Table 12.2). Noradrenaline is a more potent vasopressor than dopamine, but both dopamine and noradrenaline have specific drawbacks. Dopamine is associated with a greater risk of tachycardia than noradrenaline. Dopaminergic stimulation may also have unwanted endocrine effects via its effects on the hypothalamo-pituitary gland [32]. Noradrenaline can precipitate myocardial ischaemia and cardiac failure as a result of increased afterload.

As with fluid therapy, the choice of vasopressor agent in sepsis continues to be a topic of debate, as again there are few data consistently supporting one drug over another. A recent observational study suggested that dopamine use in patients with septic shock may be associated with worse outcomes; in a multivariate analysis, with ICU mortality as the dependent factor, dopamine administration was independently associated with a higher risk of death from shock of any cause (odds ratio 1.67; 95% confidence interval 1.19–2.35, $p = 0.003$) and septic shock (odds ratio 2.05; 95% confidence interval 1.25–3.37, $p = 0.005$) [32]. A recently completed randomised controlled study in Europe comparing noradrenaline and dopamine as first-line agent in the management of shock should help provide some further guidance on the choice of vasopressor agent. Meanwhile, current guidelines recommend either dopamine or noradrenaline as first-line vasopressor agents in patients with septic shock [22, 29]. Whichever drug is chosen, patients with septic shock are often relatively resistant to vasopressors and may require very high doses. The reasons underlying this are not fully defined but include increased production of the natural vasodilator NO via cytokine-induced induction of NO synthase, and cytokine-induced down-regulation of α_1-adrenergic receptors [34, 35].

Inotropic agents

Inotropic therapy generally aims to restore cardiac output, but in patients with fluid-resuscitated septic shock, cardiac output is usually normal or high. Hence, the goals of inotropic therapy are more difficult to define, and must focus on the adequacy of the cardiac output rather than on the cardiac output value *per se*. Inotropic therapy must, therefore, be guided by global and regional measures of tissue perfusion and oxygenation (see below).

Dobutamine is the inotropic agent of choice for patients who have received adequate fluid resuscitation but have inadequate cardiac output. Dobutamine has predominantly β_1-adrenergic properties, but its mild α-adrenergic effects help limit the increase in heart rate seen with isoproterenol, a pure β-adrenergic agent. A decrease in arterial pressure during dobutamine administration should raise the possibility of underlying fluid deficits. Dobutamine was used, in addition to fluids and red cell transfusion, to increase $ScvO_2$ to more than 70% as part of the early goal-directed therapy protocol in the study by Rivers et al. [9]; this protocol was associated with improved outcomes compared to standard care. However, despite these beneficial effects in this particular situation, dobutamine should not routinely be used to increase cardiac output or oxygen delivery (DO_2I) to so-called supranormal levels, as this approach is not beneficial in all patients [36]. Dobutamine may have additional beneficial effects on microcirculatory blood flow. Administration of dobutamine to patients with septic shock at a dose of 5 µg/kg/min for 2 hours was associated with improved capillary perfusion as assessed by orthogonal polarisation spectral imaging, but this improvement did not correlate with, and so was not dependent on, increases in cardiac index or systemic arterial pressure [23].

Dopexamine hydrochloride is a newer, synthetic catecholamine, similar to dopamine in structure, which is not licensed for clinical use in the USA. It has marked β_2 agonist activity, weak β_1-adrenergic activity, and some dopaminergic receptor activity. It has been suggested that, due to its dopaminergic effects, dopexamine may have beneficial effects on the renal or hepatosplanchnic circulations, but study results have been conflicting and a meta-analysis found no evidence to support the use of dopexamine for this purpose [37]. In addition, its use is limited by the development of marked tachycardia, particularly at higher doses.

Phosphodiesterase (PDE) inhibitors are a group of drugs that prolong or enhance the effects of physiological processes mediated by cyclic adenosine monophosphate (cAMP) or cGMP. PDEIII inhibitors, such as enoximone and milrinone, have inotropic and vasodilating properties. Due to their vasodilating properties and their long half-lives, they must be used with caution in patients who are hypotensive. Administration of very small doses of PDE inhibitors may reinforce the effects of dobutamine [38]. Some studies have suggested that these agents may also have anti-inflammatory effects and beneficial effects on hepatosplanchnic perfusion [39], but further studies are needed to determine their exact role, if any, in the routine management of patients with septic shock.

Other vasoactive agents

The potential role of arginine vasopressin in improving haemodynamic status in patients with septic shock has attracted considerable attention in recent years. Vasopressin is an endogenous hormone secreted by the neurohypophysis in response to an increase in serum osmolality or a decrease in plasma volume. In patients with septic shock vasopressin levels are unexpectedly low for the degree of hypotension [40], suggesting a potential value in administering exogenous vasopressin to restore levels to normal and by so-doing increasing arterial blood pressure. In normal individuals, administration of vasopressin has little effect on arterial pressure, but in patients with septic shock, several studies have demonstrated increased arterial pressure, increased urine output and reduced requirements for other vasopressor agents in patients receiving low doses (0.01–0.04 U/min) of vasopressin [41, 42]. Vasopressin may decrease cardiac output and this must be carefully monitored. In a clinically relevant sheep model of septic shock, vasopressin administration was associated with improved survival [43]. The recently completed multicentre VASST study, which randomised 779 patients to noradrenaline or vasopressin, suggested that in patients with less severe shock, vasopressin was associated with reduced mortality rates compared to noradrenaline treatment [44]. Interestingly, the benefit seemed to be greater when the vasopressor requirements were only limited. Hence, a reasonable statement is that vasopressin (or terlipressin) cannot be seen as a replacement for noradrenaline or dopamine but may be considered in patients with septic shock requiring vasopressors.

Other therapies in sepsis with vasoactive effects

There are many other interventions that may have useful haemodynamic effects in patients with septic shock, including corticosteroids and activated protein C.

High-dose corticosteroids were commonly used for their anti-inflammatory properties in the treatment of patients with sepsis until the end of the 1980s, when their effectiveness was questioned [45, 46]. However, more recently, as the concept of 'relative adrenal insufficiency' in patients with septic shock has emerged, prolonged courses of lower doses of corticosteroids have been found to improve shock reversal [47] and outcome in patients with septic shock [48]. Keh et al. reported that hydrocortisone treatment increased mean arterial pressure and reduced noradrenaline requirements. There was an increase in systemic vascular resistance and a reduction in cardiac index and heart rate. The underlying mechanisms are unclear but may, in part, be related to inhibition of NO formation by corticosteroids [49]. A multicentre randomised controlled French trial that included 300 patients with septic shock [48] reported that treatment with hydrocortisone (50 mg IV every 6 hours) and fludrocortisone (50 μg PO daily) was associated with a reduced mortality compared to placebo in patients with relative adrenal insufficiency (as assessed by non-response to a corticotrophin test) [48]. However, the recent international multicentre CORTICUS study failed to demonstrate an effect of hydrocortisone on outcomes, although time to shock reversal was reduced in treated patients [50]. The place of steroid therapy in patients with septic shock therefore remains unclear.

Drotrecogin alfa (activated), a recombinant form of activated protein C, has been shown to improve survival in patients with severe sepsis in a large, multicentre randomised controlled trial [51]. Patients treated with the drug had significantly less cardiovascular dysfunction (as assessed by the sequential organ failure assessment (SOFA) score) during the treatment period and faster resolution of cardiovascular and respiratory dysfunction [52]. The drug is now licensed for the treatment of adult patients with severe sepsis at a high risk of death who have no contraindications. A recent study has suggested that some of the beneficial effects of drotrecogin alfa (activated) on haemodynamic status may be related to its effects on the microcirculation, with improved microvascular perfusion in patients treated with the drug [53].

12.4 Endpoints of resuscitation

As mentioned above, the endpoints of resuscitation in patients with septic shock are difficult to define. Currently available monitoring only encompasses global indices of perfusion, yet if regional perfusion and oxygenation are indeed key components in the development of sepsis-associated organ dysfunction and multiple organ failure, then monitoring peripheral organ perfusion may provide better endpoints. Despite correction of global haemodynamic alterations, many patients still suffer from regional blood flow alterations [54, 55]. New techniques, including orthogonal polarisation spectral imaging, should soon enable us to visualise the microcirculation and to quantify changes in microcirculatory flow and oxygenation, and studies will then need to demonstrate that targeting therapies at these microcirculatory changes does indeed improve outcome. In the meantime, resuscitation must be guided by global haemodynamic variables, including mean arterial pressure and cardiac output, complemented by indicators of tissue oxygenation.

Mixed venous oxygen saturation (SvO_2) is a global measure of whole body oxygen balance, (i.e. the relationship between oxygen delivery and oxygen consumption). SvO_2 varies directly with cardiac output, haemoglobin concentration and arterial oxygen saturation (SaO_2). SvO_2 can be measured continuously using a pulmonary artery catheter (PAC) and is usually 70–75% in critically ill patients. The less invasive $ScvO_2$, measured in the superior vena cava using a central venous catheter, has been promoted since it was used as one of the endpoints of resuscitation in the study by Rivers et al. [9] in patients with severe sepsis and septic shock presenting to the emergency department. However, $ScvO_2$ reflects the venous oxygenation of blood from the upper half of the body while SvO_2 measures whole body venous oxygen saturation, and in patients with septic

Table 12.3 Possible causes of raised blood lactate levels in patients with sepsis.

Anaerobic metabolism
Increased glycolysis
Inhibition of pyruvate dehydrogenase
Altered lactate clearance due to impaired liver function or decreased liver blood flow
Regional production of lactate

shock, the relationship between $ScvO_2$ and SvO_2 is not always reliable [56]. In critically ill patients, $ScvO_2$ is slightly higher that SvO_2 [56]. The interpretation of cardiac output ideally requires assessment of SvO_2 (or $ScvO_2$). For example, if a patient has a low cardiac output but a normal or high SvO_2, these conditions may simply reflect a low oxygen demand, such as can be found in patients treated with large doses of sedatives and perhaps muscle relaxants. In such a case, any intervention to increase cardiac output is unlikely to improve the haemodynamic status. However, if SvO_2 is also low, the low cardiac output becomes a concern, as this combination may suggest acute circulatory failure. Although many people have stopped using a PAC in light of recent neutral studies regarding its benefits, its use may still be important in patients who do not rapidly improve, enabling more reliable interpretation of cardiac output.

Blood lactate levels provide a useful indication of the presence of anaerobic metabolism due to hypoperfusion, and repeated measurements can provide useful information about the adequacy of global tissue oxygenation in response to treatment. In patients with sepsis, causes of hyperlactataemia other than hypoperfusion may cloud the interpretation of blood lactate levels (Table 12.3), but the prognostic value of raised blood lactate levels is, nevertheless, well established in patients with septic shock, particularly if they are persistent [57]. Blood lactate levels persistently above 2 mmol/L suggest that tissue oxygenation may be inadequate and resuscitation suboptimal.

Importantly, and unfortunately, no single variable alone is adequate to guide resuscitation, and each patient must be assessed individually according to clinical evaluation, including the three 'windows' onto the peripheral circulation: the skin, mental status and urine output, complemented by global haemodynamic and oxygenation variables and blood lactate levels.

12.5 Conclusion

The haemodynamic management of severe sepsis is just one part of the multifaceted package of treatments for the patient with severe sepsis [22]. The key goals are to correct hypovolaemia and arterial hypotension and then to optimise oxygen delivery. Fluid resuscitation must start early and be guided by repeated fluid challenges. Vasopressor treatment should be titrated individually according to clinical evaluation and targeted to goals of regional flow. However, the specific endpoints of therapy remain under debate. Guidelines on haemodynamic management in sepsis have been published and recently updated, but clinical studies documenting improved outcome from different interventions are often lacking and considerable controversy remains regarding optimal fluid, vasopressor and transfusion regimens. Each patient is different and management must be titrated to the individual characteristics and clinical picture, complemented by global (and regional where available) haemodynamic and oxygenation variables.

Case study

A previously healthy 69-year-old man was admitted for severe right lower lobe pneumonia. On admission his arterial pressure was 95/55 mmHg and heart rate was 115/min. The patient was very dyspnoeic, with a respiratory rate of 35/min. Blood gases, on 60% non-rebreathing mask, showed PaO_2 of 8.65 kPa, pH 7.32, PCO_2 4 kPa and blood lactate 2.4 mmol/L. The trachea was quickly intubated and mechanical ventilation started.

In addition to intravenous amoxicillin-clavulanate and clarithromycin, a 1000 ml saline solution was quickly infused by a peripheral intravenous line, whilst a central venous catheter and an arterial catheter were inserted. The initial central venous pressure (CVP) was 13 mmHg, but hypotension worsened to 80/50 mmHg, so that a dopamine infusion was started at 5 μg/kg/min, and then increased to 10 μg/kg/min. With the dopamine, the mean arterial pressure rose to 65 mmHg and the CVP to 16 mmHg. Despite the relatively high CVP, we started another fluid challenge with 500 ml gelatin solution with the aim of increasing the mean arterial pressure to 75 mmHg, without changes to the dopamine infusion. The CVP rose to 18 mmHg, but the arterial pressure increased to 75 mmHg and the patient was weaned off dopamine in the subsequent hour.

This case illustrates that a relatively high CVP is not a contraindication to fluid administration provided that a fluid challenge technique is used. It also shows that vasopressors (dopamine and/or noradrenaline) may be used transiently even in patients who may eventually respond to fluids. Importantly too, starting a vasopressor infusion does not prevent the continuation or resumption of fluid administration.

References

1. Levy MM, Fink MP, Marshall JC, et al. 2001 SCCM/ESICM/ACCP/ATS/SIS International Sepsis Definitions Conference. *Crit Care Med* 2003; 31: 1250–6.
2. Vincent JL, Sakr Y, Sprung CL, et al. Sepsis in European intensive care units: results of the SOAP study. *Crit Care Med* 2006; 34: 344–53.
3. Metrangolo L, Fiorillo M, Friedman G, et al. Early hemodynamic course of septic shock. *Crit Care Med* 1995; 23: 1971–5.

4. Groeneveld AB, Nauta JJ, Thijs LG. Peripheral vascular resistance in septic shock: its relation to outcome. *Intensive Care Med* 1988; 14: 141–7.

5. Court O, Kumar A, Parrillo JE, et al. Clinical review: myocardial depression in sepsis and septic shock. *Crit Care* 2002; 6: 500–508.

6. Parker MM, McCarthy KE, Ognibene FP, et al. Right ventricular dysfunction and dilatation, similar to left ventricular changes, characterize the cardiac depression of septic shock in humans. *Chest* 1990; 97: 126–31.

7. Vincent JL, Gris P, Coffernils M, et al. Myocardial depression characterizes the fatal course of septic shock. *Surgery* 1992; 111: 660–7.

8. Weil MH, Shubin H. The 'VIP' approach to the bedside management of shock. *JAMA* 1969; 207: 337–40.

9. Rivers E, Nguyen B, Havstad S, et al. Early goal-directed therapy in the treatment of severe sepsis and septic shock. *N Engl J Med* 2001; 345: 1368–77.

10. Rackow EC, Falk JL, Fein IA, et al. Fluid resuscitation in circulatory shock: a comparison of the cardiorespiratory effects of albumin, hetastarch, and saline solutions in patients with hypovolemic and septic shock. *Crit Care Med* 1983; 11: 839–50.

11. Heughan C, Niinikoski J, Hunt TK. Effect of excessive infusion of saline solution on tissue oxygen transport. *Surg Gynecol Obstet* 1972; 135: 257–60.

12. Hunt TK. Surgical wound infections: an overview. *Am J Med* 1981; 70: 712–18.

13. Lang K, Boldt J, Suttner S, et al. Colloids versus crystalloids and tissue oxygen tension in patients undergoing major abdominal surgery. *Anesth Analg* 2001; 93: 405–9.

14. Vincent JL. Plugging the leaks? New insights into synthetic colloids. *Crit Care Med* 1991; 19: 316–18.

15. Boldt J, Ducke M, Kumle B, et al. Influence of different volume replacement strategies on inflammation and endothelial activation in the elderly undergoing major abdominal surgery. *Intensive Care Med* 2004; 30: 416–22.

16. Brunkhorst FM, Engel C, Bloos F, et al. Intensive insulin therapy and pentastarch resuscitation in severe sepsis. *N Engl J Med* 2008; 358: 125–39.

17. Cochrane Injuries Group. Human albumin administration in critically ill patients: systematic review of randomized controlled trials. *BMJ* 1998; 317: 235–40.

18. Vincent JL, Sakr Y, Reinhart K, et al. Is albumin administration in the acutely ill associated with increased mortality? Results of the SOAP study. *Crit Care* 2005; 9: R745–54.

19. Finfer S, Bellomo R, Boyce N, et al. A comparison of albumin and saline for fluid resuscitation in the intensive care unit. *N Engl J Med* 2004; 350: 2247–56.

20. Vincent JL, Navickis RJ, Wilkes MM. Morbidity in hospitalized patients receiving human albumin: a meta-analysis of randomized, controlled trials. *Crit Care Med* 2004; 32: 2029–38.

21. Dubois MJ, Orellana-Jimenez C, Melot C, et al. Albumin administration improves organ function in critically ill hypoalbuminemic patients: a prospective, randomized, controlled, pilot study. *Crit Care Med* 2006; 34: 2536–40.

22. Dellinger RP, Levy MM, Carlet JM, et al. Surviving sepsis campaign: International guidelines for management of severe sepsis and septic shock: 2008. *Crit Care Med* 2008; 36: 296–327.

23. De Backer D, Creteur J, Dubois MJ, et al. The effects of dobutamine on microcirculatory alterations in patients with septic shock are independent of its systemic effects. *Crit Care Med* 2006; 34: 403–8.

24. Weil MH, Henning RJ. New concepts in the diagnosis and fluid treatment of circulatory shock. *Anesth Analg* 1979; 58: 124–32.

25. Vincent JL, Weil MH. Fluid challenge revisited. *Crit Care Med* 2006; 34: 1333–7.

26. Meier-Hellmann A, Bredle DL, Specht M, et al. The effects of low-dose dopamine on splanchnic blood flow and oxygen uptake in patients with septic shock. *Intensive Care Med* 1997; 23: 31–7.

27. Hoogenberg K, Smit AJ, Girbes AR. Effects of low-dose dopamine on renal and systemic hemodynamics during incremental norepinephrine infusion in healthy volunteers. *Crit Care Med* 1998; 26: 260–5.

28. Bellomo R, Chapman M, Finfer S, et al. Low-dose dopamine in patients with early renal dysfunction: a placebo-controlled randomised trial. Australian and New Zealand Intensive Care Society (ANZICS) Clinical Trials Group. *Lancet* 2000; 356: 2139–43.

29. Hollenberg SM, Ahrens TS, Annane D, et al. Practice parameters for hemodynamic support of sepsis in adult patients: 2004 update. *Crit Care Med* 2004; 32: 1928–48.

30. Martin C, Papazian L, Perrin G, et al. Norepinephrine or dopamine for the treatment of hyperdynamic septic shock? *Chest* 1993; 103: 1826–31.

31. De Backer D, Creteur J, Silva E, Vincent JL. Effects of dopamine, norepinephrine, and epinephrine on the splanchnic circulation in septic shock: Which is best? *Crit Care Med* 2003; 31: 1659–67.

32. Bailey AR, Burchett KR. Effect of low-dose dopamine on serum concentrations of prolactin in critically ill patients. *Br J Anaesth* 1997; 78: 97–9.

33. Sakr Y, Reinhart K, Vincent JL, et al. Does dopamine administration in shock influence outcome? Results of the Sepsis Occurrence in Acutely Ill Patients (SOAP) Study. *Crit Care Med* 2006; 34: 589–97.

34. Hollenberg SM, Cunnion RE, Zimmerberg J. Nitric oxide synthase inhibition reverses arteriolar hyporesponsiveness to catecholamines in septic rats. *Am J Physiol* 1993; 264: H660–3.

35. Bucher M, Kees F, Taeger K, et al. Cytokines down-regulate alpha1-adrenergic receptor expression during endotoxemia. *Crit Care Med* 2003; 31: 566–71.

36. Hayes MA, Timmins AC, Yau EH, et al. Elevation of systemic oxygen delivery in the treatment of critically ill patients. *N Engl J Med* 1994; 330: 1717–22.

37. Renton MC, Snowden CP. Dopexamine and its role in the protection of hepatosplanchnic and renal perfusion in high-risk surgical and critically ill patients. *Br J Anaesth* 2005; 94: 459–67.

38. Vincent JL, Leon M, Berre J, et al. Addition of phosphodiesterase inhibitors to adrenergic agents in acutely ill patients. *Int J Cardiol* 1990; 28 Suppl 1: S7–11.

39. Kern H, Schroder T, Kaulfuss M, et al. Enoximone in contrast to dobutamine improves hepatosplanchnic function in fluid-optimized septic shock patients. *Crit Care Med* 2001; 29: 1519–25.

40. Landry DW, Levin HR, Gallant EM, et al. Vasopressin deficiency contributes to the vasodilation of septic shock. *Circulation* 1997; 95: 1122–5.

41. Landry DW, Levin HR, Gallant EM, et al. Vasopressin pressor hypersensitivity in vasodilatory septic shock. *Crit Care Med* 1997; 25: 1279–82.

42. Malay MB, Ashton RC, Jr, Landry DW, et al. Low-dose vasopressin in the treatment of vasodilatory septic shock. *J Trauma* 1999; 47: 699–703.

43. Sun Q, Dimopoulos G, Nguyen DN, et al. Low-dose vasopressin in the treatment of septic shock in sheep. *Am J Respir Crit Care Med* 2003; 168: 481–6.

44. Russell JA, Walley KR, Singer J, et al. Vasopressin versus norepinephrine infusion in patients with septic shock. *N Engl J Med* 2008; 358: 877–87.
45. Bone RC, Fisher CJJ, Clemmer TP, et al. A controlled clinical trial of high-dose methylprednisolone in the treatment of severe sepsis and septic shock. *N Engl J Med* 1987; 317: 653–8.
46. The Veterans Administration Systemic Sepsis Cooperative Study Group. Effect of high-dose glucocorticoid therapy on mortality in patients with clinical signs of systemic sepsis. *N Engl J Med* 1987; 317: 659–65.
47. Briegel J, Forst H, Haller M, et al. Stress doses of hydrocortisone reverse hyperdynamic septic shock: a prospective, randomized, double-blind, single-center study. *Crit Care Med* 1999; 27: 723–32.
48. Annane D, Sebille V, Charpentier C, et al. Effect of treatment with low doses of hydrocortisone and fludrocortisone on mortality in patients with septic shock. *JAMA* 2002; 288: 862–71.
49. Keh D, Boehnke T, Weber-Cartens S, et al. Immunologic and hemodynamic effects of 'low-dose' hydrocortisone in septic shock: a double-blind, randomized, placebo-controlled, crossover study. *Am J Respir Crit Care Med* 2003; 167: 512–20.
50. Sprung CL, Annane D, Keh D, et al. Hydrocortisone therapy for patients with septic shock. *N Engl J Med* 2008; 358: 111–24.
51. Bernard GR, Vincent JL, Laterre PF, et al. Efficacy and safety of recombinant human activated protein C for severe sepsis. *N Engl J Med* 2001; 344: 699–709.
52. Vincent JL, Angus DC, Artigas A, et al. Effects of drotrecogin alfa (activated) on organ dysfunction in the PROWESS trial. *Crit Care Med* 2003; 31: 834–40.
53. De Backer D, Verdant C, Chierego M, et al. Effects of drotrecogin alfa activated on microcirculatory alterations in patients with severe sepsis. *Crit Care Med* 2006; 34: 1918–24.
54. Poeze M, Solberg BC, Greve JW, et al. Monitoring global volume-related hemodynamic or regional variables after initial resuscitation: what is a better predictor of outcome in critically ill septic patients? *Crit Care Med* 2005; 33: 2494–500.
55. Sakr Y, Dubois MJ, De Backer D, et al. Persistent microcirculatory alterations are associated with organ failure and death in patients with septic shock. *Crit Care Med* 2004; 32: 1825–31.
56. Varpula M, Karlsson S, Ruokonen E, et al. Mixed venous oxygen saturation cannot be estimated by central venous oxygen saturation in septic shock. *Intensive Care Med* 2006; 32: 1336–43.
57. Friedman G, Berlot G, Kahn RJ, et al. Combined measurements of blood lactate concentrations and gastric intramucosal pH in patients with severe sepsis. *Crit Care Med* 1995; 23: 1184–93.

13 Acute Coronary Syndromes and Myocardial Infarction

Alex Hobson and Nick Curzen

Wessex Cardiac Unit, Southampton University Hospitals NHS Trust, Southampton and Southampton University Medical School, Southampton, UK

Take Home Messages

- Acute coronary syndromes and myocardial infarction occur frequently in critically ill patients.
- Adequate oxygenation, prompt pain relief and reversal of hypothermia, anaemia, hypotension and tachycardia can help both to prevent and to treat acute coronary syndromes and myocardial infarction.
- Many patients in critical care have co-morbidities which render guideline-based care inappropriate.
- Evidence for best treatment is scanty and management decisions are difficult: close co-operation between the critical care team, cardiologists and other specialists is essential.

13.1 Introduction

The spectrum of diseases that include acute coronary syndromes (ACS) and myocardial infarction (MI) is a major cause of morbidity and mortality, and the commonest reason for hospitalisation in many developed countries. The recent growth of both medical and invasive treatment options has contributed to increasing dilemmas regarding patient management. Nowhere are these difficulties more apparent than in critically ill patients in whom the rapidly expanding literature base is rarely directly applicable. In this chapter we examine the definition, pathophysiology and diagnosis of acute coronary syndromes and outline treatment options. We then highlight the difficulties and controversies encountered in critically ill patients, presenting either with acute coronary syndromes or with acute coronary syndromes complicating other diagnoses.

Cardiovascular Critical Care. Edited by M. Griffiths, J. Cordingley and S. Price.
© 2010 Blackwell Publishing Ltd.

Pathophysiology

ACS and MI are caused, in the majority of cases, by a common underlying pathophysiology: atherosclerotic plaque rupture or erosion. Chronic inflammation is involved in the process of atheroma formation [1]. The likelihood of plaque rupture and erosion is determined by the strength of the plaque's fibrous cap and the stresses to which it is exposed (related to wall stress and blood flow across the intimal surface of the plaque [2]), and is increasingly understood to be related to an acute inflammatory process. Plaque rupture leads to a rapidly escalating vascular inflammatory response involving the activation and aggregation of platelets, thrombus formation, the release of vasoactive mediators and microembolisation, all of which contribute to vessel occlusion. Local factors as well as factors influencing systemic hypercoagulability affect the degree of subsequent thrombosis. These factors explain why ACS is prevalent in critically ill patients, in whom, for example, increased cardiac output may increase vessel wall stress, or sepsis may lead to hypercoagulability. It is this improved understanding of the dynamic process that explains the focus of medical therapies of ACS in the form of anti-platelet agents (aspirin and clopidogrel), thrombolytics, anti-coagulants (low molecular weight heparins (LMWH)) and anti-inflammatory agents (such as high-dose statins).

Definition

ACS and MI are divided into (1) ST segment elevation MI (STEMI), (2) non-ST segment elevation MI (NSTEMI), (3) high risk ACS and (4) low risk ACS (also still known as unstable angina) on the basis of the history, electrocardiogram (ECG) and cardiac enzymes (Table 13.1). This classification is important in that it allows therapies to be tailored to fit the expected underlying pathophysiology and an assessment of risk [3].

Acute STEMI

This usually relates to complete and persistent occlusion of a major coronary artery due to thrombosis superimposed on plaque rupture or erosion. Classically, acute STEMI presents as localised ST elevation infarction, but new left bundle branch block (LBBB) and a true posterior myocardial infarct can also occur following vessel occlusion and are therefore included with STEMI for management purposes. The diagnosis is made by a history of chest pain, compatible ECG changes and a subsequent rise in cardiac enzymes.

NSTEMI

Evidence of MI (by cardiac enzyme release) without ST elevation on the ECG is defined as NSTEMI. NSTEMI is caused by transient occlusion of coronary arteries, or occlusion of arteries in areas where the ECG is less sensitive. This leads to varying degrees of infarction which can be detected by the subsequent release of cardiac enzymes. Classically, therefore, NSTEMI is defined by the presence of at least two of the following: chest pain, ECG changes or a rise in cardiac enzymes.

Table 13.1 Classification of acute coronary syndromes (ACS) and myocardial infarction (MI) on the basis of electrocardiogram (ECG) findings and cardiac enzymes.

Classification	ECG findings	Cardiac enzymes
STEMI	ST segment elevation LBBB True posterior MI	Elevated
NSTEMI	Possible changes include ST depression and T wave changes ECG can be normal	Elevated
High risk ACS	ST depression and/or T wave changes	Not elevated
Low risk ACS	Normal ECG	Not elevated

STEMI ST, segment elevation myocardial infarction; NSTEMI, non-ST segment elevation myocardial infarction; LBBB, left bundle branch block; ECG, electrocardiogram.

ACS

If there is no evidence of MI (no enzyme release) but a cardiac cause is suspected, the term ACS or unstable angina is used. ACS does not include chronic stable angina but by definition includes increasingly frequent, severe or prolonged angina, new onset angina, angina that occurs at rest and angina that is difficult to control on medication.

Diagnosis

The diagnosis of ACS and MI is based on the history, examination, ECGs and cardiac enzymes.

History

The usual history is of typical ischaemic chest pain, although atypical features are not uncommon. For example, one study revealed that acute myocardial ischaemia was found in 22% of those presenting with stabbing chest pain, 13% of those presenting with pleuritic chest pain and 7% of those with pain that was entirely reproducible on palpation [5]. Atypical features are more common in the elderly, the young and in diabetics [4]. ACS can also present as indigestion, abdominal pain and increasing dyspnoea. The history is also critical in excluding other important causes of chest pain including aortic dissection and pulmonary emboli. Communication difficulties due to language problems or patient sedation can be problematic, particularly in the intensive care unit (ICU) setting.

Examination

Physical examination is often normal. It is, however, useful in excluding other causes of chest pain such as pneumothorax, pericarditis and aortic dissection, assessing the patient for signs of haemodynamic compromise, identifying co-morbidities such as significant valvular disease or peripheral vascular disease, and identifying early complications of MI such as acute mitral regurgitation.

Investigation

An immediate ECG at presentation is essential for prompt diagnosis and for risk stratification. ST changes are the most reliable signs of ACS and MI, followed by T wave, and then non-specific changes [5]. ECGs may also give clues to alternative diagnoses such as pulmonary embolism and pericarditis. Comparison with previous ECGs is helpful, especially in patients with left ventricular hypertrophy, previous MI and in those with bundle branch block. ECGs can be normal in all ACS except STEMI, especially if the patient is pain free at the time of investigation [7]. For this reason ECGs should be repeated in patients with suspected ischaemic chest pain, especially if the pain recurs. Continuous ST segment monitoring can be useful, as some ischaemic episodes are silent (not accompanied by symptoms), particularly in the ICU setting.

Cardiac enzymes are important as an aid to diagnosis in those with non-specific ECGs and atypical symptoms and are also useful in risk stratification. The most specific markers of cardiac necrosis are the cardiac troponins [8]. In MI, levels rise in the blood within 3 or 4 hours; however, levels peak between 6 and 12 hours following an event and for that reason if the first result is negative a troponin should be repeated 12 hours after the last episode of pain, before excluding any cardiac damage. Whilst troponins are highly specific for myocardial damage they are not specific to ischaemic heart disease (IHD) as conditions such as pulmonary embolism, aortic dissection and myocarditis are associated with increased levels. Alternative causes of raised troponin levels are common in critically ill patients and will be covered in more detail later. Interpretation of troponin results can require considerable thought and experience; the test can be a mixed blessing [9]. For example, troponin levels remain elevated for up to 2 weeks, so that a single high reading does not make a definitive diagnosis, nor does it provide a specific time point for the troponin release.

Risk stratification

Risk stratification is crucial in patients with ACS and MI, enabling prompt and appropriate evidence-based treatment to be initiated in order to minimise the risk of progression and complications. In STEMI the detection of characteristic ECG changes (or new LBBB) enables prompt reperfusion strategies to be initiated in order to limit infarct size and reduce mortality. In ACS without persistent ST segment elevation the history, examination, ECG and cardiac markers all aid risk assessment, by identifying patients who have prognostic advantage from revascularisation as well as optimal medical treatment [3]. Most of the known risk factors for developing IHD are associated with an increased risk in ACS and MI. Age, male sex, diabetes and a history of congestive heart failure or IHD (in particular MI, previous bypass surgery or percutaneous intervention within 6 months) all convey increased risk [10].

Clinical presentation

A presentation with pain at rest, poor response to initial treatment and recurrent episodes of pain all increase risk [11].

Table 13.2 Risk scores for STEMI/NSTEMI.

Score	Patient group	Prediction	Factors included
TIMI score for unstable angina/NSTEMI [16]	Unstable angina/NSTEMI	Risk of all cause mortality, myocardial infarction and need for urgent revascularisation at 14 days	Age ≥ 65 years, three or more risk factors for IHD, previous angiographic stenosis > 50%, severe anginal symptoms, use of aspirin in the last 7 days, elevated cardiac markers, ST change on ECG
TIMI risk score for STEMI	STEMI patients eligible for thrombolysis	30 day mortality	Age, Killip class, heart rate, anterior MI or LBBB, systolic BP, time to thrombolysis, weight, prior angina, diabetes, hypertension
GRACE [17]	All ACS	All cause mortality at 6 months	Age, history of heart failure or MI, elevated resting heart rate, low systolic blood pressure, ST depression, elevated cardiac enzymes, elevated creatinine, not having PCI
PURSUIT [18]	Unstable angina/NSTEMI	Death and MI at 30 days	Old age, tachycardia, low systolic blood pressure, ST depression, signs of heart failure, elevated cardiac enzymes

TIMI, thrombolysis in myocardial infarction; GRACE, Global Registry of Acute Coronary Events; PURSUIT, platelet glycoprotein IIb/IIIa in unstable angina: receptor suppression using integrilin.

Examination

Evidence of significant co-morbidity, left ventricular dysfunction and haemodynamic instability on examination may increase risk directly, or by ruling out the use of optimal treatment strategies.

Investigation

The ECG is crucial for risk stratification as well as for diagnosis. ST segment changes convey the greatest risk, followed by T wave inversion and then a normal ECG [12]. ST changes on continuous ECG monitoring add independent prognostic information [13]. Raised markers of myocardial necrosis such as cardiac troponins are associated with worse outcomes. The degree of risk correlates with the extent to which troponin levels are raised [14]. Other biochemical markers such as brain natriuretic peptide (BNP) also provide powerful independent markers of risk [15].

Risk scores

Several risk scores incorporating these factors have been validated and are in common clinical use (Table 13.2).

Standard management

In all patients with ACS and MI, initial management strategies include measures to minimise the risk of progression and complications, treat pain and prevent and if necessary treat cardiac arrest (Figure 13.1). All patients

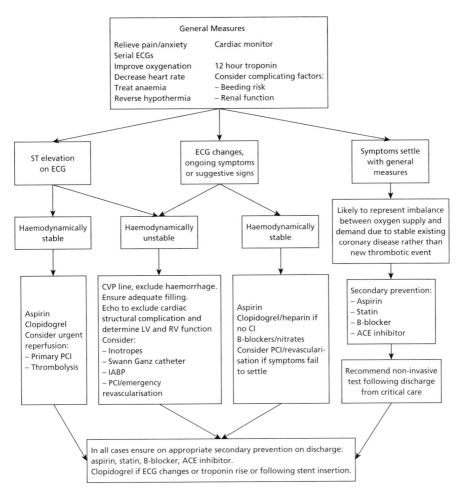

Figure 13.1 Management of ACS and MI in critical care environments. ECG, electrocardiogram; PCI, percutaneous intervention; IABP, intra-aortic balloon pump; CVP, central venous pressure; CI, cardiac index.

are managed with bed rest, oxygen and analgesia as necessary, and continuously monitored, with access to prompt defibrillation. Further treatment depends on the diagnosis. Revascularisation options are reviewed in detail in references [19, 20].

STEMI
Initial therapy
Initial therapy includes analgesia, usually morphine or diamorphine, to ease pain and anxiety. Anti-platelet agents are a mainstay of medical therapy: for example, aspirin provides almost as much benefit as thrombolysis [21]. The addition of clopidogrel confers further benefit [22, 23]. The main therapeutic aim in STEMI is prompt reperfusion.

Table 13.3 TIMI flow classification and angiographic appearances.

TIMI flow	Angiographic appearance
TIMI 0	Complete occlusion of blood flow
TIMI 1	Slow flow that never arrives at the distal end of the blood vessel
TIMI 2	Flood flow all the way down the vessel but at a slower rate than in non-infarct-related coronary vessels
TIMI 3	Complete and brisk flow of blood to the bottom of the vessel

Reperfusion strategies

At the time of presentation the infarct-related artery (IRA) is usually completely occluded. Reperfusion can therefore be defined as re-establishing blood flow down the vessel. However, the degree of reperfusion varies and has been classified according to the TIMI score (Table 13.3). Evidence from angiographic studies in STEMI patients consistently demonstrates an inverse relationship between TIMI flow level and subsequent mortality (i.e. TIMI 0 has highest mortality). Specifically, there is an outcome advantage from having TIMI 3 versus TIMI 2 flow.

Two strategies for reperfusion are available: primary percutaneous intervention (PCI) and thrombolysis. Both have been proven to save lives when performed within 12 hours of the onset of symptoms. If primary PCI can be performed within 90 minutes of presentation it is the preferred strategy for reperfusion. A meta analysis of randomised trials comparing PCI and thrombolysis shows that one additional life would be saved for each 25 patients undergoing PCI [24]. This is at the expense of an additional risk of access site bleeding with PCI, although the risk of stroke and in particular haemorrhagic stroke is reduced [24]. PCI, which usually involves implantation of a metallic stent to scaffold the material up against the vessel wall at high pressure (see case study), has the advantage of providing mechanical treatment to the underlying atherosclerotic plaque as well as of the occlusive thrombus. When combined with aggressive anti-platelet therapies including aspirin, clopidogrel and glycoprotein IIb/IIIa inhibitors such as abciximab, PCI achieves superior rates of TIMI 3 flow compared to aspirin and thrombolysis. The benefits of PCI are particularly strong in patients with cardiogenic shock, in those presenting between 3 and 12 hours from the onset of symptoms and in those with contra-indications to thrombolysis but not to PCI.

Aspirin and thrombolysis remains a very effective treatment and is preferred where PCI is logistically impossible or in patients presenting early (< 6 hours) where there is an anticipated delay to PCI. In patients presenting to a hospital without PCI facilities between 3 and 9 hours from the onset of symptoms, transfer for primary PCI can be considered if the anticipated transfer time is less than 60 minutes. In patients treated with thrombolysis the choice of thrombolytic therapy depends on a balance of the individual risks and benefits. Studies in which patients were randomised to in-hospital or pre-hospital thrombolysis show a 15–20%

reduction in mortality with pre-hospital treatment, again highlighting the importance of early reperfusion [19].

A proportion of patients fail to reperfuse adequately despite prompt thrombolysis. This is suggested by ongoing ST segment elevation and symptoms 45–60 minutes after drug administration. Angiographic studies demonstrate that even with the best modern thrombolytics TIMI 3 flow is only achieved in around 60% of patients. In this situation there is evidence suggesting a benefit from reperfusion with 'Rescue PCI' particularly if this can be performed promptly [27]. In patients who develop recurrent ST elevation, after ST segments have initially settled after thrombolysis, PCI should be performed. Current data suggest no benefit from re-thrombolysis in patients with failed reperfusion. Recent guidelines from the European Society of Cardiology recommend that patients who receive thrombolysis should undergo angiography and revascularisation where possible within 24 hours of admission even when thrombolysis was successful at achieving reperfusion [28]. This is an important recommendation, practical only in PCI centres or hospitals with excellent transfer arrangements to PCI centres. Note that the recommendation is based upon the data from studies in which routine angiography and revascularisation were performed very early, and always in less than 24 hours [29,30]. In contrast, recent data have demonstrated no long-term advantage to PCI of occluded infarct-related arteries beyond 3 days after the MI [31, 32]. In other words, patients benefit from early revascularisation in MI, even after successful thrombolysis, but do not benefit from routine PCI to persistently occluded IRA beyond 3 days. These data are consistent with the main endpoint advantage in transfer for PCI in STEMI patients compared with thrombolysis: namely a significant reduction in the incidence of re-infarction [33, 34].

The leading cause of death in patients hospitalised with MI is cardiogenic shock (e.g. 55% in GUSTO 1 (Global Utilization of Streptokinase and Tissue Plasminogen Activator for Occluded Coronary Arteries) [35]). The risks involved in these patients often influence the decision-making process, leading to erroneously conservative management. Indeed, patients with cardiogenic shock complicating MI often have the most to gain from emergency angiography with a view to revascularisation [36, 37].

Adjunctive and later drug therapy
Current guidelines recommend therapy with unfractionated heparin as an adjunct to fibrinolytic therapy, given as a continuous infusion for 48 hours. However, in one study using the LMWH enoxaparin throughout the hospital admission prevented one death or MI for each 50 patients treated when compared with unfractionated heparin [38]. This strategy was, however, associated with an increased bleeding risk, with one excess major bleed for every 150 patients treated. Fondaparinux (a synthetic factor Xa inhibitor) has also shown promise as an adjunct to thrombolysis in the treatment of STEMI, with a lower risk of bleeding, although there are concerns that higher rates of catheter-related thrombus observed during PCI in patients undergoing an early invasive strategy may lead to adverse outcomes [39].

NSTEMI/high risk ACS

The management strategy for high risk ACS shares many features with that of STEMI. Continuous monitoring and prompt treatment are essential.

Pharmacological therapy

This should be administered immediately. First, opiate analgesics are given for persistent pain. As well as their analgesic effect they are venodilators that may relieve pulmonary congestion. Second, anti-platelet therapy is essential and has been proven to reduce the risk of death and progression to MI. Aspirin is often given before hospital admission and reduces the risk of vascular death, MI and stroke by 46% [40]. There is evidence of an additional benefit from clopidogrel [41]; a 300 mg loading dose is usually given although there is evidence of an additional benefit from a 600 mg loading dose when given shortly before PCI [42]. Glycoprotein IIb/IIIa receptor inhibitors reduce the risk of death and MI in NSTEMI patients undergoing PCI [43] and are now recommended for administration to troponin-positive patients undergoing an early but not immediate (within 48 hours but not within 2.5 hours) PCI [4]. Third, whilst there is no evidence that they improve outcome, nitrates are often given to relieve symptoms. Fourth, anti-thrombin treatment should be given in all high risk patients. The LMWH enoxaparin confers additional benefit above unfractionated heparin [44, 45], although the shorter half-life and reversibility of unfractionated heparin justifies its use in selected patients. Finally, beta blockers are recommended in ACS if there are no contra-indications, especially if there are ongoing symptoms. The intravenous route is recommended in high risk patients [4]. In contrast to their use in chronic left ventricular dysfunction their use should be avoided in the acute situation in patients with clinical or radiographic signs of left ventricular dysfunction. Calcium channel blockers are often given when beta blockers are contra-indicated. They are, however, themselves contraindicated in those with left ventricular dysfunction in whom their use is associated with an increased risk of death. Standard drug therapy in high risk ACS also includes ACE inhibitors and statins, although there is little evidence that they are of additional benefit when given very early in the clinical course.

Interventional/revascularisation strategies

Despite medical therapy, NSTEMI is associated with a 30% mortality, MI, refractory angina and readmission to hospital with ACS at 6 months [46]. Historically patients with ongoing chest pain or dynamic ECG changes were considered for angiography and revascularisation. There is now good evidence that an early invasive strategy is of benefit in other ACS patients [47–49]. These randomised studies have shown that a strategy of early routine angiography with a view to revascularisation in ACS patients with ECG changes or a raised troponin reduces subsequent death and MI. A routine early revascularisation strategy is, however, not universally employed owing to inadequate access to PCI facilities [50, 51].

Low risk ACS

Patients without recurrence of chest pain, without ST segment or other dynamic ECG changes and without a rise in cardiac enzymes are considered to be at low risk. Indeed there may still be doubt as to the diagnosis. In those with a good history of ischaemic sounding chest pain or minor ECG changes (T wave flattening or inversion) treatment should be initiated with aspirin, clopidogrel, LMWH, a beta-blocker and appropriate secondary prevention. If there are no progressive ECG changes and there is no rise in cardiac enzymes (measured 12 hours after the most severe episode of pain) LMWH and clopidogrel can be discontinued, and non-invasive testing should be performed.

Factors complicating the treatment of ACS and MI

A number of factors complicate management decisions by altering the balance of risks and benefits, particularly with regard to the use of PCI, thrombolytics and potent anti-platelet therapy. These include: difficulties with vascular access, renal impairment (leading to an increased risk of contrast nephropathy), anaemia and bleeding problems leading to potential difficulties with both thrombolytics and potent anti-platelet agents and allergies to the anti-platelet agents necessary to prevent stent thrombosis following PCI and stent insertion. These high risk patients are usually excluded from clinical trials, making evidence-based management difficult. They are also among the patients most likely to require treatment in the ICU.

ACS and MI in critical care

There are clear guidelines for the management of ACS and MI [4, 52]. However, in the critical care setting patients with ACS and MI frequently have complicating factors such as respiratory failure, renal failure, anaemia, coagulopathies, recent surgery or an uncertain outcome (for example, following prolonged resuscitation or in relation to malignant disease) which necessitate compromise and greater individualisation of treatment. In addition, these patients are excluded from most trials and therefore the management of MI and ACS in this context can be challenging.

Patients with ACS and MI in critical care fall into two broad categories: those with an initial presentation of ACS and MI who require critical care because of complications relating to ACS or MI or complications of its treatment and those in whom ACS/MI complicates another condition. Finally there are critically ill patients who are found to have an elevated troponin level with no other evidence of ACS/MI.

In the early stages of ACS or MI, cardiac arrest, cardiogenic shock and pulmonary oedema can all necessitate management in ICU. Treatment with thrombolysis and potent anti-platelet agents may lead to spontaneous haemorrhage (including haemorrhagic stroke) and bleeds secondary to access site complications after PCI. Upper gastrointestinal (GI) bleeds occur in 1.2% and lower GI bleeds in 0.4% of all patients following MI [53]. Haemodynamically stable patients following ACS and MI are not at higher than usual risk from endoscopic investigation and should have standard initial management [54]. If the ACS settles and a lesion is found on endoscopy that will heal with a proton pump inhibitor, angiography with a view to revascularisation should be withheld to allow healing (usually 4 weeks). If the ACS does not settle or there is haemodynamic instability, close consultation with the gastroenterologist regarding the endoscopic findings is advised before deciding on anti-platelet therapy and angiography. In addition, acute renal failure may occur secondary to poor cardiac function, or as a reaction to medication (e.g. streptokinase, ACE inhibitors) or contrast.

Cardiology patients with AMI who require ICU admission present important dilemmas relating to their management. Assessment as to progress and prognosis requires the combined experience and expertise of both an interventional cardiologist and an intensive care specialist. Thus, the outlook of a young patient, fully revascularised by PCI after an acute anterior MI, is entirely different from an elderly patient with a post-infarct ventricular septal defect (VSD). Continuing aggressive support in the face of two or three system failures may be appropriate if there is a genuine prospect of recovery from the initial cardiac insult. Other common decisions surround the choice of inotropes, sedative and timing of intra-aortic balloon pump removal or extubation. These challenges are illustrated in the case study.

ACS is also a common occurrence in patients already in ICU as a result of another severe illness or as part of post-operative management. One series of unselected consecutive (predominantly medical) ICU admissions revealed that 25.8% had evidence of MI (from troponin levels, ECG and echocardiography) during admission [55].

Diagnosis of ACS and MI in critical care

The optimal strategy for diagnosing ACS and MI in ICU has yet to be established. Ischaemic symptoms can be difficult to evaluate in the critically ill because symptoms may be masked by analgesics or sedatives, and many patients are unable to communicate. Sweating, tachycardia and hypo- or hypertension suggests a change in status of the ventilated patient. Greater emphasis should be placed on cardiac enzymes, ECGs and additional modalities such as echocardiography. Both ECGs and cardiac enzymes, however, have important limitations in critically ill patients. Cardiac enzymes are highly specific for myocardial damage but do not indicate the underlying cause. Raised troponin levels are common in critically ill patients without any other evidence of MI, especially those with a systemic inflammatory response (up to 85% of patients with septic shock [56]). Other causes of raised troponin levels commonly seen in ICU include shock from any cause, chemotherapy, pulmonary embolism, renal failure, subarachnoid haemorrhage, stroke, cardiac contusion, myocarditis and heart failure. ECGs also have limitations: LBBB and ventricular pacing can make evaluation difficult. Other abnormalities such as subarachnoid haemorrhage, pulmonary embolus, electrolyte imbalances and hyperventilation can also cause ECG changes, and in some cases ACS is associated with a normal ECG.

These factors combine to make diagnosis difficult. Whilst a high index of suspicion is required it is important that over-diagnosis does not lead to inappropriate treatment. Echocardiography to look for regional wall abnormalities can be helpful if the diagnosis remains in doubt.

Peri-operative ACS and MI

More than 50% of peri-operative deaths are caused by cardiac events [57]. Intra-operatively myocardial ischaemia and infarction can be diagnosed on the basis of ECG changes. Indeed, 80% of significant ECG changes on a 12-lead ECG will be detected with monitoring of leads II and V5 [58]. The management of STEMI is difficult in the peri-operative period. Thrombolysis and the potent anti-platelet agents used for primary PCI can lead to significant bleeding related to the surgery and are generally contra-indicated. In many cases anti-platelet agents such as aspirin can be started immediately and heparin, after close discussion with the surgeons, often within several hours of surgery. In all cases a careful balance of the risks and benefits is required and this will depend on the size and site of the infarct as well as the extent and site of the surgery.

Ischaemic events are most likely during tracheal intubation, with initial surgical stimulation and about 2–3 days post-operatively [59]. During the peri-operative period there is an increase in myocardial oxygen demand due to increases in heart rate, myocardial contractility and wall tension. However, myocardial oxygen supply can decrease due to global factors such as severe hypotension, anaemia, hypoxia and pre-existing local factors such as coronary disease. ACS in the peri-operative period can therefore be caused not only by thrombus formation but also by the additional demands of surgery not being met due to stable coronary disease. The first necessity in treatment is therefore to optimise oxygen supply and decrease oxygen demand. Whilst there is clear evidence linking anaemia to poor outcome, there is only clear evidence that transfusion is beneficial when the haematocrit falls below 33% [60]. As well as correction of anaemia the use of adequate analgesia, sedation and beta-blockade can lead to rapid resolution in this setting.

Even if symptoms do resolve, however, it is important to ensure that MI is excluded with serial ECGs and a troponin 12 hours after the event. On-going symptoms or ECG changes despite optimising oxygen delivery and decreasing oxygen demand make ACS due to plaque rupture and thrombosis more likely. In this case further treatment with anti-platelet and anti-thrombotic agents is necessary when the surgical situation allows. Unfractionated heparin may be preferred because of its shorter half life and reversibility using protamine. Close liaison with an interventional cardiologist is required early in peri-operative patients presenting with STEMI or intractable ischaemia. Many such patients can have their prognosis improved by early PCI, without glycoprotein IIb/IIIa receptor inhibitors. This, however, demands a very rapid response to the logistical challenge of transfer to the catheter laboratory. The prevalence of peri-operative ACS and MI can be minimised by ensuring adequate oxygenation, relieving pain and anxiety, treating anaemia, reversing hypothermia and using epidurals in high risk cases.

Management of haemodynamic instability after myocardial infarction

Causes of haemodynamic instability after MI are summarised in Table 13.4. Prompt assessment with echocardiography to check for new valvular regurgitation, VSD or cardiac rupture is essential. Whilst percutaneous closure has been attempted for infarct related VSDs, urgent surgery remains the only option in the majority of cases, and as a result the mechanical complications of MI, are indications for emergency surgical review. If haemodynamic instability relates purely to the infarct, prompt PCI and intra-aortic balloon pump (IABP) insertion may be life-saving, as can emergency bypass surgery [61]. Hypotension related to treatments already received (e.g. bleeding caused by thrombolysis or a reaction to medication) must be excluded.

Table 13.4 Causes of haemodynamic instability post MI. Presentation, management and outcome.

Cause	Presentation/management
Left ventricular dysfunction	Accounts for 85% of cases. Common when > 40% of LV mass is infarcted. Usually presents within 24 hours with features of low cardiac output and LV failure. Supportive treatment with inotropes, diuretics and IABP. Emergency revascularisation can be life-saving. Prognosis, however, remains poor
Cardiac rupture	Occurs in about 3% of STEMI, usually from day 4 to 10. Usually presents with sudden death. However, can have more indolent presentation. Diagnosis confirmed with echocardiography. Prognosis almost invariably fatal without emergency surgery
Post infarct VSD	Occurs in about 2% of STEMI. Presents with signs of heart failure and a new systolic murmur. Diagnosis confirmed with echocardiography. 90% of patients die without surgery. With emergency surgery survival is about 50% and higher in anterior than inferior MI
Acute mitral regurgitation	Mild, well-tolerated MR is common. Severe in 1% of MI, usually due to rupture of postero-medial papillary muscle (in inferior MI). Presents with heart failure and new murmur. Confirmed with echocardiography. Mortality > 90% with medical therapy; 30% peri-operative mortality
Right ventricular infarction	Presents with hypotension, raised venous pressure but no pulmonary oedema. Complicates large infero-posterior MI. Treated with careful fluid administration with monitoring of wedge pressure
Arrhythmias	Atrial fibrillation complicates 10–20% of MIs. DCCV should be performed if a rapid ventricular response is associated with haemodynamic compromise. Sustained ventricular tachycardia occurs in 2% of MI. Complete heart block occurs in 6% and if associated with compromise should be treated with atropine and a temporary pacemaker if sustained
Volume depletion	Bleeding as a result of thrombolysis, anti-platelet or anti-thrombotic drugs or as a result of access site complications must be considered. Volume depletion can also occur as a result of aggressive diuretic and vasodilator therapy
Drug reaction	Streptokinase commonly causes hypotension. Aspirin and heparin have been associated with anaphylaxis

LV, left ventricular; IABP, intra-aortic balloon pump; MR, mitral regurgitation; DCCV, direct current cardioversion.

Management of ACS and MI patients following resuscitation from cardiac arrest

If there is no history available and there are no ECG changes it can be difficult to make the diagnosis of MI as it is difficult to know what emphasis to place on raised cardiac enzymes in the context of prolonged cardiac arrest and cardiac massage. In patients who are haemodynamically stable with an uncertain neurological outcome there is seldom a role for PCI. By contrast, younger patients resuscitated but unconscious with clear-cut ST elevation are usually considered candidates for emergency PCI, but will clearly demand critical care support.

Management following percutaneous intervention

Regular cardiology review is required to monitor for femoral haematomas and apply external compression devices (such as the FemoStop™) where necessary. A low index of suspicion for retroperitoneal haemorrhage is important, as is early echocardiography to exclude tamponade. In patients recovering from stent therapy it is imperative that aspirin and clopidogrel therapy are continued in the intubated patient to avoid the risk of stent thrombosis (aspirin can also be given intravenously and per rectum).

Management following surgical revascularisation

Patients undergoing emergency revascularisation have significantly increased mortality and morbidity when compared with those undergoing elective coronary artery bypass graft (CABG). However, in addition to standard post-operative care, there are many features that are common to both groups that need to be specifically addressed in this patient population [62].

Bypass graft-related issues

Specific considerations for the intensivist include: whether complete or partial revascularisation has been undertaken, whether endarterectomy was performed, the type of grafts used, the degree of ventricular impairment and whether any additional surgery has been performed, for example mitral valve annuloplasty and aortic valve replacement, as these will affect post-operative management. Patients with incomplete revascularisation are at increased risk of post-operative ischaemia particularly when inotropic agents are used, in which case IABP insertion or agents that do not increase myocardial oxygen demand (i.e. levosimendan) may be preferable. After endarterectomy, the risk of graft occlusion is greater, and early use of anti-platelet agents should be considered. The use of constrictor agents in patients with arterial grafts can precipitate graft spasm with associated ischaemia, and should be avoided where possible. Previous early use of calcium channel blockade in patients with radial arterial grafting is, however, no longer considered standard.

Graft failure is often heralded by the development of ventricular arrhythmias, the appropriate response to which is urgent echocardiography and coronary arteriography/re-exploration. ECG and biomarker interpretation in the context of recent CABG are often unhelpful; however, if gross new ECG changes are present (compared with immediately post-operatively) this is significant. Where concern exists regarding graft patency, early discussion with the surgeon and an interventional cardiologist is essential.

Ventricular dysfunction

Patients with significant left ventricular dysfunction pre-operatively would normally return from the operating theatre with an IABP *in situ*. Even where extensive hibernation is present, and recovery of ventricular function is expected following re-vascularisation, the IABP should not usually be removed until the time that the patient is being weaned from other inotropic agents. The order in which left ventricular support is removed should be tailored to the requirements of individual patients. Where the patient has undergone concomitant surgery involving left ventricular volume reduction, the ventricular volume may be very small, and therefore require relatively rapid pacing rates (up to 130 bpm) in order to maintain cardiac output. This is particularly challenging after an incomplete revascularisation. Right ventricular function is exquisitely sensitive to coronary perfusion pressure, and where significant dysfunction exists in the context of hypotension, pressor agents may be required. Further, a small pericardial collection around the right ventricle in this context can have very significant haemodynamic effects.

Echocardiography should be performed in order to exclude pericardial collection, ischaemia, MI and valve dysfunction in patients who fail to wean from mechanical ventilation post-CABG owing to hypotension or pulmonary oedema. If echocardiography at rest is unhelpful, stress echocardiography should be performed. The type of stress will depend on the suspected reason for failure to wean. Ideally, a targeted echocardiogram should be performed at the time of failure to wean. However, if this is not possible, dobutamine stress echocardiography should be performed for suspected ischaemia, and volume and pressor agent stress for suspected mitral regurgitation. In the context of left ventricular dysfunction, where patients have been successfully revascularised and there is no significant valvular pathology, they should be treated with optimal heart failure medication and assessed for their suitability for biventricular pacing.

Emergency revascularisation

After a recent MI, the post-operative mortality and morbidity rates rise sharply [62]. Additional risk is conferred by the presence of a mechanical complication of acute MI. After a significant pre-operative myocardial injury, patients often require significant cardiovascular support, whilst avoiding further ischaemia (mechanical support and inotrope selection) and pulmonary artery catheterisation (particularly in the context of right ventricular infarction). Whilst awaiting myocardial recovery, early tracheostomy may be considered, and where the patient fails to wean, or develops new haemodynamic instability, treatable causes should be aggressively excluded and treated (ischaemia, mitral regurgitation, ventricular septal defect).

Conclusion

ACS and MI are common in critical care. Optimal care ensuring adequate oxygenation, prompt pain relief and reversal of hypothermia, anaemia, hypotension and tachycardia can help both prevent and treat ACS and MI. Many patients in critical care have co-morbidities which makes guideline-based care inappropriate, evidence for best treatment is scanty and management decisions are difficult. Close co-operation between the critical care team, cardiologists and other specialists is essential.

Case study

A previously fit 48-year-old male smoker with a positive family history of ischaemic heart disease collapsed at home one evening whilst watching television. His wife was unable to detect a pulse and initiated cardio-pulmonary resuscitation. Resuscitation was continued a few minutes later by paramedics who cardioverted him out of ventricular fibrillation on two occasions on the way to hospital. On arrival at the Emergency Department he was unconscious with clinical signs of a low cardiac output. He underwent standard resuscitation and required sedation and mechanical ventilation for agitation and acute pulmonary oedema with hypoxia. An ECG demonstrated widespread ST elevation in leads V1–V6 and a cardiology opinion was sought. He was seen by the on-call interventional cardiologist and transferred to the catheter lab. During transfer he was defibrillated on two further occasions. On arrival in the lab there was pulmonary oedema fluid coming up the endotracheal tube and his systolic blood pressure was 60 mmHg. An IABP was inserted. Diagnostic angiography showed an acute thrombotic stenosis in his left main coronary artery (Figure 13.2a). He was treated with abciximab and

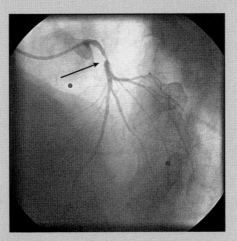

Figure 13.2a Left anterior oblique angiogram of left coronary artery showing important stenosis of distal left main stem artery (arrow).

Continued

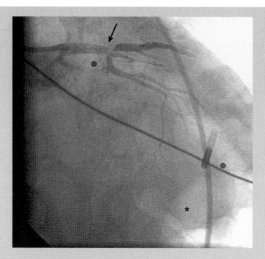

Figure 13.2b Right anterior oblique (RAO) angiogram of left coronary artery showing important stenosis of distal left main stem artery (arrow). An inflated intra-aortic balloon pump is seen (asterisk).

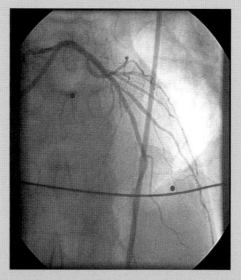

Figure 13.2c Posteroanterior (PA) cranial projection after insertion of coronary stent.

heparin, and stents were successfully inserted into his left main and left anterior descending coronary arteries, re-establishing TIMI III (normal) flow (Figures 13.2b and c). At the end of the procedure his systolic blood pressure was 95 mmHg supported with a low-dose adrenaline infusion. He was transferred to the ICU. The consultant cardiologist spoke to the patient's wife immediately after the intervention and explained that the patient was gravely ill, despite a technically successful procedure.

Continued

- Days 1 and 2: over the following 48 hours the patient remained unwell and required inotropic support in the form of adrenaline, noradrenaline and milrinone. He developed a large haematoma in the groin used for the angiogram and a FemoStop™ was applied. He woke up when the sedation was weaned and had to be resedated because of irritable behaviour and was noted to have abnormal limb movements (spontaneous extension and external rotation of his arms). Aspirin and clopidogrel were administered nasogastrically, but absorption of naso-gastric feed was intermittent.
- Days 3–7: a CT scan of the brain showed no focal abnormality and 'hypoxic brain damage with unknown prognosis' was diagnosed. Repeated attempts at waking the patient eventually produced manageable behaviour but with persistent confusion. Respiratory and cardiovascular status improved to the point where a strategy for withdrawal of inotropes, removal of IABP and extubation was required.
- Days 7–10: the patient was extubated on day 8. He remained on three inotropes and IABP but had been established on small doses of β-blocker and ACE inhibitor as well as a statin, aspirin and clopidogrel. On day 9 the patient required re-intubation for acute hypoxia diagnosed as a combination of acute pulmonary oedema and atelectasis. The following day it was decided that the IABP must be removed.
- Day 11–22: the patient was extubated and moved to HDU (high dependency unit). Patient now only confused at night but experiencing persistent short-term memory loss. Discharged from hospital on day 22. Still alive 9 months later and had returned to work.

Comment

Robust data support the use of (1) aspirin and clopidogrel to prevent stent thrombosis, (2) early use of β-blocker to reduce cardiac rupture and arrhythmia and promote ventricular remodelling and (3) early ACE inhibitor to promote remodelling. Increasing evidence suggests benefit for early statin therapy after ACS. When was it reasonable to discharge the patient from the ITU? A routine CABG operation was cancelled for every day this patient remained on the unit.

References

1. Mahmoudi M, Curzen N, Gallagher P. Atherogenesis: the role of inflammation and infection. *Histopathology* 2007;50(5):535–46.
2. Fuster V. Mechanisms leading to myocardial infarction: insights from studies of vascular biology. *Circulation* 1994;90:2126–46.
3. Archbold RA, Curzen N. The role of revascularisation in the treatment of acute coronary syndromes: who should you refer? *Clinical Med* 2004;4:32–5.
4. Bertrand ME, Simoons ML, Fox KAA, et al. Management of acute coronary syndromes in patients presenting without persistent ST-segment elevation.

The task force on the Management of Acute Coronary Syndromes of the European Society of Cardiology. *Eur Heart J* 2002;23:1809–40.

5. Lee TH, Cook EF, Weisberg M, et al. Acute chest pain in the emergency room. Identification and examination of low-risk patients. *Arch Intern Med* 1985;145:65–9.

6. Savonitto S, Ardissino D, Granger CB, et al. Prognostic value of the admission electrocardiograph in acute coronary syndromes. *JAMA* 1999;281:707–13.

7. Rouan GW, Lee TH, Cook EF, et al. Clinical characteristics and outcome of acute myocardial infarction in patients with initially normal or non-specific electrocardiograms (a report from the Multicenter Chest Pain Study). *Am J Cardiol* 1989;64:1087–92.

8. Jaffe AS, Ravkilde J, Roberts R, et al. It's time for a change to a troponin standard. *Circulation* 2000;102:1216–20.

9. Curzen N. Troponins in patients with chest pain: a mixed blessing? *BMJ* 2004;329:1357–8.

10. Campbell RWF, Turpie AGG, Maseri A, et al. Management strategies for a better outcome in unstable coronary artery disease. *Clin Cardiol* 1998;21:314–22.

11. Theroux P, Fuster V. Acute coronary syndromes: unstable angina and non-Q-wave myocardial infarction. *Circulation* 1998;97:1195–206.

12. Diderholm E, Andren B, Frostfeldt G, et al. ST depression in ECG at entry indicates severe coronary lesions and large benefits of an early invasive treatment strategy in unstable coronary artery disease. The FRISC II ECG substudy. *Eur Heart J* 2002;23:41–9.

13. Patel DJ, Holdright DR, Knight CJ, et al. Early continuous ST segment monitoring in unstable angina: prognostic value additional to the clinical characteristics and the admission electrocardiograph. *Heart* 1996;75:222–8.

14. Lindahl B, Venge P, Wallentin L. Relation between troponin T and the risk of subsequent cardiac events in unstable coronary artery disease. The FRISC study group. *Circulation* 1996;93:1651–7.

15. de Lemos JA, Morrow DA, Bentley JH, et al. The prognostic value of B-type natriuretic peptide in patients with acute coronary syndromes. *N Engl J Med* 2001;345:1014–21.

16. Antman E, Cohen M, Bernick PJ, et al. The TIMI risk score for unstable angina/non-ST elevation myocardial infarction, a method for prognostication and therapeutic decision making. *JAMA* 2000;284:835–42.

17. Granger CB, Goldberg RJ, Dabbous OH, et al. for the Global Registry of Acute Coronary Events Investigators. Predictors of hospital mortality in the global registry of acute coronary events. *Arch Intern Med* 2003;163:2345–53.

18. Boersma E, Pieper KS, Steyerbery EW, et al. for the PURSUIT Investigators. Predictors of outcome in patients with acute coronary syndromes without persistent ST-segment elevation. Results from an international trial of 9461 patients. *Circulation* 2000;101:2557–67.

19. Curzen N. Designing treatment for acute myocardial infarction in a modern health service: pre-hospital thrombolysis or primary angioplasty? *Circulation* 2006;113:89–92.

20. Bellenger N, Curzen N. Revscularisation in acute coronary syndromes. In: Keogh B, Treasure T, eds. *The Evidence Base for Cardiothoracic Surgery.* TMF Publishing, 2005, pp. 179–88.

21. ISIS-2 (Second International Study of Infarct Survival) Collaborative Group. Randomised trial of intravenous streptokinase, oral aspirin, both, or neither among 17,187 cases of suspected acute myocardial infarction: ISIS-2. *Lancet* 1988;2:349–360.

22. Sabatine MS, Cannon CP, Gibson CM, et al. Addition of clopidogrel to aspirin and fibrinolytic therapy for myocardial infarction with ST-segment elevation. *N Engl J Med* 2005;24:1248–50.

23. Chen ZM, Pan HC, Dhen YP, et al. for the COMMIT collaborative group. Addition of clopidogrel to aspirin in 45,852 patients with acute myocardial infarction: randomised placebo-controlled trial. *Lancet* 2005;366:1607–21.

24. Keeley EC, Boura JA, Grines CL. Primary angioplasty versus intravenous thrombolytic therapy for acute myocardial infarction: a quantitative review of 23 randomised trials. *Lancet* 2003;361:13–20.

25. The GUSTO investigators. An international randomised trial comparing four thrombolytic strategies for acute myocardial infarction. *N Eng J Med* 1993;329:673–82.

26. Assessment of the Safety and Efficacy of a New Thrombolytic (ASSENT-2) Investigators. Single-bolus tenecteplase compared with front-loaded alteplase in acute myocardial infarction: the ASSENT-2 double-blind randomised trial. *Lancet* 1999;354:716–22.

27. Gershlick AH, Stephens LA, Hughes S, et al. Rescue angioplasty after failed thrombolytic therapy for acute myocardial infarction. *N Engl J Med* 2005;26:2758–68.

28. Silber S, Albertsson P, Aviles FF, et al. for the ESC Taskforce. Guidelines for percutaneous coronary interventions: the task force for percutaneous coronary interventions of the European Society of Cardiology. *Eur H J* 2005;26:804–47.

29. Scheller B, Hennen B, Hammer B, et al. Beneficial effects of immediate stenting after thrombolysis in acute myocardial infarction. *J Am Coll Cardiol* 2003;42:634–41.

30. Fernandez-Aviles F, Alonso JJ, Castro-Beiras A, et al. Routine invasive strategy within 24 hours of thrombolysis versus ischaemia-guided conservative approach for acute myocardial infarction with ST-segment elevation (GRACIA-1): a randomised controlled trial. *Lancet* 2004;364:1045–53.

31. Dzavik Y, Buller CE, Lamas GA, et al. Randomised trial of percutaneous coronary intervention for subacute infarct-related coronary artery occlusion to achieve long-term patency and improve ventricular function: the Total Occlusion Study of Canada (TOSCA)-2 trial. *Circulation* 2006;114:2449–57.

32. Hochman JS, Lamas GA, Buller CE, et al. for the Occluded Artery Trial Investigators. Coronary intervention for persistent occlusion after myocardial infarction. *N Eng J Med* 2006;355:2395–407.

33. Anderson HR, Nielsen TT, Rasmussen K, et al. A comparison of coronary angioplasty with fibrinolytic therapy in acute myocardial infarction. *N Engl J Med* 2003;349:733–42.

34. Widimsky P, Budesinsky T, Vorac D, et al. Long distance transport for primary angioplasty vs immediate thrombolysis in acute myocardial infarction. *Eur Heart J* 2003;24:94–104.

35. Holmes DR Jr, Bates ER, Kleiman NS, et al. Contemporary reperfusion therapy for cardiogenic shock: the GUSTO-1 trial experience. The GUSTO-1 Investigators. Global utilization of streptokinase and tissue plasminogen activator for occluded coronary arteries. *J Am Coll Cardiol* 1995;26:668–74.

36. Hochman JS, Sleeper LA, Webb JG, et al. Early revascularisation in acute MI complicated by cardiogenic shock. *N Engl J Med* 1999;341:625–34.

37. Williams SG, Wright DJ, Tan LB. Management of cardiogenic shock complicating acute myocardial infarction; towards evidence-based medical practice. *Heart* 2000;83:621–6.

38. Antman EM, Morrow DA, McCabe CH, et al. Enoxaparin versus unfractionated heparin with fibrinolysis for ST-elevation myocardial infarction (EXTRACT-TIMI 25). *N Engl J Med* 2006;354:1477–88.

39. Yusuf S, Mehta SR, Chrolavicius S, et al. Effects of Fondaparinux on mortality and reinfarction in patients with acute ST-segment elevation myocardial infarction. *JAMA* 2006;295:1519–30.

40. Antiplatelet Trialists' Collaboration. Collaborative meta-analysis of randomised trials of antiplatelet therapy for prevention of death, myocardial infarction, and stroke in high-risk patients. *BMJ* 2002;324:71–86.

41. The Clopidogrel in Unstable Angina to Prevent Recurrent Events (CURE) trial investigators. Effects of clopidogrel in addition to aspirin in patients with acute coronary syndromes without ST-segment elevation. *N Engl J Med.* 2001;345:494–502.

42. Patti G, Colonna G, Pasceri V, et al. Randomized trial of high loading dose of clopidogrel for reduction of periprocedural myocardial infarction in patients undergoing coronary intervention. *Circulation.* 2005;111:2099–106.

43. The CAPTURE investigators. Randomised placebo-controlled trial of abciximab before and during coronary intervention in refractory unstable angina: the CAPTURE study. *Lancet* 1997;349:1429–35.

44. Antman EM, McCabe CH, Gurfinkel EP, et al. Enoxaparin prevents death and cardiac ischemic events in unstable angina/non-Q-wave myocardial infarction. Results of the thrombolysis in myocardial infarction (TIMI) 11 B trial. *Circulation* 1999;100:1595–601.

45. Antman EM, Cohen M, McCabe CH, et al. Enoxaparin is superior to unfractionated heparin for preventing clinical events at 1-year follow up of TIMI 11B and ESSENCE. *Eur Heart J* 2002;23:308–14.

46. Collinson J, Flather MD, Fox KA, et al. Clinical outcomes, risk stratification and practice patterns of unstable angina and myocardial infarction without ST elevation: prospective registry of acute ischaemic syndromes in the UK (PRAIS-UK). *Eur Heart J* 2000;21:1450–7.

47. Cannon CP, Weintaub WS, Demopoulos LA, et al. Comparison of early invasive and conservative strategies in patients with unstable coronary syndromes treated with the glycoprotein IIb/IIIa inhibitor tirofiban (TACTICS-TIMI 18). *N Engl J Med* 2001;341:1879–87.

48. FRISC II investigators. Invasive compared with non-invasive treatment in unstable coronary-artery disease. FRISC II prospective randomised multicentre study. Fragmin and Fast Revascularisation during Instability in Coronary artery disease Investigators. *Lancet* 1999;354:708–15.

49. Fox KA, Poole-Wilson PA, Henderson RA, et al. Interventional versus conservative treatment for patients with unstable angina or non-ST elevation myocardial infarction: the British Heart Foundation RITA 3 randomised trial. *Lancet* 2002;360:743–51.

50. Miller C, Lipscomb K, Curzen N. Are district general hospital patients with unstable angina at a disadvantage? *Postgrad Med J* 2003;79:93–8.

51. Bellenger N, Eichhofer J, Crone D, Curzen N. Hospital stay in patients with non-ST-elevation acute coronary syndromes. *Lancet* 2004;363:1399–400.

52. Van de Werf F, Ardessino D, Betriu A, et al. Management of acute MI in patients presenting with ST-segment elevation. *Eur H J* 2003;24:28–66.

53. Cappell MS. Gastrointestinal bleeding associated with myocardial infarction. *Gastroenterol Clin N Am* 2000;29(2):423–4.

54. Cappell MS. The safety and clinical utility of esophagogastroduodenoscopy for acute gastrointestinal bleeding after myocardial infarction: a six-year study

of 42 endoscopies in 34 consecutive patients at two university teaching hospitals. *Am J Gastroenterol* 1993;88:344–50.

55. Lim W, Qushmaq I, Cook DJ, et al. Elevated troponin and myocardial infarction in the intensive care unit: a prospective study. *Crit Care* 2005;9:636–44.

56. Ammann P, Fehr T, Minder EI, et al. Elevation of troponin I in sepsis and septic shock. *Intensive Care Med* 2001;27:965–9.

57. Mangano DT. Perioperative cardiac morbidity. *Anesthesiology* 1990;72:153–84.

58. London MJ, Hollenberg M, Wong MG, et al. Intraoperative myocardial ischaemia: localisation by continuous 12-lead electrocardiography. *Anesthesiology* 1988;69:232–41.

59. Mangano DT, Wong MG, London MJ, et al. Perioperative myocardial ischaemia in patients undergoing noncardiac surgery – II: Incidence and severity during the first week after surgery. The study of perioperative ischaemia research group. *J Am Coll Cardiol* 1991;17:851–7.

60. Wu WC, Rathore SS, Wang Y, et al. Blood transfusion in elderly patients with acute myocardial infarction. *N Engl J Med* 2001;345:1230–6.

61. Allen BS, Rosenkranz E, Buckberg GD, et al. Studies on prolonged acute regional ischaemia in MI with LV power failure: a medical/surgical emergency requiring urgent revascularisation with maximal protection of remote muscle. *J Thorac Cardiovasc Surg* 1989;98:691–703.

62. Kurki TS, Kataja M, Reich DL. Emergency and elective coronary artery bypass grafting: comparisons of risk profiles, postoperative outcomes, and resource requirements. *J Cardiothorac Vasc Anesth* 2003. 17(5):594–7.

14 Cardiogenic Shock

Divaka Perera and Gerald S. Carr-White
Guys' and St Thomas' NHS Foundation Trust, London, UK

Take Home Messages

- Cardiogenic shock remains one of the major causes of morbidity and mortality following AMI.
- Rapid revascularisation and intra-aortic balloon counterpulsation are central to improving survival.
- The rational uses of inotropes and newer emerging mechanical and pharmacological treatments should be considered in patients who fail to improve after revascularisation.
- Patients with cardiogenic shock often have more scope for recovery than previously realised.

14.1 Causes and epidemiology

Cardiogenic shock is one of the leading causes of in-hospital mortality and, despite significant recent advances, fewer than half these cases survive to hospital discharge. It is defined as inadequate tissue perfusion due to a primary cardiac pathology. The commonest cause of cardiogenic shock is acute myocardial infarction (AMI), with cardiogenic shock complicating between 5 and 10% of acute infarctions and ST-elevation myocardial infarction accounting for over 90% of these cases.

Cardiogenic shock complicating AMI

Factors such as age, blood pressure, heart rate and Killip class are predictors of the development of cardiogenic shock following AMI, but are not specific enough to be of use in risk-stratifying patients in everyday clinical practice. In acute infarction, shock is due to left ventricular (LV) failure in approximately 80% of cases; the other 20% are due to (in decreasing frequency) severe mitral regurgitation, ventricular septal rupture, isolated right ventricular failure, tamponade and other causes (e.g. prior severe valvular disease, excess beta blocker or calcium channel blocker therapy)

Cardiovascular Critical Care. Edited by M. Griffiths, J. Cordingley and S. Price.
© 2010 Blackwell Publishing Ltd.

[1]. In the setting of AMI, the overall in-hospital mortality rate is approximately 60% in medically treated patients, with higher mortality in patients older than 75 years [2].

Women account for approximately 40% of all cases of cardiogenic shock due to myocardial infarction, and in the larger American studies, mortality rates appear to be higher in Hispanics and African Americans and lower in Asians [3]. The factors most predictive of increased mortality following cardiogenic shock include age, presence of renal failure, cardiac output at presentation, time to reperfusion, ejection fraction < 30%, multivessel coronary disease and the presence of moderate to severe mitral regurgitation [4, 5].

Other causes of cardiogenic shock

As illustrated in Table 14.1, a variety of valvular and non-ischaemic myopathic processes can be complicated by cardiogenic shock, the precise clinical features and epidemiology depending on the underlying diagnosis.

Table 14.1 Causes of cardiogenic shock.

Intrinsic myocardial dysfunction	Acute myocardial infarction Acute myocardial ischaemia Cardiomyopathy (dilated or restrictive) Acute myocarditis Right ventricular failure Takotsubo cardiomyopathy
Valvular heart disease	Chronic valvular heart disease Acute aortic or mitral insufficiency
Myocardial trauma	Myocardial contusion Coronary artery dissection/rupture
Other cardiac causes	Acute ventricular septal defect Hypertrophic obstructive cardiomyopathy Other causes of LVOT obstruction Congenital heart disease Cardiac tamponade Intracardiac tumours Prolonged tachyarrhythmia/bradyarrythmia Acute pulmonary embolus
Other non-cardiac causes	Overwhelming sepsis Malignant hypertension Severe anaemia Respiratory acidosis Hypophosphataemia/hypocalcaemia
Drugs	B-blocker or calcium antagonist overdose Cardiotoxic chemotherapy agents ACE inhibitor overdose Opiate or barbiturate overdose

LVOT, left ventricular outflow tract.

When cardiogenic shock results from deterioration of a chronic dilated cardiomyopathy, the in-hospital mortality rate rises steeply with the presence of the following features: acute renal failure, requirement for inotropes, ventricular arrhythmias, history of cerebrovascular accident and significant hyponatraemia [6]. The aetiology and clinical course of myocarditis are extremely variable, but cardiogenic shock can sometimes develop rapidly in fulminant cases. As the underlying process is often reversible, management of myocarditis involves rapid and aggressive supportive therapy whenever haemodynamic compromise ensues.

14.2 Pathophysiology

The classical paradigm of cardiogenic shock is mechanical dysfunction related to the amount of non-viable myocardium, and it is generally accepted that cardiogenic shock is likely when more than 40% of the LV myocardium is infarcted or fibrosed. As such, limiting the extent of infarction by rapid revascularisation is central to managing cardiogenic shock following AMI. However, several other pathophysiological processes can compound the intrinsic mechanical dysfunction that accompanies myocardial necrosis, many of which are potentially reversible. Indeed, the SHOCK trial demonstrated that left ventricular ejection fraction (LVEF) is not always depressed in the setting of cardiogenic shock and that most survivors have only New York Heart Association (NYHA) class I congestive heart failure [7].

Irrespective of aetiology, both acute and chronic heart failure cause profound activation of the renin-angiotensin-aldosterone, sympathetic and vasopressor systems, and in the chronic phase the relevant antagonists (ACE-inhibitors, spironolactone, beta blockers and more recently vaptans) confer important benefits in terms of mortality and morbidity. These homeostatic systems are acutely activated in cardiogenic shock and can contribute to the adverse haemodynamics seen. In addition, a systemic inflammatory response syndrome-type mechanism has been implicated in the pathophysiology of cardiogenic shock [8]. Elevated levels of complement, interleukins, C-reactive protein and inflammatory nitric oxide synthetase (iNOS) are often seen in large myocardial infarctions and can also be seen in non-ischaemic cardiogenic shock. These may induce hypotension and impair directly myocardial efficiency, possibly by interfering with calcium metabolism.

Finally, ongoing myocardial ischaemia, myocardial stunning and hibernation are important mechanisms, particularly in those with multivessel coronary disease. The terms hibernation and stunning are predominantly derived from animal models and their distinction from each other and from ischaemia in acute clinical settings is difficult. From a clinical point of view, it is appropriate to group them together as reversible LV dysfunction in a territory subtended by a stenosed coronary artery. All three mechanisms reflect the presence of coronary artery disease, leading to potentially reversible local abnormalities of function; practically, they can only be classified in retrospect, based on the timing and extent of recovery of myocardial function following coronary revascularisation.

14.3 Clinical manifestations and diagnosis

The 'typical' patient with cardiogenic shock has severe systemic hypotension, signs of systemic hypoperfusion (e.g. cool extremities, oliguria), a sinus tachycardia and respiratory distress due to pulmonary congestion. However, not all patients present with this constellation and many develop shock after presentation, usually within 24 hours of admission. In clinical trials the diagnosis tends to rely on most or all of the following:

- Systemic hypotension (systemic arterial pressure < 80–90 mmHg or mean arterial pressure 30 mmHg below basal levels for 30 minutes or longer)
- Absence of hypovolaemia (pulmonary capillary wedge pressure > 15 mmHg)
- Reduced cardiac output (cardiac index < 2.2 l/min/m^2)
- Evidence of tissue hypoperfusion
  - o Low mixed venous oxygen saturations (< 60%)
  - o Reduced urine output (< 30 ml/hour or 0.5 ml/kg/hour)
  - o Rising lactate levels
  - o Cold peripheries (extremities colder than core)

However, it should be noted that hypotension may be masked by intense sympathetic activation (baroreceptor response to shock). In the SHOCK registry 5.2% of patients did not have overt hypotension (defined as a systolic pressure below 90 mmHg) despite signs of peripheral hypoperfusion [9]. These normotensive patients had an appreciable in-hospital mortality rate, although this was lower than that in the classical hypotensive cohort (43 versus 66%). In addition, pulmonary congestion may be absent at presentation in about one-third of patients, although pulmonary capillary wedge pressures are often similar in those with and without signs of pulmonary congestion. Usually, the diagnosis is suspected in a clammy patient with borderline blood pressure and oliguria. In these cases, demonstration of cardiac dysfunction by echocardiography often confirms the diagnosis, which can be further verified by invasive measurement of cardiac output, right atrial pressure and mixed venous oxygen saturations.

Routine blood tests (full blood count (FBC), renal and liver function, cardiac enzymes and inflammatory markers) are important in evaluating other organ dysfunction, the presence of infection or an inflammatory response and the degree of myocardial damage (although cardiac enzymes are not an accurate predictor of cardiogenic shock). A 12-lead ECG is obviously mandatory to document evidence of ischaemia and infarction and also to exclude dysrhythmias. A chest X-ray may help guide fluid balance by showing the presence or absence of interstitial fluid. Elevated brain natriuretic peptide (BNP) or NT-proBNP levels are not specific to cardiogenic shock but do correlate with prognosis regardless of the cause of shock [10]. These markers are most useful for their negative predictive value, as a low BNP level effectively excludes cardiogenic shock in the setting of hypotension or significant hypoxia and should lead to consideration of alternative aetiologies [11]. BNP levels should be indexed to both age- and sex-related values to minimise false positive results.

Echocardiography

Echocardiography plays a central role in the diagnosis of cardiogenic shock. It is often assumed that echocardiography is a simple way to confirm the diagnosis and exclude other complications; however, mistakes are frequently made and whilst this is covered in more detail in other chapters, it is worth highlighting some of the issues that are particularly relevant.

Assessment of regional wall motion and global LV function

In the majority of cases echocardiography will show regional wall motion abnormalities reflecting the underlying coronary abnormalities. Following myocardial infarction, abnormalities of wall movement on 2-D images are found in approximately 80% of Q wave infarcts and rather less frequently after non-transmural infarcts. The most specific abnormality to recognise is regional myocardial systolic thinning in an affected area [12]. This is a relatively robust criterion, since it is unaffected by overall motion of the heart, which occurs in the presence of any regional abnormality of function, and which compromises any attempt to document endocardial motion alone.

Generally, blood flow must be reduced to 50% in at least 5% of the myocardium for 'conventional' systolic wall motion abnormalities to occur [13]. In regions where blood supply is less compromised, wall motion characteristically becomes asynchronous, with delay in the onset of inward motion, and a corresponding delay in the onset of relaxation [14]. Overall amplitude may thus be preserved, but that supporting useful work during ejection is substantially reduced. Such abnormalities, which will be missed by simple amplitude analysis, are more liable to respond to medical or surgical interventions as they represent lesser degrees of ischaemia [15]. This scenario is often particularly pronounced in the intensive care setting with inotropic support, which frequently worsens the dysynchrony and myocardial efficiency. Often a ventricle driven by inotropes will appear to have relatively well-preserved function and it is only when the timing of wall motion is analysed that it can be seen that most of the myocardial work is taking place outside ejection.

Complications of AMI

The clinical syndrome of cardiogenic shock without evidence of significant LV dysfunction always needs explaining; right ventricular infarction, acute mitral regurgitation and a ventricular septal defect all produce the features of cardiogenic shock but with active LV wall motion. Very severe mitral regurgitation characteristically produces severe pulmonary oedema with no audible murmur, and it should always be suspected by the echocardiographic finding of a very active left ventricle in a shocked patient (see Chapter 18). In combination with a marked tachycardia, it can give rise to confusing Doppler data. If the systolic atrioventricular (AV) pressure drop is low due to the combination of systemic hypotension and the very high left atrial pressure, which results from what is effectively an absent mitral valve, the extent of regurgitation may be seriously underestimated by colour flow. For the same reason, the continuous wave Doppler profile may show a sinusoidal trace of low forward and backward velocities, often with all the energy in the envelope, indicating laminar flow to and fro between atrium and ventricle. In such patients a transoesophageal echo is often needed to demonstrate the responsible anatomy.

It is important to recognise right ventricular infarction as a cause of post-infarction cardiogenic shock. In inferior myocardial infarction, its presence increases mortality and morbidity by a factor of ten; in addition it selects a group who derive more benefit from revascularisation and whose systemic hypotension responds to increased filling rather than inotropic support. The wall of the right ventricle is thin, so that systolic thinning cannot be recognised. It is thus necessary to look for an increase in cavity size, a reduction in ejection fraction and often strikingly reversed septal motion on M-mode. Indeed in severe cases this last may be the sole basis for right ventricular contractile function. Low velocity tricuspid regurgitation, which will summate with right ventricular diastolic disease in elevating the systemic venous pressure, is also common. At the same time the left ventricle is underfilled. An additional method of diagnosing right ventricular infarction is by measuring the longitudinal movement of the tricuspid annulus towards the apex of the right ventricle.

Assessment of filling pressures

In a shocked patient, assessment of adequate filling pressures is vital and often relies on a combination of clinical signs, haemodynamic monitoring and the response of both of these to cautious fluid challenges. Echocardiography does have a role in assessing filling pressures. Indirect assessment of left atrial pressures can be made by a variety of methods described elsewhere, but the ratio of the mitral inflow E wave and tissue Doppler E prime velocity is perhaps one of the most robust, though it is less well validated in intubated patients. Right-sided filling pressures are usually assessed by measuring the size and reactivity of the inferior vena cava, but this can be misleading in patients receiving positive pressure ventilation, particularly when high end-expiratory pressures are used.

Non-ischaemic cardiogenic shock

Echocardiography can provide clues to the underlying aetiology in cardiogenic shock that is unrelated to coronary disease. In acute severe myocarditis, wall thickness and cavity size may be preserved in the presence

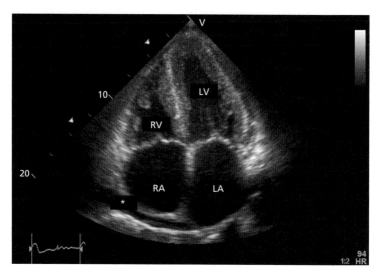

Figure 14.1 Typical echocardiogram of cardiac amyloidosis with concentric left ventricular hypertrophy and a speckled appearance to the myocardium, biatrial enlargement (LA, left atrium; RA, right atrium; LV, left ventricle; RV, right ventricle), a pericardial effusion (askerisk) and mildly thickened mitral and tricuspid valves (small arrows).

of regional or global LV dysfunction, often with an associated pericardial effusion. In Takotsubo cardiomyopathy, there is characteristic ballooning of the apex with preserved wall motion in other regions [16]. Echo contrast may need to be used as apical views are often poor in the intensive care setting. The presence of a dilated right heart may suggest a shunt at atrial or ventricular level (assessment of saturations via a pulmonary catheter can be useful in this situation), a large pulmonary embolus, right ventricular infarction or a right ventricular cardiomyopathy. Significant LV hypertrophy and a small cavity size should prompt consideration of hypertrophic cardiomyopathy, in which case an outflow tract gradient must be excluded before starting inotropic support, or infiltrative diseases such as sarcoid, storage diseases, mitochondrial cardiomyopathies, Fabry's disease or amyloid. In cardiac amyloidosis there is often a dramatic reduction in systolic thickening, usually well seen by M-mode, and you may see mitral and tricuspid valve and atrial septal thickening and a small pericardial effusion (Figure 14.1).

Invasive haemodynamic monitoring

All patients in cardiogenic shock need constant haemodynamic monitoring. An arterial line (for measurement of arterial pressures, gas exchange and acid base balance) and a central venous line (for right atrial pressures and monitoring of central venous saturations) are mandatory in such patients. More invasive monitoring can then be provided via lithium dilution cardiac output (LiDCO), pulse contour cardiac output (PICCO) or a pulmonary artery catheter. Recent evidence suggests that pulmonary artery catheters may potentially provide more harm than benefit, but the authors still believe they do play a role in patients with right ventricular or biventricular dysfunction in whom manipulating the pulmonary vascular tone is an important therapeutic goal. In the majority of patients with cardiogenic shock our preference is for the relatively less invasive LiDCO. It must be remembered that PICCO and LiDCO cardiac output measurements are unreliable in the presence of cardiac shunts or an intra-aortic balloon pump (IABP).

14.4 Management of cardiogenic shock

The key factor in the management of cardiogenic shock is rapid diagnosis and treatment before myocardial and other organ damage is irreversible. The cause should be identified and precipitants and confounding factors should be treated (such as anaemia, arrhythmias and vasodepressor drugs). The initial goal is optimisation of cardiac output and organ perfusion. It should be remembered that as many as 20% of patients with cardiogenic shock do in fact have relative hypovolaemia, and where there is doubt, small boluses of fluid should be given with intensive bedside monitoring. The use of IABPs and inotropes is described in subsequent sections. Hypoxaemia, acidosis, hyperglycaemia and uraemia should be corrected as these may cause further myocardial depression and decrease the contractile or vasopressor response to inotropic support [17].

Intra-aortic counterpulsation
Haemodynamic effects

Coronary perfusion occurs primarily during diastole and, in 1958, Harken showed that a failing heart could be supported by removing blood from the femoral artery in systole and replacing this volume rapidly during diastole [18]. Although impractical in its original form, this concept led to the development of the IABP in the 1960s [19, 20]. Aortic counterpulsation is carried out by placing a balloon catheter in the descending aorta, which is inflated early in diastole and deflated just prior to the onset of the subsequent systole. Synchronisation of inflation and deflation with the cardiac cycle is usually achieved by detection of the R wave on the electrocardiogram (ECG-triggered) but can also be linked to the patient's aortic pressure waveform (pressure-triggered).

The physiological goals of IABP therapy are to increase myocardial oxygen supply and decrease myocardial oxygen demand. Inflation of the balloon in diastole results in augmentation of aortic diastolic pressure and an increase in the aorto-coronary pressure gradient, with a consequent increase in coronary flow [21] (Figure 14.2). On the other hand, rapid deflation of the balloon just prior to the beginning of systole causes a void in the aorta, which in turn leads to a drop in *end*-diastolic pressure and subsequent systolic pressure (Figure 14.3). It should be noted that mean arterial pressure should increase with proper IABP function, as the augmentation of diastolic pressure is typically greater than the decrease in systolic pressure. The reduction in systolic pressure or afterload translates

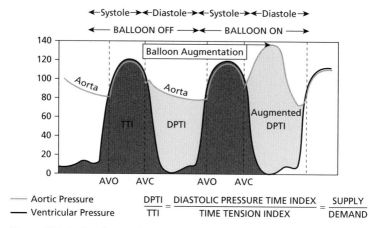

Figure 14.2 Aortic and ventricular pressure, with and without counterpulsation. Two cardiac cycles are depicted, with and without IABP respectively. The diastolic pressure time index (DPTI, the integrated aorto-coronary pressure gradient) is proportional to myocardial oxygen supply and increases with IABP therapy. The tension time index (TTI, the area under the LV pressure curve) is a primary determinant of myocardial oxygen consumption and decreases with IABP therapy. AVO, aortic valve open; AVC, aortic valve closed.

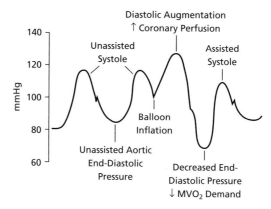

Figure 14.3 Aortic pressure waveform during counterpulsation. Assessment of the timing of counterpulsation should be carried out in a 2:1 ratio as shown. In addition to augmentation of diastolic pressure (which is a measure of enhanced coronary perfusion), counterpulsation should also reduce afterload, indicated by a lower end-diastolic pressure in the assisted beat compared to the unassisted beat.

to a drop in systolic wall tension, which is an important determinant of myocardial oxygen demand [22]. The simultaneous increase in coronary perfusion and decrease in oxygen demand is a unique feature of balloon counterpulsation and contrasts with the action of pharmacological inotropic agents, which increase cardiac output at the expense of increased myocardial oxygen demand and hence could potentially accelerate the downward spiral of cardiac function.

Aortic counterpulsation in cardiogenic shock

The impressive physiological profile of the IABP is backed by a growing body of evidence supporting its clinical efficacy. In the pre-thrombolysis era, two small randomised studies had failed to demonstrate benefit of IABP in treating cardiogenic shock [23, 24]. However, since then, several non-randomised studies have shown improved outcomes in patients with cardiogenic shock who have been treated with thrombolysis and received an IABP (Figure 14.4) [25–29]. Thrombolysis has been clearly demonstrated to reduce infarct size and improve survival in patients with ST-elevation MI, but it appears to be a less efficient treatment for patients in cardiogenic shock. Impaired coronary perfusion associated with cardiogenic shock may be responsible for the reduced efficacy of thrombolytic therapy in this setting [30] and the synergistic effect of thrombolysis and IABP in reducing mortality may be attributable to augmentation of coronary flow with counterpulsation [31]. Seven percent of the 40,000 patients enrolled in the GUSTO-1 trial developed cardiogenic shock and a quarter of these received IABP therapy. There was a strong trend in favour of reduced mortality in the group that received both treatments compared to those who only had thrombolysis (47% vs 60%, $p = 0.06$) [26]. Similarly, in NRMI-2 (one of the largest AMI registries, $n = 23{,}180$), IABP was used in a third of patients in cardiogenic shock and these patients had a substantial mortality benefit compared to those who received thrombolytic therapy (49% vs 77%) [28]. TACTICS was one of the few randomised trials of IABP use in cardiogenic shock. Twenty seven patients were randomised to receive fibrinolysis and IABP therapy and 27 patient to fibrinolysis alone. Six-month mortality was lower in the group that received IABP and fibrinolysis (34% vs 43%), but the result failed to reach statistical significance ($p = 0.23$) [29]. This trial exemplifies the difficulties in conducting randomised trials in such critically ill patients;

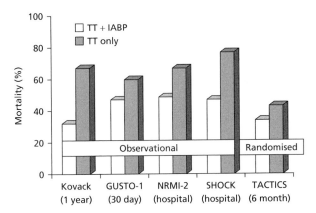

Figure 14.4 Synergy between thrombolysis and IABP in the treatment of cardiogenic shock. X axis shows percentage mortality and y axis the relevant clinical trials. TT, thrombolysis; IABP, intra-aortic balloon pump.

while the numbers recruited were low, a third of the patients in the fibrinolysis-only arm deteriorated to such an extent that they crossed over to receive IABP therapy.

Despite the paucity of randomised evidence, IABP therapy is now a Class I indication in the American College of Cardiology/American Heart Association (ACC/AHA) guidelines for management of patients with cardiogenic shock [32]. In patients not responsive to conventional medical therapy, IABP insertion should be considered early in the management of cardiogenic shock, irrespective of the reperfusion strategy used. The evidence base for IABP use in non-ischaemic cardiogenic shock is less robust and there are no randomised trials showing benefit. However, an IABP or LVAD should be considered in such patients, particularly if there is clinical deterioration with an increasing requirement of inotropes.

Contraindications and complications of the IABP

Significant aortic valve incompetence is an absolute contraindication to IABP therapy. Augmentation of diastolic pressure in the ascending aorta would exacerbate aortic regurgitation and LV dilatation, resulting in deterioration of cardiac function. If aortic regurgitation is suspected on clinical grounds, further evaluation by echocardiography is advisable prior to IABP insertion. Severe peripheral vascular disease, active bleeding and aortic aneurysm are relative contraindications and the decision on IABP insertion will depend on the clinical scenario.

The incidence of IABP complications has fallen as techniques, equipment and experience have improved. In a recent review of the Benchmark Registry (the largest IABP registry to date, including more than 22,000 patients), major IABP-related complications occurred in 2.7% of patients, including major access site bleeding (1.4%), amputation (0.1%) and death attributable to IABP therapy (0.05%) [33]. Sheathless insertion and the use of smaller gauge catheters (8 as opposed to 9.5 French) have led to a lower rate of ischaemic limb complications. Formation of thrombus on the balloon is a theoretical source of embolic complications, especially if assist ratios lower than 1:1 are used, although there is little evidence that anticoagulation reduces the risk of such events. On balance, the authors recommend intravenous anticoagulation with unfractionated heparin to maintain an activated partial thromboplastin time (APTT) ratio of 1.5–2.5, particularly when prolonged IABP use (> 24 hours) is anticipated.

Management of a patient receiving counterpulsation

A degree of access site bleeding affects up to 5% of patients requiring IABP therapy following AMI. Although usually minor, the bleeding can be severe enough to warrant transfusion in a third of these cases. The insertion site should be inspected regularly for blood loss or haematoma and clinically silent retroperitoneal bleeding suspected in the event of unexplained blood loss. Anticoagulation therapy should be monitored as above and thrombocytopenia excluded on a daily basis. Patients should also be monitored for limb ischaemia and foot pulses, and colour and capillary refill should be checked at regular intervals. Most intensive care units also continually monitor differential toe temperatures in these patients. IABP catheter migration is most likely to occur during patient transfer and should be assessed on a chest radiograph. Upward displacement is more common and may be manifest as diminution of the left radial pulse (if the balloon moves over the origin of the left subclavian artery), while downward displacement may cause a decrease in urine output if the balloon crosses the renal arteries.

A common problem encountered during counterpulsation is failure of adequate augmentation of diastolic pressure, which could be due to a variety of patient, IABP catheter or IABP console related factors. Low mean arterial and augmented diastolic pressures may reflect severely impaired stroke volume or increased heart rate, and cardioversion of tachyarrhythmias should be considered early. Failure of augmentation may also be due to migration of the IABP catheter tip, kinking of the catheter shaft, low helium levels or a balloon leak, which is often manifest as blood in the helium line. Failure of augmentation may be due to IABP timing errors, in particular late inflation (causing diastolic augmentation after the dichrotic notch) or early deflation (resulting in a sharp drop in the balloon waveform following peak diastolic augmentation). Conversely, early inflation or late deflation can result in the balloon being inflated while the aortic valve is open (with the balloon waveform being superimposed on the LV systolic component of the aortic waveform) which can actually increase afterload and decrease cardiac output further. IABP timing should be assessed regularly by comparing assisted and unassisted waveforms (Figure 14.3) in a 2:1 or 3:1 assist ratio, and inflation/deflation adjusted accordingly.

Revascularisation
Early revascularisation or medical stablisation?
Early definition of coronary anatomy, with a view to revascularisation, is at the heart of managing ischaemic cardiogenic shock. The pathophysiology of cardiogenic shock is depressed myocardial contractility due to myocardial ischaemia and necrosis, which leads to decreased cardiac output and lower coronary perfusion pressure, which in turn further exacerbates ischaemia. Resolution of ischaemia by revascularisation is a crucial step in halting this vicious spiral. The benefit of early revascularisation was firmly established by the SHOCK trial (Should We Emergently Revascularize Occluded Coronaries For Cardiogenic Shock) [7]. This was a multi-centre, prospective trial which randomly assigned patients with cardiogenic shock due to acute MI (characterised by ST-elevation, Q-wave or new left bundle branch block) to emergency revascularisation (ERV) ($n = 152$) or initial medical stabilisation (IMS) ($n = 150$). Shock was rigorously defined as systolic blood pressure persistently lower than 90 mmHg, cardiac index less than 2.2 l/min/m^2 and pulmonary capillary wedge pressure greater than 15 mmHg. Thrombolysis was used in 63% of the IMS group and IABP was used in 86% of patients overall. Early revascularisation was achieved by percutaneous coronary intervention (PCI) or coronary bypass surgery (CABG).

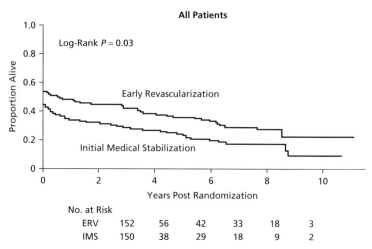

Figure 14.5 Long-term outcome following early revascularisation (ERV) compared to initial medical stabilisation (IMS) of cardiogenic shock in the SHOCK trial.

There was a trend towards decreased mortality at 30 days (the primary end-point) in the ERV group compared to IMS (46.7% vs 56%; 95% CI for difference −20.5% to 1.9%, $p = 0.11$). However, mortality at 6 months (the secondary end-point) was significantly lower with revascularisation than with medical therapy (50.3% vs 63.1%, $p = 0.027$). These findings translate to an impressive treatment benefit of 13 lives saved per 100 treated (or eight patients needing to be treated to save one life). A recent report suggests that this benefit is maintained in the long term, with 6-year survival in the revascularisation group remaining significantly better than the medically treated group (32.8% vs 19.2%) [34] (Figure 14.5).

Treatment of the elderly patient with cardiogenic shock is particularly challenging. When patients in the SHOCK trial were stratified dichotomously by age, the benefits of early revascularisation were only seen in those who were younger than 75 years of age (30-day mortality was 41.4% and 56.8% respectively, with ERV and IMS, $p = 0.02$). In fact, patients older than 75 years appeared to have a worse outcome when given early revascularisation (30-day mortality was 75% and 53.1% respectively, with ERV and IMS, $p = 0.16$). However, the number of patients in the latter group was small, and these differences were not seen on long-term follow-up [34]. Furthermore, elderly patients who received early revascularisation in the larger, non-randomised SHOCK registry were seen to derive the same magnitude of benefit as patients younger than 75 years of age [35]. Hence the elderly require individualised judgements, based on prior functional status and comorbidity, as well as the patient's own wishes.

Percutaneous or surgical revascularisation?

In stable coronary artery disease, surgical and percutaneous revascularisation are complementary treatments, the choice of technique being largely dictated by coronary anatomy. It is generally held that CABG poses a higher risk of early complications, which are offset by a better long-term outcome in certain subsets of patients. Theoretically, these differences in early complications may be magnified in patients with cardiogenic shock, whose early mortality is up to two orders of magnitude higher than in elective patients. There have been no randomised comparisons of percutaneous intervention and coronary bypass surgery for treatment of cardiogenic shock. In the SHOCK trial, the mode of revascularisation was individualised to the patient, although the protocol recommended that PCI was performed only on the infarct-related artery (IRA) and that patients with significant multi-vessel disease or left main stem (LMS) disease were treated with CABG. Of the patients receiving emergent revascularisation, 63% were treated with PCI and 37% with CABG. In this observational analysis, both treatments appeared to proffer similar mortality benefits in the short and medium term; survival was 56% vs 57% ($p = 0.86$) at 30 days and 52% vs 47% ($p = 0.71$) at 1 year in patients treated with CABG and PCI respectively [36].

Apart from selection bias that is inherent in any observational study, several caveats apply to this comparison. The protocol design resulted in the PCI group receiving less complete revascularisation than surgically treated patients, which is associated with increased mortality and morbidity in the long term. Furthermore, stents and glycoprotein IIb/IIIa inhibitors were only used in 37% and 67% of PCI patients respectively, although both interventions have subsequently been shown to reduce mortality in patients with cardiogenic shock [37]. These considerations and a reticence on the part of surgeons to undertake emergency CABG in these high-risk patients has meant that primary PCI has largely superseded CABG in the treatment of cardiogenic shock. A recent report showed that the rate of primary PCI in shock patients has doubled from 27 to 54% in the decade following publication of the SHOCK trial findings, while emergency CABG was only performed in 2–3% of such cases [1]. Nevertheless, emergency CABG surgery remains an important component (and Class IA indication [32]) of an early invasive strategy, particularly in patients with complex multi-vessel disease and in the event of mechanical complications of AMI (Figure 14.6).

PCI during uncomplicated myocardial infarction is usually restricted to the IRA, where the culprit vessel can be reliably identified [32]. In contrast, remote ischaemia in non-infarct territories plays an important role in the pathogenesis of pump failure in cardiogenic shock, as coronary autoregulation is impaired in these cases [38]. As a consequence, coronary blood flow drops linearly with decreasing mean arterial pressure, and coronary lesions in non-infarct vessels may act as a substrate for remote ischaemia and extension of the infarct zone [39]. Indeed, non-IRA coronary disease is an independent predictor of outcome following shock in the wake of an acute MI. While multi-vessel PCI would achieve more complete revascularisation and potentially halt this cascade, such a strategy needs to be tempered by an increased risk of distal embolisation and 'no-reflow' due to the pro-thrombotic and inflammatory milieu that complicates cardiogenic shock. Hence it is currently recommended that multi-vessel PCI should only be considered if treatment of the IRA fails to

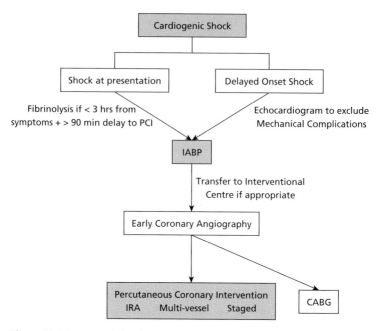

Figure 14.6 Recommendations for management of cardiogenic shock complicating acute myocardial infarction. IABP, intra-aortic ballon pump; PCI, percutaneous coronary intervention; IRA, infarct related artery; CABG, coronary artery bypass graft surgery.

improve haemodynamics in the cardiac catheterisation laboratory, when the IRA cannot be identified with certainty or CABG cannot be performed for any reason [32, 40]. In the event of multi-vessel disease, staged PCI or CABG should be carried out if the patient's condition improves following PCI to the IRA.

The benefits of platelet inhibition via glycoprotein IIb/IIIa blockade during primary PCI are well established [41, 42]. Although most studies only included haemodynamically stable patients, there is reasonable evidence to suggest that these agents may be even more effective at reducing mortality following PCI for cardiogenic shock complicating acute MI [43, 44]. GP IIb/IIIa inhibitors should be used routinely in such patients and should ideally be administered early (on coronary care or intensive care units), particularly if PCI is expected to be delayed, as is the case with patients requiring transfer to an intervention centre.

Use of inotropic and vasopressor agents

In the setting of cardiogenic shock due to acute infarction or coronary ischaemia, intra-aortic counterpulsation is nearly always preferable to pharmacological vasopressor or inotropic agents. However, in practice, these agents are often used as an adjunct, or prior to insertion of an IABP. Inotropic agents will increase myocardial oxygen demand during ischaemia and will also exacerbate dysynchrony, thereby reducing the efficiency of energy transfer to the circulation. These dual mechanisms will potentially worsen ischaemic ventricular dysfunction and must be balanced against any beneficial effect due to increased coronary perfusion. It should also be noted that coronary perfusion does not equate to mean arterial pressure, but is a product of coronary lumen area, cardiac output, diastolic filling time and coronary perfusion pressure (which in turn is most closely linked to diastolic aortic pressure). So in ischaemic cardiogenic shock the aim is to maximise cardiac output and diastolic aortic pressure whilst preserving diastolic filling time (by preventing tachycardia) and minimising any increase in myocardial oxygen demand. Whilst most patients with cardiogenic shock are relatively vasoconstricted, a substantial minority will have a vasodilatory response due to systemic inflammation or infection. Where there is clinical doubt, measurement of the systemic vascular resistance with catheter-based devices may be useful.

Detailed pharmacology of the various agents is beyond the scope of this chapter but the guiding principles are summarised below. There is no good scientific data showing superiority of any particular agent; the following are the authors' preferences in different scenarios. When arterial pressure is very low (i.e. systolic pressure is below 75 mmHg), a vasopressor (such as low dose noradrenaline) or dopamine is usually the first-line treatment to increase diastolic aortic pressure. Where arterial pressures are only mildly reduced but there is evidence of end organ dysfunction and a low measured cardiac index, the choices are between dobutamine (+/− dopamine), milrinone or levosimendan. In the presence of a significant tachycardia, dopamine and higher doses of dobutamine should be avoided to prevent increasing the heart rate further (and reducing coronary filling time). In patients on beta blockers, beta agonists (dopamine and dobutamine) are less preferable to milrinone or levosimendan. In those with a raised pulmonary vascular resistance, milrinone is often tried earlier due to its pulmonary vasodilator properties.

Levosimendan is a relatively new pharmacological agent acting via calcium-dependent binding to cardiac troponin C and ATP-dependent K+ channel activation, and preliminary data suggest that it may have less detrimental effects on ventricular relaxation and oxygen consumption when compared to beta agonists [45]. The first two trials comparing levosimandan with dobutamine (LIDO and CASINO) suggested there was a mortality advantage with levosimandan. However, the larger European SURVIVE trial with 1,327 patients showed no significant difference, though it has been argued that some of the adverse events seen with levosimandan could have been avoided by not giving the loading dose [46].

Nesiritide is a recombinant DNA form of human B-type natriuretic peptides. It binds to particulate guanylate cyclase receptor of vascular smooth muscle and endothelial cells, dilating veins and arteries. It reduces pulmonary capillary wedge pressure and improves dyspnea in patients with acutely decompensated congestive heart failure. However, it has been shown to increase mortality and renal dysfunction and until further clinical trial data are presented should probably be avoided.

One condition seen in patients on high doses of inotropes which must be recognised is that of left ventricular outflow tract (LVOT) obstruction. Classically this is seen in an underfilled and often hypertrophied left ventricle driven by inotropes. It can also be seen after mitral repair, particularly where there is a long posterior leaflet, and after aortic valve surgery where there is significant LV hypertrophy. Typically the patient has a low cardiac output state, oliguria and a systolic murmur at the left sternal edge. The condition can only be reliably diagnosed with echo, with typically a small active left ventricle, sometimes systolic anterior motion of the mitral valve and a typical scimitar-shaped high LVOTgradient. The treatment is adequate fluid resuscitation, avoidance of any tachycardia and if necessary peripheral vasoconstrictors such as phenylephrine. If left undiagnosed a viscious cycle can evolve with increasing inotropes being used to try to augment the cardiac output which will worsen the obstruction and ultimately lead to multi-organ failure and death.

Other therapies
Ventilation strategies
A detailed discussion of ventilation in cardiogenic shock is beyond the scope of this chapter. In brief, there is good evidence that treatment with CPAP or bi-level positive airway pressure (BiPAP) significantly reduces the need for subsequent invasive ventilation, compared to standard therapy (including oxygen via face mask, diuretics and nitrates). In a recent meta-analysis of 23 trials involving non-invasive ventilation in cardiogenic pulmonary oedema, CPAP was also associated with significant mortality benefits compared to standard therapy, with a trend to benefit with BiPAP [47]. In practice, the mode of ventilation will be influenced by these considerations, as well as the ease and efficacy of non-invasive ventilation in individual patients, many of whom may be nursed in a supine position due to an indwelling IABP catheter.

Pacing
The indications for temporary pacing following an acute infarction are well established [32]. However, the detrimental effects of right ventricular apical pacing are becoming increasingly evident and in the setting of cardiogenic shock this should be avoided where possible. In those with sinus node disease a temporary atrial wire should be used, and in those with AV block AV sequential temporary pacing should be considered. In these patients, the AV interval should then be optimised with echocardiography to maximise diastolic filling time.

In patients without bradycardic indications for pacing but with a low LVEF and left bundle branch block on their ECG, temporary biventricular pacing can be considered when weaning from a ventilator is otherwise impossible, and this is certainly backed up by case reports of efficacy [48]. In patients with a low ejection fraction and RV apical pacing in whom a low cardiac output is preventing weaning, a temporary upgrade to biventricular pacing could also be considered; there are no specific criteria to guide selection, apart from a paced QRS complex that is greater than 220 msec.

Left ventricular assist devices and transplantation
Cardiac transplantation should be considered in patients who fail to improve following revascularisation (or have unfavourable coronary anatomy) or

have a non-ischaemic cause of cardiogenic shock, particularly in those who do not have multi-organ failure. Although mortality rates are very high in this group, aggressive haemodynamic support with a left ventricular assist device (LVAD) can be a bridge to recovery or dramatically improve the chances of survival to transplantation. There is increasing interest in percutaneous LVADs which can be inserted in the cardiac catheterisation laboratory, especially in patients who are too haemodynamically unstable for transfer to a transplant unit. In contrast to IABPs, these devices actively augment cardiac output and could potentially provide complete replacement of LV function in the short term. In animal models, LVADS have been shown to reduce infarct size and improve microvascular function compared to IABP support [49] and randomised clinical trials of LVAD vs IABP support for patients in cardiogenic shock are currently underway. At the time of writing, two types of percutaneous LVAD are available for clinical use: the TandemHeart® (CardiacAssist Inc, USA) (which injects blood drawn from the left atrium into the femoral artery by means of a centrifugal pump) and the Impella® catheters (Abiomed, USA) (which aspirate blood directly from the left ventricle and inject up to 5.5 l/min into the ascending aorta via a microaxial pump) (see Chapter 8).

14.5 Specific conditions

Right ventricular failure

In the setting of an inferior infarct, right ventricular failure increases the mortality by a factor of 10, but also (as one would expect) increases the benefit from revascularisation. The medical treatment of right ventricular failure, however, is often fairly disappointing. The key factor is to ensure adequate right-sided filling pressures, and ventilation parameters should be optimised accordingly. When pulmonary pressures are elevated milrinone (Levosimendan), nitric oxide, prostaglandin and even sildafenil can be empirically tried. Beta agonists are often relatively ineffective.

Diastolic disease

Restrictive ventricular disease can be very difficult to treat. Beta agonists are often ineffective and can worsen the situation. Adrenaline in particular should nearly always be avoided, as it often exacerbates the diastolic dysfunction. In the hypertensive patient with pulmonary oedema and a low cardiac output, aggressive diuresis must be avoided as these patients often have depleted intravascular volume. Instead, they should be treated with aggressive vasodilatation, often with very high doses of nitrates. In all causes of diastolic dysfunction sinus rhythm is often beneficial, although in those with very high LV diastolic pressures, restoration of sinus rhythm can occasionally worsen the situation, with left atrial contraction causing predominantly retrograde flow down the pulmonary veins. Dynamic LV outflow obstruction can often be generated, especially with the use of intropes and diuretics, and this should be treated as detailed above. Theoretically levosimendan may be beneficial, though no robust scientific data support its use in this setting.

Cardiac tamponade

This is an important differential diagnosis in a hypotensive patient with poor peripheral perfusion, particularly as it is a readily reversible condition. The diagnosis is based on clinical features and not echocardiography, although the latter may be helpful in delineating the amount of fluid present, its location and whether it can be drained percutaneously. In particular, echocardiographic signs of tamponade are either absent or unreliable in post-operative patients. In those with a low cardiac output and oliguria, all effusions should be considered for drainage even in the absence of 'classical' features of tamponade.

Case study

A 74-year-old man presented to his local hospital with a 4 day history of intermittent chest pain at rest and progressive exertional dyspnoea. He was a smoker and had a history of hypertension, for which he had been prescribed a thiazide diuretic. On admission, he was clammy and his pulse rate was 115 bpm and blood pressure 120/80 mmHg. His respiratory rate was 25 per minute and SpO_2 on air was 89%. Heart sounds were normal, jugular venous pressure was elevated by 3 cm and auscultation of his chest revealed basal crepitations in both lung fields. The 12-lead ECG showed a sinus tachycardia, with 2–3 mm depression of the ST segments across leads V_2–V_5.

A diagnosis of an acute coronary syndrome was made and he was treated with aspirin, clopidogrel, low-molecular-weight heparin and an intravenous infusion of glyceryl trinitrate. As there was clinical evidence of pulmonary oedema, he was also treated with an intravenous bolus of a loop diuretic and his FiO_2 was increased to 0.60. The SpO_2 increased to 92% but the heart rate increased to 120 bpm, and he passed 20 ml of urine in the following hour. The ST segments remained depressed on serial ECG monitoring. The arterial blood pH was 7.3, base deficit 7 mmol/L, lactate 4 mmol/l, while mixed venous SvO_2 was 50%. Echocardiography showed akinetic antero-apical segments, a hypokinetic inferior wall and an LVEF of 30% with a Doppler-calculated cardiac index of 2.1 l/min/m².

In view of the low mixed venous oxygen saturations, low cardiac index and evidence of tissue hypoperfusion a diagnosis of cardiogenic shock was made. The patient was transferred emergently to the cardiac catheter laboratory, where an IABP was inserted via his left femoral artery. Coronary angiography showed subtotal ostial occlusion of the left anterior descending (LAD) artery, a critical lesion in the mid-dominant right coronary artery (RCA) and diffuse circumflex artery disease. At this point his blood pressure fell to 80/55 mmHg. The LAD was reopened by angioplasty and stenting, following which the blood pressure improved to 100/70 mmHg, with a persistent sinus tachycardia of 110 bpm. Given his haemodynamic state, the non-infarct-related RCA was also treated by PCI, following which his blood pressure increased to 110/80 mmHg and his heart rate decreased to 90 bpm, with resolution of the ST segment changes. During the subsequent 24 hours, his condition improved steadily, with the aid of IABP therapy which was removed 48 hours later.

References

1. Babaev A, Frederick PD, Pasta DJ, et al. Trends in management and outcomes of patients with acute myocardial infarction complicated by cardiogenic shock. *JAMA* 2005;294:448–54.

2. Hochman JS, Boland J, Sleeper LA, et al. Current spectrum of cardiogenic shock and effect of early revascularization on mortality. Results of an International Registry. SHOCK Registry Investigators. *Circulation* 1995;91:873–81.

3. Palmeri ST, Lowe AM, Sleeper LA, et al. Racial and ethnic differences in the treatment and outcome of cardiogenic shock following acute myocardial infarction. *Am J Cardiol* 2005;96:1042–9.

4. Hands ME, Rutherford JD, Muller JE, et al. The in-hospital development of cardiogenic shock after myocardial infarction: incidence, predictors of occurrence, outcome and prognostic factors. The MILIS Study Group. *J Am Coll Cardiol* 1989;14:40–6.

5. Hochman JS, Buller CE, Sleeper LA, et al. Cardiogenic shock complicating acute myocardial infarction – etiologies, management and outcome: a report from the SHOCK Trial Registry. Should We Emergently Revascularize Occluded Coronaries for Cardiogenic Shock? *J Am Coll Cardiol* 2000;36:1063–70.

6. Chen MC, Chang HW, Cheng CI, et al. Risk stratification of in-hospital mortality in patients hospitalized for chronic congestive heart failure secondary to non-ischemic cardiomyopathy. *Cardiology* 2003;100:136–42.

7. Hochman JS, Sleeper LA, Webb JG, et al. Early revascularization in acute myocardial infarction complicated by cardiogenic shock. SHOCK Investigators. Should We Emergently Revascularize Occluded Coronaries for Cardiogenic Shock. *N Engl J Med* 1999;341:625–34.

8. Kohsaka S, Menon V, Lowe AM, et al. Systemic inflammatory response syndrome after acute myocardial infarction complicated by cardiogenic shock. *Arch Intern Med* 2005;165:1643–50.

9. Menon V, Slater JN, White HD, et al. Acute myocardial infarction complicated by systemic hypoperfusion without hypotension: report of the SHOCK Trial Registry. *Am J Med* 2000;108:374–80.

10. Tung RH, Garcia C, Morss AM, et al. Utility of B-type natriuretic peptide for the evaluation of intensive care unit shock. *Crit Care Med* 2004;32:1643–7.

11. Januzzi JL, Morss A, Tung R, et al. Natriuretic peptide testing for the evaluation of critically ill patients with shock in the intensive care unit: a prospective cohort study. *Crit Care* 2006;10:R37.

12. Tennant R and Wiggers CJ. The effect of coronary occlusion on myocardial contraction. *Am J Physiol* 1935;112:351–61.

13. Wyatt HL, Forrester JS, Tyberg JV, et al. Effect of graded reductions in regional coronary perfusion on regional and total cardiac function. *Am J Cardiol* 1975;36:185–92.

14. Weyman AE, Franklin TD, Jr, Hogan RD, et al. Importance of temporal heterogeneity in assessing the contraction abnormalities associated with acute myocardial ischemia. *Circulation* 1984;70:102–12.

15. Koh TW, Pepper JR and Gibson DG. Early changes in left ventricular anterior wall dynamics and coordination after coronary artery surgery. *Heart* 1997;78:291–7.

16. Gianni M, Dentali F, Grandi AM, et al. Apical ballooning syndrome or takotsubo cardiomyopathy: a systematic review. *Eur Heart J* 2006;27: 1523–9.

17. van den Berghe G, Wouters P, Weekers F, et al. Intensive insulin therapy in the critically ill patients. *N Engl J Med* 2001;345:1359–67.

18. Harken DE. The surgical treatment of acquired valvular disease. *Circulation* 1958;18:1–6.

19. Moulopoulos SD, Topaz S and Kolff WJ. Diastolic balloon pumping (with carbon dioxide) in the aorta – a mechanical assistance to the failing circulation. *Am Heart J* 1962;63:669–75.

20. Kantrowitz A, Tjonneland S, Freed PS, et al. Initial clinical experience with intraaortic balloon pumping in cardiogenic shock. *JAMA* 1968;203:113–8.

21. Kern MJ, Aguirre F, Bach R, et al. Augmentation of coronary blood flow by intra-aortic balloon pumping in patients after coronary angioplasty. *Circulation* 1993;87:500–11.

22. Williams DO, Korr KS, Gewirtz H, et al. The effect of intraaortic balloon counterpulsation on regional myocardial blood flow and oxygen consumption in the presence of coronary artery stenosis in patients with unstable angina. *Circulation* 1982;66:593–7.

23. O'Rourke MF, Norris RM, Campbell TJ, et al. Randomized controlled trial of intraaortic balloon counterpulsation in early myocardial infarction with acute heart failure. *Am J Cardiol* 1981;47:815–20.

24. Flaherty JT, Becker LC, Weiss JL, et al. Results of a randomized prospective trial of intraaortic balloon counterpulsation and intravenous nitroglycerin in patients with acute myocardial infarction. *J Am Coll Cardiol* 1985;6: 434–46.

25. Kovack PJ, Rasak MA, Bates ER, et al. Thrombolysis plus aortic counterpulsation: improved survival in patients who present to community hospitals with cardiogenic shock. *J Am Coll Cardiol* 1997;29:1454–8.

26. Holmes DR, Jr, Bates ER, Kleiman NS, et al. Contemporary reperfusion therapy for cardiogenic shock: the GUSTO-I trial experience. The GUSTO-I Investigators. Global Utilization of Streptokinase and Tissue Plasminogen Activator for Occluded Coronary Arteries. *J Am Coll Cardiol* 1995;26:668–74.

27. Sanborn TA, Sleeper LA, Bates ER, et al. Impact of thrombolysis, intra-aortic balloon pump counterpulsation, and their combination in cardiogenic shock complicating acute myocardial infarction: a report from the SHOCK Trial Registry. Should We Emergently Revascularize Occluded Coronaries for Cardiogenic Shock? *J Am Coll Cardiol* 2000;36:1123–9.

28. Barron HV, Every NR, Parsons LS, et al. The use of intra-aortic balloon counterpulsation in patients with cardiogenic shock complicating acute myocardial infarction: data from the National Registry of Myocardial Infarction 2. *Am Heart J* 2001;141:933–9.

29. Ohman EM, Nanas J, Stomel RJ, et al. Thrombolysis and counterpulsation to improve survival in myocardial infarction complicated by hypotension and suspected cardiogenic shock or heart failure: results of the TACTICS Trial. *J Thromb Thrombolysis* 2005;19:33–9.

30. Bates ER and Topol EJ. Limitations of thrombolytic therapy for acute myocardial infarction complicated by congestive heart failure and cardiogenic shock. *J Am Coll Cardiol* 1991;18:1077–84.

31. Kono T, Morita H, Nishina T, et al. Aortic counterpulsation may improve late patency of the occluded coronary artery in patients with early failure of thrombolytic therapy. *J Am Coll Cardiol* 1996;28:876–81.

32. Antman EM, Anbe DT, Armstrong PW, et al. ACC/AHA guidelines for the management of patients with ST-elevation myocardial infarction: a report of the American College of Cardiology/American Heart Association Task Force

on Practice Guidelines (Committee to Revise the 1999 Guidelines for the Management of Patients with Acute Myocardial Infarction). *Circulation* 2004;110:e82–292.

33. Stone GW, Ohman EM, Miller MF, et al. Contemporary utilization and outcomes of intra-aortic balloon counterpulsation in acute myocardial infarction: the benchmark registry. *J Am Coll Cardiol* 2003;41:1940–5.

34. Hochman JS, Sleeper LA, Webb JG, et al. Early revascularization and long-term survival in cardiogenic shock complicating acute myocardial infarction. *JAMA* 2006;295:2511–5.

35. Dzavik V, Sleeper LA, Cocke TP, et al. Early revascularization is associated with improved survival in elderly patients with acute myocardial infarction complicated by cardiogenic shock: a report from the SHOCK Trial Registry. *Eur Heart J* 2003;24:828–37.

36. White HD, Assmann SF, Sanborn TA, et al. Comparison of percutaneous coronary intervention and coronary artery bypass grafting after acute myocardial infarction complicated by cardiogenic shock: results from the Should We Emergently Revascularize Occluded Coronaries for Cardiogenic Shock? (SHOCK) Trial. *Circulation* 2005;112:1992–2001.

37. Chan AW, Chew DP, Bhatt DL, et al. Long-term mortality benefit with the combination of stents and abciximab for cardiogenic shock complicating acute myocardial infarction. *Am J Cardiol* 2002;89:132–6.

38. Beyersdorf F, Acar C, Buckberg GD, et al. Studies on prolonged acute regional ischemia. III. Early natural history of simulated single and multivessel disease with emphasis on remote myocardium. *J Thorac Cardiovasc Surg* 1989;98:368–80.

39. Okuda M. A multidisciplinary overview of cardiogenic shock. *Shock* 2006;25:557–70.

40. Hochman JS. Cardiogenic shock complicating acute myocardial infarction: expanding the paradigm. *Circulation* 2003;107:2998–3002.

41. Montalescot G, Barragan P, Wittenberg O, et al. Platelet glycoprotein IIb/IIIa inhibition with coronary stenting for acute myocardial infarction. *N Engl J Med* 2001;344:1895–903.

42. Stone GW, Grines CL, Cox DA, et al. Comparison of angioplasty with stenting, with or without abciximab, in acute myocardial infarction. *N Engl J Med* 2002;346:957–66.

43. Hasdai D, Harrington RA, Hochman JS, et al. Platelet glycoprotein IIb/IIIa blockade and outcome of cardiogenic shock complicating acute coronary syndromes without persistent ST-segment elevation. *J Am Coll Cardiol* 2000;36:685–92.

44. Huang R, Sacks J, Thai H, et al. Impact of stents and abciximab on survival from cardiogenic shock treated with percutaneous coronary intervention. *Catheter Cardiovasc Interv* 2005;65:25–33.

45. Moiseyev VS, Poder P, Andrejevs N, et al. Safety and efficacy of a novel calcium sensitizer, levosimendan, in patients with left ventricular failure due to an acute myocardial infarction. A randomized, placebo-controlled, double-blind study (RUSSLAN). *Eur Heart J* 2002;23:1422–32.

46. Mebazaa A, Nieminen MS, Packer M, et al. Levosimendan vs dobutamine for patients with acute decompensated heart failure: the SURVIVE Randomized Trial. *JAMA* 2007;297:1883–91.

47. Peter JV, Moran JL, Phillips-Hughes J, et al. Effect of non-invasive positive pressure ventilation (NIPPV) on mortality in patients with acute cardiogenic pulmonary oedema: a meta-analysis. *Lancet* 2006;367:1155–63.

48. Guo H, Hahn D and Olshansky B. Temporary biventricular pacing in a patient with subacute myocardial infarction, cardiogenic shock, and third-degree atrioventricular block. *Heart Rhythm* 2005;2:112.

49. Meyns B, Stolinski J, Leunens V, et al. Left ventricular support by catheter-mounted axial flow pump reduces infarct size. *J Am Coll Cardiol* 2003;41:1087–95.

15 Peri-operative Care of the Heart Transplant Recipient

Keith McNeil[1] and John Dunning[2]
[1]The Prince Charles Hospital, Brisbane, Australia
[2]Papworth Hospital, Cambridge, UK

Take Home Messages

- Heart transplantation usually occurs in the context of complex medical and surgical co-morbidities, which impact significantly in the post-transplant period.
- Early post-transplant haemodynamic instability is predominantly related to right ventricular (RV) dysfunction, and cardiac support algorithms must take this into consideration.
- Afterload reduction is key to effective support of a failing RV.
- Cardiac dysrhythmia or haemodynamic instability occurring after 72 hours post transplant must prompt active exclusion of acute cell mediated allograft rejection.
- Pericardial tamponade should be considered in all cases of early post-transplant haemodynamic instability and cardiac dysfunction.

15.1 Introduction

The peri-operative management of heart transplant recipients presents a formidable challenge to critical care and transplant physicians. A complex array of medical and surgical issues is presented in the context of a patient with significant co-morbidities, undergoing a major surgical procedure involving the implantation of a vital organ, damaged from the outset by the effects of brainstem death and ischaemia. The improvements in survival following heart transplantation seen in more recent years have resulted predominantly from improved outcomes in the early post-transplant period (Figure 15.1) [1], highlighting the critical importance of the peri-operative care of these patients.

The intensive care phase of managing these patients commences with optimal care of the donor, and continues in the operating theatre, through

---

Cardiovascular Critical Care. Edited by M. Griffiths, J. Cordingley and S. Price.
© 2010 Blackwell Publishing Ltd.

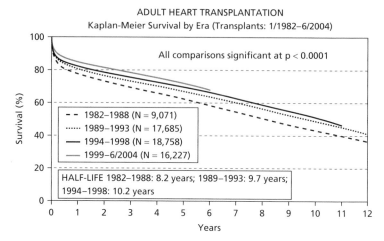

ADULT HEART TRANSPLANTATION
Kaplan-Meier Survival by Era (Transplants: 1/1982–6/2004)

Figure 15.1 Analysis of survival following heart transplantation by era. Note improvement in early outcomes in modern eras with stable attrition rate after 3 months.

to the intensive therapy/treatment unit (ITU) proper. The principles of care relating to any ITU patient apply equally to a cardiac transplant recipient; however, there are a number of specific transplant-related issues which will form the basis of the ensuing discussion.

15.2 General principles

In the immediate post-operative period, heart transplant recipients often have residual pulmonary oedema with a concomitant increase in the risk of post-operative pneumonia. In combination with adequate analgesia, patients should therefore be extubated and mobilised early to facilitate effective sputum clearance and to prevent atelectasis.

Patients should be rewarmed as soon as possible, but hyperthermia should be avoided. This hastens the resolution of lactic acidosis and aids in correction of coagulopathy. Coagulopathy occurs as a consequence of cardio-pulmonary bypass (increased fibrinolysis, platelet dysfunction and heparin) and pre-operative warfarin therapy. Blood products, vitamin K and protamine should be used as indicated by bleeding and coagulation tests. Anti-fibrinolytic agents (e.g. aprotinin) are widely used intra- and post-operatively in these patients. If significant bleeding continues after rewarming and correction of coagulopathy, re-exploration should be performed. Activated factor VII has been effective in helping to stop otherwise uncontrollable non-surgical bleeding [2].

Cardiac dysrhythmias are common after transplantation. The transplanted heart is denervated, and temporary pacing (typically sequential – dual chamber pacing, sensing and response (DDD) at 90–110 min^{-1} for the first 48–72 hours) or isoprenaline is frequently required for bradyarrhythmias associated with sinus node dysfunction and/or atrioventricular dissociation. The incidence of these conduction abnormalities is related to the ischaemic time and the surgical technique used for implantation, with a lower incidence reported for the bicaval anastamosis [3]. Any dysrhythmia should prompt investigation and correction of electrolyte disturbances (hypokalaemia and hypomagnesaemia are common post transplant). The onset of sustained atrial fibrillation or flutter beyond the first 72 hours should trigger investigation for acute rejection. Atrial tachyarrhythmias are treated with either amiodarone and/or electrical cardioversion. Digoxin and atropine are ineffective because of the autonomic denervation in these patients. Ventricular dysrhythmias are uncommon. Electrolyte abnormalities should be corrected and treatment should follow standard protocols.

15.3 Haemodynamic management

Cardiac dysfunction early post transplant ranges from mild right ventricular (RV) impairment through to severe biventricular failure, termed 'primary allograft failure'. 'Graft failure' accounts for 40% of deaths within 30 days of transplant [1]. It also plays a significant role in the other major reported causes of 30-day mortality – multi-organ failure (14%) and non-cytomegalovirus (CMV) infection (13%) [1].

Cardiac dysfunction after heart transplantation is multifactorial. Impaired RV contractility is a direct consequence of brainstem death in the donor [4] and the ischaemia-reperfusion injury that occurs during organ retrieval and preservation [5]. Pericardial tamponade must be actively excluded in all cases of post-transplant cardiac dysfunction. Other causes include the injudicious use of inotrope and pressor agents and, rarely, hyperacute (antibody-mediated) rejection (see below).

Patients with long-standing heart failure have co-morbidities which complicate the treatment of post-transplant RV dysfunction. Low systemic vascular resistance (SVR) as a consequence of ACE inhibitor therapy compromises systemic blood pressure and therefore coronary perfusion pressure post-operatively. Pulmonary vascular resistance (PVR) is increased in heart failure patients as a consequence of long-standing raised left atrial pressure (LAP), which may further compromise RV performance and cardiac output. Many patients with long-standing heart failure have co-existing renal impairment, resulting in volume overload. Thus, in the early post-transplant period, heart transplant recipients may present the complex clinical scenario of a low SVR coupled with acute RV dysfunction secondary to the combination of decreased contractility, suboptimal preload and increased afterload (PVR). The principles of managing these patients are therefore to optimise these factors.

Optimising right ventricular function

The above scenario has implications for the choice of management strategies initially used to wean patients from cardio-pulmonary bypass, and subsequently applied in the ITU. This situation is not analogous to supporting a patient where left ventricular (LV) dysfunction dominates the clinical picture. Indeed, the algorithms used to support the LV are different (and may be deleterious) to those used for optimal support of the RV, which has a very different physiology [6–8].

The RV functions in a low-resistance circuit and has a limited capacity to increase stroke volume. The RV thus relies on increased heart rate to augment cardiac output in the short term, and maintenance of sinus or a paced atrial rhythm at a rate of around 110 beats per minute is required for optimal RV performance in this setting. Equally, atrial tachyarrhythmias are poorly tolerated as RV filling (and therefore Starling haemodynamics and contractility) is impaired in this situation.

RV function is exquisitely sensitive to changes in afterload. It is therefore important when choosing inotropes not to increase the PVR. Traditionally, dopamine has been the inotrope of choice, in combination with isoprenaline, which itself has a modest pulmonary vasodilating and positive chronotropic effect [9]. In a 'straightforward' heart transplant where only mild RV dysfunction is present, this combination, with appropriate fluid management, will allow the RV to recover whilst maintaining an adequate cardiac output. Dobutamine, which has minimal alpha agonist activity, can be used as an alternative to dopamine; however, this agent may result in inappropriate tachycardia or atrial dysrhythmia, and can lower SVR, particularly if used in combination with isoprenaline.

In situations where RV dysfunction is more significant, treatment becomes much more complex. Achievement of optimal Starling effects may actually require volume loading (analogous to the treatment of RV infarction). Optimal RV filling can be assessed either by direct visualisation of the RV at surgery or via transoesophageal echocardiography. Once filling has been optimised, an intra-aortic balloon pump should be considered. This will improve proximal aortic pressure and coronary perfusion, potentially allowing for reduction of vasopressors, which may contribute to an increase in the PVR [6, 7, 9].

The choice of pharmacologic circulatory support in the setting of RV failure is based on knowledge of the RV pathophysiology outlined above. Adrenaline and noradrenaline increase PVR, and although seemingly effective at maintaining blood pressure, in this context they are usually counterproductive in the longer term, with requirements for escalating doses in the face of increasing RV dysfunction related to the increased PVR. In addition, lactic acidosis after cardiac transplantation, which reduces myocardial performance in its own right, has been shown to correlate with the use of these agents [10]. Adrenaline has also been shown in animal models and an isolated human myocardium model [11] to significantly reduce myocardial contractility, and catecholamine injury has been identified as one of the major factors causing reduced myocardial contractility in brainstem death [4]. Inotropic agents that do not increase and may lower PVR include the phosphodiesterase (PDE) 3 inhibitors (milrinone [12] and enoximone [13]) and levosimendin [14, 15]. PDE 3 inhibitors exert their pharmacologic action via cAMP, resulting in both a positive inotropic effect and (vascular) smooth muscle relaxation. Unlike catecholamines, PDE 3 inhibitors do not increase myocardial oxygen demand, possibly as a result of reduced afterload [9, 12]. The smooth muscle relaxing effects of PDE 3 inhibition are not selective for the pulmonary circulation, however, and thus low SVR may result from the use of these agents, particularly where co-existing renal dysfunction leads to impaired drug clearance. Levosimendan, a calcium sensitising agent, appears to reduce PVR and increase myocardial contractility without increasing myocardial oxygen demand [7, 16, 17]. Experience with this class of drugs is limited, but their mode of action makes them theoretically attractive for use in RV failure [7].

Tri-iodothyronine (T_3) has acute inotropic effects [18, 19], and is used in the active management of the brainstem dead donor [20, 21]. The biologically active forms of thyroid hormone are decreased by brainstem death and cardiopulmonary bypass [22, 23], and T3 improves immediate post-transplant myocardial contractility [11, 24]. In the authors' experience, T_3 has proven a valuable adjunct to therapy for severe post-transplant RV dysfunction. Similarly, post-transplant myocardial function may be enhanced by insulin therapy, which protects cardiomyocytes from re-oxygenation-induced hypercontracture, a hallmark of acute reperfusion injury. This protective mechanism is independent of metabolic modulation, and works via a so-called survival pathway, which involves activation of a variety of enzyme systems with enhanced calcium sequestration into the sarcoplasmic reticulum [25, 26].

A pressor agent may be necessary to maintain systemic blood pressure. If allograft function is acceptable, small doses of noradrenaline are effective and well tolerated. Noradrenaline, however, is a potent pulmonary vasoconstrictor and will inevitably increase RV afterload; thus its use in association with significant RV dysfunction must be considered carefully. An alternative or adjunct to noradrenaline (allowing dose reduction) is arginine vasopressin (AVP). AVP is used in the management of the cardiac donor both for its antidiuretic and systemic vasoconstrictor effects [20, 21]. AVP is effective in cardiac arrest, and in a variety of advanced shock states including vasodilatory shock post-cardiac surgery and peri-operative hypotension secondary to ACE inhibitor therapy [27]. In the authors' experience, AVP displays little (if any) pulmonary vasoconstrictor activity, and for this reason it is the preferred agent for maintaining systemic vascular tone in the setting of RV dysfunction of any cause.

Pericardial tamponade

Pericardial tamponade should be actively excluded in any case of early cardiac allograft dysfunction. Initial signs of tamponade include reduced peripheral perfusion, decreasing urine output and progressive hypoxaemia. These signs may present before signs of overt haemodynamic compromise manifest. If clinical deterioration occurs, or where progressive post-operative improvement does not occur, echocardiography should be performed. Any pericardial fluid collection visualised in these circumstances should be considered for drainage, regardless of whether or not traditional echocardiographic signs of tamponade are present.

In particular, small pericardial collections localised over the right or left atrium can limit atrial filling and lead to significant haemodynamic compromise.

Pulmonary vasodilators

Afterload reduction is the most effective treatment of RV dysfunction. The agents are those employed in the treatment of pulmonary arterial hypertension, and include inhaled nitric oxide (NO), intravenous or inhaled prostacyclin and oral sildenafil. NO has the advantage of not only lowering PVR but also (by virtue of the inhaled route) optimising ventilation/perfusion matching [6, 7]. Intravenous prostacyclin (epoprostenol) is a powerful pulmonary vasodilator, but also causes significant systemic vasodilatation, and as such may be associated with systemic hypotension [6]. Additionally, as prostacyclin is delivered intravenously, it can worsen ventilation:perfusion matching [28]. Sildenafil, a PDE 5 inhibitor, works by augmenting the activity of cGMP (the pathway by which NO exerts its vasodilatory action) and has been shown to be effective in treating PAH [29]. No formal trials of any of these agents have been performed in cardiac transplantation, but all have been used to support the RV in the early post-operative period.

Mechanical assist devices

In situations where severe refractory cardiac dysfunction occurs, short-term mechanical support should be considered to provide adequate support whilst allowing sufficient time for the transplanted heart to recover (see Chapter 8). Devices designed for longer-term placement are not generally used in this situation because if recovery does not occur in the short term, the prognosis is poor. Furthermore, re-transplantation in the setting of primary graft failure is generally associated with poor outcomes.

Difficulty weaning from CPB should prompt early insertion of an intra-aortic balloon pump. Extra-corporeal membrane oxygenation (ECMO) has the added advantage of allowing reduction in mechanical ventilatory support which has positive benefits in terms of reducing the PVR and improving diastolic right heart filling [30]. Short-term mechanical assist devices such as the Abiomed® have been employed as a bridge to recovery in this setting. There are no hard and fast rules as to when mechanical assistance should be used. As a general rule, however, once it is obvious that conventional pharmacological support is ineffective, mechanical support should be considered early before either the RV is irreparably damaged or other organ failure ensues.

15.4 Immunosuppression after heart transplantation

A detailed discussion of transplant immunology and individual immunosuppressive agents is outside the scope of this chapter. The reader is referred to one of the excellent review articles for more detail [31, 32].

Acute, cell-mediated rejection is not likely to be encountered in the ITU as it rarely occurs within the first week unless the immunosuppressive protocol has been compromised; however, it should always be considered in any case of unexplained haemodynamic instability. Hyperacute, antibody-mediated rejection occurs directly following reperfusion and is a rare cause of primary allograft failure. It is caused by circulating pre-formed (anti-HLA) antibodies, which activate complement leading to rapid destruction of the allograft. Pre-operative immunological screening and prospective cross-matching are used to prevent this fatal complication. Treatments with high-dose intravenous immunoglobulin, plasma exchange and anti-B cell therapies such as cyclophosphamide or rituximab have been applied with variable results.

Standard immunosuppressive therapy is started pre-operatively and continued throughout the peri-operative period (Table 15.1). The aim of immunosuppression in the ITU setting is to minimise T-cell alloreactivity. This is achieved with a combination of complementary strategies involving T-cell depletion, blocking of T-cell proliferation signals and inhibition of T-cell proliferation via inhibition of DNA synthesis. Typically, a combination of a calcineurin inhibitor (CNI), either cyclosporine or tacrolimus, mycophenolate and predinisolone is used initially. Currently there are trials assessing the role and efficacy of mTOR (mammalian target of rapamycin) inhibitors (sirolimus and everolimus) as adjuncts to or replacements for the traditional agents.

The major early side-effects of immunosuppression are renal dysfunction associated with CNI therapy, and an increased risk of infection. The anti-IL-2 receptor blocking monoclonal antibodies (dacluzimab and basiliximab) are being used increasingly in induction protocols to minimise

Table 15.1 Typical immunosuppression regimen (no induction).

Timing	Drug	Dose
Acceptance of organs	Mycophenolate	3 g orally
Induction of anaesthesia	Methylprednisolone	500 mg IV infusion over 30 minutes
Reperfusion	Methylprednisolone	500 mg IV infusion over 30 minutes
Immediate post-op period	Methylprednisolone	125 mg IV bolus, 3 doses given 8, 16 and 24 hours post-op.
Maintenance therapy		
	Prednisolone	1 mg/kg/day in 2 divided doses, reducing by 5 mg/day to 0.2 mg/kg/day
	Mycophenolate	3 g/day in 2 divided doses. Maintain WCC $\geq 4 \times 10^9$/l
	Cyclosporin (Neoral®)	Commence 50 mg, increase 50 mg per dose to total 10 mg/kg/day in two divided doses. Aim for cyclosporin level of ≥ 350 ng/l (EMIT assay) by day 7 depending on kidney function (some units now dose based on C_2 levels)

early exposure to CNIs; however, formal trials of this strategy are currently lacking. It is important to administer this antibody therapy after bleeding has been controlled, unlike the practice in renal transplantation where it is administered pre-operatively.

15.5 Anti-infective therapy

Prophylactic antibiotics are started pre-operatively, aiming to cover *Staphylococcus* and community acquired respiratory pathogens. A combination of vancomycin and a third-generation cephalosporin (such as ceftriaxone) is typically employed. Antibiotics are generally continued until methicillin-resistant *Staphylococcus aureus* (MRSA) and other cultures are negative, drains have been removed and the patient is mobile. Anti-viral (CMV and herpes viruses) and antifungal prophylaxis is usually commenced on day 1 or 2, as per unit protocols.

15.6 Conclusion

The peri-operative period is a critical phase for every heart transplant recipient, as it is complicated by complex pathophysiology revolving predominantly around RV dysfunction. Optimal care of the donor is the first step in optimising the function of the cardiac allograft. A sound knowledge of the principles outlined above is essential for a satisfactory outcome, and in particular recognition that the algorithms used are subtly different from those employed in the conventional support and management of post-cardiotomy LV dysfunction.

Case study

A 48-year-old female with a 25 pack year smoking history presented in cardiogenic shock following a large anterior myocardial infarct. Percutaneous revascularisation was successful in restoring flow, but there was no subsequent improvement in myocardial function. She was managed initially with conventional inotrope and pressor support with the addition of an intra-aortic balloon pump (IABP). Despite this therapy, progressive renal and respiratory dysfunction ensued, requiring haemofiltration and ventilatory support.

She was assessed and listed for urgent heart transplantation, but given that she was a small blood group O, implying a long wait on the transplant waiting list, she progressed to insertion of a left ventricular assist device (LVAD: extracorporeal Thoratec™) 72 hours after her initial presentation. The procedure was relatively uncomplicated but did require two returns to theatre for bleeding. Following restoration of

Continued

haemodynamic stability there was progressive improvement in her renal and respiratory function.

She remained stable over the next 3 months on the LVAD, beta blocker therapy and anti-coagulation (warfarin). Approximately 3 months after insertion of the LVAD a donor heart became available from a 55-year-old female ex-smoker suffering a subarachnoid haemorrhage. No hormonal resuscitation was applied to the donor and the ischaemic time was predicted to be 5 hours.

The explant procedure was predictably difficult, with multiple adhesions leading to significant bleeding. The total ischaemic time was slightly more than 6 hours and the heart limped off bypass with significant inotrope (adrenaline) and pressor (noradrenaline) support, and an IABP. Echocardiographic assessment of the transplanted heart revealed severe right ventricular dysfunction with only mildly abnormal left ventricular dysfunction. No pericardial collection was identified. Pulmonary vascular resistance was 180 dynes/sec/cm^5. Following transfer back to the intensive care unit (ICU), pharmacological support was changed with commencement of dopamine, milrinone and vasopressin, with weaning of the adrenaline and noradrenaline. Atrial pacing was employed at 110 beats per minute. IABP support was continued and inhaled nitric oxide was commenced. Bolus followed by a 6 hour infusion of T3 was administered, along with usual supportive therapy.

There was gradual improvement over the ensuing 48 hours. Nitric oxide was weaned on day 3 post transplantation, enabling extubation. Renal function recovered and inotropic support was reduced to low-dose dopamine (5 μg/kg/minute). Oral sildenafil (25 mg TDS) was commenced following discontinuation of the inhaled nitric oxide. Immunosuppression consisted of basiliximab (monoclonal antibody that prevents T cell proliferation), two doses 4 days apart, with the first dose given on day 2 following control of bleeding. Standard doses of methyl prednisolone and mycophenolate were administered, but cyclosporine was withheld until day 6 following improvement in renal function, aiming for a trough level of between 150 and 200 μg/L by day 8.

The patient was discharged from the ICU to the ward on day 8 post transplant with ongoing moderate but haemodynamically stable right ventricular dysfunction, which would be expected to continue to improve over the following 6–12 weeks.

This case demonstrates the typical problems in the modern era of cardiac transplantation, that is patients with increasing levels of morbidity presenting for transplantation with the immediate post-transplant course being dominated by right ventricular dysfunction. In these situations it is necessary to tailor immunosuppressive requirements to the specific clinical situation, taking into account post-operative bleeding, renal dysfunction and control of the alloimmune response.

References

1. Taylor DO, Edwards LB, Boucek MM, et al. Registry of the International Society for Heart and Lung Transplantation: Twenty-third Official Adult Heart Transplantation Report – 2006. *J Heart Lung Transplant* 2006; 25: 869–79.

2. Walsham J, Fraser JF, Mullany D, et al. The use of recombinant activated factor VII for refractory bleeding post complex cardiothoracic surgery. *Anaes Intensive Care* 2006; 34(1): 13–20.

3. Scott C, Dark JH, McComb JM. Arrhythmias after acrdiac transplantation. *Am J Cardiol* 1992; 70: 1061–3.

4. Smith M. Physiologic changes during brain stem death – lessons for management of the organ donor. *J Heart Lung Transplant* 2004; 23: S217–22.

5. Renner A, Sagstetter MR, Götz ME, et al. Heterotopic rat heart transplantation: severe loss of glutathione in 8-hour ischaemic hearts. *J Heart Lung Transplant* 2004; 23: 1093–102.

6. McNeil K, Dunning J, Morrell NW. The pulmonary physician in critical care (13): the pulmonary circulation and right ventricular failure in the ITU. *Thorax* 2003; 58: 157–62.

7. Piazza G, Goldhaber SZ. The acutely decompensated right ventricle. pathways for diagnosis and management. *Chest* 2005; 128: 1836–52.

8. Voelkel NF, Quaife RA, Leinwand LA, et al. Right ventricular function and failure: report of a National Heart, Lung and Blood Institute working group on cellular and molecular mechanisms of right heart failure. *Circulation* 2006; 114(17): 1883–91.

9. Stobierska-Dzierzek B, Awad H, Michler RE. The evolving management of acute right-sided heart failure in cardiac transplant recipients. *J Am Coll Cardiol* 2001; 38: 923–31.

10. Mohacsi P, Pedrazzinia G, Tanner H, et al. Lactic acidosis following heart transplantation: a common phenomenon? *Eur J Heart Failure* 2002; 4(2): 175–9.

11. Timek T, Bonz A, Dillmann R, et al. The effect of triiodothyronine on myocardial contractile performance after epinephrine exposure: implications for donor heart management. *J Heart Lung Transplant* 1998; 17(9): 931–40.

12. Levy HJ, Bailey JM, Deeb GM. Intravenous milrinone in cardiac surgery. *Ann Thorac Surg* 2002; 73: 325–30.

13. Bauer J, Dapper F, Demirakca S, et al. Perioperative management of pulmonary hypertension after heart transplantation in childhood. *J Heart Lung Transplant* 1997; 16: 1238–47.

14. Petaja LM, Sipponen JT, Hammainen PJ, et al. Levosimendan reversing low output syndrome after heart transplantation. *Ann Thorac Surg* 2006; 82(4): 1529–31.

15. Raja SG, Rayen BS. Levosimendan in cardiac surgery: current best available evidence. *Ann Thorac Surg* 2006; 81(4): 1536–46.

16. Mebazza A, Karpati P, Renaud E, et al. Acute right ventricular failure: from pathophysiology to new treatments. *Intensive Care Med* 2004; 30: 185–96.

17. Slawsky MT, Colucci WS, Gottlieb SS, et al. Acute hemodynamic and clinical effects of levosimendan in patients with severe heart failure: study investigators. *Circulation* 2000; 102: 2222–7.

18. Holland FW II, Brown PS Jr, Clark RE. Acute severe postischemic myocardial depression reversed by triiodothyronine. *Ann Thorac Surg* 1992; 52: 301–5.

19. Klemperer JD, Zelano J, Helm RE, et al. Triiodothyronine improves left ventricular function without oxygen wasting effects after global hypothermic ischaemia. *J Thorac Cardiovasc Surg* 1995; 109: 457–65.

20. Ullah S, Zabala L, Watkins B, et al. Cardiac organ donor management. *Perfusion* 2006; 21(2): 93–8.

21. Rosendale JD, Kauffman HM, McBride MA, et al. Hormonal resuscitation yields more transplanted hearts, with improved early function. *Transplantation* 2003; 75(8): 1336–41.

22. Klemperer JD, Klein I, Gomez M, et al. Thyroid hormone treatment after coronary-artery bypass surgery. *N Engl J Med* 1995; 333: 1522–7.

23. Bennett-Guerrero E, Kramer DC, Schwinn DA. Effect of chronic and acute thyroid hormone reduction on perioperative outcome. *Anesth Analg* 1997; 85: 30–6.

24. Novitzky D, Cooper DK, Chaffin JS, et al. Improved cardiac allograft function following triiodothyronine therapy to both donor and recipient. *Transplantation* 1990; 49: 311–16.

25. Yellon DM, Sack MN. Insulin therapy as an adjunct to reperfusion after acute coronary ischaemia: a proposed direct myocardial cell survival effect independent of metabolic modulation. *JACC* 2003; 41(8): 1404–7.

26. Abdallah Y, Gkatzoflia A, Gligorievski D, et al. Insulin protects cardiomyocytes against reoxygenation-induced hypercontracture by a survival pathway targeting SR Ca^{2+} storage. *Cardiovasc Res* 2006; 70(2): 346–53.

27. Jochberger S, Wenzel V, Dunser MW. Arginine vasopression as a rescue vasopressor agent in the operating room. *Curr Opin Anaesthesiol* 2005; 18: 396–404.

28. Otulana B, Higgenbottam T. The role of physiological dead space and shunting the gas exchange of patients with pulmonary hypertension: a study of exercise and prostacyclin infusion. *Eur Resp J* 1988; 1: 732–7.

29. Galie N, Ghofrani HA, Torbicki A, et al. Sildenafil use in pulmonary arterial hypertension (SUPER) study group. Sildenafil citrate therapy for pulmonary arterial hypertension. *NEJM* 2005; 353(20): 2148–57.

30. Jardin F, Vieillard-Baron A. Right ventricular function and positive pressure ventilation in clinical practice: from hemodynamic subsets to respirator settings. *Intensive Care Med* 2003; 29; 1426–34.

31. Taylor DO. Cardiac transplantation: drug regimens for the 21st century. *Annal Thoracic Surg* 2003; 75(6 Suppl): S72–8.

32. Hopkins PMA. (2006) Pharmacological manipulation of the rejection response. In: Hornick P, Rose M, eds. *Methods in Molecular Biology, vol. 333: Transplantation Immunology: Methods and Protocols.* Humana Press.

16 Adult Congenital Heart Disease Syndromes

Antonia Pijuan Domènech[1,2], Katerina Chamaidi[1,3] and Michael A. Gatzoulis[1,4]

[1]Adult Congenital Heart Centre and Centre for Pulmonary Hypertension, Royal Brompton & Harefield NHS Foundation Trust, London, UK
[2]Adult Congenital Heart Disease Unit, Hospital Vall d´Hebron, Barcelona, Spain
[3]General Hospital of Trikala, Greece
[4]National Heart & Lung Institute, Imperial College, London, UK

Take Home Messages

- There are few data regarding the evaluation of pre-operative risk factors in adult patients with congenital heart disease (ACHD).
- Physicians in charge of the post-operative management of ACHD patients must be familiar with the specific conditions and associated haemodynamics.
- A knowledge of any previous interventions is essential.
- Although data exist regarding primary repair of CHD in infancy and its peri-operative complications, these data cannot be extrapolated to the adult CHD population.

16.1 Introduction

Advances in paediatric cardiology and cardiac surgery have enabled more than 85% of patients with congenital heart disease (CHD) to survive into adulthood [1]. Despite the impact of interventional cardiology, the total number of surgical procedures for patients with CHD has been maintained, if not increased, in the past decade. The majority of the lesions, including the complex ones, can be repaired in infancy, but residual sequelae are considerable [2]. The complexity of the surgery in adults with CHD has increased, particularly with redo operations [3]. Although some similarities with surgery for acquired heart disease do exist, there are several significant factors to take into account regarding the operative risk assessment and the post-operative course of adults with CHD [4].

The objective of this chapter is to discuss the most frequent indications for surgical intervention in adult patients with CHD, and the pre-operative factors that may influence their post-operative course. Aortic and mitral

---

Cardiovascular Critical Care. Edited by M. Griffiths, J. Cordingley and S. Price.
© 2010 Blackwell Publishing Ltd.

valve replacement and surgery for the ascending or descending aorta are not discussed there as they are included in other chapters.

16.2 Pre-operative risk assessment

Despite the relative youth of the adult congenital heart disease (ACHD) population undergoing cardiac surgery, co-morbidity and other organ involvement are common [4]. However, post-operative mortality is relatively low, but varies with complexity of the underlying disease [4]. A retrospective study that analysed all patients with ACHD that were admitted to the adult intensive care unit (ICU) of Royal Brompton Hospital over a 5-year period showed a total ICU mortality of 4.4% [4]. The 32% of patients classified as having simple ACHD (Canadian Consensus Conference definition, Appendix 1) had APACHE II scores of 18.4, zero mortality, a short ICU stay (1.8 ± 2 days) and a low rate of ICU therapeutic interventions. Patients with complex ACHD (68%), however, had similar APACHE II scores but a significantly higher ICU mortality (10.6%), and a relatively prolonged ICU stay. In the patients undergoing cardiac surgery, retrospective analysis of risk factors using the logistic EuroSCORE demonstrated that this overestimates the risk in patients with simple lesions and underestimates the risk in complex lesions. The predictors of mortality and length of hospital stay from this study are shown in Table 16.1.

Although there are few data regarding the pre-operative risk assessment of adult patients with CHD, there are several factors that merit specific consideration. The more commonly performed surgical procedures are shown in Table 16.2.

Redo-sternotomy

Prior to undertaking re-sternotomy it is necessary to establish the relationship of great vessels, conduit or right ventricle to the inner surface of the sternum. Although historically a lateral chest X-ray (CXR) was performed, cardiac magnetic resonance (CMR) is now regarded as the imaging modality of choice. In some cases a clear space can be seen between the sternum and the

Table 16.1 Predictors of mortality and morbidity in ACHD patients undergoing cardiac surgery.

Predictors of ICU and hospital mortality
Pre-operative abnormal thyroid function
Pre-operative elevated plasma creatinine levels
Pre-operative elevated plasma bilirubin levels
Predictors of ICU and hospital length of stay
Complexity of underlying cardiac disease
History of cardiac arrhythmia
Previous need for emergency admission
Pre-operative abnormal thyroid function
Pre-operative elevated plasma bilirubin levels

Table 16.2 Surgical procedures in adults with congenital heart disease.

Blalock–Taussig: palliative procedure that involves the creation of an anastomosis between a subclavian artery and the ipsilateral pulmonary artery

Waterston: palliative procedure that involves connection between the ascending aorta and the right pulmonary artery

Pulmonary artery banding: surgically created stenosis of the main pulmonary artery performed as a palliative procedure to protect the lungs against high blood flow and pressure when a definite surgical correction is not immediately advisable, for example in the setting of non-restrictive ventricular septal defect

Mustard and Senning operations: surgical palliation for TGA in the past consisted in atrial switch where the venous return is redirected to the contralateral ventricle, allowing the relief of extreme cyanosis, but implying that the RV will be systemic

Rastelli: surgical correction for TGA with VSD that includes re-direction of the LV to aorta, closure of the VSD and connection of the RV to the PA.

Arterial switch: corrective surgery for TGA that includes reattachment of great arteries to the contralateral ventricles and coronary artery reimplantation, resulting in the left ventricle supporting the systemic circulation

Fontan procedure: a palliative operation for patients with a univentricular circulation, involving diversion of the systemic venous return to the pulmonary artery without the interposition of a subpulmonary ventricle. A classic Fontan includes placement of a valved conduit between the right atrium and the pulmonary artery

Total cavopulmonary connection: the IVC flow is directed by a baffle within the right atrium into the lower portion of the divided SVC which is connected to the pulmonary artery. The upper part of the SVC is connected to the superior aspect of the pulmonary artery as in the bidirectional Glenn procedure

TGA, Transposition of the great arteries; RV, right ventricle; IVC, inferior vena cava; SVC, superior vena cava; VSD, ventricular septal defect; LV, left ventrical; PA, pulmonary artery.

heart. Conversely there may be either no discernible space or distortion or erosion of the sternum, particularly by a dilated right ventricle or an extra-cardiac conduit. Of additional concern is the presence retrosternally of a thin-walled right ventricular aneurysm or dilated ascending aorta.

Conduit replacement

In several conditions in which repair of right ventricular outflow tract obstruction is not possible, a conduit between the sub-pulmonary ventricle and the pulmonary arteries is required (see Table 16.3) [5]. The requirement for repeat surgery 20 years after the initial operation is high, and it may not be possible to avoid damaging the conduit on re-opening the chest [6, 7].

Table 16.3 Conditions in which conduit replacement may be required.

TOF with intramural coronary artery
Pulmonary atresia with VSD
Double outlet RV (Rastelli procedure)
TGA with large VSD (Rastelli procedure)

TOF, Tetralogy of Fallot; VSD, ventricular septal defect; RV, right ventricle; TGA, transposition of the great arteries.

Arrhythmia-targeting surgery

CHD that causes right heart dilatation is commonly associated with atrial flutter or fibrillation, and intra-atrial re-entry tachycardia. A concomitant right atrial Maze procedure is performed in many centres in patients undergoing right-sided surgery [8]. Although the Maze procedure may restore sinus rhythm, complications such as junctional rhythm that may require temporary pacing and a tendency to fluid retention due to atrial appendage removal and decrease in natriuretic peptide release may occur. These are more common if left-sided atrial intervention is added.

Cyanosis

Long-standing cyanosis carries specific additional risks to patients undergoing surgery. These include: intrinsic haemostatic and haematologic abnormalities, congenital and/or acquired collateral vessels, renal dysfunction and an increased risk of intra-operative myocardial injury.

16.3 Simple congenital heart disease

Coarctation of the aorta

Native coarctation of the aorta has a biphasic clinical presentation. It may present as an arterial patent ductus dependent lesion, where cardiac output is maintained primarily by flow through a patent ductus arteriosus, in infancy or later in childhood or adult life (Figures 16.1a and b). If left untreated, 90% of patients do not survive beyond the age of 50 due to cardiovascular or cerebrovascular complications related to the profound increase in afterload, or proximal hypertension.

Indications for surgical repair of primary coarctation in adults are decreasing as endovascular angioplasty and stenting has improved [9]. When surgical repair is required, end-to-end anastomosis is the preferred method. The immobility of the aorta in the adult patient and the presence of multiple intercostal collaterals present challenges to the surgeon. Long segment stenosis may be repaired with resection and an interposition tube graft. This requires cross clamping of the aorta that carries an inherent risk of paraplegia. The indications for redo surgery include recoarctation and aneurysm formation.

Atrial septal defect (ASD)

Percutaneous closure of ostium secundum ASD is the current treatment of choice. If percutaneous closure is not feasible, surgical closure is indicated at any age when right ventricular dilatation is present [10]. In all types of ASD, atrial arrhythmias are a relatively common feature, and predict late post-operative arrythmia [11]. The surgical outcomes of ASD repair are, however excellent with very low peri-operative mortality. Certain types of ASD warrant specific mention:

- Sinus venosus ASD is associated with a higher incidence of sick sinus syndrome and the need for pacemaker implantation.

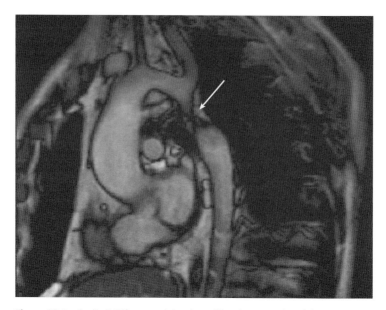

Figure 16.1a Cardiac MRI from an adult patient with native coarctation of the aorta presenting with systemic hypertension and weak, delayed femoral pulses. Note discrete, severe coarctation beyond the aortic isthmus (arrowed) with some post-stenotic dilatation of the descending intrathoracic aorta. Note also a rather dilated left subclavian artery (feeding the bronchial collaterals) and dilated ascending aorta (a feature of coexisting bicuspid aortic valve, seen in up to 70% of patients with coarctation).

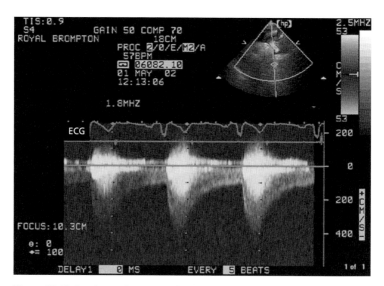

Figure 16.1b Doppler continuous wave (CW) sample in the area of coarctation from the same patient, showing a peak velocity at the excess of 4 m/sec (pressure gradient more than 64 mmHg) and increased velocity throughout systole and diastole (diastolic tail), both indicative of significant, severe coarctation. (See also colour plate 16.1)

- Patients with complete AVSD present early in life, and unless treated expediently develop irreversible pulmonary vascular disease, contraindicating reparative surgery in adulthood.
- Reoperation can be required for relief of late post-operative subaortic stenosis due to the elongated left ventricular outflow tract in AVSD.

Ventricular septal defect (VSD)

Large VSDs can result in right ventricular overload and pulmonary arterial hypertension. If diagnosed in adulthood, in the presence of severe pulmonary artery hypertension, surgery is contraindicated. By contrast, small, restrictive VSDs generally do not require intervention. In particular:

- Subaortic perimembranous VSDs with associated prolapse of the aortic valve cusp into the VSD may result in aortic regurgitation. In which case, although the VSD may be small, elective VSD closure may be considered to preserve the integrity of the aortic valve and avoid replacement in the future [12].
- A specific complication related to VSD closure is the development of complete heart block, although the incidence is lower since introduction of the trans-atrial approach.
- Double chambered right ventricle associated with a small restrictive VSD. VSD repair in this situation is a low risk operation with low recurrence rates.

Subaortic stenosis

Recurrence of subaortic stenosis can occur in adults with several types of congenital heart disease [13]. Specific post-surgical complications are iatrogenic VSD and complete heart block.

16.4 Moderately complex congenital heart disease

Tetralogy of Fallot (TOF)
Pulmonary valve replacement

Pulmonary regurgitation is common after surgical or percutaneous relief of pulmonary stenosis as part of repair of TOF. Long-term studies have demonstrated that pulmonary regurgitation results in progressive right ventricular dilatation, dysfunction, exercise intolerance, ventricular tachycardia and sudden cardiac death [14]. Pulmonary regurgitation is more frequent where a transannular patch has been used to reconstruct the right ventricular outflow tract. Patients with progressive right ventricular dilatation should be referred for elective pulmonary valve replacement before symptoms develop. Although the peri-operative risk is low, redo-sternotomy and right ventricular dysfunction are potential complicating factors.

Late primary repair of tetralogy of Fallot

Some patients with favourable anatomy survive to adulthood with unrepaired TOF. The natural history of unrepaired TOF is, however, 40% mortality in the first year, 70% in the first 10 years and 95% in the first

40 years. Patients presenting in adulthood with an unrepaired TOF (Figures 16.2a and b) may have raised pulmonary artery pressures despite severe right ventricular outflow tract obstruction, due to either chronic cyanosis or LV dysfunction.

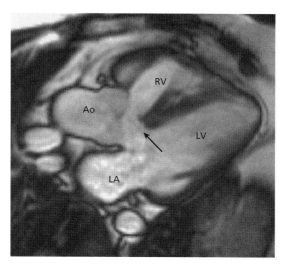

Figure 16.2a Cardiac MRI from an adult patient with unrepaired tetralogy of Fallot (four chamber view). Note hypertrophied right ventricle and a large unrestrictive ventricular-septal defect (arrowed). LV, left ventricle; RV, right ventricle; Ao, aorta; LA, left atrium.

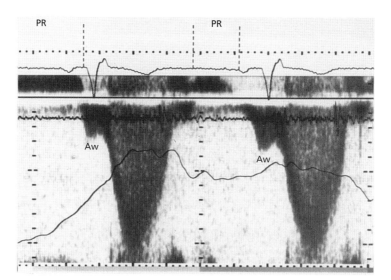

Figure 16.2b Doppler (pulsed wave) sample in the main pulmonary artery of same patient after repair. Note forward flow (Aw) in the pulmonary artery in late diastole, coinciding with the P wave of the ECG and atrial systole, which is present throughout respiration and contributes to pulmonary blood flow and cardiac output and counteracts the effect of pulmonary regurgitation (PR). This is a marker of right ventricular restrictive physiology.

Early mortality for late primary repair has been reported between 0 and 15% in most recent surgical series [4, 15, 16]. Post-operative morbidity in this patient population is significant, however [4]. The risk factors for late repair include: severe cyanosis, impaired ventricular function, significant tricuspid regurgitation and RV diastolic dysfunction, evaluated by the presence of antegrade diastolic flow in the main pulmonary artery, coinciding with atrial systole (A wave), throughout the respiratory cycle (Figure 16.2b). More recently, the level of haemoglobin (reflecting the degree of cyanosis) and the need for reconstruction with a right ventricular outflow patch were reported as additional risk factors.

Ebstein's anomaly of the tricuspid valve

Indications for cardiac surgery in adults with Ebstein's anomaly are the presence of severe tricuspid regurgitation in symptomatic patients, cyanosis due to right to left shunt through an ASD and paradoxical emboli [18]. Where possible, valve repair is preferable to valve replacement [19], and plication of the atrialised right ventricle as well as a right-sided Maze procedure are required in most cases [20]. Although mortality is low, post-operative morbidity is not insignificant, and relates to low cardiac output due to the right ventricular dysfunction and the presence after surgery of a relatively small functional right ventricle (Figure 16.3) [4, 21]. In such cases, a Glenn anastamosis may be considered at the time of surgery (see Chapter 10, Figures 10.3a and b) [21].

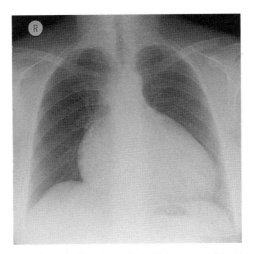

Figure 16.3 Chest radiograph of a patient with Ebstein's anomaly of the tricuspid valve (postero-anterior projection). Note marked cardiomegaly, a very large right atrium and a small pedicle of the heart. The aortic knuckle is also small, indicative of a lifelong low-systemic cardiac output status and underdevelopment of the aorta (common in many congenital heart conditions).

Double outlet right ventricle

In this lesion, more than 50% of both great arteries arise from the right ventricle. The main indication for cardiac surgery during adulthood is conduit replacement. Late repair is rarely seen in this condition, but can be achieved provided that pulmonary stenosis has protected the pulmonary vasculature and that significant right ventricular hypoplasia is not present.

16.5 Complex congenital heart disease

Congenitally corrected TGA (ccTGA)

The indications for surgery in ccTGA (Chapter 10, Figure 10.1b) include the presence of a large VSD and left ventricular outflow tract (LVOT) obstruction with progressive cyanosis. The classical approach is VSD closure plus LV to pulmonary artery conduit. Direct relief of pulmonary stenosis is rarely achieved due to the high risk of complete heart block that this procedure carries. Following surgery, due to changes in geometry of the right ventricle, tricuspid regurgitation may develop necessitating tricuspid valve repair or replacement.

Transposition of the great arteries (TGA)

Patients with simple TGA (Chapter 10, Figure 10.1a) that survive to adulthood have had previous palliative (atrial switch, Mustard or Senning) or corrective (arterial switch) surgery. Indications for intervention in this patient population depend upon the preceding surgery. Patients with palliative surgery may require relief of baffle obstruction (usually a percutaneous procedure) or tricuspid valve surgery for tricuspid regurgitation (associated with failure of the systemic right ventricle). In those who have undergone arterial switch, repeat surgery may be required for neo-aortic regurgitation, supra-pulmonary stenosis or coronary artery disruption.

Fontan circulation

Fontan completion for univentricular hearts is usually performed in childhood, although it can also be contemplated in adulthood (Chapter 10, Figure 10.3c). Patients with previous atrio-pulmonary Fontan and atrial arrhythmias are increasingly considered for total cavopulmonary conversion in adulthood (Chapter 10, Figure 10.4). In both situations, the immediate post-operative morbidity is high, and comprehensive knowledge of Fontan physiology is essential.

The effects of a Fontan-type circulation are extreme. Blood flow from the systemic venous circulation through the lungs is entirely passive and systemic venous hypertension is an inevitable consequence (Figure 16.4). Despite a number of modifications in surgical technique that have favourably influenced the early post-operative course, the chief cause of morbidity and mortality in this group remains the low cardiac output state. Factors that may limit cardiac output in this patient population include:

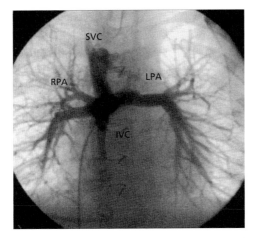

Figure 16.4 Angiogram from a patient with single ventricle physiology and total cavopulmonary connection (TCPC). Note direct anastomosis of the superior vena cava (SVC) with the right pulmonary artery (RPA) and the catheter through the inferior vena cava (IVC) and lower part of the TCPC anastomosis to the underside of the right pulmonary artery (RPA).

increase in pulmonary vascular resistance (contributed to by, for example, positive pressure ventilation and atelectasis), hypovolaemia and loss of sinus rhythm. At the time of surgery, fenestration between the right and left atrium may be performed. The resultant right-left shunt in the presence of raised systemic venous pressures allows decompression of the right atrium, and in children has been shown to increase post-operative survival. The benefits in adulthood are not clearly defined.

16.6 Conclusion

The ACHD patient population represents a significant challenge to the ICU physician, as the underlying pathophysiology may be very complex. As more of these patients are surviving to adulthood, they will inevitably increasingly require ICU input. Current recommendations are that such patients be managed in specialist units; however, emergency admissions do occur, and these will not always be primarily to such a centre. An understanding of the diagnosis, associated pathophysiological features, previous interventions and possible complications is crucial. The management of such patients in the ICU setting is described in Chapter 10.

Case study

A 22-year-old man with tetralogy of Fallot (TOF) was referred with dyspnoea and marked cyanosis for primary surgical repair (Figures 16.2a and b). He had undergone a Waterston shunt aged 5 years, after which he was lost to follow up for a number of years. At operation, surgery performed consisted of transection of the aorta at the level of right pulmonary artery anastomosis and takedown of the Waterston anastomosis. The main pulmonary artery was incised and a pulmonary valve comissurotomy performed. The right ventricle was opened longitudinally, muscular bundles were excised and the VSD was closed with a patch. The patient was re-warmed and came off bypass with a low dose infusion of dopamine.

The post-operative course was prolonged and stormy. The patient developed atrial flutter in the immediately post-operative period with a ventricular rate of 150 beats/min. Due to haemodynamic compromise direct current (DC) cardioversion was performed promptly with concomitant loading with intravenous amiodarone. The patient remained in a low cardiac output state requiring haemofiltration and inotropic support with milrinone. Left atrial pressure was 10 mmHg, with a right atrial pressure of 20 mmHg.

Progressive hypoxia ensued and the patient developed acute respiratory distress syndrome, requiring increasing positive pressure ventilation. Transoesophageal echocardiography showed no tamponade and a hypertrophied RV with impaired long axis function. No residual pulmonary valve stenosis or VSD was seen. There was mild pulmonary regurgitation. Left ventricular systolic function was preserved. Pulsed waved Doppler in the main pulmonary artery showed A waves throughout the respiratory cycle (Figure 16.2b), allowing for the diagnosis of RV restriction to be made.

Inotropic requirements were gradually decreased and the patient became easier to ventilate over the following 7 days. The chest radiograph showed resolution of the interstitial oedema. The patient was ultimately extubated on the 12th post-operative day, transferred to the cardiology ward on day 16 and made a full recovery, leaving the hospital on the 23rd post-operative day.

Comment

Late primary repair or redo-surgery for congenital heart disease is often complicated by a low cardiac output state, which can be refractory to conventional therapy. This low cardiac output state is often not related to systolic dysfunction of the systemic ventricle, but rather due to impaired transpulmonary blood flow and thus reduced systemic ventricular filling. Impaired transpulmonary blood flow, in turn, can be due to the absence of a subpulmonary ventricle (Fontan circulation), systolic dysfunction of the RV (Ebstein's anomaly of the tricuspid valve), diastolic dysfunction

Continued

of the RV (as shown in this case) or pulmonary arterial hypertension. In the presence of restrictive, RV disease, atrial contraction and its contribution to forward pulmonary blood flow may be crucial. This forward pulmonary arterial flow, coincident with atrial systole, makes a further contribution towards the total cardiac output by counteracting the effects of pulmonary regurgitation. Maintaining or restoring sinus rhythm, therefore, and avoiding as much as possible high airway pressures associated with mechanical ventilation (that interacts with diastolic flow) and drugs that alter RV compliance are the priorities for supporting such a patient. Furthermore, lung reperfusion injury is common following reparative surgery in patients with congenital heart disease associated with severe and chronic depletion of pulmonary blood flow and marked cyanosis. However, this is usually a transient phenomenon and patients respond well to positive pressure ventilation.

References

1. Wren C, O'Sullivan JJ. Survival with congenital heart disease and need for follow up in adult life. *Heart* 2001;85:438–43.
2. Engelfriet P, Boersma E, Oechslin E, et al. The spectrum of adult congenital heart disease in Europe: morbidity and mortality in a 5 year follow up period. *Eur Heart J* 2005;26:2325–33.
3. Niwa K, Perloff JK, Webb GD, et al. Survey of specialized tertiary care facilities for adults with congenital heart disease. *Int J Cardiol* 2004;96:211–16.
4. Price S, Trenfield S, Jagger S, et al. Intensive care in adults with congenital heart disease: cost implications of a changing patient population. *Crit Care* 2005;9(Suppl 1):P212.
5. Cho JM, Puga F, Danielson G, et al. Early and long term results of the surgical treatment of tetralogy of Fallot with pulmonary atresia with or without major aortopulmonary collaterals. *J Thorac Cardiovasc Surg* 2002;124:70–81.
6. Caldarone C, McCrindle B, Van Asdell G, et al. Independent factors associated with longevity of prosthetic pulmonary valves and valved conduits. *J Thorac Cardiovasc Surg* 2000;120:1021–31.
7. Khambadkone S, Coats L, Taylor A, et al. Percutaneous pulmonary valve implantation in humans: results in 59 consecutive patients. *Circulation* 2005;112:1189–97.
8. Stulak J, Dearani J, Puga F, et al. Right-sided maze procedure for atrial tacyarrythmias in congenital heart disease. *Ann Thorac Surg* 2006;81:1780–5.
9. Carr J. The results of catheter-based therapy compared with surgical repair of adult aortic coarctation. *J Am Coll Cardiol* 2006;47:1101–7.
10. Webb GD, Gatzoulis MA. Atrial septal defects in the adult: recent progress and overview. *Circulation* 2006;114:1645–53.
11. Gatzoulis MA, Freeman M, Siu SC, et al. Atrial arrythmia after surgical closure of atrial septal defects in adults. *N Engl J Med* 1999;340:839–46.
12. Brauner R, Birk E, Sahar G, et al. Surgical management of ventricular septal defect with aortic valve prolapse: clinical considerations and results. *Eur J Cardiothorac Surg* 1995;9(6):315–9.

13. Oliver JM, Gonzalez A, Gallego P, et al. Discrete subaortic stenosis in adults: increase prevalence and slow rate of progression of the obstruction and aortic regurgitation. *J Am Coll Cardiol* 2001;38:835–42.

14. Bouzas B, Kilner PJ, Gatzoulis MA. Pulmonary regurgitation: not a benign lesion. *Eur Heart J* 2005;26:433–9.

15. Atik FA, Atik E, da Cunha CR. Long-term results of correction of tetralogy of Fallot in adulthood. *Eur J Cardiothorac Surg* 2004;25:250–5.

16. Hu DC, Seward JB, Puga FJ, et al. Total correction of tetralogy of Fallot at age 40 years and older: long term follow up. *J Am Coll Cardiol* 1985;5:40–4.

17. Horer J, Friebe J, Schreiber C, et al. Correction of tetralogy of Fallot and of pulmonary atresia in adults. *Ann Thorac Surg* 2005;80:2285–92.

18. Chauvaud S, Berrebi A, d'Atellis N, et al. Ebstein's anomaly: repaired based on functional status. *Eur J Card Surg* 2003;23:525–31.

19. Kiziltan H, Theodoro D, Warnes C, et al. Late results of bioprosthetic tricuspid valve replacement in Ebstein's anomaly. *Ann Thorac Surg* 1998;66:1539–45.

20. Sarris GE, Giannopoulos NM, Tsoutsinos AJ, et al. Results of surgery for Ebstein anomaly: a multicenter study from the European Congenital Heart Surgeons Association. *J Thorac Cardiovasc Surg* 2006;132(1):50–7.

21. Chavaud S. Ebstein's malformation. Surgical treatments and results. *Thorac Cardiovas Surg* 2000;48(4):220–3.

17 Management of Arrhythmias in Adults with Congenital Heart Disease

Barbara J. Deal

Feinberg School of Medicine, Northwestern University, Children's Memorial Hospital, Chicago, Il, USA

Take Home Messages

- Arrhythmia is a common and dangerous complication of adult congenital heart disease (ACHD).
- Delay in diagnosis is common and contributes to the associated morbidity.
- Certain lesions are associated with a higher incidence of and risk from arrhythmia.
- Although the principles of acute anti-arrhythmic therapy are similar to those employed for patients without ACHD, the acuity of care needs to be accelerated, with recognition of the potential haemodynamic and neurological risks.
- Treatment of the acute arrhythmia needs to be coordinated with a plan for addressing the underlying haemodynamic abnormalities in a definitive manner, in addition to catheter ablations and device therapy for the arrhythmia.

17.1 Introduction

Due to improved survival, there are now more adults than children with congenital heart disease (CHD), the majority aged between 20 and 40 years. Arrhythmias are the most common complication encountered by this population, occurring in 18–20% of all adult congenital heart disease (ACHD) patients [1, 2], with the incidence increasing from roughly 22% at 40 years to greater than 40% by 55 years [2]. The general methods used to treat arrhythmias in ACHD patients in the intensive care setting are similar to those with acquired heart disease, and have been well described [3]. This chapter focuses on issues specific to the ACHD population.

Cardiovascular Critical Care. Edited by M. Griffiths, J. Cordingley and S. Price.
© 2010 Blackwell Publishing Ltd.

Table 17.1 General principles of arrhythmia care in adults with congenital heart disease.

Recognition of presence of arrhythmia
- Tachycardia: ventricular rate > 100 bpm
- Non-specific symptoms; congestive heart failure
- Lack of heart rate variability

Highest risk lesions
- Cyanotic heart disease
- Ebstein's anomaly of the tricuspid valve, with atrial level shunt
- Single ventricle, tricuspid atresia (Fontan repairs)
- Senning/Mustard repairs of transposition of the great arteries
- Hypertrophic cardiomyopathy
- Left ventricular or right ventricular outflow tract obstructive lesions

Diagnosis of mechanism of arrhythmia
- Lesion-specific arrhythmias
- Electrocardiographic indicators of SVT versus VT
- Adenosine as a diagnostic manoeuvre

Acute treatment
- Immediate cardioversion/defibrillation for haemodynamic instability
- Acute rate-control to achieve ventricular rate < 130 bpm: temporising only
- Conversion to sinus/atrial rhythm rather than rate control is the goal
- Avoidance of multi-drug regimens and delay in conversion
- Assessment for thrombus formation

Appropriate follow-up
- Evaluate haemodynamics prior to planning any intervention
- Assess potential benefits of:
  medication/ablation/reoperation/pacing/resynchronisation/defibrillator
- Social issues of obtaining care after discharge
- Health care directives

SVT, Supraventricular tachycardia; VT, ventricular tachycardia.

The presence of CHD alters the haemodynamic consequences of arrhythmias, the potential risks to the patient and the required acuity of treatment. The challenges of managing arrhythmias in the ACHD population relate first to recognition of the existence of an arrhythmia, and then responding with appropriate rapidity . Thereafter management is directed to resolving any predisposing haemodynamic abnormalities, and optimising the follow-up care for the patient relative to the arrhythmia. Table 17.1 summarises the general principles of arrhythmia care in ACHD patients.

17.2 Tachycardia

Recognition of arrhythmia

Recognising the presence of arrhythmia is often the most difficult aspect of a patient's care, with delayed recognition and treatment contributing to patient morbidity and mortality. Supraventricular tachycardia (SVT) frequently presents as fatigue, dizziness, malaise or congestive heart failure. Further, SVT or paroxysmal atrioventricular block may result in syncope or near-syncope, with spontaneous resolution of the arrhythmia prior to presentation. In ACHD patients with a prior midline sternotomy, regardless of the type of cardiac repair, the presence of a ventricular rate greater than 100 bpm should be considered to be an SVT until proven otherwise. In the intensive care setting the diagnosis is more complex, with the presence of many predisposing causes for sinus tachycardia, such as fever, infection, blood loss and the use of sympathomimetic drugs. The presence of 2:1 atrioventricular conduction during SVT superimposed on an abnormal electrocardiogram (ECG) further confounds ECG interpretation; thus, the usual ventricular rate during SVT in Fontan or Mustard/Senning patients is 90–140 bpm. Lack of variability of the heart rate should always raise suspicion of supraventricular tachycardia with atrioventricular block, particularly in ACHD patients with congestive heart failure.

Recognising the haemodynamic complications of an arrhythmia for patients with congenital heart lesions is essential to determining the rapidity and level of intervention. Clearly, a haemodynamically unstable patient with any cardiac lesion is an emergency, but with certain types of congenital cardiac lesions, the transition to instability may occur rapidly. The highest-risk patients include those with cyanosis, Ebstein's anomaly (due to increased risk of right-to-left atrial shunting during tachycardia), those with univentricular physiology (including prior Fontan-type repairs), a systemic right ventricle (particularly those with atrial repairs for transposition of the great arteries), and those with left or right ventricular outflow tract obstruction (Table 17.1). In these ACHD patients, the luxury of delaying intervention for even a number of hours is not available, as congestive heart failure, neurological disturbance or abrupt deterioration of the rhythm may occur. Additional high risk factors include faster ventricular rates (greater than 180 bpm), prolonged duration of tachycardia, and the presence of findings indicative of congestive heart failure, such as hepatomegaly, oedema and pulmonary congestion.

Certain congenital heart lesions are more commonly associated with specific mechanisms of tachycardia [4], although it should be noted that any arrhythmia can occur in an ACHD patient at any given time. For example, although tetralogy of Fallot patients received early and extensive interest due to the development of ventricular tachycardia (VT), supraventricular arrhythmias occur with three- to four-fold greater incidence in this condition (12–34% versus 4–7%) [5–7]. Electrocardiographic discriminators between VT and SVT in the setting of a wide QRS rhythm have been well documented [8]. In addition to the presence of atrioventricular dissociation, VT is more commonly associated with a more prolonged QRS duration, left axis deviation, concordant QRS pattern across the precordial leads, and a slurred downstroke or prolongation of the R to S nadir (> 70 msec) in right precordial leads. In the intensive care setting, the use of adenosine as a diagnostic tool in wide QRS tachycardia is valuable; a 2:1 or greater atrioventricular relationship

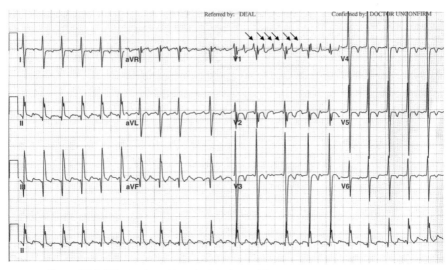

Figure 17.1 ECG of patient with repaired single ventricle. Note 2:1 atrioventricular conduction of atrial tachycardia, atrial epicardial pacing wires have been attached to lead V1 in order to highlight the periodicity of the atrial impulse (arrows).

indicating atrial tachycardia (Figure 17.1). A defibrillator should be present due to the risk of pro-arrhythmia, or the development of antidromic conduction of SVT over an additional accessory connection.

17.3 Acute treatment

The optimal treatment of any tachycardia is guided by specific knowledge of the mechanism of arrhythmia (Table 17.2). In the intensive care setting, the management goal for arrhythmia in ACHD patients is almost always the prompt restoration of sinus/atrial rhythm. In those who are haemodynamically stable but with a rapid ventricular response during SVT, transient rate-control with calcium-channel or beta-blocking medication may be achieved while preparations for definitive therapy are made.
In refractory atrial fibrillation, only rarely is rate control an acceptable compromise for longer-term treatment. Of note, such patients often have significant residual haemodynamic lesions that may be amenable to additional surgical intervention. In ACHD patients, the unpredictable response to both anaesthetic and sedative agents and to DC cardioversion, and the difficulty of obtaining access to the heart for trans-venous pacing means that cardioversion is not without significant risk. It cannot be over-emphasised, however, that delaying conversion to sinus rhythm for more than a very short period of time in the high-risk patients listed above may have disastrous consequences.

In patients with tachycardia duration of less than 48 hours, it is generally assumed that it is safe to proceed with attempts for rhythm conversion without the need for prior anticoagulation. Transthoracic

Table 17.2 Congenital heart lesions commonly associated with specific arrhythmias.

Supraventricular tachycardia

Atrioventricular reciprocating, utilising an accessory connection

- Ebstein's anomaly
- Atrial septal defect
- Congenitally corrected L-transposition of the great arteries (ccTGA)
- Hypertrophic cardiomyopathy

Atrial re-entry tachycardia

- Atrial septal defect
- Single ventricle, especially tricuspid atresia (Fontan repairs)
- Mustard/Senning repairs of transposition of the great arteries
- Common atrioventricular canal defects
- Tetralogy of Fallot
- Total anomalous pulmonary venous connection

Atrioventricular nodal re-entry tachycardia

- Mustard/Senning repairs of transposition of the great arteries
- Left ventricular outflow tract obstructive lesions

Atrial fibrillation

- Mitral valve disorders
- Ebstein's anomaly of the tricuspid valve
- Single ventricle, especially tricuspid atresia (Fontan repairs)
- Atrial septal defects
- Tetralogy of Fallot
- Hypertrophic cardiomyopathy
- Eisenmenger's syndrome

Ventricular tachycardia

Tetralogy of Fallot/double outlet right ventricle

Aortic stenosis

Ventricular septal defects

Ventricular fibrillation

Aortic stenosis

Hypertrophic cardiomyopathy

Mustard/Senning repair of transposition of the great arteries

Sinus bradycardia

Mustard/Senning repair of transposition of the great arteries

Single ventricle: Fontan repair

Atrial septal defects

Common atrioventricular canal

Anomalous pulmonary venous return

Atrioventricular block

Congenitally corrected transposition of the great arteries

Tetralogy of Fallot

Common atrioventricular canal, especially Trisomy 21

Ventricular septal defects

Left ventricular outflow obstruction

echocardiography should be performed to assess for the presence of intracardiac thrombus. Transthoracic echocardiogram may not adequately assess the presence of thrombus in patients with massive right atrial enlargement; these patients may require transoesophageal echocardiogram prior to cardioversion. In patients with a longer or uncertain duration of tachycardia, assessment with transoesophageal echocardiography is advised to assess the possibility of cardiac thrombus formation. In the presence of thrombus, anticoagulation for at least 3 weeks' duration is advised, together with rate control. However, in certain haemodynamic situations where prolongation of even mild degrees of tachycardia will be seriously detrimental (high risk lesions, significant heart failure), the difficult decision to proceed with cardioversion may need to be made. Electrical cardioversion for atrial tachycardia in ACHD patients may be optimised by an anteroposterior thoracic pad configuration to direct the electrical current over the often enlarged atrial chambers. Finally, the presence of dextrocardia will require reversal of pad placement (left upper sternum and right apex for anterior configuration, and right sternal border, right infrascapular region for anteroposterior configuration). In all cases, basic principles need to be followed including electrolyte assessment (especially potassium and magnesium), measurement of QTc intervals, both initially and serially with changes in medication, and treatment of congestive heart failure or respiratory compromise with inotropic and ventilatory support as indicated.

Excellent reviews of therapy of atrial arrhythmias in CHD [4, 12, 13] and arrhythmias in the adult intensive care patient with specifics of medication dosages are available [3]. The need to avoid the administration of multiple anti-arrhythmic medications in the critically ill ACHD population cannot be overemphasised. A cocktail of anti-arrhythmic medications in succession may exacerbate electrolyte abnormalities or heart failure, or promote torsades des pointes by prolongation of the QT interval. In low-risk patients who are haemodynamically stable a trial of one anti-arrhythmic medication (in addition to adenosine) may be attempted before proceeding with cardioversion. As stated in one review [14], 'the key to management is not to make things worse (multiple or inappropriate drug therapies) and to be prepared to observe a hemodynamically stable patient with tachycardia until DC cardioversion can be undertaken safely'.

For atrial fibrillation in the intensive care setting, intravenous amiodarone has been shown to achieve conversion in 55–70% of patients [9]; however, hypotension may necessitate termination or slowing of infusion. Although intravenous ibutilide preceded by magnesium will convert up to 75% of atrial flutter, and a lesser percentage of atrial fibrillation, there is very little information available specific to ACHD patients, although it is generally accepted that its use should be avoided in the presence of QT prolongation. A small bolus of intravenous amiodarone (150 mg over 2 hours) followed by magnesium (1 g) and ibutilide (1 mg) intravenously has been reportedly highly effective in achieving conversion in a small number of adult patients without CHD [10]; however, the use of this combination in ACHD patients has not been fully evaluated and the risk of pro-arrhythmia in structurally abnormal hearts may be significantly increased.

Adenosine in appropriate doses should effectively terminate SVT due to accessory connections or atrioventricular nodal re-entry, and is effective in some atrial (and less often, ventricular) tachycardias. Adenosine may also unmask atrial tachycardia by blocking the ventricular response, allowing visualisation of atrial activity. In atrial tachycardia (atrial macro-re-entry, atrial flutter) a judicious trial of calcium channel-blocking medication as a single bolus, such as diltiazem, may be effective, although its use may be precluded by impaired ventricular function. Rapid atrial over-drive pacing for tachycardia termination is highly effective, and may avoid the risk of profound bradycardia sometimes associated with direct-current cardioversion. This may be carried out using atrial epicardial pacing wires in patients recovering from surgery or in centres where transoesophageal pacing is available.

For wide QRS tachycardia, a trial of adenosine may be diagnostic and sometimes therapeutic. The American College of Cardiology/American Heart Association/European Society of Cardiology (ACC/AHA/ECS) guidelines recommend intravenous amiodarone as the intravenous medication of choice; however, the significant risk of hypotension may be augmented in patients with structural heart disease and compromised ventricular function [11]. Here, either intravenous lidocaine or procainamide may be administered as alternative therapy. For high-risk patients, proceeding directly to cardioversion may be the most beneficial approach.

17.4 Bradycardia

There are many specific structural cardiac defects that predispose to the development of bradycardia and may result in admission to the cardiac intensive care unit, or mean that the patient is unable to mount a tachycardia appropriate to his or her clinical status. Thus, those with atrial repairs of transposition of the great arteries may present with profound bradycardia as adults, with ventricular rates of 25–35 bpm while awake. Other lesions at increased risk of developing late sinus node dysfunction include Fontan-type repairs of a single ventricle, atrial septal defects and repair of anomalous pulmonary venous drainage. The incidence of hypothyroidism is increased in patients with structural heart disease and Trisomy 21, and should be screened for in the setting of bradycardia. The late development of paroxysmal complete atrioventricular block may present as recurrent syncope in patients with repaired tetralogy of Fallot, or complete atrioventricular canal defects (especially in association with Trisomy 21) [16]. Risk factors for late atrioventricular block include bifascicular block with PT prolongation, and perioperative complete heart block, although this information is rarely available with adult patients. Although most bradycardia is attributed to the results of atrial surgery, recently there has been recognition of the role of gene defects such as NKX

2.5 in the development of progressive bradycardia and conduction defects, most notably in association with atrial and ventricular septal defects [15].

Permanent pacemakers are indicated for symptomatic bradycardia, and may be needed for significant bradycardia in patients requiring chronic anti-arrhythmic medications, as well as post-operative second- or third-degree atrioventricular block [17]. Temporary transvenous pacing may be required for acutely symptomatic patients prior to permanent pacemaker implantation; however, consideration of the cardiac anatomy is clearly important in ACHD patients, where standard venous access to the ventricular and atrial chambers may not be available. Intravenous isoproterenol infusion may be used to augment the junctional or ventricular response rate as a temporising measure, but peripheral vasodilatation and hypotension or increased ventricular ectopy may limit this use.

17.5 Post-acute treatment care

The development of tachycardia in ACHD is frequently associated with residual haemodynamic lesions, and optimal treatment should focus on identifying and correcting the underlying structural or functional abnormalities, which may be amenable to catheter or surgical intervention. Cardiac catheterisation may therefore be required but possibly will need to be delayed until congestive heart failure symptoms have improved with a few days of medical therapy. Catheter ablation of SVT in patients with repaired CHD has produced very good results with the exception of those with a Fontan circulation with atriopulmonary connections [4, 18, 19]. Note, however, that repeated attempts at catheter ablation in patients with haemodynamic abnormalities may allow progression of ventricular dysfunction or promote thrombus. There is now sizeable experience with incorporating arrhythmia surgery into re-operations for structural abnormalities, with reduction in arrhythmia recurrence to less than 10% during mid-term follow-up [20–24]. With current techniques, re-operation for patients with associated atrial tachycardia/fibrillation should not be undertaken without concurrent arrhythmia intervention.

Patients with chronotropic incompetence, such as atrial repairs of transposition of the great arteries or atrial septal defects, may benefit from maintenance of an appropriate atrial rate by atrial pacing combined with anti-tachycardia pacing and/or a defibrillator in high-risk patients. The development of atrial tachycardia in Mustard/Senning patients is significantly associated with an increased risk of sudden death [25, 26], and such patients should receive implantable defibrillators. Patients with ventricular dysfunction, QRS prolongation and bradycardia may benefit from ventricular resynchronisation at the time of anti-bradycardia pacing. The presence of such patients on the intensive care unit should prompt close liaison with pacing and echocardiography technicians to determine optimal pacemaker settings for the current clinical status. With rapid changes in loading conditions, medication and ventilatory support, these pacing settings may need to be repeatedly re-optimised.

In determining care following intensive care discharge, the ACHD patient is particularly challenging. There should therefore be comprehensive planning of ongoing care after the emergent arrhythmia is treated to avoid re-admission. Finally, but probably initially as well, the development of arrhythmias should prompt discussion and documentation of a living will for health care directives.

17.6 Summary

The growing population of ACHD patients is at significant risk for developing arrhythmias, with an ever-increasing incidence of arrhythmias with age. Detection of the presence of arrhythmias is often challenging, and delay in recognition and appropriate therapy contributes to morbidity and mortality. Certain congenital heart defects are associated with particular types of arrhythmia, as well as increased haemodynamic risk during tachycardia. Highest risk patients include those with cyanosis, Ebstein's anomaly of the tricuspid valve, single ventricle repairs (Fontan), systemic right ventricles (atrial switch for transposition of the great arteries) and right and left heart obstructive lesions. Although the principles of acute anti-arrhythmic therapy are similar to those employed for patients without CHD, the urgency of care needs to be accelerated, with recognition of the potential haemodynamic and neurological risks.

In ACHD patients the development of arrhythmias is often accompanied by residual haemodynamic problems, which may benefit from catheter or surgical intervention. Treatment of the acute arrhythmia needs to be coordinated with a plan for addressing the underlying haemodynamic abnormalities in a definitive manner, in addition to catheter ablations and device therapy for the arrhythmia. The ACHD patient presents particular challenges when planning appropriate post-discharge care.

Case study

A 27-year-old man presented to the emergency department with a 30-minute history of racing heart beat. Past medical history was remarkable for repair of transposition of the great arteries with a Mustard procedure at 5 days of age. He had a resting sinus bradycardia of 50–60 bpm, and had developed sustained episodes of palpitations from 26 years of age. He was treated with digoxin, and after presenting with sustained supraventricular tachycardia, was treated with oral sotalol, as well as warfarin, and scheduled for electrophysiology study and potential catheter ablation. Due to work commitments, he delayed the procedure.

Continued

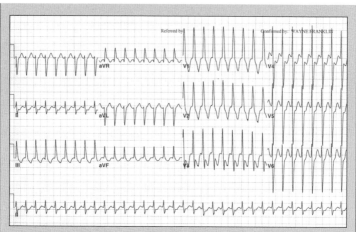

Figure 17.2 ECG of case history.

He returned with palpitations after missing his evening dose of sotalol. In the emergency department, his electrocardiogram showed a rate of 204 bpm, with right axis deviation and marked right ventricular hypertrophy, with QRS duration of 100 msec and QTc of 440 msec (Figure 17.2). Adenosine 12 mg was administered intravenously, resulting in 2:1 atrioventricular conduction for 2 beats, followed by resumption of 1:1 conduction. Low amplitude P waves at a rate of 200 bpm were discerned with difficulty during adenosine administration.

He was admitted to the intensive care unit. He was alert and anxious, with blood pressure 140/80, heart rate 200 bpm, respiratory rate 18 and oxygen saturation 97%. Lungs were clear. Cardiac examination revealed an increased right ventricular impulse, a loud second heart sound, a 3/6 systolic murmur at the lower left sternal border and no diastolic murmur or gallop appreciable. Liver was palpable 2 cm below the right costal margin. Laboratory data revealed a potassium of 3.6 mmol/L and magnesium of 2.0 mmol/L. Magnesium sulphate (1 g) was administered intravenously over 10 minutes. Ibutilide (1 mg) was infused over 10 minutes. Heart rate decreased to 100 bpm, with marked QTc prolongation to 570 msec. A second dose of intravenous magnesium was given, followed by an oral dose of propranolol 20 mg. Low amplitude P waves were difficult to discern. Following propranolol, heart rate gradually slowed over the next 60 minutes to 60 bpm.

Subsequent electrophysiology testing induced atrial re-entry tachycardia, with earliest activation between the atrial baffle and the tricuspid valve. Successful ablation was performed with access from both the systemic and pulmonary venous atrium. Ventricular stimulation study induced sustained ventricular fibrillation. He underwent implantation of a transvenous dual chamber anti-tachycardia pacemaker/defibrillator.

References

1. Immer FF, Althaus SM, Berdat PA, et al. Quality of life and specific problems after cardiac surgery in adolescents and adults with congenital heart diseases. *Eur J Cardiovasc Prev Rehabil* 2005;12:138–43.
2. van der Velde ET, Vriend JW, Mannens MM, et al. CONCOR, an initiative towards a national registry and DNA-bank of patients with congenital heart disease in the Netherlands: rationale, design, and first results. *Eur J Epidemiol* 2005;20:549–57.
3. Trappe HJ, Brandts B, Weismueller P. Arrhythmias in the intensive care patient. *Curr Opin Crit Care* 2003;9:345–55.
4. Walsh EP. Arrhythmias in patients with congenital heart disease. *Card Electrophysiol Rev* 2002;6:422–30.
5. Harrison DA, Siu SC, Hussain F, et al. Sustained atrial arrhythmias in adults late after repair of tetralogy of Fallot. *Am J Card* 2001;87:584–8.
6. Roos-Hesselink J, Perlroth MG, McGhie J, et al. Atrial arrhythmias in adults after repair of tetralogy of Fallot. Correlations with clinical, exercise and echocardiographic findings. *Circulation* 1995;91:2214–19.
7. Gatzoulis MA, Balaji S, Webber SA, et al. Risk factors for arrhythmia and sudden cardiac death late after repair of tetralogy of Fallot: a multicentre study. *Lancet* 2000;356:975–81.
8. Tipple MA. Usefulness of the electrocardiogram in diagnosing mechanisms of tachycardia. *Pediat Cardiol* 2000;21:516–21.
9. Delle Karth G, Geppert A, Neunteufl T, et al. Amiodarone versus diltiazem for rate control in critically ill patients with atrial tachyarrhythmias. *Crit Care Med* 2001;29:1149–53.
10. Hennersdorf MG, Perings SM, Zuhlke C, et al. Conversion of recent-onset atrial fibrillation or flutter with ibutilide after amiodarone has failed. *Intensive Care Med* 2002;28:925–9.
11. American Heart Association in collaboration with International Liaison Committee on Resuscitation, 2005 International Consensus on Cardiopulmonary Resuscitation and Emergency Cardiovascular Care Science with Treatment Recommendations. Part 7.3: Management of symptomatic bradycardia and tachycardia. (Advanced Cardiovascular Life Support). 2005 AHA Guidelines for Cardiopulmonary Resuscitation and Emergency Cardiovascular Care. *Circulation* 2005;112 (suppl):IV-67–77.
12. Balaji S, Harris L. Atrial arrhythmias in congenital heart disease. *Cardiol Clin* 2002;20:459–68.
13. Triedman JK. Arrhythmias in adults with congenital heart disease. *Heart* 2002;87:383–9.
14. Wiseman MN, Tavel ME. Wide-complex tachycardia: management in patient with a history of congenital heart disease. *Chest* 2000;117:268–71.
15. Prall OW, Elliott DA, Harvey RP. Developmental paradigms in heart disease: insights from tinman. *Ann Med* 2002;34:148–56.
16. Banks MA, Jenson J, Kugler JD. Late development of atrioventricular block after congenital heart surgery in down syndrome. *Am J Cardiol* 2001;88:A7,86–9.
17. Gregoratos G, Abrams J, Epstein AE, et al. ACC/AHA/NASPE 2002 guideline update for implantation of cardiac pacemakers and antiarrhythmia devices: summary article. A report of the American College of Cardiology/American Heart Association Task Force on Practice Guidelines (ACC/AHA/NASPE Committee to Update the 1998 Pacemaker Guidelines). *J Cardiovasc Electrophysiol* 2002;13:1183–99.

18. Triedman JK, Bergau DM, Saul JP, et al. Efficacy of radiofrequency ablation for control of intraatrial reentrant tachycardia in patients with congenital heart disease. *J Am Col Cardiol* 1997;30:1032–8.

19. Kannankeril PJ, Anderson ME, Rottman JN, et al. Frequency of late recurrence intra-atrial reentry tachycardia after radiofrequency catheter ablation in patients with congenital heart disease. *Am J Cardiol* 2003;92:879–81.

20. Deal BJ, Mavroudis C, Backer CL, et al. Impact of arrhythmia circuit cryoablation during Fontan conversion for refractory atrial tachycardia. *Am J Cardiol* 1999;83:563–8.

21. Deal BJ, Mavroudis C, Backer CL. Beyond Fontan conversion: surgical therapy of arrhythmias including patients with associated complex congenital heart disease. *Ann Thorac Surg* 2003;76:5 542–53.

22. Backer CL, Deal BJ, Mavroudis C, et al. Conversion of the failed Fontan circulation. *Cardiol Young* 2006;16 Suppl 1:85–91.

23. Karamlou T, Silber I, Lao R, et al. Outcomes after late reoperation in patients with repaired tetralogy of Fallot: the impact of arrhythmia and arrhythmia surgery. *Ann Thorac Surg* 2006;81:1786–96.

24. Ashburn DA, Harris L, Downar EH, et al. Electrophysiologic surgery in patients with congenital heart disease. *Semin Thorac Cardiovasc Surg Pediatr Card Surg Annu* 2003;6:51–8.

25. Dos L, Teruel L, Ferreira IJ, et al. Late outcome of Senning and Mustard procedures for correction of transposition of the great arteries. *Heart* 2005;91:652–6.

26. Kammeraad JA, van Deurzen CH, Sreeram N, et al. Predictors of sudden cardiac death after Mustard or Senning repair for transposition of the great arteries. *J Am Coll Cardiol* 2004;44:1095–102.

18 Mitral Valve Disease

Susanna Price and Derek Gibson

Royal Brompton & Harefield NHS Foundation Trust, London, UK

Take Home Messages

Mitral regurgitation:
- As a primary cause of ICU admission it is likely to be severe.
- Physical signs and investigations may be atypical.
- It may present as a failure to wean from ventilatory support.

Mitral stenosis:
- ICU admission is usually precipitated by the onset of atrial fibrillation
- Physical signs and investigations are usually classical.

Mitral valve replacement:
- Failure may present with pulmonary oedema.
- Significant regurgitation is easily diagnosed using M-mode transthoracic echocardiography.

18.1 Introduction

Although mitral valve (MV) disease alone rarely necessitates general intensive care admission, treatment is usually effective and the diagnosis should therefore not be missed. The rapidly changing haemodynamics of critically ill patients may make the diagnosis of important mitral valve disease difficult. Further, the physiological abnormalities seen vary significantly, both between individual patients and in the same patient over time. The ability to use invasive and non-invasive monitoring of such patients allows disturbed physiology to be characterised in some detail, thus enabling individualised management. The investigation and management of mitral valve disease in critical care is therefore largely determined by experience and anecdote, as there is little in the way of controlled data for this patient population.

Cardiovascular Critical Care. Edited by M. Griffiths, J. Cordingley and S. Price.

18.2 Mitral regurgitation

Severe primary mitral regurgitation

Primary mitral regurgitation (MR) in its most severe form presents as left ventricular (LV) failure, often of sudden onset with pulmonary oedema and/or cardiogenic shock. In the absence of infective endocarditis, mitral valve replacement or acute myocardial infarction, the cause is likely to be chordal rupture, or much less commonly papillary muscle rupture [1]. Rarer reported causes of severe MR include blunt trauma and bullet or stab wounds to the chest.

Diagnosis of severe primary mitral regurgitation

Unlike patients with less severe disease, the physical examination may be actively misleading (Table 18.1). The expected pansystolic murmur may be very short or absent, and the presence of a loud third heart sound may appear to confirm the diagnosis of severe LV disease. In addition, both radiographic and echocardiographic features may be atypical and thus bedside assessment and haemodynamic monitoring are frequently unreliable for the diagnosis and quantification of regurgitation.

In addition, invasive haemodynamic monitoring can also be misleading, as although characteristically patients will have a high pulmonary capillary wedge pressure (PCWP) with significant pulmonary capillary v-waves, these are often absent (33%) and right-sided filling pressures are frequently normal (82%) [2]. In such cases, where the patient presents with bilateral pulmonary infiltrates, differentiation from adult respiratory distress syndrome (ARDS) may be difficult, and the two pathologies may co-exist.

The crucial finding in these conditions is to demonstrate a very active LV in a patient with a low cardiac output state. Echocardiography will characteristically show a hyper-dynamic LV with a normal end-diastolic and reduced end-systolic volume, associated with tachycardia (unless the patient is taking a beta-blocking drug). The M-mode pattern is also characteristic, with large amplitude reciprocal motion of the septum and posterior LV wall. The end-systolic volume may be so low as to suggest, erroneously, the diagnosis of hypertrophic cardiomyopathy.

Table 18.1 Clinical features of mitral regurgitation causing critical illness.

Clinical feature	Notes
Low cardiac output/cardiogenic shock	Both may be present
Pulmonary oedema	May be asymmetrical
Tachycardia	May be absent if patient beta-blocked
Displaced apex	May be normal if very acute
High JVP	May not be elevated
Hyperdynamic left ventricle	May be absent after myocardial infarct
Pan-systolic murmur	If very severe, may be absent, or S3 heard
Loud P2	May be absent

The next stage is to demonstrate anatomical evidence of MV disease, usually in the form of a flail cusp with associated ruptured chords or papillary muscle stump. Alternatively, vegetations may be demonstrated, the size and distribution of which should be determined, as the greater the total mass of infected material, the more likely are direct toxaemic effects on the circulation (independent of the severity of the MR). These anatomical echocardiographic findings should be confirmed using trans-oesophageal echocardiography (TOE), as the precise abnormalities are crucial in planning surgical management.

Doppler echocardiography should be undertaken, but the results in very severe MR are quite different from those in patients in whom the condition is stable. With the loss of an effective MV, the resistance to backward blood flow from the LV into the left atrium (LA) may be similar to that of forward flow into the aorta. This directly influences the morphology of the continuous wave (CW) MR trace, which comes to resemble that of mild LV outflow tract obstruction (LVOTO) (Figure 18.1). At the same time, LA pressure may equilibrate with that in the LV by end-ejection, so the velocities are correspondingly low. Indeed, they may be so low that on the colour flow Doppler the characteristic regurgitant jet is not apparent in the LA. Instead, there are low velocity sinusoidal blood flow velocities to and fro across the valve orifice.

In addition to the features mentioned, quantification of MR in the intensive care unit (ICU) is particularly challenging as positive pressure ventilation, sedation and vasoactive drugs influence the degree of regurgitation. Patients may thus have little or no MR when they are fully sedated and ventilated, presenting with failure to wean from ventilatory

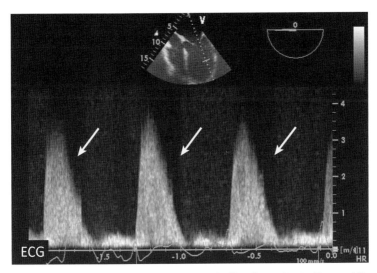

Figure 18.1 TOE showing continuous wave trans-mitral Doppler consistent with severe MR. For reference, a 2D image is shown at the top of the figure, with the cursor positioned across the mitral valve. Note the low velocities (< 4 m/sec) and short, triangular-shaped pattern (v-wave cutoff sign), arrowed.

support. In ischaemic MR the increased myocardial oxygen demand resulting during the stress of weaning from ventilatory support can induce acute ischaemic MR. In such cases, a targeted trans-thoracic study performed at the time that the patient is haemodynamically compromised or dobutamine stress echocardiography with dynamic afterload testing may be crucial in making the diagnosis [3].

Management of severe primary mitral regurgitation

The treatment of patients with severe MR is surgical unless there are very strong contraindications. Once the diagnosis has been made, every effort should be made to transfer the patient to a surgical centre, and medical treatment should be directed at providing support until the patient reaches the operating table. Supportive management of severe MR includes positive pressure mechanical ventilation and renal replacement therapy as required. The patient's haemodynamics may be improved by a reduction in afterload with an intra-aortic balloon (IABP) counterpulsation and/or intravenous vasodilators for acute MR after myocardial infarction, and inotropic support [4]. These measures merely serve to support the patient, resolve pulmonary oedema, correct acid-base disturbance and improve cardiac output while awaiting surgery to replace or repair the mitral valve.

The timing of surgery is controversial. In patients with a ruptured papillary muscle in particular, the earliest possible surgery is essential [5]. With ruptured chordae, the position is different if the patient can be stabilised, since LV function may begin to improve 24–48 hours after chordal rupture, as the LV adapts to the volume load. It is unlikely, however, that either vasodilators or counterpulsation affect this process to any great degree, and where the patient fails to respond, surgery should not be delayed.

Left ventricular disease complicated by mitral regurgitation
Ischaemic mitral regurgitation

This is probably a more common clinical problem than severe primary MR, though, like much of acute medicine, all is not straightforward. Not uncommonly, patients with apparently mild functional MR who are stable when sedated and mechanically ventilated develop pulmonary oedema associated with worsening MR on attempting to wean from ventilatory support. Although the volume load of the LV may not be greatly increased, the underlying mechanism appears to be a small increase in LV cavity size associated with an abrupt rise in LA pressure caused by the relatively small regurgitant volume into a non-compliant cavity. Frequently, there is underlying myocardial ischaemia, and dobutamine stress echocardiography may reveal the diagnosis (Chapter 4). In the presence of severe ischaemic MR, surgical mortality is particularly high [6, 7], and percutaneous coronary revascularisation should be considered, especially where other patient features make the surgical risk prohibitive. Although data regarding the impact of emergent balloon angioplasty are conflicting, some studies show dramatic success [8]. However, the use of anti-platelet agents following angioplasty may increase the peri-operative risk should surgery subsequently be undertaken.

Where surgical or percutaneous intervention is not an option, additional measures known to be of use in chronic severe mitral regurgitation may have a role in the management of these patients. However, due to the severity of regurgitation, this treatment is often unsuccessful. Management is thus limited to afterload reduction (acutely with the use of IABP, intravenous sodium nitroprusside) and more chronically with an angiotensin converting enzyme inhibitor. In ischaemic MR, this may be combined with anti-ischaemic agents such as beta blockers and oral nitrates. In patients with significant LV dysfunction, biventricular pacing may reduce the severity of MR [9], but predicting which patients will benefit is difficult. On occasion, the degree of regurgitation may be increased and therefore echocardiography should be used to determine the effects of any intervention and optimise the pacemaker settings [10, 11].

Left ventricular disease associated with left bundle branch block and mild mitral regurgitation

In a small group of patients with left bundle branch block (LBBB) and LV disease, MR may be very prolonged. Whilst not severe in terms of volume, this has the effect of reducing the time available for forward flow across the MV, and thus in extreme cases of limiting stroke volume and increasing LA pressure (Figure 18.2). Furthermore, with increasing heart rate the duration of MR does not change, so filling time is shortened further. These

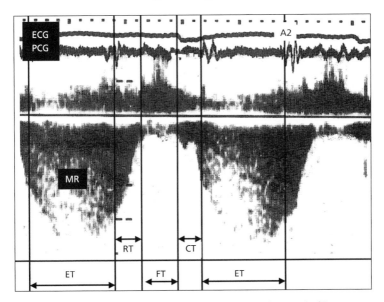

Figure 18.2 ECHO demonstrating mild MR temporally limiting left ventricular filling. Here, the MR is long and continues after the aortic component of the second heart sound (A2), allowing only a short time for ventricular filling (FT). ECG, electrocardiogram; PCG, phonocardiogram; MR, mitral regurgitation; ET, ejection time; RT, isovolumic relaxation time; FT, filling time; CT, isovolumic contraction time.

haemodynamic effects may be severe enough to cause cardiogenic shock, particularly when the heart rate increases, for example on weaning from mechanical ventilation.

This condition can be readily diagnosed using trans-thoracic echocardiography (TTE) and should be suspected when the duration of the MR on the CW Doppler trace exceeds 500 ms, or when LV filling time measured by pulsed wave (PW) Doppler falls below 200 ms. Once diagnosed, treatment is by ventricular pacing: simple right ventricular (RV) dual chamber (DDD) pacing is often effective, although biventricular pacing may be more so. In a minority of patients the severity of MR itself can be altered by biventricular pacing; however, this is unpredictable, and even if successful, given the rapidly changing dynamics in the critically ill, may not be maintained.

18.3 Mitral stenosis

As with severe MR, significant mitral stenosis (MS) may mimic ARDS, presenting with poor gas exchange and bilateral pulmonary infiltrates; however, the history will usually suggest the underlying diagnosis, clinical features are typical and echocardiographic findings characteristic. A precipitant for acute deterioration may be the onset of atrial fibrillation, which may mask the classic clinical signs, such as the mid-diastolic murmur. Prompt and adequate anticoagulation is essential to avoid the development of intracardiac thrombus.

Where the patient is admitted to the ICU in extremis, with pulmonary oedema, cardiogenic shock or cardiac arrest, emergent balloon valvotomy has been performed with good effect although mortality remains significant [12]. In addition, successful percutaneous intervention for critically ill patients with severe MS has been reported using either the Inoue balloon or the metallic valvulotome [13–15].

18.4 Prosthetic mitral valve disease

With improved surgical techniques and patient survival, patients with previous valve replacement will increasingly present to the ICU, either with valve dysfunction or co-existent disease. In patients with a prosthetic MV, adequate and appropriate anticoagulation is critical, and must be adjusted according to the valve implanted [16]. Sub-therapeutic anticoagulation, even for 24 hours, may lead to acute thrombosis presenting as acute, severe cardiovascular collapse, particularly in patients with Bjork–Shiley or Sorin valves. The differential diagnosis is pannus formation. Thrombosis is suggested by a more acute presentation, more severe symptoms and associated embolic phenomena. On TTE with MV obstruction the pattern of LV wall motion is characteristic: the amplitude of posterior wall motion is often normal, but the septal motion is strikingly reversed, so that the LV dimension is almost fixed throughout the cardiac cycle. In addition, although stroke volume is low, very high (up to 3 m/sec) velocities may be recorded on Doppler across the MV prosthesis, which are maintained throughout diastole. This pattern has been mistaken for the Doppler of mild aortic regurgitation and its significance therefore not recognised. TOE may be used to differentiate pannus from thombus, which is of lower echo intensity and tends to extend into the LA. Patients with MV prosthesis thrombosis may be managed with either surgery or thrombolysis. Although surgical mortality is high (0–69%), and treatment with intravenous thrombolysis guided by serial echocardiography is possible, there is a significant risk of cerebral thromboembolism (12%), and current recommendations are that thrombolysis is reserved only for patients in extremis in whom surgery is contra-indicated [17].

Severe prosthetic MR may be caused by tissue valve disintegration, strut fracture, disc malfunction or paraprosthetic regurgitation, usually associated with infective endocarditis. Xenograft rupture may occur very rapidly with cusp dehiscence in a degenerating prosthesis, presenting with pulmonary oedema and cardiogenic shock. Here the clinical history and examination, combined with echocardiographic features, usually suggest the diagnosis. Severe mitral paraprosthetic regurgitation presents as acute heart failure with a raised JVP and a soft systolic murmur of functional TR. There is characteristically no MR murmur. Severe paraprosthetic MR occurring long after implantation must be assumed to be infective in origin. The organisms are usually found in the sutures which rot, leading to dehiscence of a large part or even the entire ring. Vegetations are not usually present on a mechanical valve and may be difficult to detect on echocardiography due to artefact from the high-intensity echoes from metal or plastic. If the valve ring is radio-opaque a rocking motion may be demonstrated by screening, although this is sometimes inappropriately diagnosed when it is simply a function of increased amplitude of LV wall motion. The characteristic echocardiographic findings of severe paraprosthetic MR are of a very active LV with associated normalisation of septal motion (Figure 18.3).

18.5 Post-operative management of mitral valve surgery

Post-operative management following MV surgery is frequently uncomplicated; however, there are certain associated conditions that, when present, are particularly challenging. These relate to the valve itself, the ventricles, the coronary arteries and pulmonary vasculature (Table 18.2).

Valve-related post-operative complications

In 1–16% of cases, mitral valve repair may be associated with a degree of LV outflow tract obstruction (LVOTO) due to systolic anterior motion (SAM) of the MV. Associations are the presence of a small annuloplasty ring, a tall posterior leaflet and/or hypertrophy of the LV affecting the septum.

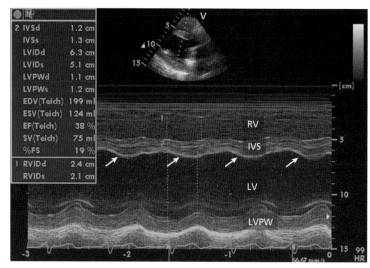

Figure 18.3 Parasternal long axis M-mode echocardiogram demonstrating a dilated left ventricle and reversed paradoxical movement of the interventricular septum (arrowed), indicating volume overload of the left ventricle. IVS, interventricular septum; RV, right ventricle; PW LV, posterior wall left ventricle; ECG, electrocardiogram. RV, right ventricle; IVS, interventricular septum; LV, left ventricle; LVPW, left ventricular posterior wall; IVSd, interventricular septum (diastole); IVSs, interventricular septum (systole); LVIDd, left ventricular internal diameter (diastole); LVIDs, left ventricular internal diameter (systole); LVPWd, left ventricular posterior wall (diastole); LVPWs, left ventricular posterior wall (systole); EDV(Teich), end-diastolic volume (Teicholz method); ESV(Teich), end-systolic volume (Teicholz method); EF (Teich), ejection fraction (Teicholz method); SV(Teich), stroke volume (Teicholz method); %FS, fractional shortening; RVIDd, right ventricular internal diameter (diastole); RVIDs, right ventricular internal diameter (systole).

Table 18.2 Post-operative complications.

Valve-related complications	General complications
MV repair	Generalised left ventricular dysfunction
Left ventricular outflow tract obstruction	Circumflex coronary artery disruption
Acute failure	Pulmonary hypertension
MV replacement	Right ventricular dysfunction
Paraprosthetic regurgitation	Tamponade
Prosthetic block	

Post-operatively, this presents as progressively worsening cardiac output despite escalating inotropic support, and is readily diagnosed with echocardiography. Treatment is conservative, with fluid resuscitation and afterload increase. In the unusual event that medical therapy fails, surgical revision may be necessary.

Acute MR due to failure of a mitral repair causes a low cardiac output and pulmonary oedema associated with a new pan-systolic murmur. A comprehensive TOE assessment of the MV is essential to determine the severity and mechanism of regurgitation, and to guide surgical intervention.

Valve obstruction occurring within the first 48 hours of surgery is unusual but potentially life-threatening, and presents with intermittent severe MS. This condition requires urgent surgical revision [18]. Following MV replacement in the context of endocarditis, particularly with reconstruction of the posterior annulus, paraprosthetic regurgitation may develop early following surgery. Where the paraprosthetic leak is small, initial management includes limitation of systolic blood pressure and tight control of anticoagulation. However, repeat surgery may be necessary as the paraprosthetic leak may progressively worsen. The timing of surgical revision should be determined by the clinical status of the patient together with serial echocardiographic studies.

General post-operative complications

Left ventricular failure following MV repair/replacement is not uncommon, particularly in the context of myocardial ischaemia/infarction, and the ICU management of this is standard. In patients with LV dysfunction and LBBB who are undergoing MV surgery, where LV and RV epicardial leads have been placed, biventricular pacing may be used to optimise synchrony and cardiac output. If unexpected RV or LV failure arises following surgery, TOE may be used to diagnose iatrogenic coronary artery stenosis by the presence of aliasing in the proximal coronary artery. Following MV surgery specifically, there are two scenarios that warrant particular attention. Firstly, where there has been no preservation of sub-valvar apparatus the LV dysfunction may appear disproportionately severe and require a high level of mechanical and inotropic support. Second, where there has been extensive surgery relating to the posterior annulus, there may result direct or indirect (from localised haematoma) disruption of the circumflex coronary artery, resulting in significant regional wall motion abnormality and LV failure. Prompt intervention to restore coronary flow is imperative.

Pulmonary hypertension is common in patients undergoing mitral valve surgery. Indeed, in patients with MS, pulmonary hypertension increases both the risk and benefits of surgical intervention. The pulmonary hypertension is often severe, and improves rapidly post-operatively, requiring no specific intervention where RV function and cardiac output are adequate. Diagnosis of RV failure in the post-operative state is relatively simple [19], and although it will normally recover over a period of 7–10 days, where RV failure is severe ICU mortality approaches 50%. Management of RV failure in the presence of pulmonary hypertension is limited to positive inotropy and reduction in afterload. However, where a fall in pulmonary arterial pressures is seen, care should be taken to ensure that this reflects a successful therapeutic intervention (i.e. cardiac function has improved and/or the pulmonary vascular resistance has decreased), rather than progressive RV failure. Although maintenance of an adequate preload is essential, the high central venous pressure required to maintain LV filling predisposes to the development of a 'tight pericardium' and here stenting the chest open may help. Paralysis, use of the lowest possible airway pressures whilst avoiding hypercapnia, aggressive treatment of bronchospasm, drainage of any pleural effusions and early extubation where possible can also improve RV function. Where RV failure occurs despite normal PA pressures, intra-aortic balloon counterpulsion or occasionally right ventricular assist device implantation may be necessary as a bridge to RV recovery.

18.6 Conclusions

Primary mitral valve disease requiring admission to the general ICU is relatively unusual. The intensive care physician should, however, be aware of the specific challenges that this patient population presents in terms of diagnosis, and also the treatment options available. Where operated, patients may require a high degree of post-operative support, and knowledge of specific complications (both general and valve-related) together with close surgical liaison are essential.

Case study

A 45-year-old man was transferred from his local ICU for management of acute respiratory distress syndrome (ARDS). His only past medical history was of mitral valve replacement for ruptured chordae 10 years previously, at which time he was noted to have significantly impaired left ventricular function. Regular medication included warfarin, lisinopril and frusemide.

He had visited his general practitioner 2 weeks previously complaining of a productive cough, and was started on broad-spectrum antibiotics. Despite this, he became increasingly unwell and was admitted to the local hospital 4 days later with pyrexia, hypotension, oliguria and confusion. On examination there were no stigmata of endocarditis, he was pyrexial (38.5), his pulse rate of 124 (SR) was of normal volume, character and waveform, the jugular venous waveform was normal, and recorded blood pressure was 80/40 mmHg. The apex of the heart was displaced downwards and to the left, and there was a palpable RV lift. On auscultation, normal mitral valve prosthetic heart sounds were associated with a soft pan-systolic murmur, and bilateral coarse inspiratory crackles were noted. Initial investigations revealed an elevated white cell count, C-reactive protein and a chest X-ray consistent with bilateral pneumonia. All blood and sputum cultures were negative. TOE was reported as showing good biventricular function and a normally functioning mitral valve prosthesis. The patient was treated with fluid resuscitation, pressor agents, intravenous antibiotics and non-invasive ventilation, but continued to deteriorate, requiring invasive mechanical ventilation.

After 10 days of treatment, he was apyrexial; however, his gas exchange remained poor (FiO_2 0.8, PO_2 7.2) and a diagnosis of ARDS was made.

Continued

Because of continued deterioration in arterial blood gases, he was transferred for management of lung injury.

Repeat trans-thoracic echocardiography demonstrated the LV to be dilated, with normalisation of septal motion (Figure 18.3) consistent with volume overload of the left heart. Aortic regurgitation was mild, with an end-diastolic velocity of 2.8 m/sec, consistent with an elevated LVEDP (Figure 18.4). The forward velocities of the mitral valve

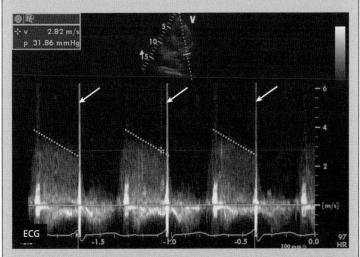

Figure 18.4 Continuous wave Doppler of aortic regurgitation showing end-diastolic velocity of 2.8 m/sec, consistent with an elevated LVEDP. Artefact from prosthetic mitral valve opening is arrowed.

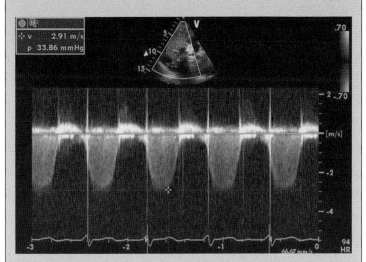

Figure 18.5 Continuous wave Doppler of tricuspid regurgitation demonstrating a peak velocity of 2.9 m/sec (pressure drop 34 mmHg). (See also colour plate 18.1).

Continued

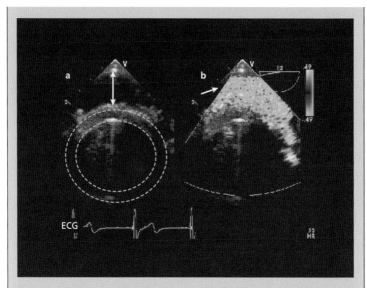

Figure 18.6 TOE (mid-oesophageal view) demonstrating severe paraprosthetic regurgitation. In the left side of the figure (**a**) outline of the valve leaflets (inner circle) and sewing ring (outer circle) are highlighted. Arrow indicates the space between the sewing ring and annulus. In the right side of the figure (**b**) colour Doppler demonstrates flow between the sewing ring and annulus in systole (arrowed). (See also colour plate 18.2).

prosthesis were higher than had been recorded previously on CW Doppler at 2.2 m/sec; however, no paraprosthetic regurgitation was seen on colour Doppler. Tricuspid regurgitation was mild, with a peak velocity of 2.9 m/sec, giving an estimated right ventricular systolic pressure (RVSP) of 40–45 mmHg (half systemic) (Figure 18.5).

As TTE features were all suggestive of a significant mitral regurgitation, TOE was performed and demonstrated a significant paraprosthetic leak (Figure 18.6).

The patient underwent redo-surgery, at which findings were consistent with endocarditis, with significant dehiscence of approximately 40% of the sewing ring from the annulus. The mitral valve was re-replaced, and after 2 weeks admission, the patient was discharged home to complete a full course of antibiotics.

Comment

Patients with previous mitral valve replacement or repair are at risk of endocarditis. Where significant mitral regurgitation resulting in pulmonary oedema ensues, the clinical features may mimic pneumonia.

The treating ICU physician and echocardiographer must be aware that the features of severe MR may be atypical in this patient population, and the echocardigoraphic features may not be typical of severe regurgitation. Where reversed septal motion is seen in a patient who has undergone previous MV surgery, there should be a high index of suspicion of valve malfunction, and TOE should be undertaken.

References

1. Jouan J, Tapia M, Cook R, et al. Ischemic mitral valve prolapse: mechanisms and implications for valve repair. *Eur J Cardiothorac Surg* 2004;26(6):1112–7.
2. Horstkotte D, Schulte HD, Niehues R, et al. Diagnostic and therapeutic considerations in acute, severe mitral regurgitation: experience in 42 consecutive patients entering the intensive care unit with pulmonary edema. *J Heart Valve Dis* 1993;2(5):512–22.
3. Dion R, Benetis R, Elias B, et al. Mitral valve procedures in ischemic regurgitation. *J Heart Valve Dis* 1995;4 Suppl 2:S124–9; discussion S129–31.
4. Bardet J, Masquet C, Kahn JC, et al. Clinical and hemodynamic results of intraortic balloon counterpulsation and surgery for cardiogenic shock. *Am Heart J* 1977;93(3):280–8.
5. Nishimura RA, Gersh BJ, Schaff HV. The case for an aggressive surgical approach to papillary muscle rupture following myocardial infarction: 'From paradise lost to paradise regained'. *Heart* 2000;83(6):611–3.
6. Chen Q, Darlymple-Hay MJ, Alexiou C, et al. Mitral valve surgery for acute papillary muscle rupture following myocardial infarction. *J Heart Valve Dis* 2002;11(1):27–31.
7. Tavakoli R, Weber A, Vogt P, et al. Surgical management of acute mitral valve regurgitation due to post-infarction papillary muscle rupture. *J Heart Valve Dis* 2002;11(1):20–5; discussion 26.
8. Shawl FA, Forman MB, Punja S, et al. Emergent coronary angioplasty in the treatment of acute ischemic mitral regurgitation: long-term results in five cases. *J Am Coll Cardiol* 1989;14(4):986–91.
9. Breithardt O, Sinha AM, Schwammenthal E, et al. Acute effects of cardiac resynchronisation therapy on functional mitral regurgitation in advanced systolic heart failure. *J Am Coll Cardiol* 2003;41:765–70.
10. Kindermann M, Frohlig G, Doerr T, et al. Optimizing the AV delay in DDD pacemaker patients with high degree AV block: mitral valve Doppler versus impedance cardiography. *Pacing Clin Electrophysiol* 1997;20:2453–62.
11. Sogaard P, Egeblad H, Pedersen AK, et al. Sequential versus simultaneous biventricular resynchronization for severe heart failure: evaluation by tissue Doppler imaging. *Circulation* 2002;106:2078–84.
12. Lokhandwala YY, Banker D, Vora AM, et al. Emergent balloon mitral valvotomy in patients presenting with cardiac arrest, cardiogenic shock or refractory pulmonary edema. *J Am Coll Cardiol* 1998;32(1):154–8.
13. Goldman JH, Slade A, Clague J. Cardiogenic shock secondary to mitral stenosis treated by balloon mitral valvuloplasty. *Cathet Cardiovasc Diagn* 1998;43(2):195–7.
14. Trehan VK, Nigam A, Mukhopadhyay S, et al. Bedside percutaneous transseptal mitral commissurotomy under sole transthoracic echocardiographic guidance in a critically ill patient. *Echocardiography* 2006;23(4):312–4.
15. Ward DE, Tanner MA. Percutaneous mitral commissurotomy using the metallic valvulotome technique in a critically ill adult. *Clin Cardiol* 2004;27(6):369–70.
16. Butchart EG, Gohlke-Bärwolf C, Antunes MJ, et al. Recommendations for the management of patients after heart valve surgery. *Eur Heart J* 2005;26(22):2463–71.
17. Kumar S, Garg N, Tewari S, et al. Role of thrombolytic therapy for stuck prosthetic valves: a serial echocardiographic study. *Indian Heart J* 2001;53(4):451–7.

18. Santé P, Renzulli A, Festa M, et al. Acute postoperative block of mechanical prostheses: incidence and treatment. *Cardiovasc Surg* 1994;2(3):403–6.
19. Carr-White GS, Kon M, Koh TW, et al. Right ventricular function after pulmonary autograft replacement of the aortic valve. *Circulation* 1999;100(19 Suppl):II36–41.

19 Aortic Valve Disease

Susanna Price and Derek Gibson

Royal Brompton & Harefield NHS Foundation Trust, London, UK

> **Take Home Messages**
>
> - In patients with aortic stenosis, it is preferable to avoid decompensation than to have to try to rescue the patient.
> - Critical aortic stenosis is a surgical disease – even when the patient is in extremis.
> - Catastrophic aortic regurgitation should not be managed expectantly.

19.1 Introduction

Minor forms of aortic valve disease are generally irrelevant to the intensive care unit (ICU) patient population, except where considering the need for antibiotic prophylaxis. However, when severe enough to warrant ICU admission, clinical features are often atypical. Moreover, more severe forms of aortic valve disease are important, as they will often impact significantly on the management of the patient. A striking example is critical aortic stenosis (AS), as the clinical manifestations are almost never improved by pharmacology, patients are unusually challenging to resuscitate when cardiac arrest occurs, and it may be relieved by one of the most effective operations in cardiac surgery – aortic valve replacement.

19.2 Aortic stenosis

Aetiology

The aetiology of aortic valve disease changes with patient age [1]. In patients less than 70 years of age AS is mainly associated with a congenitally bicuspid aortic valve, in contrast to patients more than 70 years, where degenerative aortic valve disease prevails [1, 2] (Figure 19.1a and b). In both patient populations, there may be sub-aortic stenosis that is equally

---

Cardiovascular Critical Care. Edited by M. Griffiths, J. Cordingley and S. Price.
© 2010 Blackwell Publishing Ltd.

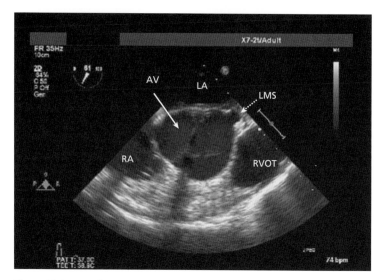

Figure 19.1a Two-dimensional trans-oesophageal echocardiography (mid-oesophageal view) in a young patient with bicuspid aortic valve disease. This demonstrates a short-axis view of a bicuspid aortic valve (AV), with the eccentric closure line indicated by the solid arrow. LA, left atrium; RA, right atrium; LMS, left main stem coronary artery (broken arrow); RVOT, right ventricular outflow tract.

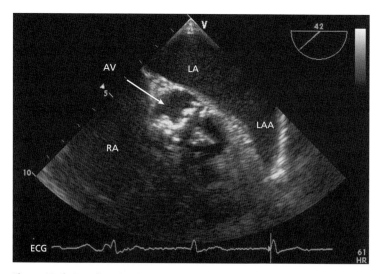

Figure 19.1b Two-dimensional trans-oesophageal echocardiography (short-axis, mid-oesophageal view) in an elderly patient with degenerative, calcific aortic valve disease. The extensive leaflet calcification is seen as bright, white echogenic areas. LA, left atrium; RA, right atrium; LAA, left atrial appendage; AV, aortic valve (arrowed); ECG, electrocardiogram.

or more important than the associated valvular stenosis. This includes the presence of a sub-aortic 'membrane' in patients with congenital heart disease (see Case study), and/or ventricular obstruction (either cavity or sub-aortic) in patients with severe left ventricular (LV) hypertrophy. Identification of these associated features may crucially affect patient management.

Associated manifestations and co-morbidity
Left ventricular disease
LV disease that occurs in association with AS is variable, may be severe and ranges from dilatation to hypertrophy (Figures 19.2a and b). In patients with LV dilatation, it may be indistinguishable from that seen in dilated cardiomyopathy (DCM). Indeed, the patient may even be erroneously diagnosed as DCM with clinically unimportant AS. LV hypertrophy (LVH) has a variable relationship to the severity of AS, and may also be severe, even mimicking hypertrophic cardiomyopathy. LVH presents particular challenges to the intensivist as patients tolerate atrial fibrillation and hypotension very poorly, and the LV readily becomes ischaemic when inotropic agents are used.

Co-morbidity
In the elderly with AS, coronary artery disease co-exists in up to 30–50% of patients [3–5]. This may contribute to the patient's symptoms by exacerbating the mismatch between myocardial oxygen delivery and consumption, and is clinically indistinguishable from ischaemia due to severe LVH alone. Where significant coronary artery disease co-exists, resultant ongoing ischaemia may exacerbate LV dysfunction and lead to overestimation of its severity.

Respiratory disease is also relatively common in elderly patients and may co-exist with aortic stenosis. In patients with severe emphysema, dyspnoea as a result of pulmonary disease may limit exercise tolerance, thus protecting them from the more malignant symptoms of critical AS. In contrast, where chronic pulmonary oedema is present as a result of critical AS, pulmonary function tests may be affected by chronic pulmonary venous congestion or remodelling of the alveolar-capillary membrane, and should not preclude surgery *per se*.

Indications for ICU admission
Patients with severe AS may be admitted to the ICU either as a result of haemodynamic instability, or with AS as an incidental but important finding, or following valve replacement.

AS resulting in ICU admission is usually critical, and often previously undiagnosed owing to the insidious onset of symptoms [6]. Low cardiac output may be related to many factors including late or mis-diagnosis, onset of arrhythmia (atrial fibrillation/flutter, ventricular tachycardia, resuscitated ventricular fibrillation) or myocardial infarction (with disproportionately severe heart failure). The other important clinical presentations include the syncopal elderly patient, who may present with

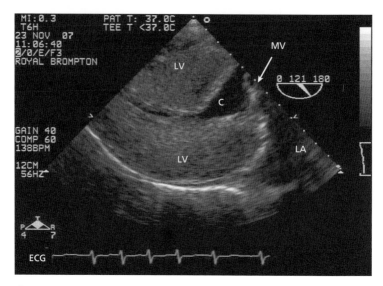

Figure 19.2a Two-dimensional trans-oesophageal echocardiography (long-axis, transgastric view) in a patient with severe left ventricular hypertrophy undergoing aortic valve replacement. The markers to the right of the image indicate 1-cm divisions. LV, left ventricular walls; C, left ventricular cavity; MV, mitral valve leaflets (arrowed); LA, left atrium; ECG, electrocardiogram.

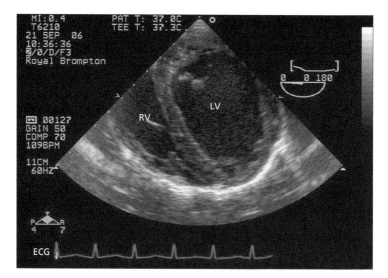

Figure 19.2b Two-dimensional trans-oesophageal echocardiography (short-axis, transgastric view) in a patient with severe left ventricular dilatation undergoing aortic valve replacement. Note the marked contrast in wall thickness when compared with the patient shown in Figure 19.2a. Both patients had aortic valve stenosis of the same severity. LV, left ventricle; RV, right ventricle; ECG, electrocardiogram.

head injury or trauma as a result of their collapse, and the pregnant patient with congenital AS. With an ageing population, the incidence of significant AS is increasing [2]. When these patients are admitted to the ICU for other indications, 'incidental' but important AS may be diagnosed, which will significantly alter patient management.

Diagnosis
The diagnosis of AS (as with other valve disease) in the ICU may be challenging. However, the ICU physician should have a high index of suspicion particularly in the elderly patient. Diagnosis relies upon history, examination and echocardiography.

History
The history obtained from the patient or relative will typically include dyspnoea, syncope and/or chest pain (+/– a history of murmur). At the extremes of age, symptoms are often well tolerated and either not noticed (adolescent/young adults) or attributed to the normal process of ageing.

Clinical findings
The clinical findings of AS include an audible, highly characteristic, long systolic murmur in the second left intercostal space. Once recognised, its presence alone suggests severe AS, requiring confirmation by echocardiography. Less clinically robust features include a slow rising pulse and a soft A2 heart sound. These findings may be either present or absent depending upon the cardiac output (CO) at the time of examination, making diagnosis in ICU particularly challenging. First, the intensity of individual heart sounds is notoriously difficult to assess in the relatively noisy environment of the ICU. Second, in order to achieve a pulse that is palpably slow rising, the CO must be adequate. Third, although the murmur of critical AS is characteristic, when the CO falls, this may be inaudible. In practical terms:
- In the presence of an adequate CO, if there is an audible AS murmur, concern should be raised. Subsequently, if the pulse is slow rising, and the patient is appropriately symptomatic, the patient should be regarded as having significant AS. If the murmur is audible but there are no other features, the patient may have moderate AS, and this should be excluded using echocardiography.
- If the CO is low and the patient shocked, the absence of any or all of these clinical signs does not exclude critical AS. The question can be simply settled by echocardiography.

Echocardiography
When AS is suspected or the patient is in a low CO state an urgent echocardiogram (either trans-thoracic or trans-oesophageal) should be performed. The features noted will include: aortic valve calcification and leaflet mobility, severity of stenosis, left ventricular function, right heart function and other significant valvular pathology.

Level of obstruction

Echocardiography will demonstrate the level and aetiology of obstruction (see Case study). Of particular relevance to intensivists is the sub-population of elderly patients (usually female) who may have high velocities across the left ventricular outflow tract whilst in the ICU, related not to critical AS, but to the presence of a small underfilled LV, with obstruction due to either LV cavity obliteration and/or systolic anterior motion (SAM) of the mitral valve. In these patients treatment should be directed towards ensuring adequate LV filling, reduction in inotropic support and beta-blockade if possible.

Severity of stenosis

According to international guidelines, the severity of AS is graded according to either the peak velocity across the valve and/or the aortic valve area (AVA) measured by the continuity equation [4–7]. With normal LV function, standard guidelines apply; however, when the LV is impaired both the peak velocity and AVA may underestimate the severity of stenosis. A more useful measure of severity is therefore the ratio of peak sub-aortic velocity and peak velocity across the valve (Figure 19.3). In practice, where doubt exists, if the peak velocity is < 3 m/sec and the aortic valve appears immobile and heavily calcified, AS should be regarded as important. Formal stress echocardiography (or even the fortuitous observation of the gradient at a post-ectopic beat) may clarify the diagnosis.

Associated features

Echocardiographic assessment of LV function and hypertrophy should be performed as standard, but on the ICU one must take into account the level of inotropic support. In particular, the long axis function of the LV may be markedly in-coordinate, even with a well-preserved ejection fraction, and may suggest additional ischaemia, particularly when the patient has LVH, is hypotensive or is on a high level of inotropic support. Associated features that increase the patient's operative risk include impaired right ventricular function, elevated pulmonary artery pressure and resistance, and additional significant valvular pathology.

Management
AS as the primary indication for ICU admission

AS is a mechanical disease, for which there is a mechanical solution. Usually (unless there is an overriding contraindication) the patient with critical AS requiring ICU admission will need aortic valve replacement (AVR) [4, 5]. If, however, the patient is not a candidate for surgical or percutaneous valve replacement, the prognosis is extremely poor. In this small number of patients, palliative care is appropriate. Whilst awaiting surgery the ICU patient with critical AS and cardiovascular collapse requires careful haemodynamic support. The consequences of severe AS result from an imbalance of oxygen supply and demand, raised ventricular diastolic pressures and an inability to increase CO to the level required. Patients with severe AS can deteriorate rapidly, so fast decision-making is necessary.

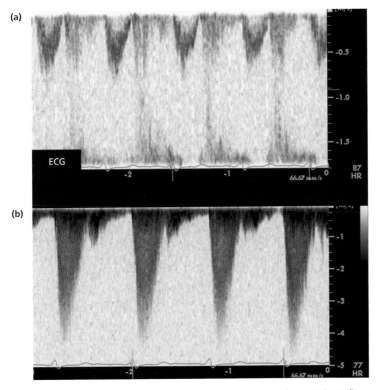

Figure 19.3 Doppler echocardiography showing step-up across the left ventricular outflow tract and aortic valve in a patient with significant aortic stenosis when comparing pulse wave (**a**) and continuous wave (**b**) Doppler. On the x axis is time, with systolic flow (away from the ventricle, towards the ascending aorta) shown below the line. In (**a**) (pulsed wave Doppler) peak velocity is 0.5 m/sec, representing the velocity of blood below the aortic valve. In (**b**) (continuous wave Doppler) this has increased to > 4 m/sec, representing severe aortic stenosis. ECG, electrocardiogram.

Supportive therapy

All patients will require standard invasive monitoring, and in addition either pulmonary artery catheterisation or echocardiographic monitoring to determine the effects of therapeutic manoeuvres (Chapter 3). Patients with critical AS that has resulted in ICU admission are at risk when given any drug that may cause systemic vasodilatation, and this should be avoided if possible, with potentially some exceptions [8]. In general, inotropic agents worsen the imbalance between myocardial oxygen supply and demand, and this is further aggravated in the presence of severe LVH. The resultant LV ischaemia may worsen CO, an effect that is further exacerbated in the presence of co-existing coronary artery disease, in which case, insertion of an intra-aortic balloon pump (IABP) may be helpful. There are three clinical scenarios where the balance may be in favour of inotropic/inodilator usage: hypotension, severely elevated systemic vascular resistance, and during tracheal intubation and mechanical ventilation.

Hypotension in severe AS is poorly tolerated, particularly in the patient with significant LVH, as coronary artery perfusion is severely compromised. Here, inotropic and/or pressor agents may be required to increase the mean arterial pressure to ensure adequate end-organ perfusion, and diastolic pressure to ensure adequate coronary perfusion. In the presence of a very high systemic vascular resistance inodilators/dilators may be used, but with great caution due to the potential for hypotension and fall in afterload [8]. Finally, if the patient requires sedation and ventilation for pulmonary oedema on the ICU, this should be performed by a senior cardiothoracic anaesthetist where possible. Unnecessary vasodilatation and radical changes in heart rate should be avoided, and where possible vascular access with invasive monitoring obtained prior to induction. On occasion, rescue cardiopulmonary bypass may be required. In addition to the general measures described, other factors that should be considered include exclusion of coronary artery disease and avoidance of arrhythmias (including careful electrolyte control and early institution of intravenous amiodarone therapy).

AS as an 'incidental' finding
Requiring emergency non-cardiac surgery
Critical AS is major risk factor for any GA other than AVR [9]. In general, if the patient needs emergency surgery, anaesthesia should be undertaken by the most senior cardiac anaesthetist available, with full invasive monitoring, and if possible with TOE guidance; hypotension is poorly tolerated in such patients as it may rapidly result in irreversible cardiac arrest. The patient with critical AS is therefore not suitable for spinal or epidural anaesthesia owing to the potential for sudden loss of vasomotor tone. In addition, the surgeon undertaking such an emergency procedure must be made aware of this, as requests for periods of controlled hypotension may prove impossible. If significant LV disease is present or coronary artery disease suspected, elective insertion of an IABP may be indicated. Minimally invasive (trans-apical/trans-femoral) AVR performed at short notice will become available in the near future, and may change significantly the management of such patients.

Medical/surgical ICU admission not requiring surgery
In the presence of severe AS, when the patient is progressing adequately, the ICU physician should continue to move the patient forward, but cautiously, particularly if the patient has had previous syncope or pulmonary oedema. Once the patient is well enough, however, early AVR should be considered. Where the patient is not progressing due to limited CO, pulmonary oedema or life-threatening arrhythmias, urgent AVR should be considered.

19.3 Aortic regurgitation

Unlike AS, aortic regurgitation (AR) is generally well tolerated unless it is very severe or of sudden onset into a hypertrophied ventricle. The clinical consequences of severe AR relate to changes in coronary artery flow, left ventricular size and function, and the conducting system [4, 5].

Severe AR: indications for ICU admission

AR as a primary indication for ICU admission due to haemodynamic instability is likely to be 'ultra' severe (effectively an absent aortic valve), occurring as a result of endocarditis (Chapter 20), dissection (Chapter 22) or sudden failure of a prosthetic valve. Endocarditis and aortic dissection, unlike prosthetic AVR failure, may result in ICU admission for less severe AR.

Diagnosis

Review of the history may suggest the underlying cause for severe AR. The management will depend in some cases purely on the severity of AR (catastrophic prosthesis failure) and in others on the underlying condition (dissection, endocarditis). In all cases with severe AR, initial management will include valve replacement or resuspension, unless surgery is contraindicated. In these rare cases, the prognosis is grave. Where a patient is being managed on the ward for infective endocarditis of the aortic valve, sudden deterioration requiring ICU admission should raise the suspicion of formation of a fistula, complete heart block or myocardial infarction secondary to coronary embolism.

Clinical features

The major clinical feature suggesting a patient with a low cardiac output has catastrophic AR is the finding of a normal volume pulse in a tachycardic, shocked patient. When the patient is in extremis, however, the pulse volume will be reduced. Other classical findings may also mislead, as the pulse may not be collapsing and the early diastolic murmur may be absent (due to a very short murmur and diastolic time). Patients may have an S3 (associated with premature mitral valve closure) and pulmonary oedema. Additional clinical features relate to the underlying aetiology, for example the unequal pulses in dissection and peripheral stigmata of endocarditis. When a previously haemodynamically stable patient undergoing treatment for aortic valve endocarditis suddenly deteriorates, additional clinical features should be sought (Table 19.1).

Echocardiography

All patients with AR resulting in ICU admission must undergo urgent echocardiography – either TTE or TOE. The choice of imaging will depend upon the underlying aetiology, patient status, echogenicity and local expertise. Important echocardiographic features suggestive of catastrophic AR include: demonstration of an active left ventricle, premature closure of the mitral valve on M-mode echocardiography and a low regurgitant end-diastolic velocity (Figure 19.4). These findings are explained by the underlying pathophysiology and are important, as their appearance is associated with increased operative mortality.

Coronary artery perfusion occurs during diastole, and is supported by the diastolic pressure difference between the aortic root and the left

Table 19.1 Important signs in severe aortic regurgutation secondary to infective endocarditis.

Severe AR	Fistula – right heart	CHB	Fistula – left heart
Cardiogenic shock + normal volume pulse	Sudden elevation of central venous pressure	Abrupt fall in heart rate	Sudden pulmonary oedema
Pulmonary oedema S3 Duroisier's sign +ve	Continuous murmur*	Worsening of AR	Continuous murmur*

AR, aortic regurgitation; CHB, complete heart block; S3, third heart sound.
*Continuous murmur may be difficult to differentiate from the combination of mitral regurgitation plus aortic regurgitation.

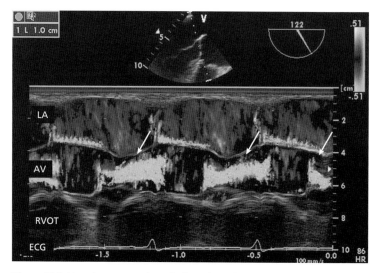

Figure 19.4 M-mode trans-oesophageal echocardiography (mid-oesophageal, left ventricular outflow tract view) in a patient with severe aortic valve endocarditis. Here, the colour jet represents blood flow back into the left ventricle during diastole (arrowed), and is 10 mm in depth, representing severe aortic regurgitation. For reference, a two-dimensional picture is shown at the top of the image. LA, left atrium; AV, aortic valve; RVOT, right ventricular outflow tract; ECG, electrocardiogram. (See also colour plate 19.1).

ventricle. Thus, when end-diastolic AR velocity is less than 2 m/sec (16 mmHg), AR is severe and coronary artery perfusion likely to be compromised. This, combined with increased LV work and the prolongation of systole (by up to 30%), further limits the diastolic time available for coronary flow. Premature AV opening implies aortic and LV pressures have equilibrated at end-diastole, and there is very low pressure supporting coronary artery flow. In extreme cases, the MR may be pre-systolic – again due to very high left ventricular diastolic pressures.

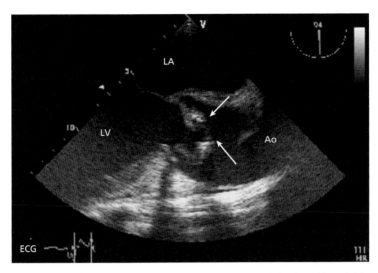

Figure 19.5 Two-dimensional trans-oesophageal echocardiography (mid-oesophageal, left ventricular outflow tract view) in a patient with severe aortic valve endocarditis undergoing aortic valve and root replacement. The valve leaflets are thickened, with excessive tissue due to vegetations (arrowed). LA, left atrium; LV, left ventricle; Ao, ascending aorta; ECG, electrocardiogram.

Pre-operative coronary arteriography

This is often indicated by the age of the patient [3–5]. However, when severe AR occurs due to infective endocarditis, the risks of vegetation embolisation during catheter manipulation may outweigh the potential benefits (Figure 19.5). In general, in the presence of severe AR, where there is active LV function and no evidence of myocardial ischaemia, it is unlikely the patient has significant coronary artery disease. Each patient must, however, be managed on an individual basis.

Management of severe AR

Unlike regurgitation of any other valve, AR directly compromises coronary flow at the same time as it increases myocardial oxygen demand. The more severe the AR, the more significant the reduction in coronary artery flow, and the worse the patient outcome. Indeed, once premature closure of the MV is identified, performance of emergency surgery reduces mortality from 80 to 20%. Hence, where catastrophic AR is diagnosed, urgent referral to a cardiothoracic surgeon is crucial, even if the patient's condition is sub-optimal.

Pharmacological support of severe AR

Similar to severe AS, there is little pharmacological support that is helpful. In general, vasodilatation may worsen the situation by causing coronary steal, and pressor agents increase AR as a result of the increase in afterload. If the patient has previously been taking beta-blockers, and as a result has significant bradycardia (once CHB has been excluded) atropine may be used to increase heart rate and thereby reduce the duration of regurgitation. Aminophylline and milrinone have also been used in this situation with good effect; however, in catastrophic AR, isoprenaline may worsen haemodynamic instability.

Aortic root abscess

In a patient with aortic valve endocarditis, aortic root abscess should be assumed to be present until proven otherwise by TOE. Features suggestive of aortic root abscess include increasing PT interval, broadening of the QRS axis and a change in the heart axis on 12-lead ECG. These patients are at risk of sudden progression to a high grade AV block. If the patient develops these changes and surgery is not imminent a temporary transvenous pacing wire must be inserted. With the diagnosis of aortic root abscess, urgent surgical consultation is indicated.

Moderate AR

Moderate AR is generally well tolerated. Clinical features and echocardiographic findings are usually characteristic. The major concern for the ICU clinician is to avoid the AV becoming infected as it is at relatively higher risk for development of infective endocarditis. When the underlying condition requiring ICU admission has resulted in sub-optimal haemodynamics, management should include avoidance of bradycardia and reduction in afterload whilst maintaining diastolic blood pressure to ensure adequate coronary perfusion pressure. If, however, the patient becomes haemodynamically unstable, and this is not due to deterioration in the underlying condition, the AR may be more severe than previously thought and should be re-evaluated by echocardiography.

19.4 Aortic valve replacement

With an increasingly elderly population, more patients will present to the ICU having previously undergone AVR. These patients may be admitted either with AVR as an incidental clinical complication or directly as a result of valve failure or infection [10–12]. In addition, in cardiothoracic centres, a large number of patients will be admitted to the ICU for their immediate post-operative management.

Patients with previous AVR

Where the aortic prosthesis is functioning well, ICU physicians must ensure that scrupulous asepsis is observed with all vascular cannulation (central or peripheral), and indwelling lines and catheters are removed as soon as possible. Although the risk of infective endocarditis is small, indwelling lines are a recognised risk factor, and all intensivists should be vigilant, particularly with patients with mechanical prostheses, where the risk of infection is possibly higher [10–12]. In such patients, oral anticoagulation may only be interrupted for short periods without substituting therapeutic doses of heparin.

Where the aortic prosthesis is not functioning normally, urgent, expert echocardiography should be performed. The diagnosis of 'heart failure' in a patient with any valvular prosthesis must always be assumed to be prosthesis malfunction until proven otherwise. The commonest cause for valve dysfunction after bioprosthetic valve degeneration (either regurgitation or stenosis, and mechanical or bioprosthetic valves) is infection. Thus, where a patient is admitted to a general ICU with haemodynamic instability and an AVR in situ, the ICU physician should discuss the case with a cardiothoracic centre.

Mechanical prosthetic AVR malfunction

All mechanical prosthetic valves have a degree of regurgitation related to the normal functioning of the valve (wash jets) designed to avoid thrombus developing and causing valve malfunction. Thus, a minor degree of regurgitation between the leaflets is normal. The wash jets of each type of AVR are characteristic and easily identified by echocardiographers. If haemodynamically significant regurgitation is detected, this implies dehiscence of the sewing ring, and infection should be suspected until proven otherwise. Urgent TOE should be performed and commonly demonstrates paraprosthetic regurgitation, but vegetations are not usually seen (Figure 19.6). These patients should have haemodynamic management appropriate for the severity of their AR. However, as they

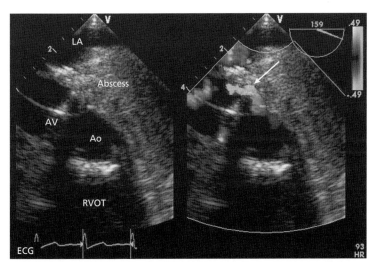

Figure 19.6 Two-dimensional trans-oesophageal echocardiography (mid-oesophageal, left ventricular outflow tract view) in a patient with previous St Jude aortic valve replacement and an aortic root abscess. Note the small paraprosthetic jet (arrowed in the figure on the right) and the absence of vegetations on the valve. At operation the abscess was found to extend to the level of the pulmonary artery bifurcation, providing the only continuity between the ascending aorta above this level and the aortic root. LA, left atrium; AV, aortic valve; Ao, ascending aorta; RVOT, right ventricular outflow tract; ECG, electrocardiogram. (See also colour plate 19.2).

are at risk of complete dehiscence with valve embolisation, they should be regarded as a surgical emergency, even if the regurgitation is only moderate.

All mechanical valves have a degree of stenosis that is not usually haemodynamically significant. When a patient develops AS related to mechanical valve malfunction, this is usually chronic and due to pannus, a combination of fibrosis and thrombosis. This is likely to be sterile and can be readily detected using TOE. In patients with significant AS as a result of prosthetic valve malfunction, prompt surgical referral is indicated.

Bioprosthetic AVR malfunction

In contrast to mechanical valve prostheses, severe regurgitation and stenosis in bioprosthetic AVRs relate more frequently to the natural lifetime of the valve, and infective endocarditis is less common.

When severe AR is seen this is usually through the valve leaflets as a result of cusp rupture or perforation. If AVR was performed for AS, and in the presence of a small, stiff LV, this regurgitation is tolerated poorly, and the patient may present with severe pulmonary oedema. Patients with previous bioprosthetic AVR should have close follow-up in outpatients and early signs of valve degeneration should prompt surgical referral, thus avoiding emergency admission for severe regurgitation. In parallel, where a patient with moderate AR through a bioprosthetic AVR is admitted to the ICU for other reasons, this AR differs from native AR and should not be ignored. Discussion with the responsible surgeon is required, with a plan for early surgery. Although infective endocarditis on a bioprosthetic AVR is less common than with mechanical valves, it does occur. In these cases, TOE may demonstrate vegetations with or without valve leaflet destruction, and paraprosthetic regurgitation is much less usual.

As with mechanical AVR, most bioprosthetic AVRs have a minor degree of stenosis. Once the valve starts to degenerate, however, leaflet calcification may increase the degree of stenosis rapidly. It is unusual for such patients to develop AS to a degree that necessitates ICU admission. Once AS is recognised, as with bioprosthetic AV regurgitation, surgical referral is indicated.

19.5 Management of the patient immediately post AVR

Post-operatively, the cardiovascular factors specific to AVR that influence patient progression generally relate to the underlying ventricular disease rather than the valve replacement itself. It is difficult to predict pre-operatively how the LV will respond to the change in afterload following AVR for AS. Certain features render patient populations at risk for significant haemodynamic instability post-operatively:

- Severe LV systolic dysfunction
- Extensive calcification
- Significant pulmonary hypertension and right ventricular dysfunction
- Small volume, hypertrophied and restrictive LV, with slow wall thinning in diastole.

Severe LV systolic dysfunction pre-operatively may be improved, unchanged or worsened post bypass. ICU management may include the use of multiple inotropic agents, IABP, ventricular assist devices and advanced pacing (single/dual chamber or multi-site). Where possible, pacing should be optimised using echocardiography.

AS may be associated with extensive calcification (ascending aorta, aortic root, inter-ventricular septum, anterior mitral valve leaflet). Acute heart block is common and indicates the placement and maintenance of epicardial pacing wires, including daily recording of the ventricular wire thresholds. In patients with an inadequate underlying rhythm/rate, some centres insert a temporary transvenous ventricular pacing wire as further backup. If a complete heart block (CHB) lasts for > 24 hours or appears after this time, the integrity of the conducting system must be questioned with an electrophysiologist, as permanent pacemaker insertion may be indicated.

Significant pulmonary hypertension is not uncommon in AS, and the pressures do not normalise immediately upon replacing the aortic valve. Where this co-exists with RV dysfunction, post-operatively the patient may require significant support. Further, these patients tolerate even small collections in the pericardial space poorly. Where haemodynamic instability occurs, TOE should be performed with a low threshold for re-exploration.

The function of a small, hypertrophied LV may also be worsened post bypass due to deficiencies in myocardial protection, a sudden reduction in afterload or smaller ventricular size. By contrast the LV may be restrictive, with a short filling time. Such patients tolerate bradycardia poorly and pacing (optimised using echocardiography) may be indicated with rates of up to 130 bpm. Inotropes used to support systolic function may induce myocardial ischaemia or cause a left ventricular outflow tract obstruction (LVOTO) and worsen any mitral regurgitation. The most challenging patient population also have significant RV dysfunction. Here, supporting the RV with inotropes may cause significant LVOTO and lower cardiac output and echo guidance is essential to monitor the effects of inotropes, dilators, pressors, pulmonary artery dilators and to optimise the patient's haemodynamic status. Although these patients generally require rapid pacing, extreme tachycardia is detrimental and atrial fibrillation tolerated very poorly. Amiodarone may be used if the patient is considered high risk of post-operative AF, and where persistent and the rate cannot be controlled pharmacologically, early discussion with an electrophysiologist is important.

19.6 Conclusion

Management of patients with aortic valve disease, like so much of ICU practice, depends on identification of risk, understanding of physiological disturbances and balancing of priorities. All cases are different and it is unlikely that decisions regarding ICU management will ever be made on the basis of large randomised trials. The potential benefits of optimal management on outcome are particularly large in this group of patients.

Case study

A 76-year-old man was admitted for elective aortic valve replacement for AS. Pre-operative echocardiography demonstrated severe AS (gradient 120 mmHg peak), mild AR, significant left ventricular dysfunction and moderate TR due to permanent pacing wires, associated with secondary severe right ventricular dysfunction. Pulmonary artery systolic pressure was estimated at two-thirds systemic. Additional co-morbidity included mild chronic obstructive pulmonary disease from previous smoking, and significant renal impairment.

Surgery was uneventful (23 mm perimount AVR) and the patient was successfully weaned from cardiopulmonary bypass on noradrenaline 0.02 µg/kg/min, milrinone 0.4 µg/kg/min and dual chamber pacing.

Over subsequent hours the patient was stable; however, the following day he developed progressive hypotension, oliguria and a low cardiac output state, requiring increasing inotropic support. TOE demonstrated severe right ventricular dysfunction, dynamic LVOTO (Figure 19.7) and evidence of global left ventricular ischaemia. In order to minimise LVOTO, milrinone was reduced to 0.2 µg/kg/min, the patient filled and pressor dosage increased (noradrenaline 0.18 µg/mg/min). An intra-aortic balloon pump was inserted. In order to support the right ventricle, the patient was started on inhaled nitric oxide (15 ppm).

Continued

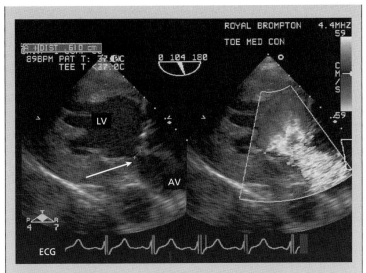

Figure 19.7 Two-dimensional trans-oesophageal echocardiography (trans-gastric left ventricular outflow tract view) in a patient with bicuspid aortic valve and sub-aortic stenosis (arrowed). In the figure on the right, colour Doppler reveals flow acceleration and aliasing of the colour jet, indicating high velocity blood flow due to the sub-aortic membrane. LV, left ventricle; AV, aortic valve; ECG, electrocardiogram. (See also colour plate 19.3).

The infusion rate of pressors and inodilators was adjusted using concurrent cardiac output monitoring and TOE in order to minimise the dynamic LVOTO, whilst maintaining optimal right ventricular support.

References

1. Rapaport E. Natural history of aortic and mitral valve disease. *Am J Cardiol* 1975; 35(2): 221–7.
2. Cowell S, Newby DE, Boon NA, et al. Calcific aortic stenosis: same old story? *Age Ageing* 2004; 33: 538–544.
3. Morrison GW, Thomas RD, Grimmer SF, et al. Incidence of coronary artery disease in patients with valvular heart disease. *Br Heart J* 1980; 44(6): 630–7.
4. Bonow RO, Carabello BA, Chatterjee K, et al. ACC/AHA 2006 guidelines for the management of patients with valvular heart disease: a report of the American College of Cardiology/American Heart Association Task Force on Practice Guidelines. *Circulation* 2006; 114(5): e84–231.
5. Vahanian A, Baumgartner H, Bax J, et al. Guidelines on the management of valvular heart disease: the Task Force on the Management of Valvular Heart Disease of the European Society of Cardiology. *Eur Heart J* 2007; 28(2): 230–68.
6. Chambers J. Low 'gradient', low flow aortic stenosis. *Heart* 2006; 92(4): 554–8.
7. Fiegenbaum FH, Armstrong WF. *Fiegenbaum's Echocardiography*, 6th edn. Lippincott Williams & Wilkins, Philadelphia.

8. Umesh N, Khot MD, Gian M, et al. Nitroprusside in critically ill patients with left ventricular dysfunction and aortic stenosis. *New Engl J Med* 2003; 348: 1756–63.

9. Christ M, Sharkova Y, Geldner G, et al. Preoperative and perioperative care for patients with suspected or established aortic stenosis facing noncardiac surgery. *Chest* 2005; 128: 2944–53.

10. Nishimura RA, Carabello BA, Faxon DP, et al. ACC/AHA 2008 guideline update on valvular heart disease: focused update on infective endocarditis. *J Am Coll Cardiol* 2008; 52: 676–85.

11. Horstkotte D, Follath F, Gutschik E, et al. Guidelines on prevention, diagnosis and treatment of infective endocarditis. *Eur Heart J* 2004; 25(3): 267–76.

12. NICE Short Clinical Guidelines Technical Team. *Prophylaxis Against Infective Endocarditis: Antimicrobial Prophylaxis Against Infective Endocarditis in Adults and Children Undergoing Interventional Procedures.* National Institute for Health and Clinical Excellence, London. 2008.

20 Infective Endocarditis

David Hunter and John Pepper

Royal Brompton & Harefield NHS Foundation Trust, London, UK

Take Home Messages

- Infective endocarditis (IE) has a high mortality and morbidity.
- Fifty percent of patients suffer a serious complication: heart failure, stroke or paravalvular abscess.
- Take blood cultures before starting antibiotics.
- Twenty-five percent of patients with hospital-acquired *Staphylococcus aureus* bacteraemia will have evidence of IE.
- Involve a microbiologist and cardiac surgeon at an early stage.
- Use transthoracic echocardiography (TTE) and transoesophageal echocardiography (TOE) to exclude vegetations, abscess or fistulae.
- Examine the patient daily and stay vigilant.

20.1 Introduction

Infective endocarditis (IE) is a lethal disease if untreated. It accounts for up to 1% of all severe hospital sepsis and despite advances in diagnostic and treatment methods, hospital mortality is still up to 33% [1]. The incidence of IE has remained static over the last 30 years at 3–4 per 100,000 per year, increasing with age and peaking at more than 15 per 100,000 for those aged over 65 years [2]. This static incidence of IE and the increase in prevalence with age in spite of medical advances has been attributed to the reduction in developed countries of rheumatic heart disease, increased intravenous drug use, an ageing population with degenerative valvular disease, increasing numbers of patients with intravascular prostheses, increasing exposure to nosocomial disease and more haemodialysis patients [3]. Previous emphasis on antibiotic prophylaxis for dental procedures to reduce IE incidence has now changed. Current thinking is that more cases of IE are related to other types of medical procedures than are related to dental work [3]. The changing epidemiology and microbiology of the disease places demands on the critical care team to maintain a high index of suspicion for

---

Cardiovascular Critical Care. Edited by M. Griffiths, J. Cordingley and S. Price.
© 2010 Blackwell Publishing Ltd.

IE in susceptible patients; especially those with catheter or IV line-based bacteraemia, diabetes mellitus, human immunodefiency virus (HIV), immunosuppressive treatment and prosthetic valves or other intravascular devices.

20.2 Definition and incidence

IE is an endovascular microbial infection of cardiovascular structures frequently occurring at areas of damaged endothelium caused by turbulent flow or foreign bodies. These may occur within the heart or as an endarteritis of large intrathoracic vessels. Common sites of IE include: native valve tips, prosthetic valve rings (particularly if associated with para-prosthetic leak), patent ductus arteriosus, coarctation of the aorta, ventriculo-septal defect, and other surgically formed intra- and extra-cardiac shunts. Whilst strictly speaking infection associated with pacing wires, or lines placed in the heart but not connected to endocardial structures, should not be termed IE, for all diagnostic and therapeutic purposes they are considered as such.

IE is not a reportable disease and this hampers collection of accurate figures for its incidence. In one unpublished but reported review of 26 publications published between 1993 and 2003 the median incidence of IE was 3.6 per 100,000 per year (range 0.3 to 22.4). The male to female ratio was about 2:1, and the median in-hospital mortality rate was 16% (range 11–26%). The mean age of patients varied between 36 and 69 years and the incidence increased with age [2]. The incidence of IE in children is very low in countries where there is little rheumatic fever.

20.3 Pathogenesis

The endothelial lining of the heart and valves is usually resistant to bacterial or fungal infection. Endocarditis arises from a complex interaction between the host (vascular endothelium, immune system, haemostatic mechanisms, cardiac anatomy) and the invading microorganisms (enzyme and toxin production) and the peripheral events that have caused the bacteraemia. Animal studies suggest that endothelial damage appears to be the initial event, followed by platelet-fibrin deposition which provides a milieu for bacterial colonisation. Endothelial damage may be either mechanical or inflammatory. Valve inflammation can arise in several clinically silent situations; up to 25% of patients aged > 40 years have degenerative valve lesions that harbour micro-ulcerations and local inflammation, resembling arteriosclerosis [4].

The likelihood that endothelial damage is the inciting event is also demonstrated by the observation that the areas of vegetation formation are similar to those where blood flow injury is most likely to occur: on the ventricular side of semilunar valves and the atrial side of atrio-ventricular valves. Jet lesions may also damage endothelium and vegetations may form on such sites of injury, for example, the anterior mitral leaflet in aortic regurgitation, the atrial wall in mitral regurgitation and the septal leaflet of the tricuspid in a ventriculo-septal defect (VSD). This endothelial damage creates a predisposition for deposition of platelets and fibrin on the surface of the endothelium, which results in the formation of non-bacterial thrombotic endocarditis (NBTE), previously termed marantic endocarditis. This, followed by an episode of bacteraemia, allows adherence of the bacteria in the bloodstream to the NBTE and their subsequent proliferation.

Endothelial adhesion molecules are recognised by surface components of certain bacteria. For example, streptococci that produce surface glycans and dextran appear to be more likely to cause IE than those that do not [5]. Endothelial cells, fibroblasts and platelets at the site of endothelial injury produce fibronectin that enhances adherence of microorganism to the vegetation. Receptors for fibronectin and adhesion molecules have been described on the surface of *Staph. aureus*, *Streptococuss viridans*, *Strep. pneumoniae* and *Candida albicans*. Bound fibronectin acts as a bridging molecule towards host cell integrins, which in turn initialise the uptake process that leads to streptococcal internalisation. Once inside the cell, the streptococci can persist, protected from antibiotics and host defence [5]. Similarly, staphylococci and streptococci that bind to platelets and stimulate the clotting cascade appear more virulent than other organisms that are simply shed into the bloodstream [6]. The invasion of the endothelium that occurs with infection disrupts the endothelial surface, further promoting platelet-fibrin deposits. Extremely high concentrations of bacteria (10^9 to 10^{11} bacteria per gram of tissue) may accumulate within the vegetation. Interestingly, *Staph. aureus* may also induce tissue factor production by endothelial cells, which may partially explain why this organism can adhere to relatively normal valves.

This cycle of adherence, organism growth and platelet-fibrin deposition repeats itself many times as the vegetation enlarges. Attempts have been made to interfere with this binding process; in order to prevent organisms from binding to the prosthetic valve ring, a silver-coated polyester ring was developed and subjected to clinical trials. Unfortunately concerns regarding increased peri-valvular leak and emboli led to its withdrawal in 2000 [7].

Following treatment, capillaries and fibroblasts may appear in the vegetation, but untreated, the lesions tend to be avascular. Even after successful antibiotic treatment, many sterile vegetations persist indefinitely [8]. Vegetation growth often results in leaflet perforation and may cause chordal rupture, leading to severe valvular regurgitation. Infection may also extend outside the valve leaflets into the surrounding structures such as the sinotubular junction, the annulus, the myocardium or the conduction system. Cavitation in the aortic wall may result in a peri-aortic abscess that usually remains in communication with the lumen. Rarely, these abscesses can erode into the pericardial cavity or another cardiac chamber such as the left atrium. In bioprosthetic valve IE, the valvular tissue itself is frequently involved as well. Vegetations can grow large enough to interfere directly with leaflet function and result in both valvular stenosis and regurgitation. Mechanical valves have a slightly greater risk for IE in the early post-operative period, but by 5 years there is probably no difference in the incidence of IE between mechanical and bioprostheses [9–11]. In developed countries, about a quarter of cases of IE involve prosthetic valves (PVE). The cumulative risk of PVE is 1–3% at 1 year and 2–6% at 5 years after valve implantation [12].

20.4 Susceptible patients

Cardiac factors

Patients with abnormal heart valves, or prosthetic valves, have an increased risk of IE (Table 20.1). Patients with prosthetic valves have two risk phases for IE, early and late. Early PVE (occurring within 1 year of implantation) is more likely to be nosocomial and therefore have a different causative organism than late PVE, which is usually community acquired. There appears to be no difference in risk of IE, either early or late, between patients receiving mechanical or bioprosthetic valve replacements [13]. Overall, patients with prosthetic valves have a risk of IE approximately 5–10 times that in patients with native valve disease [9] and account for 7–25% of IE cases in developed countries [12].

The greatest risk of IE occurs after prosthetic valve replacement for native valve endocarditis (NVE), or prosthetic valve endocarditis (PVE) or valvular damage resulting from a previous episode of IE [14]. About 75% of cases of IE have a pre-existing structural abnormality of a cardiac valve, and while rheumatic disease is the most common lesion in the third world, mitral valve prolapse is now reported in around 25% of cases in Northern Europe and North America. There is, however, general agreement now that patients with mitral valve prolapse do not present an increased risk of IE without either valve thickening or regurgitation [15]; indeed the risk is probably proportional to degree of regurgitation [14].

Congenital heart disease (CHD) is also a risk factor for IE, not only because of increased turbulence in various congenital lesions leading to endothelial damage, for example aortic stenosis or untreated VSD, but also because many CHD patients have previously undergone surgical repair,

Table 20.1 Patients at increased risk of infective endocarditis [29].

Acquired valvular heart disease with stenosis or regurgitation
Prosthetic heart valve
Structural congenital heart disease, including surgically corrected or palliated structural conditions, but excluding isolated atrial septal defect, fully repaired ventricular septal defect or fully repaired patent ductus arteriosus, and closure devices that are judged to be endothelialised
Previous infective endocarditis
Hypertrophic cardiomyopathy

often involving the use of prosthetic valves or shunts. In a large series of paediatric patients, VSD, tetralogy of Fallot (TOF) and aortic stenosis were the most frequently encountered congenital abnormalities predisposing to IE [16, 17]. Biscuspid aortic valve is one of the most common congenital cardiac abnormalities, with an incidence between 0.9 and 2% of the adult population [18]; it is also an important risk factor for the development of IE [19]. However, whilst patients with aortic valve disease account for 15–30% of IE cases, only 10–20% have pre-existing CHD [20].

Non-cardiac factors

Non-cardiac risk factors for IE can be divided into four groups:

1. Factors promoting NBTE, considered a pre-requisite for bacterial adhesion, include: leukaemia, hepatic cirrhosis, hypercoagulability states, inflammatory bowel disease, systemic lupus erythematosis and steroid medication.
2. Compromised immune defence, either humoral (e.g. corticosteroids) or cellular. Chronic alcoholism is associated with increased infection rates and there is a low incidence of predisposing cardiac lesions in alcoholic patients with IE [21, 22]. HIV infection probably independently increases the risk of IE [23]; however, in this group of patients IE is also often associated with intravenous drug use or long-term intravenous catheters.
3. Compromised local non-immune defence mechanisms such as increased transmucosal permeability associated with inflammatory bowel disease and reduced capillary clearance of bacteria in patients with AV fistulae for haemodialysis.
4. Increased frequency of bacteraemias from broken skin (e.g. burns, bed sores), or intensive care patients (central lines), haemodialysis patients or intravenous drug use.

20.5 Prevention

General measures

Prevention of iatrogenic bacteraemia is vital. Simple measures such as hand washing, using full barrier precautions during line insertion, cleaning the skin with 2% chlorhexidine, avoiding the femoral insertion site and removing unnecessary catheters have an important role in reducing bloodstream infection [24, 25]. Other simple measures include adequate treatment of infections that could lead to bacteraemia or fungaemia, and effective management of conditions that can lead to repeated or prolonged infections, such as bed sores. Finally, appropriate and prompt treatment of suspected bacteraemia to prevent the development of IE is fundamental.

Antibiotic prophylaxis

Whilst in the past antibiotic prophylaxis for IE was focused on dental procedures in susceptible individuals, this strategy has not demonstrably reduced the incidence of IE. The focus of IE prophylaxis has changed with the concept that bacterial load from cumulative bacteraemia over the course of a year is many orders of magnitude greater than that from a dental extraction [26]. Whether antibiotic prophylaxis is effective in reducing the incidence of IE when given before an invasive procedure is a question for which there is limited available evidence. Thus the efficacy of antibiotic prophylaxis in the prevention of IE remains controversial [27]. Successive guidelines from the European Society of Cardiology (ESC 2004) [15], the British Society for Antimicrobial Chemotherapy (BSAC 2006) [28] and the American Heart Association (AHA 2007) [3], whilst agreeing upon individuals who are at highest risk of IE (Table 20.1), successively reduce the number of procedures for which antimicrobial prophylaxis is recommended. Recently, the National Institute for Health and Clinical Excellence (NICE) in England recommended that at-risk patients undergoing interventional procedures should no longer be given antibiotic prophylaxis against IE [29]. This new advice is given on the basis that there is insufficient evidence that antibiotic prophylaxis before dental, or non-dental, treatments reduces the incidence of IE even if the duration of bacteraemia post procedure is reduced. There are, however, known risks associated with antibiotic administration.

The applicability of the NICE guidance to the specific ICU population remains controversial. For patients in intensive care it seems prudent to follow the American Heart Association guidance [3], targeting antibiotic prophylaxis at those with the greatest risk of a poor outcome from IE undergoing those procedures most likely to produce a significant bactereraemia (Table 20.2).

20.6 Diagnosis

Clinical features

The most important factor for the diagnosis of endocarditis is a high index of suspicion. In 1994, a group at Duke University proposed standardised criteria for assessing patients with suspected IE [30]. These criteria have been validated in subsequent series [31, 32]. However, a modification of the Duke criteria proposed in 2000 [33] is more helpful clinically, given the increased use of transoesophageal echocardiography (TOE) and the recognised importance of *Staph. aureus* bacteraemia [34]. The proposed modification also included the new major criterion of positive culture for *Coxiella burnetii* (the agent of Q fever) or an anti-phase 1 immunoglobulin G antibody titre > 1:800. Table 20.3 lists these modified diagnostic criteria. Of the clinical criteria, heavy weight is given to new valvular regurgitation or positive echocardiographic findings. It is vital that as well as regular clinical examination, repeat echocardiographic examination of at-risk long-stay ICU patients is conducted if fever is unresolved or recurrent.

It is vital to collect appropriate microbiological data prior to starting antibiotics for IE. This may require repeated collections of blood cultures together with serological and polymerase chain reaction-based testing,

Table 20.2 Prophylaxis for infective endocarditis.

Patients with

Prosthetic cardiac valve or prosthetic material used for cardiac valve repair.

Previous infective endocarditis.

Congenital heart disease (CHD):

- Unrepaired cyanotic CHD, including palliative shunts and conduits
- Completely repaired congenital heart defect with prosthetic material or device, whether placed by surgery or catheter intervention, during the first 6 months after the procedure (i.e. prior to complete endothelialisation)
- Repaired CHD with residual defects at the site or adjacent to the site of a prosthetic patch or prosthetic device (which inhibits endothelialisation).

Cardiac transplantation recipients who develop cardiac valvulopathy.

Procedures

Dental procedures:

- All dental procedures that involve manipulation of gingival tissue or the peri-apical region of teeth or perforation of the oral mucosa.

Respiratory tract procedures:

- All invasive procedures that involve incision or biopsy of the respiratory mucosa (e.g. tonsillectomy/adenoidectomy).
- Bronchoscopy only where incision of respiratory tract mucosa is involved.
- Drainage of abscess or empyema.

Gastro-intestinal (GI) or genito-urinary (GU) procedures:

- Cystoscopy.
- Oesophagogastroduodenoscopy and colonosocopy (only when established infection).

Cardiac procedures:

- Surgery for placement of prosthetic valves or insertion of intravascular/intracardiac material.

Adapted from Wilson et al. [3].

which may be particularly valuable where blood cultures are negative and where fastidious organisms are involved [35–39].

Echocardiographic evidence of infective endocarditis

Echocardiography has become the most important tool used in diagnosing IE. Both transthoracic echocardiography (TTE) and TOE have important roles in the diagnosis and management of patients with IE. TTE is rapid and cheap; however, views may be inadequate for physical reasons in up to 20% of adult patients, and in any event spatial resolution is much less than TOE, and so overall sensitivity for vegetations using TTE may be less than 60% [12]. TOE utilises higher frequency ultrasound (6–7 MHz) and has a better spatial resolution than TTE and can depict structures as small as 1 mm in diameter, whereas TTE can only resolve to approximately 5 mm. Moreover, due to the proximity of the probe to the left atrium, TOE is disproportionately better at acquiring images of the mitral valve and views of prosthetic valves.

Echocardiographic examination for IE is focused upon visualising mobile masses, perivalvular abscesses or 'rocking' of prosthetic valve rings.

Table 20.3 Modified Duke criteria for diagnosis of IE [33]. IE is confirmed in the presence of two major criteria, or one major + three minor criteria, or five minor criteria. Possible IE is diagnosed in the presence of one major + one minor criterion, or three minor criteria.

Major criteria		
Blood culture positive for IE	Typical IE microorganisms from two separate blood cultures	*Strep. viridans*, *Strep. bovis*, HACEK group, *Staph. aureus*, or community acquired enterococci
	Microorganisms consistent with IE from persistently positive blood cultures	At least two positive blood cultures drawn > 12 hours apart; or All of three or a majority of ≥ four separate blood cultures drawn ≥ 12 hours apart
	Single positive blood culture for *Coxiella burnetii* or antiphase I IgG antibody titre > 1:800	
Echocardiogram positive for IE	Oscillating intracardiac mass: ● on valve or supporting structures ● in path of regurgitant jet ● on implanted material ● abscess ● new partial dehiscence of prosthetic valve	TOE recommended in patients with prosthetic valves with clinical suspicion of IE or complicated IE (paravalvular abscess); otherwise TTE initially
New valvular regurgitation	Worsening or changing of pre-existing murmur is not sufficient	
Minor criteria		
Predisposition	Predisposing heart condition Injection drug use	
Fever	Temperature > 38°C	
Vascular phenomena	Major arterial emboli Septic pulmonary infarcts Mycotic aneurysm Intracranial haemorrhage Conjunctival haemorrhages Janeway's lesions	
Immunologic phenomena	Glomerulonephritis Osler's nodes Roth's spots Rheumatoid factor	
Microbiological evidence	Positive blood culture not meeting major criteria above Serological evidence of active infection with organism consistent with IE	This excludes single positive cultures for coagulase-negative *Staphylococcus* and organisms that do not cause IE

Spectral and colour flow Doppler ultrasound are also used to detect valvular regurgitation, particularly leaflet perforations or para-valvular regurgitation by prosthetic valve rings. In all patients a complete echo examination, including all visible intra-thoracic vessels, must take place. In patients who have previously undergone cardiac surgery this includes cannulation sites, e.g. ascending aorta, cavae and pulmonary veins, as well as the operative site and intracardiac structures, as IE has been described in all these areas. It is vital that images are stored for later comparison, especially if small mobile masses are visualised in patients who do not fulfil other criteria for IE, as a change in conformation over time will increase suspicion of active infection.

Intracardiac devices such as pacemaker and implantable cardiac defibrillators are increasingly used in cardiac units. It is impossible echocardiographically to distinguish benign thrombus on an intracardiac device from infected thrombus. It is important to follow the device throughout its course in the cardiac chambers, and special attention must be paid where the device crosses a valve. When there is documented evidence of IE in these patients, there is a high likelihood of device infection, and thus these should be replaced if valve surgery subsequently becomes necessary.

Myocardial abscess formation from perivalvular extension of infection is one of the most serious complications of IE, and is associated with an approximate doubling of the mortality rate. Although ECG changes may occur such as prolongation of the PT interval or new interventricular conduction defects, TOE is the investigation of choice for assessment of abscess. These lesions are most commonly associated with the aortic valve. Mechanical disruption can occur between the aortic annulus and the left ventricle, due to the enlargement of a subannular abscess cavity which gradually encircles the left ventricular outflow tract, separating it from the aorta.

Several studies have shown that multiple echocardiographic examinations may be useful in determining the prognosis of patients with IE during therapy; for example, failure of a vegetation to shrink during antibiotic treatment is an adverse sign [40].

20.7 Causative organisms (Table 20.4)

Staph. aureus is the major causative agent in intravenous drug users (IVDU), with *Pseudomonas aeruginosa* also commonly seen in this group. Fungal endocarditis is also principally seen in IVDU and patients who have recently undergone vascular surgery or prolonged antibiotic intravenous therapy. Patients with hospital-acquired *Staph. aureus* bacteraemia are particularly susceptible to IE and should undergo TOE, as up to 25% will have evidence of IE [34]. This approach has been shown to be cost-effective in patients with catheter-associated bacteraemia in determining the appropriate length of therapy [41].

Table 20.4 The commonest micro-organisms causing infective endocarditis.

Organism	Incidence (%)
Streptococci	60–80
Viridans streptococci	5–18
Enterococci	5–18
Other streptococci	15–25
Staphlococci	20–35
Coagulase-negative	10–27
Coagulase-positive	1–3
Gram-negative organisms	1–3
Fungi	2–4
HACEK organisms	5–10

HACEK: H – *Haemophilus aphrophilus, parainfluenzae, paraphrophilus, influenzae;*
A – *Actinobacillus actinomycetemcomitans;* C – *Cardiobacterium hominis;* E – *Eikenella
corrodens;* K – *Kingella kingae.*

HACEK is an acronym (Table 20.3) for a group of slow-growing
fastidious gram-negative bacteria which account for approximately 5–10%
of all community-acquired IE. They are the most common cause of gram-
negative IE in non-IVDUs. Because of their fastidious nature they are a
common cause of culture-negative IE and have a reputation for producing
large vegetations leading to macroembolic events. Whether this association
is due to the nature of the organisms or to delay in diagnosis, or a
combination of the two, is unknown.

20.8 Complications

The most frequent complication is heart failure, which also has the
greatest impact upon prognosis [42–44]. In native valve IE, acute heart
failure occurs more frequently in aortic valve infections (29%) than
with mitral (20%) or tricuspid (8%) disease [42]. The ability of the
heart to withstand volume overload associated with valvular regurgitation
depends on several factors: its severity and speed of onset, which valve is
involved, and the size and function of the heart chamber receiving the
volume overload. Mitral regurgitation presents both a volume overload
and an afterload decrease to the left ventricle, which explains why it is
often better tolerated than acute aortic regurgitation (AR), which results
in both volume overload and an afterload increase. Tricuspid valve
regurgitation is best tolerated of all. Heart failure may develop acutely
from perforation of a native or bioprosthetic valve leaflet, rupture of
infected mitral chordae, valve obstruction by bulky vegetations, or sudden
intracardiac shunts from fistulous tracts or prosthetic dehiscence. The
rapid increase in LV diastolic pressure in acute AR may lead to premature
closure of the mitral valve before the end of ventricular diastole. This
'preclosure' can be documented by echocardiography and has been used as

a sign that the LV cannot handle the increased volume and that operative intervention is indicated.

The next most frequent complication is embolisation. Up to 65% of embolic events in IE involve the central nervous system, and neurologic complications develop in 20–40% of all patients with IE [45, 46]. Stroke is the most common consequence of emboli from vegetations; the risk appears to be much greater for mitral, particularly with involvement of the anterior mitral leaflet, than aortic valve IE [47], and increases with increasing vegetation size in fungal and staphlococcal but not streptococcal IE [48]. In two more recent studies, TOE assessment of vegetation length (> 10 mm) and mobility predicted the risk of embolism, most commonly stroke [49, 50]. It should be remembered that stroke due to either emboli or mycotic aneurysm may be the presenting sign of IE. The rate of embolic events decreases rapidly after starting effective antibiotics, going from 13 events per 1000 patient-days in the first week of treatment to < 1.2 events per 1000 patient-days after 2 weeks of treatment [46]. Right-sided IE, most commonly in IVDU, can lead to mycotic pulmonary embolism, resulting in lung abscess or empyema, either of which may be the presenting feature. Emboli may involve other organs including the liver, spleen, kidney and gut. Splenic abscess may develop from bacteraemic seeding of a previously infarcted area or direct seeding of the spleen by an infected embolus. Splenic abscess can be a cause of prolonged fever and may cause diaphragmatic irritation with pleuritic or left shoulder pain; abdominal pain and splenomegaly may be absent. Abdominal ultrasound may be useful in the diagnosis of splenic abscess, though computed tomography (CT) and magnetic resonance imaging (MRI) have the highest sensitivity and specificity. Peripheral emboli can produce metastatic abscesses (Figure 20.1). Finally, rarely, coronary emboli can result in myocardial infarction and heart failure.

Renal failure is common in IE. While often attributed to immune complex glomerulonephritis (GN), a recent study of 62 patients revealed that localised infarction was present in 31% and acute GN in 26% [51]. The commonest type of GN was vasculitic, without deposition of immunoproteins in glomeruli. Of the renal infarcts, over 50% were septic emboli, especially in patients with *Staph. aureus*. Renal failure in many cases is multi-factorial and complicates pre-existing dysfunction. Pre-renal causes and toxicity associated with antibiotics occur commonly.

Extension of the infection outside the valve annulus is a particularly worrying development, predicting a higher mortality, and almost always requires surgical intervention [52]. It is most common in aortic valve IE (Figure 20.2a and b). Periannular abscesses may initially not communicate with the lumen of the aorta or a cardiac chamber, but usually progress to break through to such areas. TOE is the best modality to detect perivalvular abscess, and can readily detect flow into and out of the abscess using colour flow Doppler. Rarely, abscesses may form directly on valve leaflets, a feature of severe mitral IE.

(a)

(b)

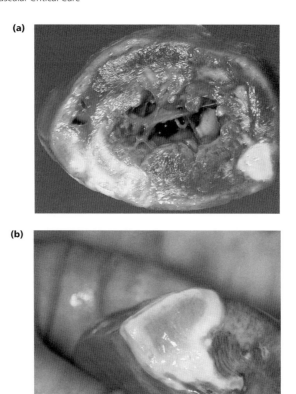

Figure 20.1 Post-mortem findings in a patient with *Staph. aureus* endocarditis with multiple abscesses. (**a**) Myocardial abscess. (**b**) Renal abscess. (See also colour plate 20.1).

20.9 Management

Medical

In uncomplicated cases (rare on ICU) treatment should be started only when the results, including antibiotic sensitivities, of the initial blood cultures are obtained. This may require re-culturing and waiting up to 8 days in a patient who has recently received antibiotics. In cases complicated by active sepsis, severe valvular dysfunction, conduction defects or infective emboli, empirical bacteriocidal antibiotic therapy should be started after three blood cultures have been taken. Infectious disease specialists should be involved to help with the antibiotic decision-making, and a cardiac surgeon should be informed at an early stage, especially if there is a suspicion of an aortic root abscess or in PVE.

A carefully documented initial physical examination, particularly focusing on the cardiopulmonary, dermatological and neurological systems, is important to detect new embolic phenomena. Common clinical signs found are splinter haemorrhages, conjunctival petechiae, Osler's nodes (tender subcutaneous nodules often in the pulp of digits) and Janeway's lesions (non-tender erythematous haemorrhagic or pustular

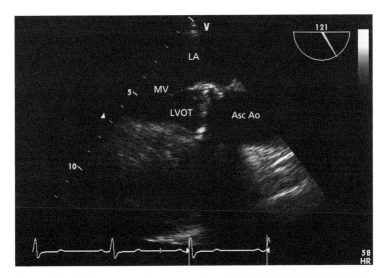

Figure 20.2a TOE long-axis aortic view of a patient with calcific aortic stenosis. The aortic valve is shown heavily calcified between the left ventricular outflow tract (LVOT) and ascending aorta (Asc Ao). The mitral valve (MV) and left atrium (LA) are also annotated.

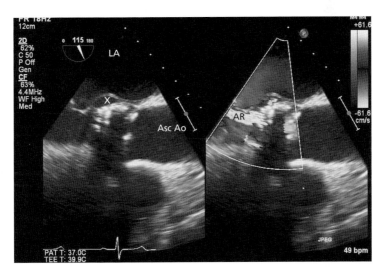

Figure 20.2b TOE of same patient as Figure 20.2a, but after 3 months ICU care with MRSA-infected bed-sores. Note the development of aortic root abscess (X) in the left panel. Note flow in and out of the abscess on colour flow Doppler in the right panel, together with a jet of aortic regurgitation (AR). (See also colour plate 20.2).

lesions often in the palms or soles). Whilst not pathomneumonic, the retinae should be carefully examined for Roth spots (retinal haemorrhages with a white centre). Baseline full blood count and measurement of renal and liver function should be obtained, and repeated with a surveillance blood culture obtained at 72 hours.

C-reactive protein (CRP) should be measured at the start of therapy and levels followed for the first week of therapy, as patients with high CRP (> 122 mg/l) or whose levels fail to fall after 1 week of therapy have a higher risk of poor outcome [53]. Whilst CRP should fall rapidly during the first 2 weeks of treatment, it may remain slightly elevated for 6 weeks or longer.

Most patients become afebrile within 5–10 days of the start of appropriate antibiotic treatment. Persistent fever beyond the first week of therapy often indicates the development of a complication such as valve destruction or extension of infection into the myocardium with abscess formation. Late fever may also indicate localised infection from septic emboli or a drug fever. Other signs of inadequate control of the infection are a persistently elevated CRP or white cell count. Erythrocyte sedimentation rate (ESR) is not a useful measure of treatment response.

The management of anticoagulation in patients with IE is difficult. There is no proven advantage of anticoagulation, including aspirin, in the treatment of native valve IE. Patients with PVE anticoagulated with warfarin should have their warfarin changed to intravenous heparin therapy, as surgical intervention is more likely to be required. Patients with PVE who have suffered a cerebral event should have all anticoagulation stopped as mortality is markedly increased, particularly if associated with *Staph. aureus* [54].

Surgical

Early cardiac surgical input regarding indications for operation is essential (Table 20.5). The rapidly rising incidence of antibiotic resistance requires a multidisciplinary approach with infectious disease consultation. The need to intervene quickly once heart failure occurs cannot be overemphasised.

Heart failure is considered the strongest indication for early cardiac surgery in the setting of IE. The propensity analysis of Vikram suggests that patients with moderate or severe heart failure in the setting of complicated left-sided native valve IE showed the greatest reduction in mortality with operation (14% vs. 51%), although surgery was associated with a reduction in overall 6-month mortality in all the study patients [44]. However, a more recent propensity study conducted on a similar group of patients contests this result [55]. Operation to prevent embolisation is controversial. The incidence of embolic complications falls dramatically over 2 weeks after

Table 20.5 Indications to consider surgery in active endocarditis.

Heart failure from aortic or mitral regurgitation
Early prosthetic valve endocarditis
Haemodynamically significant prosthetic valve dysfunction
Perivalvular abscess
Persistent infection after 7–10 days of appropriate antibiotic therapy
Difficult to treat organisms, e.g. fungi, *Brucella* spp, *Coxiella* ssp., *Staph. lugdunensis*, resistant *Enterococcus* ssp.
Large mobile vegetation in first week of therapy
Recurrent emboli despite appropriate antibiotic therapy
Obstructive vegetations

commencing appropriate antibiotics [46–56]. Therefore, it is suggested that prophylactic surgery for large (> 10 mm) anterior mitral leaflet vegetations is most likely to be beneficial if undertaken within the first week after presentation.

A neurological complication from IE markedly increases the risk of cardiac surgery. In a retrospective study of 181 patients with cerebral complications in this setting, 44% had further neurological deterioration if an embolic cerebral event had occurred within 7 days of the surgery, compared to 16.7% who had new neurological damage if operation was delayed between 8 and 14 days, and only 2.3% experienced deterioration if surgery was delayed for 4 weeks [57]. The situation was different for haemorrhagic stroke, where the risk persisted for up to 4 weeks. Therefore, it is wise to delay valve surgery for 2–3 weeks after an embolic cerebral episode, but for a month after a cerebral bleed.

Surgery may also be required to drain abscesses from septic emboli. This can include drainage of empyema in right-sided IE or abdominal abscesses (mainly splenic) in left-sided IE. Abscesses should be drained prior to cardiac surgery to prevent re-infection of a new valve repair or prosthesis.

Post-operative management

A large systemic inflammatory response is frequently seen following cardiac surgery for IE, often requiring the use of pressor agents and cardiac output monitoring. The inflammatory response also frequently leads to coagulopathy. Renal function is also usually impaired and it is not unusual for a period of renal replacement therapy to be required.

Usually, removal of the infected valve and all surrounding infected tissue combined with a new valve results in a dramatic improvement in the patient's clinical condition. If this does not occur, it is important to check the integrity of the valve replacement, or repair, with echocardiography. These patients should be managed in conjunction with a consultant microbiologist and usually require at least 1 month of intravenous antibiotics.

20.10 Outcome and prognosis

In general, native valve IE has a lower rate of surgical intervention and better survival than PVE. Streptococcal IE diagnosed early with treatment started before complications occur should have a good outcome. However, if the diagnosis is delayed, or other causative organisms are involved, particularly *Staph. aureus*, the need for surgical intervention is greater, complications, particularly embolic are more likely, and overall outcome is worse. Long-term survival following hospital discharge is good, with 81% survival at 10 years in one series, although 47% of those treated medically during the active phase required surgery later, the majority within 2 years [58]. The spectrum of patients presenting with IE is changing. Patients are now older, more likely to have a nosocomial infection, more IVDUs and increasingly resistant bacteria; for these reasons, despite improving antimicrobials and medical care, IE remains a disease with high mortality, requiring constant vigilance for diagnosis and treatment in the ICU population.

20.11 Summary

Despite medical advances the incidence of IE has remained static for the past 20 years. This is due in part to an ageing population and increasing numbers of patients with indwelling cannulae and catheters. Antibiotic prophylaxis prior to dental and other procedures in high-risk patients has not been proven to be of benefit and its use is now contentious. However, there is increasing understanding of the methods of adherence of bacteria to damaged endothelium in IE, which may lead to novel methods of IE prophylaxis in the future. In the ICU simple measures to reduce the incidence of bacteraemia associated with invasive procedures have been shown to be effective in reducing bloodstream infection which can lead to IE in susceptible patients. Use of the modified Duke criteria and the increasing availability of TOE on the ICU help with early diagnosis of IE, but a high index of suspicion is the mainstay of diagnosis. Repeated clinical and echocardiographic examinations are required to exclude IE in patients with unresolving or recurrent pyrexias. Once a diagnosis has been made, prompt targeted antibiotic therapy and involvement of a multidisciplinary team including a microbiologist and cardiac surgeon are vital to a successful outcome.

Case study

A previously fit 53–year-old female presented with intestinal obstruction. At emergency laparotomy a gangrenous terminal ileum was removed. She was metabolically unstable during the operation. Subsequently she spent 6 days in ITU where she required inotropes and recovered from a severe neutropenia.

On the general ward she appeared to be making progress, but on the 13th day she developed pleuritic chest pain and noticed loss of visual acuity. She was hypotensive and had a tachycardia of 125 bpm in sinus rhythm. A spiral CT scan revealed a small pulmonary embolus. Her left foot was mottled with absent pulses and she was oliguric with a serum creatinine of 150 μmol/l. Microbiological examination revealed a growth of MRSA from an internal jugular line, and blood cultures grew Gram-positive cocci which subsequently proved to be *Staph. aureus*. For the next 16 days she remained in ITU critically ill. On admission, a small mobile mass had been noted by TTE, on the anterior leaflet of the mitral valve. Two weeks later, a combination of TTE and TOE revealed large vegetations on the mitral and aortic valves.

At this point a cardiac surgical opinion was sought and she was transferred to a tertiary cardiac unit on the same day. On arrival a second TOE examination revealed a septal abscess. She subsequently underwent emergency aortic valve and root replacement with repair of the anterior leaflet of the mitral valve, but did not survive due to overwhelming sepsis and coagulopathy and low cardiac output. At autopsy, abscesses were found at several sites in the left ventricle, the kidney, spleen and liver (see Figures 20.1a and b).

This case illustrates the lethal nature of IE and the need to take expeditious action to make the diagnosis and involve a cardiac surgeon at an early stage.

Acknowledgement
We thank Professor Mary Sheppard for the pathology illustrations.

References
1. Angus DC, Linde-Zwirble WT, Lidicker J, et al. Epidemiology of severe sepsis in the United States: analysis of incidence, outcome, and associated costs of care. *Crit Care Med* 2001;29(7):1303–10.
2. Moreillon P, Que Y-A. Infective endocarditis. *Lancet* 2004;363:139–49.
3. Wilson W, Taubert KA, Gewitz M, et al. Prevention of infective endocarditis: guidelines from the American Heart Association: a guideline from the American Heart Association Rheumatic Fever, Endocarditis, and Kawasaki Disease Committee, Council on Cardiovascular Disease in the Young, and the Council on Clinical Cardiology, Council on Cardiovascular Surgery and Anesthesia, and the Quality of Care and Outcomes Research Interdisciplinary Working Group. *Circulation* 2007;116(15):1736–54.
4. Stehbens WE, Delahunt B, Zuccollo JM. The histopathology of endocardial sclerosis. *Cardiovasc Pathol* 2000;9(3):161–73.
5. Kreikemeyer B, Klenk M, Podbielski A. The intracellular status of *Streptococcus pyogenes*: role of extracellular matrix-binding proteins and their regulation. *Int J Med Microbiol* 2004;294(2–3):177–88.
6. Moreillon P, Que YA, Bayer AS. Pathogenesis of streptococcal and staphylococcal endocarditis. *Infect Dis Clin North Am* 2002;16(2):297–318.
7. Grunkemeier GL, Wu Y. The Silzone effect: how to reconcile contradictory reports? *Eur J Cardiothorac Surg* 2004;25(3):371–5.
8. Vuille C, Nidorf M, Weyman AE, et al. Natural history of vegetations during successful medical treatment of endocarditis. *Am Heart J* 1994;128(6 Pt 1):1200–9.
9. Calderwood SB, Swinski LA, Waternaux CM, et al. Risk factors for the development of prosthetic valve endocarditis. *Circulation* 1985;72(1):31–7.
10. Arvay A, Lengyel M. Incidence and risk factors of prosthetic valve endocarditis. *Eur J Cardiothorac Surg* 1988;2(5):340–6.
11. Ivert TS, Dismukes WE, Cobbs CG, et al. Prosthetic valve endocarditis. *Circulation* 1984;69(2):223–32.
12. Mylonakis E, Calderwood SB. Infective endocarditis in adults. *N Engl J Med* 2001;345(18):1318–30.
13. Grover FL, Cohen DJ, Oprian C, et al. Determinants of the occurrence of and survival from prosthetic valve endocarditis. Experience of the Veterans Affairs Cooperative Study on Valvular Heart Disease. *J Thorac Cardiovasc Surg* 1994;108(2):207–14.
14. Steckelberg JM, Wilson WR. Risk factors for infective endocarditis. *Infect Dis Clin North Am* 1993;7(1):9–19.
15. Horstkotte D, Follath F, Gutschik E, et al. Guidelines on prevention, diagnosis and treatment of infective endocarditis. Executive summary; the task force on infective endocarditis of the European Society of Cardiology. *Eur Heart J* 2004;25(3):267–76.
16. Johnson DH, Rosenthal A, Nadas AS. A forty-year review of bacterial endocarditis in infancy and childhood. *Circulation* 1975;51(4):581–8.
17. Horstkotte D, Paselk C, Bircks W, et al. Clinical long-term results after corrective surgery of tetralogy of Fallot. *Z Kardiol* 1993;82(9):552–62.
18. Yener N, Oktar GL, Erer D, et al. Bicuspid aortic valve. *Ann Thorac Cardiovasc Surg* 2002;8(5):264–7.
19. Leport C. Antibiotic prophylaxis for infective endocarditis. *Clin Microbiol Infect* 1998;4 Suppl 3:S56–61.

20. Michel PL, Acar J. Native cardiac disease predisposing to infective endocarditis. *Eur Heart J* 1995;16 Suppl B:2–6.

21. Snyder N, Atterbury CE, Pinto Correia J, et al. Increased concurrence of cirrhosis and bacterial endocarditis. A clinical and postmortem study. *Gastroenterology* 1977;73(5):1107–13.

22. Buchbinder NA, Roberts WC. Alcoholism. An important but unemphasized factor predisposing to infective endocarditis. *Arch Intern Med* 1973;132(5):689–92.

23. Manoff SB, Vlahov D, Herskowitz A, et al. Human immunodeficiency virus infection and infective endocarditis among injecting drug users. *Epidemiology* 1996;7(6):566–70.

24. Mermel LA. Prevention of intravascular catheter-related infections. *Ann Intern Med* 2000;132(5):391–402.

25. Pronovost P, Needham D, Berenholtz S, et al. An intervention to decrease catheter-related bloodstream infections in the ICU. *N Engl J Med* 2006;355(26):2725–32.

26. Roberts GJ. Dentists are innocent! 'Everyday' bacteremia is the real culprit: a review and assessment of the evidence that dental surgical procedures are a principal cause of bacterial endocarditis in children. *Pediatr Cardiol* 1999;20(5):317–25.

27. Prendergast BD. The changing face of infective endocarditis. *Heart* 2006;92(7):879–85.

28. Gould FK, Elliott TS, Foweraker J, et al. Guidelines for the prevention of endocarditis: report of the Working Party of the British Society for Antimicrobial Chemotherapy. *J Antimicrob Chemother* 2006;57(6):1035–42.

29. NICE. *Prophylaxis Against Infective Endocarditis.* 2008.

30. Durack DT, Lukes AS, Bright DK. New criteria for diagnosis of infective endocarditis: utilization of specific echocardiographic findings. Duke Endocarditis Service. *Am J Med* 1994;96(3):200–9.

31. Habib G, Derumeaux G, Avierinos JF, et al. Value and limitations of the Duke criteria for the diagnosis of infective endocarditis. *J Am Coll Cardiol* 1999;33(7):2023–9.

32. Perez-Vazquez A, Farinas MC, Garcia-Palomo JD, et al. Evaluation of the Duke criteria in 93 episodes of prosthetic valve endocarditis: could sensitivity be improved? *Arch Intern Med* 2000;160(8):1185–91.

33. Li JS, Sexton DJ, Mick N, et al. Proposed modifications to the Duke criteria for the diagnosis of infective endocarditis. *Clin Infect Dis* 2000;30(4):633–8.

34. Fowler VG, Jr, Li J, Corey GR, et al. Role of echocardiography in evaluation of patients with *Staphylococcus aureus* bacteremia: experience in 103 patients. *J Am Coll Cardiol* 1997;30(4):1072–8.

35. Rice PA, Madico GE. Polymerase chain reaction to diagnose infective endocarditis: will it replace blood cultures? *Circulation* 2005;111(11):1352–4.

36. Breitkopf C, Hammel D, Scheld HH, et al. Impact of a molecular approach to improve the microbiological diagnosis of infective heart valve endocarditis. *Circulation* 2005;111(11):1415–21.

37. Fenollar F, Raoult D. Molecular diagnosis of bloodstream infections caused by non-cultivable bacteria. *Int J Antimicrob Agents* 2007;30 Suppl 1:S7–15.

38. Naber CK, Erbel R. Infective endocarditis with negative blood cultures. *Int J Antimicrob Agents* 2007;30 Suppl 1:S32–6.

39. Vassalos A, Dancer SJ, MacArthur KJ. Polymerase chain reaction diagnosis in culture-negative prosthetic valve methicillin-resistant *Staphylococcus aureus* endocarditis in a patient with chronic liver disease. *Interact Cardiovasc Thorac Surg* 2004;3(2):240–2.

40. Rohmann S, Erbel R, Darius H, et al. Prediction of rapid versus prolonged healing of infective endocarditis by monitoring vegetation size. *J Am Soc Echocardiogr* 1991;4(5):465–74.

41. Rosen AB, Fowler VG, Jr, Corey GR, et al. Cost-effectiveness of transesophageal echocardiography to determine the duration of therapy for intravascular catheter-associated *Staphylococcus aureus* bacteremia. *Ann Intern Med* 1999;130(10):810–20.

42. Sexton DJ, Spelman D. Current best practices and guidelines. Assessment and management of complications in infective endocarditis. *Cardiol Clin* 2003;21(2):273–82, vii–viii.

43. Mills J, Utley J, Abbott J. Heart failure in infective endocarditis: predisposing factors, course, and treatment. *Chest* 1974;66(2):151–7.

44. Vikram HR, Buenconsejo J, Hasbun R, et al. Impact of valve surgery on 6-month mortality in adults with complicated, left-sided native valve endocarditis: a propensity analysis. *JAMA* 2003;290(24):3207–14.

45. Roder BL, Wandall DA, Espersen F, et al. Neurologic manifestations in *Staphylococcus aureus* endocarditis: a review of 260 bacteremic cases in non drug addicts. *Am J Med* 1997;102(4):379–86.

46. Heiro M, Nikoskelainen J, Engblom E, et al. Neurologic manifestations of infective endocarditis: a 17-year experience in a teaching hospital in Finland. *Arch Intern Med* 2000;160(18):2781–7.

47. Anderson DJ, Goldstein LB, Wilkinson WE, et al. Stroke location, characterization, severity, and outcome in mitral vs aortic valve endocarditis. *Neurology* 2003;61(10):1341–6.

48. Vilacosta I, Graupner C, San Roman JA, et al. Risk of embolization after institution of antibiotic therapy for infective endocarditis. *J Am Coll Cardiol* 2002;39(9):1489–95.

49. Thuny F, Di Salvo G, Belliard O, et al. Risk of embolism and death in infective endocarditis: prognostic value of echocardiography: a prospective multicenter study. *Circulation* 2005;112(1):69–75.

50. Di Salvo G, Habib G, Pergola V, et al. Echocardiography predicts embolic events in infective endocarditis. *J Am Coll Cardiol* 2001;37(4):1069–76.

51. Majumdar A, Chowdhary S, Ferreira MA, et al. Renal pathological findings in infective endocarditis. *Nephrol Dial Transplant* 2000;15(11):1782–7.

52. Brecker SJ, Pepper JR, Eykyn SJ. Aortic root abscess. *Heart* 1999;82(3):260–2.

53. Verhagen DW, Hermanides J, Korevaar JC, et al. Prognostic value of serial C-reactive protein measurements in left-sided native valve endocarditis. *Arch Intern Med* 2008;168(3):302–7.

54. Tornos P, Almirante B, Mirabet S, et al. Infective endocarditis due to *Staphylococcus aureus*: deleterious effect of anticoagulant therapy. *Arch Intern Med* 1999;159(5):473–5.

55. Tleyjeh IM, Ghomrawi HM, Steckelberg JM, et al. The impact of valve surgery on 6-month mortality in left-sided infective endocarditis. *Circulation* 2007;115(13):1721–8.

56. Steckelberg JM, Murphy JG, Ballard D, et al. Emboli in infective endocarditis: the prognostic value of echocardiography. *Ann Intern Med* 1991;114(8):635–40.

57. Eishi K, Kawazoe K, Kuriyama Y, Kitoh Y, et al. Surgical management of infective endocarditis associated with cerebral complications. Multi-center retrospective study in Japan. *J Thorac Cardiovasc Surg* 1995;110(6):1745–55.
58. Tornos MP, Permanyer-Miralda G, Olona M, et al. Long-term complications of native valve infective endocarditis in non-addicts. A 15-year follow-up study. *Ann Intern Med* 1992;117(7):567–72.

21 Pulmonary Hypertension and Right Ventricular Failure

Alain Vuylsteke

Royal Brompton & Harefield NHS Foundation Trust, London and Cardiothoracic Anaesthesia and Intensive Care, Papworth Hospital, Cambridge, UK.

Take Home Messages

- The right ventricle matters most in pulmonary hypertension: the aim of treating pulmonary hypertension is to maintain right ventricular function and cardiac output, rather than treating vascular injury.
- Management strategies are becoming more complex with the development of new drugs and better understanding of pulmonary physiology.
- Chronic thromboembolic pulmonary hypertension (CTPH) is an underdiagnosed cause of pulmonary hypertension. Surgery is curative for patients with proximal disease.

21.1 Introduction

Pulmonary hypertension (PH) is a life-threatening condition that can be associated with a great variety of both pulmonary and extra-pulmonary diseases. PH complicating critical illness usually occurs secondary to relatively common conditions, including acute respiratory failure, left heart failure and pulmonary embolism. Regardless of its aetiology and presentation, insidious or acute, significant PH is often accompanied by right ventricular (RV) dysfunction caused by increased RV afterload. RV failure occurs when increases in pulmonary vascular resistance overwhelm the ventricle's compensatory mechanisms, either abruptly or gradually in the case of chronic cor pulmonale. Ventricular interdependence (with high right-sided pressures and RV failure affecting left ventricular function), progressive RV fibrosis and systemic organ hypoperfusion (caused by antegrade and retrograde heart failure) will ultimately either cause or contribute to multiple organ failure.

Cardiovascular Critical Care. Edited by M. Griffiths, J. Cordingley and S. Price.
© 2010 Blackwell Publishing Ltd.

Pulmonary vascular remodelling, pulmonary vasoconstriction and pulmonary venous hypertension may all contribute to the development of PH, depending upon the underlying aetiology [1]. Although there is no universal cure for chronic PH, newer medical therapies improve a variety of clinically relevant end-points including survival, exercise tolerance, functional class, haemodynamics, echocardiographic parameters and quality of life. Management of acute or chronic PH associated with critical illness is a major challenge. The recent availability of drugs such as endothelin receptor antagonists, prostanoids and phosphodiesterase-5 inhibitors should not detract from the fact that conventional supportive therapy is still the basis of management of these patients in the intensive care unit (ICU). However, as the number of medications available for PH continues to increase, treatment decisions regarding first-line therapy, combination treatments and add-on strategies are becoming more complex [2].

21.2 Definitions

Pulmonary arterial hypertension (PAH) is a term used to classify a variety of conditions that share in common an injury to the pulmonary vasculature that produces elevation in pulmonary arterial pressure. It is noteworthy that the definition of PH has been the subject of debate for many years, and various numbers or indices have been proposed to define it. It is now generally accepted that PH can be defined as a sustained elevation of pulmonary arterial *mean* pressure to more than 25 mmHg at rest or 30 mmHg with exercise. It is defined as PAH if in addition the mean-capillary wedge pressure and LV end-diastolic pressure are less than 15 mmHg [3]. It is important to remember that where acute elevation in pulmonary vascular resistance occurs, acutely the RV is unable to generate very high pressures. Thus, measurement of pulmonary arterial systolic pressures of > 50–60 mmHg implies a chronic process (or acute-on-chronic) and may be the result of combined pathology.

In the critical care setting, PH is a condition in which the increase in the RV afterload leads to organ dysfunction, as a consequence of either hypoxia and/or decreased cardiac output. The aim of treating PH is to maintain RV function and cardiac output, rather than treating the vascular injury [4]. Thus, pulmonary hypertension in the presence of adequate cardiac output does not require treatment *per se*.

21.3 Classification of pulmonary hypertension

In 1998, the Second World Symposium proposed a clinical classification of PH based on pathophysiology, clinical presentation and therapeutic options. The Third World Symposium in 2003 decided to maintain the general architecture and philosophy of the classification. However, the term 'primary pulmonary hypertension' was replaced with 'idiopathic pulmonary hypertension' (Table 21.1) [5]. This classification is now

Table 21.1 Clinical classification of PH based on pathophysiology, clinical presentation and therapeutic options.

1. Pulmonary arterial hypertension	1. Idiopathic 2. Familial 3. Associated with: 3.a. Collagen vascular disease 3.b. Congenital systemic-to-pulmonary shunts 3.c. Portal hypertension 3.d. HIV infection 3.e. Drugs and toxins 3.f. Other (thyroid disorders, glycogen storage disease, Gaucher disease, hereditary haemorrhagic telangiectasia, haemoglobinopathies, myeloproliferative disorders, splenectomy) 4. Associated with significant venous or capillary involvement 4.a. Pulmonary veno-occlusive disease (PVOD) 4.b. Pulmonary capillary haemangiomatosis (PCH)
2. Pulmonary hypertension with left heart disease	1. Left-sided atrial or ventricular heart disease 2. Left-sided valvular heart disease
3. Pulmonary hypertension associated with lung diseases and/or hypoxaemia	1. Chronic obstructive pulmonary disease 2. Interstitial lung disease 3. Sleep-disordered breathing 4. Alveolar hypoventilation disorders 5. Chronic exposure to high altitude 6. Developmental abnormalities
4. Pulmonary hypertension due to chronic thrombotic and/or embolic disease	1. Thrombotic obstruction of proximal pulmonary arteries 2. Thrombotic obstruction of distal pulmonary arteries 3. Non-thrombotic pulmonary embolism (tumour, parasites, foreign material)
5. Miscellaneous	Sarcoidosis, histiocytosis X, lymphangiomatosis, compression of pulmonary vessels (adenopathy, tumour, fibrosing mediastinitis)

generally accepted and widely used, and has been used by the US Food and Drug Administration and the European Agency for Drug Evaluation for the labelling of newly approved medications in PH.

21.4 Pathophysiology

The pathophysiology of PH can be simplified to include vasoconstriction, thrombosis and remodelling of the pulmonary vasculature. These often happen concomitantly, following an initial trigger, and may be determined by genetic predisposition.

- *Vasoconstriction*: decreased activity of potassium channels causes membrane depolarisation, leading to calcium influx. Elevated cytoplasmic calcium concentrations cause pulmonary vasoconstriction and stimulate vascular smooth muscle proliferation. Dysfunctional potassium channels have also been linked to inhibition of apoptosis and contribute further to the medial hypertrophy [6, 7].

The production of vasodilators nitric oxide and prostacyclin is impaired and over-expression of vasoconstrictors such as endothelin is observed.

- *Thrombosis*: changes in local blood flow, activation of inflammatory cascades, endothelial dysfunction and co-existing coagulation disorders favour the development of local intravascular thrombosis.
- *Vascular remodelling*: morphological changes in the pulmonary vasculature that accompany PH are referred to as pulmonary vascular remodelling. Chronic hypoxia is well known to cause pulmonary vascular remodelling and PH, and it is the major mechanism implicated for the development of PH in patients with lung disease. Hypoxia-driven gene regulation in pulmonary artery fibroblasts results in mitogenic stimulation of adjacent smooth muscle cells causing pulmonary artery smooth muscle cell hyperplasia [8]. Remodelling accounts for sustained PH even after elimination of the primary causative factor, for example in drug-induced or chronic thromboembolic PH.
- *Genetic factors*: a region on chromosome 2 encoding bone morphogenetic receptor type 2 (BMPR2) underlies a small proportion of familial and idiopathic PH [9]. BMPR2 signalling appears essential in regulating growth functions in pulmonary vascular cells, inhibiting the proliferation and possibly enhancing apoptosis in smooth muscular cells as well as endothelial cells [10].

Pathophysiology of right ventricular failure associated with pulmonary hypertension

Pulmonary arteries have very little vascular tone and the pulmonary circulation has a great capacity to recruit vessels when required. This capacity enables it to handle large changes in blood flow with only small changes in pressure: a low pressure, low resistance circuit. The main function of the RV is to propel deoxygenated blood through this low impedance circulation. The resistance of the circulation is one-tenth that of the systemic circulation and requires a perfusion gradient of only 5 mmHg. Hence, the RV is thinner-walled than the LV and the complex architecture makes assessment of function difficult. In the critically ill, assessment of ventricular function is usually performed using echocardiography. Under normal circumstances the interventricular septum is functionally part of the LV; consequently the RV free wall contributes most to ejection through its long axis shortening. The thin wall and crescent shape make the RV highly compliant and therefore able to accommodate a large increase in preload with minimal change in end diastolic pressure. The primary compensatory mechanism of the RV is dilatation. RV volume overload is therefore well tolerated, with the RV becoming ellipsoid with increasing volume.

By contrast the RV is less tolerant to increases in afterload. An acute pressure increase above 50 mmHg is beyond the capacity of the RV and will

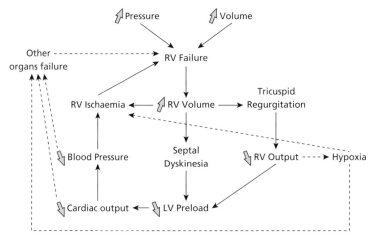

Figure 21.1 Pathophysiology of right ventricular (RV) failure.

result in rapid RV dilatation and failure (Figure 21.1) [11]. In the face of increased pressure, the interventricular septum will be displaced to the left. In addition, the RV prolongs its isovolumic contraction period, which may exceed that of the LV. This results in late systolic displacement of the interventricular septum from right to left, which is readily identifiable on M-mode echocardiography. Prolongation of systole (if there is no interventricular communication) will also result in tricuspid regurgitation of long duration. Thus, these patients are poorly tolerant of tachycardia. RV dysfunction can also occur as a consequence of direct myocardial injury, most commonly during cardiac surgery, but is also seen as a result of ischaemia, stunning or contusion.

Pathophysiology of specific causes of pulmonary hypertension
Acute lung injury (ALI)
ALI is characterised by the sudden onset of severe hypoxemia and diffuse bilateral pulmonary infiltrates in the absence of left atrial hypertension. PH and RV dysfunction are common in ALI and ARDS and are an adverse prognostic indicator in those patients [12, 13]. Underlying mechanisms of PH in this syndrome include increased levels of circulating vasoactive mediators, increased discharge from the sympathetic nervous system, acute endothelial injury, thromboemboli and pulmonary vascular remodelling. RV afterload is commonly further increased by the high airway pressures required to ventilate these patients.

Chronic obstructive pulmonary disease (COPD)
Cor pulmonale is an important consequence of COPD. Although the incidence is not precisely known, it is seen more frequently in patients

with hypoxaemia, carbon dioxide retention and severe airflow limitation. It limits peripheral oxygen delivery, increases shortness of breath and reduces exercise endurance. It is also associated with higher mortality rates independent of other prognostic variables. Numerous factors may contribute to the development of cor pulmonale in patients with COPD, but its primary cause is chronic alveolar hypoxia resulting in pulmonary vasoconstriction, vascular remodelling and pulmonary hypertension.

Among the lung diseases associated with PH, the incidence and clinical course of PH is best known for patients with COPD. It is, however, evident that the pathophysiology and treatment of these disorders is generally distinct from that of PAH disorders. However, PH due to lung diseases shares some common pathophysiologic features with PAH [14].

Acute pulmonary embolism

Pulmonary embolism (PE) is a major health problem, whose incidence is systematically underestimated. The prevalence of PE at autopsy has not changed in the last decades [3] and is approximately 15% of hospitalised patients. It is mostly caused by emboli detached from thrombus located in the venous system.

PE can be classified as (1) *massive* if it leads to shock and/or hypotension; (2) *submassive* if it is identified by echocardiographic signs of right ventricular hypokinesis; or (3) *non massive* in all other situations [15]. The diagnosis is difficult and often missed. If untreated, mortality is approximately 30%, but can be reduced to 2–8% if adequate treatment is promptly instituted. In massive PE, the acute increase in RV afterload leads to increased RV myocardial work and O_2 consumption. The cardiac index falls and the RV pressure increases as the systemic pressure falls, leading to decreased coronary perfusion of the RV. In addition, pericardial constraint in the face of RV dilatation and a leftward shift of the interventricular septum contribute to RV failure and decreased LV output. Hypoxaemia is caused by (1) increased ventilation/perfusion mismatch; (2) opening of shunts such as patent formen ovale; and (3) decreased cardiac output leading to decreased venous oxygen saturation.

Chronic thromboembolic disease (CTEPH)

This is an underdiagnosed cause of PH [16]. While up to 5% of patients develop the condition after an acute PE, only 50% suffering from CTEPH have previously been diagnosed with PE. Approximately half of these patients have a clotting abnormality, such as Factor V Leiden deficiency in protein C or S or lupus anticoagulant.

Surgery is curative for patients with proximal disease and mortality is as low as 4% in experienced centres. Specific peri-operative management is required as the operation entails long bypass times and deep hypothermic circulatory arrest for most patients with poor physiological reserve due to chronic RV failure. Finally there is a high incidence of pulmonary reperfusion injury. Survival is highly dependent on the quality of the operation and the post-operative management [17].

21.5 Diagnosis

In intensive and general care, identification of the underlying cause is imperative in order to initiate the right treatment. The initial cause is rarely completely irreversible, for example lymphangiomatosis. Evaluation of the severity of a newly discovered or long-standing problem requires, from the intensivist's viewpoint, integration of both pulmonary pressure and right ventricular function. Signs of RV failure include jugular venous engorgement, pulsatile hepatomegaly, lower limb oedema and ascites. Visual disturbances associated with papilloedema and delirium due to cerebral venous hypertension mimicking cavernous sinus thrombosis may occur. Chest X-ray and electrocardiogram can show evidence of right atrial enlargement and right ventricular hypertrophy. Unfortunately, both sensitivity and specificity are deficient. Biochemical evidence of renal and hepatic dysfunction is common resulting from systemic hypotension and venous hypertension.

Echocardiography

In PH, the characteristic echocardiographic findings are RV dilatation, hypertrophy, diastolic septal flattening, tricuspid regurgitation and pulmonary hypertension. The LV is small, compressed and D-shaped, and function is usually reduced due to paradoxical movement of the septum and distortion of normal left/right dynamics (Figure 21.2). In addition, Doppler may be used to estimate pulmonary artery systolic pressure, pulmonary vascular resistance and the severity of tricuspid valvular regurgitation (Figure 21.3). Although echocardiographic estimation of pulmonary artery systolic pressure is usually accurate, in patients with severe lung disease, pulmonary artery pressure measured by echocardiography tends to overestimate the degree of PH [18]. The added benefit of echocardiography is that it will also enable evaluation of left

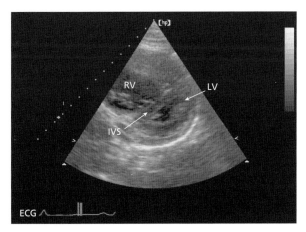

Figure 21.2 Trans-thoracic echocardiogram in a patient with severe pulmonary hypertension (parasternal short axis view). Note the dilated right ventricle and the D-shaped, small left ventricle. ECG, electrocardiogram; RV, right ventricle; LV, left ventricle; interventricular septum, arrowed.

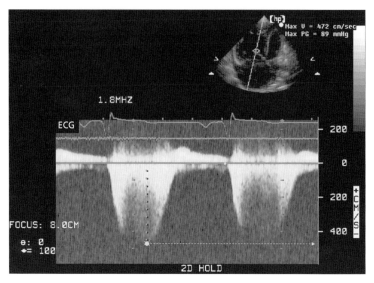

Figure 21.3 Continuous wave (CW) Doppler across the tricuspid valve in a patient with severe pulmonary hypertension. For clarity, a minaturised 2D image is shown in the right upper part of the figure, showing the cursor placed across the tricuspid valve in the apical four-chamber position. The peak velocity between right ventricle and right atrium is 4.7 m/sec, which equates to a pressure drop of 89 mmHg.

heart pathology where it may be the cause of, or contributing to, PH (for example, severe mitral regurgitation). The echocardiographic modality of choice is transthoracic echocardiography; however, where the patient is intubated, and where specific pathology that cannot be evaluated using this modality is suspected, transoesophageal echocardiography (TOE) may be required. In suspected pulmonary thromboembolism, central pulmonary artery thrombus may be demonstrated with embolus with a high sensitivity and specificity (86%) [19].

Pulmonary artery catheter

Despite the ongoing controversy concerning its use in intensive care, pulmonary artery catheter is a mainstay of the management of complicated haemodynamics in expert hands and complements the information gained by echocardiography. When performed in experienced centres, right heart catheter procedures in patients with pulmonary hypertension are associated with low morbidity and mortality rates [20]. Pulmonary artery catheterisation will confirm a low cardiac output, increased RV filling pressure and pulmonary vascular resistance. A low pulmonary artery occlusion pressure excludes the LV as the cause of PH and low cardiac output state.

Computed tomography (CT) angiography

Difficult to obtain in critically ill patients for logistic reasons, spiral CT angiography is the investigation of choice for the diagnosis of acute central

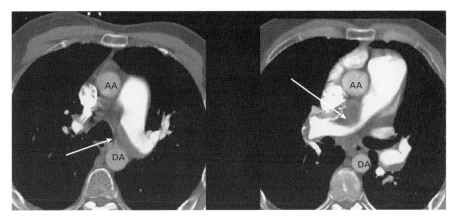

Figure 21.4 CT pulmonary angiogram in a patient with bilateral massive pulmonary emboli, which show as dark-filling defects in the opacified pulmonary arteries (arrowed). AA, ascending aorta; DA, descending aorta.

pulmonary embolism, having a positive and negative predictive value greater than 90% [21] (Figure 21.4). It also provides valuable information about the state of the lungs and techniques are under development to refine the diagnostic usefulness of this tool [22].

Other methods of diagnosis

Measurement of circulating endogenous B-type natriuretic peptide (BNP) has proven to be a sensitive and specific test for heart failure if used in conjunction with standard diagnostic procedures [23]. It is, however, not always applicable at the bedside and is more useful for cohort evaluations.

Radionuclide analysis of the right ventricle by blood-pool imaging allows accurate determination of ejection fraction and wall motion. In addition, it may be possible to estimate pulmonary artery pressure. Use of short-acting radionuclides allows for serial imaging of the RV after pharmacologic intervention or exercise. Perfusion scanning can show evidence of exercise-induced ischemia, although applicability to the RV is somewhat limited.

CT scanning of the heart is at present of limited clinical utility because cardiac motion occurs too rapidly for accurate imaging. The advent of the cine-CT may overcome this problem and allow evaluation of RV volumes and wall motion. Digital subtraction imaging allows for accurate video densitometric calculation of ejection fractions, but offers no advantage over currently available techniques.

Magnetic resonance imaging may prove to be the methodology of choice for analysis of RV function, because it enables assessment of wall motion, ejection fraction and (similar to Doppler flow studies) some indication of flow within the right-sided chambers. It may soon be possible to gain information concerning the biochemical state of the RV myocardium, perhaps providing early evidence of hypertrophy and myopathy [24].

21.6 Treatment

General principles
The commonest causes of PH in the critically ill are left heart disease and hypoxaemia. Treatment should be directed in these cases at the underlying cardiac or respiratory disease. In the minority where there is a primary increase in pulmonary pressure, treatments are either specific (e.g. thrombolysis for acute pulmonary embolism) or generic (e.g. pulmonary vasodilators) [25].

Standard measures aimed at avoiding respiratory acidosis, correcting metabolic acidosis, recruiting lung units to avoid ventilation perfusion mismatch and reduce pulmonary vascular resistance, avoiding catecholamine release by ensuring adequate analgesia and sedation, and avoiding of shivering are all important.

Inhaled oxygen is a selective pulmonary vasodilator in patients with pulmonary hypertension, regardless of primary diagnosis, baseline oxygenation or RV function.

Anticoagulation is desirable (as with any low CO state) and should be instituted at the earliest opportunity.

Pharmacology
Numerous treatments have been proposed, mostly based on vasodilation as the core of the treatment of PH. All suggested therapies should be reserved for patients with refractory PH, instituted cautiously and their effects monitored closely.

Inhaled therapies
Inhaled vasodilators only access areas of the vasculature in contact with aerated alveoli, ventilation:perfusion matching and oxygenation. Nitric oxide (NO) is a ubiquitous naturally occuring gas that functions as a vasodilator and a secondary messenger. NO has a very short half-life in the circulation because it is inactivated by haemoglobin, conferring pulmonary selectivity of this inhaled vasodilator.

The introduction of easy-to-use clinical delivery systems led to its widespread use in patients with PH and refractory hypoxaemia in intensive care, as the effective administration of NO requires a closed circuit. While effective in two-thirds of patients at improving oxygenation and decreasing pulmonary artery pressures (at doses ranging from 1 to 40 ppm), NO has never been proven to be effective in decreasing morbidity or mortality, although large randomised controlled studies have been carried out in patients with ALI where the primary aim of inhaled NO is to improve oxygenation. No large studies have examined the effects of using inhaled NO to lower pulmonary vascular resistance and improve RV function after complicated cardiac surgery, although this is one of the commonest uses of this expensive medication currently. The physiological benefits of inhaled NO only last for 24–48 hours possibly. The failure to decrease the dose of NO daily, a fault of all of the large studies, may account for the fall off in its efficacy and increased toxicity with prolonged inhalation.

Inhaled prostacyclin and derivatives such as iloprost may be given intermittently either through a ventilator circuit or in a spontaneously breathing patient. Their efficacy and response rate are similar to inhaled NO. Awake patients may not tolerate high doses owing to an unpleasant vasodilation in the mouth. Higher doses are also more likely to decrease systemic vascular pressure because the circulating half life is longer than that of NO.

Oral and intravenous medication

All systemically administered vasodilators tend to impair ventilation:perfusion matching and oxygenation. Standard vasodilators, such as glyceryl nitrate or nitroprusside, decrease pulmonary artery pressure. Most of the newer therapies used in ICU are inherited from chronic PH. Systemic side effects, such as systemic hypotension, always require a slow dose titration, often over several weeks. However, they can be used to wean patients from inhaled therapies started in the acute phase. More importantly, they cannot be interrupted in patients suffering from chronic PH.

Continuous intravenous prostacyclin (or derivatives) results in sustained clinical and haemodynamic improvement and probably in improved survival in patients with severe idiopathic hypertension. Despite potentially serious complications, long-term prostacyclin may be especially helpful in seriously ill patients awaiting transplantation [26–28]. Apart from anti-platelet effects, these agents may have anti-proliferative properties as well [29]. Oxidant stress decreases with epoprostenol therapy and is associated with haemodynamic and clinical improvement [30].

Phosphodiesterase-5 (PDE5) inhibitors, such as sildenafil, are potent acute pulmonary vasodilators in experimental models that partially reverse established pulmonary arterial hypertension. In addition, PDE5 inhibitors work in concert with NO by enhancing intracellular cGMP and cGMP-mediated vasodilator effects [31, 32]. For example, sildenafil increased the response to inhaled NO. Following reduction in mean pulmonary artery pressure and pulmonary vascular resistance with inhaled NO, crossover to sildenafil therapy maintained control of PH, facilitating discontinuation of respiratory and cardiovascular organ support [33]. The relative pulmonary vascular specificity of oral sildenafil makes it an attractive therapeutic alternative to inhaled NO and warrants further study [34]. Long-term therapy of PH with sildenafil alone or in combination with other agents is safe and well tolerated [35]. Sildenafil improves exercise capacity, WHO functional class and haemodynamics in patients with symptomatic PH [36].

Endothelin (ET) is a potent vasoconstrictor with mitogenic effects for mesenchymal cells. Therapeutic efforts at interrupting ET's pathologic effects have focused on endothelin receptor antagonists (ERAs), of which two, bosentan and sitaxsentan, are effective treatments of both primary and secondary PH [37]. Combination therapy of an ERA with a prostanoid or phosphodiesterase-5 inhibitor, two drug classes that have different mechanisms of action, is conceptually appealing, but the evidence for its efficacy and safety are still being investigated [38].

Inodilators, such as milrinone, are the most useful inotropes to use in the presence of PH and RV failure. The induced systemic vasodilation may require the addition of vasopressor therapy (noradrenaline), without a major impact on the pulmonary circulation, perhaps owing to the relative paucity of $\alpha 1$ receptors in pulmonary arteries. The calcium sensitiser levosimendan increases cardiac contractility without increasing myocardial oxygen demand, and reduces pulmonary and systemic vascular resistance. Its use in support of the left ventricle post cardiac surgery and in heart failure is now well established; however, use in support of RV function in the presence of PH is largely anecdotal [39].

Mechanical support and surgery

The most common cause of acute severe PH is massive central pulmonary embolism. The overall mortality from massive PE is 6–8%, increasing to 30% if complicated by severe hypotension. A significant number of deaths occur within hours after the onset of symptoms and initial supportive therapy has a major role in those patients. Oxygen and analgesia should be given immediately. Inadequate filling compromises RV haemodynamics – overfilling may cause excessive RV dilatation and tricuspid regurgitation – so optimal fluid therapy is still a subject of debate and no studies have so far helped to define the best fluid management. Inotropic support may or may not be beneficial [15].

Pharmacological (thrombolysis) or surgical de-obstruction should always be considered in massive PE. As the risk of thrombolysis may outweigh its benefit, careful consideration should be given and recent evidence reviewed [15].

Surgical and interventional therapies have the potential to significantly improve PH in appropriately selected patients. These interventions include atrial septostomy as a palliative procedure or bridge to transplantation in patients with refractory right heart failure, pulmonary endarterectomy for CTEPH, and closure of congenital systemic-pulmonary shunts in patients with PH without significant pulmonary vascular disease. Atrial septostomy has been used to decompress the right-sided chambers and augment left-sided filling, with concomitant increase in cardiac output. The resulting reduction in RV end diastolic pressure and wall tension is postulated to improve haemodynamics and RV contractility. Care must be taken to first exclude significant LV disease, and also to ensure the size of the fenestration is not such that it causes significant desaturation.

The use of intra-aortic balloon counter-pulsation as short-term support of the RV remains controversial; however, its use in patients with obstructive coronary artery disease around the time of revascularisation may be of benefit. Mechanical assist to support right ventricular

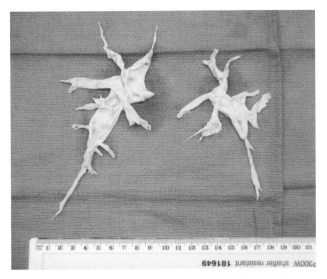

Figure 21.5 Surgically removed obstruction in patients having undergone pulmonary thromboendarterectomy.

dysfunction may be considered – the type and duration depending upon the underlying aetiology and prognosis. When lung function is compromised, extra-corporeal membrane oxygenation (ECMO) may provide effective rescue therapy particularly when RV failure and ALI coincide because higher airway pressure required to recruit injured lung may further increase RV afterload. An artificial lung perfused by the RV in parallel with the pulmonary circulation reduces ventricular load and improves cardiac output in the setting of PH [40].

Pulmonary endarterectomy offers the possibility of a cure for a minority of patients suffering from CTEPH (Figure 21.5). Although traditional preoperative testing and currently available tools are adequate in identifying the presence of proximal disease in CTEPH, they provide only limited information on the status of the microvasculature. Because persistent PH is the most important determinant of outcome, the preoperative identification of patients with CTEPH with concomitant small-vessel disease and/or microvascular disease is crucial. Lung transplantation should be considered for patients with all forms of PH who demonstrate advanced or progressive disease, but this is unfortunately not available to most patients in ICU [41].

21.7 Summary

Treating pulmonary hypertension in intensive care generally comprises supporting the right ventricle.

Case study

A 54-year-old woman was admitted to intensive care following mitral valve repair surgery. Her medical history included insulin-dependent diabetes and several episodes of transient ischaemic attacks in the last 3 years, attributed to transient atrial fibrillation for which she received warfarin. Her diabetes was well controlled with subcutaneous insulin. One week before surgery, she was instructed by her general practitioner to stop warfarin (3 mg/day INR 2.2) and take aspirin (75 mg/day). The operation was uneventful. Cardiopulmonary bypass time was 69 minutes, and she was weaned from support very easily, but with atrio-ventricular pacing. A perioperative TOE indicated that her LV was good and the repair satisfactory.

On admission to critical care, her haemodynamic parameters were satisfactory: HR 100 (paced DDD), 95/55 (65) mmHg, CVP 6 mmHg. She was sedated with a propofol infusion and ventilated with intermittent positive pressure ventilation (FiO_2 0.6, tidal volume 600 ml, respiratory rate 10 breaths per minute). Her PaO_2 was 18.41 kPa and $PaCO_2$ 4.39 kPa. Over the following 2 hours, and unnoticed by the bedside staff, her systemic blood pressure progressively decreased to reach 69/35 (55) mmHg, with a parallel slow increase in CVP (from 6 to 18 mmHg). The patient's urine output decreased to less than 20 ml/hour. Her fluid balance had been managed conservatively and she had received 200 ml of fluid in excess of losses. A transthoracic echocardiography was quickly obtained and ruled out a major pericardial effusion, but suggested right ventricular dysfunction. A pulmonary artery catheter was inserted showing an elevated pulmonary artery pressure (50/20 (34) mmHg) with a normal pulmonary capillary wedge pressure (10 mmHg), cardiac index 1.8 l/min/m^2. A dopamine infusion (5 µg/kg/min) and isoprenaline (0.004 µg/kg/min) was initiated, coupled with the administration by inhalation of 3.3 µg of iloprost. This lead to a decrease in CVP (from 18 to 8 mmHg) and pulmonary artery pressure (from 50/20 (34) to 25/14 (18) mmHg), with an increase in systemic pressure (70/40 (55) mmHg to 110/45 (65) mmHg). Her cardiac index increased to 2.3 l/min/m^2. Oral administration of sildenafil (20 mg/day) allowed a progressive wean of the isoprenaline and iloprost, and the patient was eventually discharged to the ward on day 5.

References

1. Martin KB, Klinger JR, Rounds SI. Pulmonary arterial hypertension: new insights and new hope. *Respirology* 2006;11(1):6–17.
2. Lee SH, Rubin LJ. Current treatment strategies for pulmonary arterial hypertension. *J Intern Med* 2005;258(3):199–215.
3. Gaine SP, Rubin LJ. Primary pulmonary hypertension. *Lancet* 1998;352(9129):719–25.
4. Chin KM, Kim NH, Rubin LJ. The right ventricle in pulmonary hypertension. *Coron Artery Dis* 2005;16(1):13–8.

5. Simonneau G, Galie N, Rubin LJ, et al. Clinical classification of pulmonary hypertension. *J Am Coll Cardiol* 2004;43(12 Suppl S):5S–12S.
6. Mandegar M, Remillard CV, Yuan JX. Ion channels in pulmonary arterial hypertension. *Prog Cardiovasc Dis* 2002;45(2):81–114.
7. Mauban JR, Remillard CV, Yuan JX. Hypoxic pulmonary vasoconstriction: role of ion channels. *J Appl Physiol* 2005;98(1):415–20.
8. Rose F, Grimminger F, Appel J, et al. Hypoxic pulmonary artery fibroblasts trigger proliferation of vascular smooth muscle cells: role of hypoxia-inducible transcription factors. *Faseb J* 2002;16(12):1660–1.
9. Adatia I. Recent advances in pulmonary vascular disease. *Curr Opin Pediatr* 2002;14(3):292–7.
10. Stewart DJ. Bone morphogenetic protein receptor-2 and pulmonary arterial hypertension: unraveling a riddle inside an enigma? *Circ Res* 2005;96(10):1033–5.
11. Barnard D, Alpert JS. Right ventricular function in health and disease. *Curr Probl Cardiol* 1987;12(7):417–49.
12. Leeman M. Pulmonary hypertension in acute respiratory distress syndrome. *Monaldi Arch Chest Dis* 1999;54(2):146–9.
13. Villar J, Blazquez MA, Lubillo S, et al. Pulmonary hypertension in acute respiratory failure. *Crit Care Med* 1989;17(6):523–6.
14. Presberg KW, Dincer HE. Pathophysiology of pulmonary hypertension due to lung disease. *Curr Opin Pulm Med* 2003;9(2):131–8.
15. Task Force on Pulmonary Embolism, European Society of Cardiology. Guidelines on diagnosis and management of acute pulmonary embolism. *Eur Heart J* 2000;21(16):1301–36.
16. Fedullo PF, Auger WR, Kerr KM, et al. Chronic thromboembolic pulmonary hypertension. *N Engl J Med* 2001;345(20):1465–72.
17. Valchanov K, Vuylsteke A. Pulmonary endarterectomy. *Eur J Anaesthesiol* 2006;23(10):815–23.
18. Arcasoy SM, Christie JD, Ferrari VA, et al. Echocardiographic assessment of pulmonary hypertension in patients with advanced lung disease. *Am J Respir Crit Care Med* 2003;167(5):735–40.
19. Wittlich N, Erbel R, Eichler A, et al. Detection of central pulmonary artery thromboemboli by transesophageal echocardiography in patients with severe pulmonary embolism. *J Am Soc Echocardiogr* 1992;5(5):515–24.
20. Hoeper MM, Lee SH, Voswinckel R, et al. Complications of right heart catheterization procedures in patients with pulmonary hypertension in experienced centers. *J Am Coll Cardiol* 2006;48(12):2546–52.
21. Remy-Jardin M, Remy J, Deschildre F, et al. Diagnosis of pulmonary embolism with spiral CT: comparison with pulmonary angiography and scintigraphy. *Radiology* 1996;200(3):699–706.
22. Beiderlinden M, Kuehl H, Boes T, Peters J. Prevalence of pulmonary hypertension associated with severe acute respiratory distress syndrome: predictive value of computed tomography. *Intensive Care Med* 2006;32(6):852–7.
23. Berkowitz R. B-type natriuretic peptide and the diagnosis of acute heart failure. *Rev Cardiovasc Med* 2004;5 Suppl 4:S3–16.
24. Johnson RA, Rubin LJ. Noninvasive evaluation of right ventricular function. *Clin Chest Med* 1987;8(1):65–80.
25. Peil ML, Rubin LJ. Therapy of secondary pulmonary hypertension. *Heart Lung* 1986;15(5):450–6.

26. Barst RJ, Rubin LJ, McGoon MD, et al. Survival in primary pulmonary hypertension with long-term continuous intravenous prostacyclin. *Ann Intern Med* 1994;121(6):409–15.

27. Barst RJ, Rubin LJ, Long WA, et al. A comparison of continuous intravenous epoprostenol (prostacyclin) with conventional therapy for primary pulmonary hypertension. The Primary Pulmonary Hypertension Study Group. *N Engl J Med* 1996;334(5):296–302.

28. Bresser P, Fedullo PF, Auger WR, et al. Continuous intravenous epoprostenol for chronic thromboembolic pulmonary hypertension. *Eur Respir J* 2004;23(4):595–600.

29. Clapp LH, Finney P, Turcato S, et al. Differential effects of stable prostacyclin analogs on smooth muscle proliferation and cyclic AMP generation in human pulmonary artery. *Am J Respir Cell Mol Biol* 2002;26(2):194–201.

30. Robbins IM, Morrow JD, Christman BW. Oxidant stress but not thromboxane decreases with epoprostenol therapy. *Free Radic Biol Med* 2005;38(5):568–74.

31. Steiner MK, Preston IR, Klinger JR, et al. Pulmonary hypertension: inhaled nitric oxide, sildenafil and natriuretic peptides. *Curr Opin Pharmacol* 2005;5(3):245–50.

32. Matot I, Gozal Y. Pulmonary responses to selective phosphodiesterase-5 and phosphodiesterase-3 inhibitors. *Chest* 2004;125(2):644–51.

33. Bigatello LM, Hess D, Dennehy KC, et al. Sildenafil can increase the response to inhaled nitric oxide. *Anesthesiology* 2000;92(6):1827–9.

34. Ng J, Finney SJ, Shulman R, et al. Treatment of pulmonary hypertension in the general adult intensive care unit: a role for oral sildenafil? *Br J Anaesth* 2005;94(6):774–7.

35. Preston IR, Klinger JR, Houtches J, et al. Acute and chronic effects of sildenafil in patients with pulmonary arterial hypertension. *Respir Med* 2005;99(12):1501–10.

36. Galie N, Ghofrani HA, Torbicki A, et al. Sildenafil citrate therapy for pulmonary arterial hypertension. *N Engl J Med* 2005;353(20):2148–57.

37. Kim NH, Rubin LJ. Endothelin in health and disease: endothelin receptor antagonists in the management of pulmonary artery hypertension. *J Cardiovasc Pharmacol Ther* 2002;7(1):9–19.

38. Lee SH, Channick RN. Endothelin antagonism in pulmonary arterial hypertension. *Semin Respir Crit Care Med* 2005;26(4):402–8.

39. Mebazaa A, Karpati P, Renaud E, et al. Acute right ventricular failure – from pathophysiology to new treatments. *Intensive Care Med* 2004;30(2):185–96.

40. Haft JW, Montoya P, Alnajjar O, et al. An artificial lung reduces pulmonary impedance and improves right ventricular efficiency in pulmonary hypertension. *J Thorac Cardiovasc Surg* 2001;122(6):1094–100.

41. Olsson JK, Zamanian RT, Feinstein JA, et al. Surgical and interventional therapies for pulmonary arterial hypertension. *Semin Respir Crit Care Med* 2005;26(4):417–28.

22 Aortic Dissection

Maninder S. Kalkat[1], Vamsidhar B. Dronavalli[3], David Alexander[2] and Robert S. Bonser[3]

[1]Birmingham Heartlands Hospital, Birmingham, UK
[2]Royal Brompton & Harefield NHS Foundation Trust, London, UK
[3]University Hospital Birmingham NHS Trust, Birmingham, UK

Take Home Messages

- Survival and outcome following aortic dissection is dependent on making a rapid and accurate diagnosis.
- Surgery in type A dissection confers overwhelming benefit compared with the natural history of the disease.
- Medical management is recommended initially in type B dissection – complication-specific approach to be followed.
- Close follow-up for aortic dissection by a specialised team to assess the signs of aortic expansion and aneurysm formation by serial imaging is pertinent.
- Endovascular stent graft placement for type B aortic dissection compares favourably with surgical treatment, but further studies to compare it with medical treatment are warranted.

22.1 Introduction

Dissection is the most common catastrophic event affecting the aorta, occurring two to three times more frequently than rupture of a degenerative abdominal aortic aneurysm. A dissection is characterised by the presence of a tear in the intima of the aorta through to the muscular media, allowing cleavage and separation within a medial plane. This creates a false channel or lumen within the aorta. The plane of cleavage may be propagated proximally and distally along the length of the aorta under the force of left ventricular ejection, generating excruciating pain. Those afflicted by dissection are at risk of aortic rupture and malperfusion phenomena as the origin of major branch arteries of the aorta are compromised by dissection propagation. If the ascending aorta is affected, the dissection may compromise coronary perfusion and carotid artery perfusion, aortic valve function and, if rupture occurs, death by cardiac

---

Cardiovascular Critical Care. Edited by M. Griffiths, J. Cordingley and S. Price.
© 2010 Blackwell Publishing Ltd.

tamponade [1]. Thus the disease is associated with high morbidity and mortality. Dissection has an incidence and prevalence of approximately 20–40 per million per annum [2, 3] and is more common in males (male:female ratio 5:1) [4]. The incidence of aortic dissection displays peaks at three age ranges. Proximal dissection (involving the ascending aorta) has a peak incidence at 50–60 years of age, whereas distal dissection (only involving the descending aorta) peaks at 60–70 years [5]. Dissection of the proximal aorta in patients with Marfan's syndrome or predisposing causes accounts for the third peak at 20–40 years [6, 7].

Despite advances in diagnosis and medical, surgical and endovascular management of aortic dissection, the morbidity and mortality remain significant [8] and early recognition with prompt expert management is necessary if outcomes are to be improved. A thorough understanding of the clinical presentation, classification and pathological anatomy of aortic dissection is essential to planning management.

22.2 Aetiology, pathology and pathophysiology

Aetiology

Risk factors for aortic dissection include certain congenital heart defects, connective tissue disorders, inflammatory diseases and environmental factors (Table 22.1). The greatest risk in pregnancy occurs in the third trimester when hormone-induced changes in connective tissue and hypertension are maximal. Dissection associated with pregnancy is most prevalent in Marfan's syndrome and consideration should be given to prophylactic aortic root surgery prior to pregnancy. An association with the use of cocaine and pregnancy result at least in part from transient surges in blood pressure [9, 10].

Deceleration trauma usually causes a transection injury of the aorta, but rare cases of dissection have been reported. More commonly trauma is iatrogenic, occurring either at the time of surgical manipulation of the ascending aorta during cardiac surgery or during the passage of intravascular catheters. Chronic dissection at the site of previous aortotomy for cannulation, valve access or proximal coronary bypass anastomosis has been reported.

Histological features

The aortic wall comprises three layers, the intima, tunica media and adventitia, and is approximately 2 mm thick in the ascending portion. The tunica media is the strongest component and comprises layers of elastic and collagen fibres and obliquely (ascending) or circularly (distal) orientated smooth muscle cells (5%). The media is thickest in the ascending aorta due to increased elastic fibres. Elastin appears to be deposited around microfibrillar fibres of the glycoprotein fibrillin which serves as a scaffold for the organised structure of the wall. Absence or mal-production of fibrillin is the basis of Marfan's syndrome and arises due to an inherited or spontaneous mutation of the fibrillin gene on the long arm of chromosome

Table 22.1 Aetiological conditions in acute dissection.

	Condition or factor associated with dissection
Congenital, inherited or acquired connective tissue disorders	Marfan's syndrome Ehlers–Danlos syndrome Loeys–Dietz syndrome Turner's syndrome Noonan's syndrome Cystinosis Osteogenesis imperfecta Pseudoxanthoma elasticum Menkes' syndrome
Other cardiac associations	Unicuspid and bicuspid aortic valves Coarctation of the aorta Pseudo-coarctation Supra-valvar aortic stenosis
Hypertension	Essential hypertension Phaeochromocytoma Pregnancy Body-building Cocaine abuse
Inflammatory diseases	Syphilis Polymyalgia rheumatica Giant cell arteritis Behçet's syndrome Takayasu arteritis Ormond's disease
Trauma	Deceleration injury Vascular catheter-induced Iatrogenic during cardiac surgery

15 (15q) [10]. In non-Marfan's patients with an apparent predilection to dissection, there is a degeneration of the medial elastic skeleton termed cystic medial necrosis. In this condition, the elastic lamellae become stretched, depleted and fragmented. The resulting cystic defects are filled with chondroitin sulphate, a mucopolysaccharide. The process appears to be an expression of accelerated degeneration without elastic tissue replacement and is associated with increased levels of matrix metalloproteinase within the aortic wall.

Dissection propagation

The ascending aorta, which has the highest fraction of elastic tissue, is the aortic segment that shows the greatest predilection to dissection (50–80%). There remains uncertainty whether the initiating process represents a spontaneous intimal tear with medial cleavage or whether a spontaneous bleed develops in the media breaking through into the lumen. The dissection plane propagates distally, leaving a true lumen and generating a false lumen. The propagation affects mainly the areas of greatest longitudinal and radial curvature. In the ascending aorta this leads to false luminal expansion to the right and anteriorly, which may disrupt the right coronary ostium and the non-coronary sinus of Valsalva, and along the convexity of the aortic arch, jeopardising the origins of the epi-aortic vessels. The primary entry tear is usually transverse and approximately 60% arise within 2 cm of the left main coronary ostium. The dissection plane usually propagates along the left posterolateral aspect of the descending aorta, creating a false lumen separated by an intimal flap and a relatively thinner adventitial layer on the outside. False luminal patency is maintained by fenestrations in the intima generated by the shearing of intercostal origins or secondary re-entry tears generated by the intra-luminal rupture of the pressurised false channel [1].

Malperfusion phenomena

Malperfusion phenomena due to branch artery compromise are seen in a third of cases of aortic dissection and may arise by a variety of mechanisms. The most common form occurs when the true lumen is compressed by a pressurised false lumen. This may compromise branch arteries or even the whole aorta, leading to acute lower body hypoperfusion and an acute Leriche syndrome, manifesting as impotence, fatigue and pallor affecting the lower limbs. Extension of a dissection into a branch artery may also occur, leading to a similar phenomenon without re-entry. Alternatively, the intima of the whole vessel origin may be sheared, leading to intussusceptions of the inner intimo-medial layer. The mobile intimal flap can also occlude a branch vessel, acting like a lid forced closed under pressure. Thrombosis beyond the compromised vessel ostium may further worsen ischaemia. The incidence of clinically important malperfusion phenomena is reported to be: lower limb 12–25%, cerebral 8–12%, coronary 7–10% and renal or mesenteric 5–10%.

22.3 Classification

Aortic dissections are classified according to location and acuity (Table 22.2, Figure 22.1). These classifications are pragmatic. A dissection involving the ascending aorta is managed differently from one involving the descending aorta alone. A chronic dissection will have undergone a degree of wall healing and theoretically should be more amenable to surgical intervention.

22.4 Clinical presentation

The main challenge in the management of acute aortic dissection is to make an accurate diagnosis as soon as possible [11]. About a third of the patients with dissection are initially diagnosed as having acute coronary syndromes, pulmonary embolism and abdominal emergencies (Table 22.3). As the predominant symptom of dissection is chest pain, there is a large differential diagnosis (Table 22.2). A fraction of patients will have a history

Table 22.2 Classification of aortic dissection.

Location
1. Debakey Classification [37]
   Type I: originating in the ascending aorta and extending through the aortic arch and into the descending aorta or abdominal aorta for a varying distance
   Type II: originating in and confined to the ascending aorta
   Type III: originating in the descending thoracic aorta
   (*Type IIIa* is limited to thoracic aorta and *Type IIIb* involves variable extents of abdominal aorta)
2. Stanford Classification [38]
   Type A: Dissection involving the ascending aorta irrespective of the site of origin
   Type B: Dissection originating in and confined to descending and distal aorta

Acuity
1. A dissection becomes chronic 14 days after the acute event.

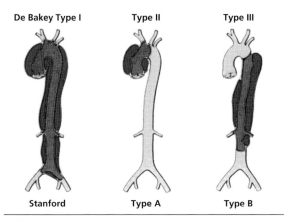

De Bakey
Type I Originates in the ascending aorta, propagates at least to the aortic arch and often beyond it distally.
Type II Originates in and is confined to the ascending aorta.
Type III Originates in the descending aorta and extends distally down the aorta or, rarely retrograde into the aortic arch and ascending aorta.

Stanford
Type A All dissections involving the ascending aorta, regardless of the site of origin.
Type B All dissections not involving the ascending aorta.

Figure 22.1 The common classifications of acute aortic dissection. (Reproduced from [39], with permission from *Circulation*.)

of Marfan's syndrome or other predisposing risk factors for dissection, while two-thirds of patients will give a history of treated hypertension.

Symptoms
Pain is the chief presenting symptom, described as sharp, tearing, ripping or stabbing in nature with a variable location. In proximal dissections the

Table 22.3 Differential diagnosis of acute dissection.

• Cardiac causes
  Myocardial infarction
  Acute coronary syndrome
  Aortic regurgitation without dissection
  Pericarditis
• Pulmonary causes
  Pleurisy
  Pulmonary embolism
  Pneuomthorax
	• Abdominal causes
	  Acute cholecystitis
	  Duodenal ulcer
	  Pancreatitis
	  Reflux oesophagitis
	• Miscellaneous
	  Musculoskeletal pain

pain is usually located anteriorly behind the sternum, whereas distal dissections are characterised by inter-scapular and back pain. Chest pain may occasionally be absent especially in cases of chronic dissection. The absence of pain substantially decreases the probability of acute dissection.

Syncope is seen in 5–10% of cases of acute type A dissection and may occur as a result of severe pain, activation of aortic baroreceptors, leakage from the aorta, cardiac tamponade or involvement of the brachiocephalic vessels with transient brain malperfusion. These patients are more likely to have type A dissection, suffer a stroke and die in hospital. Some patients present with stroke. Breathlessness may follow pain as a manifestation of acute heart failure or pleural effusion. On rare occasions, symptoms such as vocal chord paralysis (caused by compression of the left recurrent laryngeal nerve), haemoptysis or haematemesis (due to haemorrhage into the tracheobronchial tree or perforation into the oesophagus), upper airway obstruction (due to compression), superior vena cava syndrome, Horner's syndrome (due to compression of the superior cervical sympathetic ganglion) or signs of mesenteric or renal ischaemia may be encountered. Paraplegia or paraparesis from interruption of intercostal vessels occurs more commonly in patients with type B dissection and is seen in 2–3% of cases [5]. Similarly, patients may complain of transient limb weakness or numbness as a manifestation of malperfusion phenomena.

Physical signs

Hypertension is common at presentation in both type A and B dissection. Hypotension is more common in type A dissection and may be due to acute heart failure as a result of aortic regurgitation or coronary malperfusion or cardiac tamponade [12]. Examination of all pulses is critical and may identify a collapsing pulse with wide pulse pressure due to aortic regurgitation (AR), evidence of pulsus paradoxus or pulse deficits. Pulse or pressure differentials between carotid, radial or femoral arteries are common and occur in 30–50% of the patients. These patients are more likely to develop complications including neurological deficits, coma and hypotension and are at an increased risk of dying. Carotid pulse deficits are strongly related to fatal strokes. The clinical course of peripheral ischaemia can be quite variable, with a third of these patients demonstrating spontaneous resolution [5]. Refractory hypertension despite medical management is commonly seen in the patients with type B dissection. Involvement of the brachiocephalic vessels can result in differential blood pressure between the arms. In type A dissection, an early diastolic murmur of aortic regurgitation can be heard in about a third of cases.

Initial investigations
Electrocardiogram (ECG)
Many patients have non-specific T wave or ST segment changes and a few have clear evidence of coronary malperfusion, most usually with inferior ST elevation. Thus, an ECG alone may not distinguish dissection from acute myocardial infarction and a number of patients erroneously receive thrombolysis. A normal ECG is present in one-third of patients with coronary disease, whilst some patients with acute dissection involving the coronary ostia may have ECG evidence of ischaemia or infarction.

Chest X-ray
The chest X-ray is normal in about 1 in 8 cases and the classical description of a widened mediastinum only occurs in approximately 60%. Other features may include an abnormal aortic or cardiac contour and there may be apparent displacement of intimal calcification at the aortic knuckle into the vessel lumen. Pleural effusion may be an exudative reaction, a consequence of heart failure or an indication of rupture.

Laboratory investigations
Creatine kinase may be elevated due to muscle injury, but cardiac troponin may be more discriminatory provided coronary malperfusion is absent. Patients with dissection may have a moderate leukocytosis, raised C-reactive protein, serum bilirubin and lactic dehydrogenase. An elevated concentration of smooth muscle myosin heavy chain has been associated with aortic dissection [13]. A consumption coagulopathy with prolonged prothrombin and partial thromboplastin times, reduced platelet count, reduced fibrinogen and elevated D-dimers commonly accompanies dissection. At present, no biochemical test has sufficient specificity or sensitivity to aid diagnosis.

Imaging
Transthoracic/transoesophageal echocardiography
Transthoracic echocardiography (TTE) is a useful screening investigation while definitive investigations are awaited. It will provide information regarding left ventricular function, regional wall motion abnormality, aortic valve competence, and the presence of pericardial fluid, and allows a limited examination of the proximal ascending aortic wall. Approximately 60% of acute type A dissections can be confidently diagnosed using TTE, but the absence of an intimal flap is a poor indicator that dissection is not

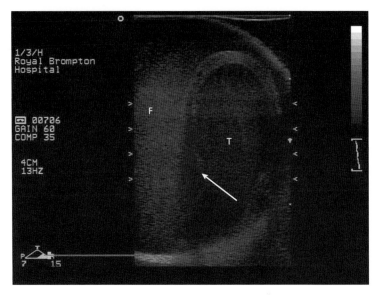

Figure 22.2 Epiaortic echocardiography of the ascending aorta in a patient with acute aortic dissection (dissection flap arrowed). Note the increased echo-density in the false lumen compared with the smaller true lumen. T, true lumen; F, false lumen.

present (high false negative). Transoesophageal echocardiography (TOE) (Figure 22.2) improves the sensitivity and can provide valuable additional advice regarding the site of entry and re-entry tears and false lumen blood flow. Small intimal tears can be detected by colour Doppler, registering jets traversing the dissection membrane. Echo-free spaces around the aorta may be evidence of peri-aortic haematoma. The sensitivity and specificity of TOE for aortic dissection diagnosis are each approximately 90%.

Computed tomography (CT)

Contrast-enhanced fine-cut CT is currently the most commonly used imaging modality in patients with suspected aortic dissection. The diagnosis is based on the demonstration of an intimal flap which separates the true from the false lumen. The flap is identified as a low attenuation linear structure in the aortic lumen (Figure 22.3). Secondary findings include internal displacement of intimal calcifications, delayed enhancement of the false lumen and aortic widening. The finding of greatest significance is the observation of false lumen being larger than true lumen in more than 90% of cases. The sensitivity and specificity of CT scan are each in the region of 90% [14].

Magnetic resonance imaging (MRI)

MRI may have the highest overall sensitivity and specificity for detection of aortic dissection [15]. However, the technique is often not available on an emergency basis and examination of haemodynamically unstable patients

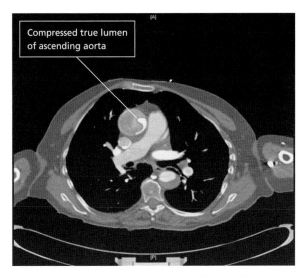

Compressed true lumen of ascending aorta

Figure 22.3 Contrast CT scan of patient showing type A dissection. The true lumen is compressed as the dissection propagates along the greater curvature of the aorta.

may be difficult. As with TOE, MRI allows localisation of entry and re-entry tears and, in addition, flow in false and true lumen can be quantified using phase contrast cine MRI or by tagging techniques. MRI may also allow visualisation of the proximal coronary arteries.

Aortography

Aortography used to be the gold standard for diagnosis, but its role has been taken over by less invasive investigations. Its use is now restricted to a component of percutaneous intervention in endovascular management of dissection and malperfusion. Contrast aortography accurately identifies branch vessel involvement, especially of renal or mesenteric vessels. The specificity of aortography for diagnosing aortic dissection is > 95%, but its sensitivity is lower than that of other techniques.

Coronary angiography

Although coronary atherosclerotic disease may be present in a quarter of patients with acute dissection and may worsen the surgical outcome, coronary angiography is rarely used as it may delay emergency surgery and has potential to cause propagation of the dissection. Its use is reserved for those cases with a definite history of ischaemic heart disease or previous surgery, particularly coronary artery bypass surgery. Coronary angiography has not been shown to improve hospital survival [16].

Intravascular ultrasound (IVUS)

IVUS is a novel, invasive technique that can directly visualise the vessel wall architecture from inside the aortic lumen, therefore allowing the accurate recognition of aortic wall characteristics and pathology. It provides visualisation of the intimal-medial flap, its movement, its circumferential and longitudinal extent and the degree of luminal compromise. Branch vessel involvement and false lumen thrombosis may be better defined with IVUS than with TOE. Although sensitivities and specificities approaching 100% have been reported, IVUS is not yet in widespread diagnostic use [17].

22.5 Management

Medical treatment

As soon as the diagnosis is made the patient should be moved to a critical care unit and invasive arterial blood pressure monitoring instituted. All type A dissections should be immediately transferred to cardiac surgical centre. There is a strong argument for also transferring cases of type B dissection, but at present, transfer is usually reserved for those patients with complications such as malperfusion phenomena. Systolic blood pressure (BP) should be reduced to ≤ 110 mmHg, but in the presence of aortic regurgitation, a mean BP of 60–75 mmH should also be targeted. Effective pain relief will help to control BP. Beta blockers are the initial drug of choice as they decrease the force of left ventricular contraction (dP/dT). Intravenous beta blockers like labetolol (both alpha and beta blocker) and esmolol are suitable for this purpose (Chapter 24).

Pleural effusions should be drained. The presence of a pericardial effusion in the presence of dissection should be assumed to be due to intra-pericardial rupture and is an indication for emergency surgery. Pericardiocentesis may be used as a holding manoeuvre during transfer in shocked patients, but this is controversial [18].

Surgical management of type A dissection

The presence of ascending aortic involvement is an indication for operative management in all but the highest risk cases [19]. Neurological status at presentation can influence the decision to operate. Obtundation, coma, stroke or paraplegia present for less than a few hours may represent malperfusion phenomena that may improve with reperfusion. However, established deficits with corresponding lesions on CT scanning may become haemorrhagic during cardiopulmonary bypass and so individualised management plans with deferment of surgery may be appropriate. The presence of mesenteric or bilateral renal ischaemia are both treatment priorities, but initial management should be directed at closing the initial entry tear surgically or endovascularly prior to a direct approach such as laparotomy, as re-institution of true luminal flow may lead to reperfusion of the affected viscera [5]. However, endovascular peripheral revascularisation may still be necessary [20].

The objectives of surgery in type A dissection are: prevention of intra-pericardial rupture, protection of the coronary artery ostia and other major vessels from malperfusion, restoration of the competence of the

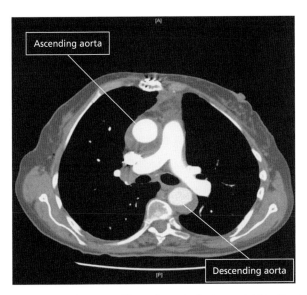

Figure 22.4 Post-operative contrast CT scan demonstrating the re-established true luminal flow in the ascending and descending aorta.

aortic valve and elimination of a distal false lumen (Figure 22.4). The reported outcomes for acute type A dissection repair vary, with reported early mortalities between 6 and 30%. In the International Registry of Aortic Dissection database, the overall hospital mortality was 25.1%. Mortality is higher in patients with instability or malperfusion phenomena. Longer-term outcomes are satisfactory, with 5- and 10-year survival for patients undergoing immediate surgical repair of 71% and 54% respectively [21, 22].

Surgical management of type B dissection

Early surgery is reserved for cases with complications, including leakage, distal malperfusion, prompt expansion, continuing pain and inability to control BP. Such emergency procedures are inevitably high risk and mortality rates are approximately 30% [23]. More recently, endovascular stenting of complicated dissections has shown great promise in reducing mortality and morbidity. Deployment of a covered endovascular stent to exclude the entry tear in the distal aortic arch may restore perfusion to organs in jeopardy. Both surgery and stenting can be combined with other percutaneous catheter-based techniques to deal with branch vessel occlusion including intimal flap fenestration and branch vessel stenting [24]. In a meta-analysis of endovascular stent graft placement in type B dissections, successful stent deployment was achieved in > 95% of cases with a neurological complication rate of 3% [25]. Survival at 2 years was 90%, but stenting failed to abolish the false lumen in about a quarter of patients.

Most uncomplicated type B aortic dissections are treated conservatively, with similar survival rates approaching 90% [26]. Medical therapy is directed towards the control of hypertension and at least 60–70% continue to be free of aortic complications in the long term. The role of endovascular treatment for all cases remains an issue of debate [27].

Anaesthetic management

Many patients present as an emergency, which necessitates rapid sequence induction. In these and elective cases, the choice of anaesthetic technique should confer cardiac stability, with particular attention to blunting the haemodynamic response to intubation. In the emergency setting, careful control of the blood pressure with beta blockade and/or intravenous venodilators may prevent progression of the dissection (see Chapter 24).

Line placement is crucial and should be guided by a discussion regarding the proposed surgical technique. Arterial monitoring should be established via a femoral artery (leaving one side for surgical access) and a radial artery. The left radial is preferentially used to avoid loss of the arterial blood pressure wave form if the dissection flap extends to the innominate artery or the surgeon cannulates the right axillary artery for perfusion access. Other routine monitoring includes 5-lead ECG, saturation probe (left hand), central venous pressure (via right internal jugular) and a nasopharyngeal temperature probe. The measurement of core temperature is essential if deep hypothermic arrest is to be used, and the nasopharyngeal route equates most closely with the cerebral temperature. Further evidence of adequate cerebral metabolic suppression may be obtained by monitoring the jugular bulb venous saturation using a retrogradely inserted jugular bulb line. A jugular bulb saturation of ≥ 95% implies that the cerebral metabolic rate is less than 25% of the rate at 37°C and this can be used as a guide for commencing circulatory arrest. Most centres advocate intra-operative TOE during aortic dissection surgery, which necessitates a 'second operator'.

Two issues of specific concern during thoracic aortic surgery are cerebral protection during deep hypothermic arrest and the maintenance of spinal perfusion. Deep hypothermic arrest is usually at 16–18°C. Cerebral perfusion may be maintained via anterograde or retrograde flow, though some surgeons advocate neither [28]. Twenty minutes is a safe period of arrest in adults, though longer periods are used in children. An absolute value is difficult to establish. It is advisable to check pupil size and reaction prior to arrest, and institute bispectral index monitoring. A variety of methods have been used to confer cerebral protection including thiopentone, propofol, isoflurane, corticosteroids and topical cooling [29]. Thiopentone will cause burst suppression and does reduce the cerebral metabolic requirement for oxygen, but the doses needed for clinical protection are high (3–10 mg/kg confers 5 minutes of electroencephalography (EEG) suppression) and necessitate increased use of vasopressors and inotropes. Propofol may be used to maintain anaesthesia during bypass and may confer an advantage during hypothermic arrest. Isoflurane cannot be administered during arrest. Corticosteroids are only of proven value in reducing cerebral oedema, and have not been shown to confer cerebral protection *per se*. The only proven method of protection is ice packing the head. Care must be taken not to cause hypothermic injuries to the face and eyes. Slow cooling and slow rewarming are also advisable during cardio-pulmonary bypass; slow rewarming allows wash-out of metabolites and free radicals at a time when the brain is particularly sensitive to permanent cellular damage. Glucose-containing solutions should be avoided as they may worsen cellular damage.

The spinal cord is largely supplied by a series of arteries which are branches of the descending thoracic aorta. Damage to these vessels may result in cord ischaemia and subsequent paralysis, affecting 5–20% of cases. Injury is also possible when hypoperfusion is prolonged. If the pressure within the cerebrospinal fluid (CSF) containing spaces is reduced, supply to the cord may be preserved even during periods of relative hypoperfusion. It is on this basis that spinal drains are advocated for cord protection during thoracic aortic surgery. The insertion technique is simple and involves dural puncture with a Thuoy needle and placement of an indwelling spinal catheter under strict aseptic conditions. Debate regarding the risk of bleeding and subsequent cord compression during full heparinisation complicates the use of spinal drains. The CSF pressure is measured and maintained using a closed manometer and drain. Both excessive and inadequate drainage of CSF may have disastrous consequences and spinal drains need careful monitoring and vigilance during the intra-operative and post-operative period. The use of shunts or partial bypass during thoracic aortic surgery does not guarantee distal perfusion or confer spinal protection. It is advisable to check motor function in the lower limbs as soon as possible post-operatively, and remove the spinal drain once adequate motor function is documented. In patients who have not had a spinal drain inserted prior to surgery but subsequently develop neurological signs of lower limb motor dysfunction post-operatively, a spinal drain may then be used for cord protection [30]. Corticosteroids may also be used to reduce spinal cord oedema.

Post-operatively, a major concern is maintenance of perfusion whilst protecting the surgical sites from surges in blood pressure. Systolic pressures of 80–100 mmHg should ensure adequate spinal cord perfusion and renal blood flow. Excessive systemic pressures may be controlled by ensuring adequate sedation and analgesia combined with anti-hypertensive therapy, for example intravenous glyceryl trinitrate. Central neuraxial blockade may be complicated by full heparinisation for bypass and the use of a spinal drain.

Post-operative complications that may occur and require vigilance include renal, mesenteric and spinal hypoperfusion. Coagulopathy following massive transfusion is common and should be aggressively corrected. Blood glucose should be closely controlled (6–8 mmol/l) as poor control worsens outcome [31].

22.6 Outcomes

Type A dissection
Untreated type A aortic dissection carries a mortality of 20% by 24 hours after presentation, 30% at 48 hours, 40% by day 7 and at least 50% at 1 month with medical management alone (Figure 22.5) [19]. Mortality is attributable to rupture, malperfusion phenomena and intractable heart failure due to severe aortic regurgitation. The most common causes of post-operative mortality are cardiac failure, intra-operative haemorrhage, multiple organ failure and major neurological injury [32]. Surgical repair does not consistently eliminate the flow and pressure in the distal false lumen.

Type B dissection
Patients with uncomplicated type B dissection have a 30-day mortality rate of 10% [8]. Patients with leg ischaemia, renal failure, visceral ischaemia or contained rupture have a 30-day mortality rate of 25%. Advanced age, rupture, shock and malperfusion are important predictors of mortality [26, 33]. The majority of patients with type B dissection are uncomplicated and can be managed medically [8].

Late complications
Both proximal and distal dissection may be complicated by late aneurysm formation, which is seen in 25–40% of the patients surviving the acute event despite adequate treatment [5]. Late aneurysm formation appears to be related to persistence of a patent false lumen, higher initial aortic

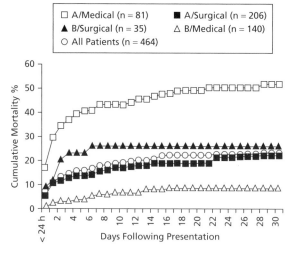

Figure 22.5 The mortality of acute dissection with and without intervention. (Reproduced from [40], with permission from *JAMA*.)

dimension and poor BP control within the first weeks of the dissection [34]. Long-term beta blockade leads to a reduction in late aneurysmal complications [35]. About 10–20% of patients with dissection experience late aneurysm rupture [36]. Hence, it is essential to follow up such cases with serial imaging.

22.7 Other acute aortic syndromes

Intra-mural haematoma (IMH)
Aortic IMH is considered a precursor of dissection, originating from ruptured vasa vasorum in medial wall layers and resulting in an aortic wall infarct that may provoke a secondary tear, causing a classic aortic dissection. IMH may progress to dissection, aneurysm formation or rupture, but a significant fraction will reabsorb with good BP control. Most IMH cases (50–85%) occur in the descending aorta and are typically associated with hypertension. Clinical manifestations of IMH are similar to acute aortic dissection. Chest pain is more common with ascending (type A) IMH; upper or lower back pain is more common with descending (type B) lesions. The diagnosis of IMH versus acute aortic dissection cannot be made clinically and is dependent on tomographic imaging. Type B IMH is treated like a type B dissection. A high fraction of type A IMHs may progress to full dissection or wall rupture and therefore these lesions are managed surgically.

Penetrating atherosclerotic ulcer (PAU)
Deep ulceration of atherosclerotic aortic plaques can lead to IMH, aortic dissection or perforation. PAU most often complicates IMH and appears as an ulcer-like projection into the aortic wall haematoma. Symptomatic ulcers or those with signs of deep erosion appear more prone to rupture, and in these patients endovascular stenting is emerging as an attractive therapeutic modality.

22.8 Summary

The possibility of aortic dissection should be considered for every patient presenting with severe chest pain. The key to achieving the best outcome is early recognition and diagnosis and prompt expert management. Patients with type A dissections should be immediately transferred to a cardiac surgical centre. There is a strong argument for also transferring cases of type B dissection, but at present this is usually reserved for those patients with complications such as malperfusion phenomena. Blood pressure control is key to preventing proliferation of the dissection flap and malperfusion syndromes. Type A dissections are managed surgically in most cases, whereas early surgery is reserved for only type B dissections associated with complications.

Case study

A 67-year-old female, a current smoker, presented to the Emergency Department with central anterior chest pain radiating to the back associated with shortness of breath and a left-sided weakness. The patient was found collapsed by a relative who then brought her to hospital, where she had an episode of profound bradycardia which was treated with atropine. Past medical history included cerebral aneurysm treated 13 years ago and she was under investigation for a breast lump. There was a family history of type B aortic dissection affecting her son.

On examination, the patient's circulation was adequate clinically but a diastolic murmur of severe aortic regurgitation was heard and the radial and brachial pulses on the left were impalpable. There were signs of a left hemiparesis. A CT scan of the head, thorax and abdomen demonstrated a type A dissection (Figure 22.3) and the decision to perform emergency repair was made. Informed consent was secured quoting a mortality of 50% (increased because of the pre-operative malperfusion), stroke rate of 10% and paraplegia of 10%. Ten units of cross-matched blood were requested, 10 units of fresh frozen plasma (FFP), 10 units of platelets and 10 units of cryoprecipitate.

Surgery commenced within 2 hours of referral. At operation a near-circumferential type A dissection with disruption of non-left and non-right commissures leading to aortic regurgitation was evident. A small transverse intimal tear 1 cm distal to the left main coronary artery was identified, with the dissection involving the right coronary ostium and in the arch involving the ostia of the innominate and left carotid artery. The ascending aorta was excised, the aortic valve resuspended and an interposition graft was anastomosed between the transected proximal and distal aorta.

The patient returned to the intensive treatment unit (ITU). Where on waking there was no movement in the legs, cerebrospinal fluid drainage was performed through a drain inserted at the L4/L5 level. Physiotherapy was instigated on the first post-operative day, at which point there were no plantar or knee reflexes. In the pursuing days the patient maintained good haemodynamic parameters and progressively improved from a respiratory aspect, with all drains and invasive monitoring having been removed by the ??8th day post surgery.

The main concern was the lack of recovery from neurological symptoms. She maintained a flaccid paralysis of the lower limbs and the impression was that there was significant injury of the spinal cord following a malperfusion injury. Unfortunately due to the cerebral aneurysmal clipping she had performed 13 years ago, an MRI could not be performed to delineate the level of spinal cord injury. Despite a small amount of recovery of power in the left leg there was no significant improvement in the lower limb neurology. The patient was discharged to a long-term rehabilitation centre for intensive neuro-rehabilitation on anti-hypertensive medication and with a planned follow-up surveillance scanning.

References

1. Borst HG, Heinemann MK, Stone CD. *Surgical Treatment of Aortic Dissection*. 1996. Churchill Livingstone, New York.
2. Fowkes FG, Ruckley CV. Increasing incidence of aortic aneurysms in England and Wales. *BMJ* 1989; 298(6665): 33–5.
3. Fuster VHJ. Aortic dissection: a medical perspective. *J Card Surg* 1994; 9(6): 713–28.
4. Larson EW. Risk factors for aortic dissection: a necropsy study of 161 cases. *Am J Cardiol* 1984; 53(6): 849–55.
5. Atkins MD, Black JH, III, Cambria RP. Aortic dissection: perspectives in the era of stent-graft repair. *J Vasc Surg* 2006; 43(Suppl A): 30A–43A.
6. Nienaber C, Eagle K. Aortic dissection: new frontiers in diagnosis and management. Part 1: From etiology to dagnostic strategies. *Circulation* 2003; 108: 628–35.
7. Nienaber C, Eagle K. Aortic dissection: new frontiers in diagnosis and management. Part 2: Therapeutic management and follow-up. *Circulation* 2003; 108: 772–8.
8. Hagan PG, Isselbacher EM, Bruckman D, et al. The International Registry of Acute Aortic Dissection (IRAD): new insights into an old disease. *JAMA* 2000; 283(7): 897–903.
9. Hsue PY, Bolger AF, Benowitz NL, et al. Acute aortic dissection related to crack cocaine. *Circulation* 2002; 105(13): 1592–5.
10. Robicsek F. Hemodynamic considerations regarding the mechanism and prevention of aortic dissection. *Ann Thorac Surg* 1994; 58(4): 1247–53.
11. Klompas M. Does this patient have an acute thoracic aortic dissection? *JAMA* 2002; 287(17): 2262–72.
12. Lauterbach SR, Brewster DC, Gertler JP, et al. Contemporary management of aortic branch compromise resulting from acute aortic dissection. *J Vasc Surg* 2006; 33(6): 1185–92.
13. Suzuki T, Nagai R. Biochemical diagnosis of aortic dissection: from bench to bedside. *Jpn Heart J* 1999; 40(5): 527–34.
14. Sommer T, Holzknecht N, Smekal AV, et al. Aortic dissection: a comparative study of diagnosis with spiral CT, multiplanar transesophageal echocardiography, and MR imaging. *Radiology* 1996; 199(2): 347–52.
15. Panting JR, Baker C, Nicholson AA. Feasibility, accuracy and safety of magnetic resonance imaging in acute aortic dissection. *Clin Radiol* 1995; 50(7): 455–8.
16. Motallebzadeh R, Valencia O, Chandrasekaran V, et al. The role of coronary angiography in acute type A aortic dissection. *Eur J Cardiothorac Surg* 2004; 25(2): 231–5.
17. Yamada E, Kyo S, Omoto R. Usefulness of a prototype intravascular ultrasound imaging in evaluation of aortic dissection and comparison with angiographic study, transesophageal echocardiography, computed tomography, and magnetic resonance imaging. *Am J Cardiol* 1995; 75(2): 161–5.
18. Isselbacher EM, Eagle KA. Cardiac tamponade complicating proximal aortic dissection. Is pericardiocentesis harmful? *Circulation* 1994; 90(5): 2375–8.
19. Nienaber CA. Aortic dissection: new frontiers in diagnosis and management: Part II: therapeutic management and follow-up. *Circulation* 2003; 108(6): 772–8.
20. Deeb GM, Bolling SF, Quint LE, et al. Surgical delay for acute type A dissection with malperfusion. *Ann Thorac Surg* 1997; 64(6): 1669–75.
21. Trimarchi S, Rampoldi V, Myrmel T, et al. Contemporary results of surgery in acute type A aortic dissection: the International Registry of Acute Aortic Dissection experience. *J Thorac Cardiovasc Surg* 2005; 129(1): 112–22.

22. Tsai TT, Fattori R, Trimarchi S, et al. Long-term survival in patients presenting with type A acute aortic dissection: insights from the International Registry of Acute Aortic Dissection (IRAD). *Circulation* 2006; 114(1_Suppl): I-350–6.

23. Svensson LG. How to obtain hemostasis after aortic surgery. *Ann Thorac Surg* 1999; 67(6): 1981–2.

24. Hartnell GG. Aortic fenestration: a why, when, and how-to guide. *Radiographics* 2005; 25(1): 175–89.

25. Eggebrecht H, Neuhauser M, Baumgart D, et al. Endovascular stent-graft placement in aortic dissection: a meta-analysis. *Eur Heart J* 2006; 27(4): 489–98.

26. Suzuki T, Ince H, Nagai R, et al. Clinical profiles and outcomes of acute type B aortic dissection in the current era: lessons from the International Registry of Aortic Dissection (IRAD). *Circulation* 2003; 108(Suppl 1): II312–17.

27. Estrera AL, Miller CC, Hazim JS, et al. Outcomes of medical management of acute type B aortic dissection. *Circulation* 2006; 114(1_Suppl): I-384–9.

28. Gega A, Rizzo JA, Johnson MH, et al. Straight deep hypothermic arrest: experience in 394 patients supports its effectiveness as a sole means of brain preservation. *Ann Thorac Surg* 2007; 84: 759–66; discussion 766–7.

29. Murkin JM. Attenuation of neurologic injury during cardiac surgery. *Ann Thorac Surg* 2001; 72: S1838–44.

30. Estrera AL, Miller CC, Chen EP. Descending thoracic aortic aneurysm repair: 12-year experience using distal aortic perfusion and cerebrospinal fluid drainage. *Ann Thorac Surg* 2005; 80: 1290–6; discussion 1296.

31. Finney SJ. The insulin, glucose, ischemia, and inflammation conundrum. *Crit Care Med* 2008; 36: 1673–4.

32. Van Arsdell GS, Butany J. Autopsies in acute type A aortic dissection. Surgical implications. *Circulation* 1998; 98(19 Suppl): II299–302.

33. Mehta RH, Bossone E, Nienaber CA, et al. Acute type A aortic dissection in the elderly: clinical characteristics, management, and outcomes in the current era. *J Am Coll Cardiol* 2002; 40(4): 685–92.

34. Marui A, Mitsui N, Koyama T, et al. Toward the best treatment for uncomplicated patients with type B acute aortic dissection: a consideration for sound surgical indication. *Circulation* 1999; 100(Suppl 19): II275–80.

35. Genoni M, Jenni R, Graves K, et al. Chronic beta-blocker therapy improves outcome and reduces treatment costs in chronic type B aortic dissection. *Eur J Cardiothorac Surg* 2001; 19(5): 606–10.

36. Panneton JM. Dissecting descending thoracic and thoracoabdominal aortic aneurysms: Part II. *Ann Vasc Surg* 1995; 9(6): 596–605.

37. DeBakey ME, Creech O. Surgical consideration of dissecting aneurysm of the aorta. *Ann Surg* 1995; 142: 586–612.

38. Crawford ES, Coselli JS, Safi HJ, et al. Surgical treatment of aneurysm and/or dissection of the ascending aorta and transverse aortic arch. Factors influencing survival in 717 patients. *J Thorac Cardiovasc Surg* 1989; 98: 659–74.

39. Tsai TT, Nienaber CA, Eagle KA. Acute aortic syndromes. *Circulation* 2005; 112(24): 3802–13.

40. Hagan PG, Nienaber CA, Isselbacher EM, et al. The International Registry of Acute Aortic Dissection (IRAD): new insights into an old disease. *JAMA* 2000; 283(7): 897–903.

23 Emergency Management of Cardiac Trauma

James Napier and Mark Messent

Intensive Care Unit, St Bartholomew's Hospital, London, UK

Take Home Messages

- There is a high level of suspicion of blunt cardiac/aortic trauma in the multiply injured patient.
- Chest X-ray/transoesophageal echocardiogram (TOE)/troponin measurements are needed to exclude damage.
- Emergency department thoracotomy is indicated in both blunt and penetrating injury if there has been witnessed recent loss of cardiac activity.
- Cardio-pulmonary bypass is associated with less neurological impairment than 'clamp and sew' when repairing penetrating aortic injuries.
- Endovascular stent graft is associated with better outcome for aortic repair than conventional techniques, but long-term outcome data are lacking.

23.1 Introduction

Cardiac trauma is commonly encountered in the multiply injured patient. It may be caused by either blunt injury to the chest wall or penetration of the thoracic cavity. This chapter discusses the management of these two groups of injuries.

Blunt trauma has a wide variety of presentations. It is prevalent in young children because their height puts their chest at car bumper level. It occurs in motor vehicle accidents through the transmission of force by the seatbelt, dashboard or steering wheel if the occupant is unrestrained or if there is significant deformation of the vehicle with intrusion into the passenger compartment. It also occurs in sporting injuries and in industrial accidents, mainly those involving falls.

Cardiovascular Critical Care. Edited by M. Griffiths, J. Cordingley and S. Price.
© 2010 Blackwell Publishing Ltd.

Penetrating trauma by contrast is prevalent in urban young male adults and in conflict zones. Indeed much of the management of penetrating trauma has evolved from the battlefield. The level of injury depends on the mass (M) and velocity (V) of the penetrating object, with the kinetic energy being $1/2\,MV^2$, and the injury can be classified in terms of low, medium and high velocity. Low velocity injuries are often caused by hand-held weapons such as knives, and cause localised damage, determined by the length and width of the weapon, as well as the path taken. Medium velocity wounds are caused by hand-held guns, and cause potentially deeper injuries with limited tissue damage along the track of the bullet. High velocity injuries caused by rifles and shrapnel from exploding ordinance cause widespread tissue destruction with the kinetic energy of the missile dissipated through the tissue planes and the temporary formation of large cavities along the missile path. The shape of the missile, along with tumble and yaw are additional factors that increase tissue destruction by spreading the dissipation of energy over a larger area.

The effects on the cardiovascular system of thoracic trauma are usually detectible in the primary and secondary surveys, although a high degree of suspicion is required as a few injuries may be slow to declare themselves, especially in the face of hypovolaemia. This may mask significant underlying problems which only manifest once the patient has been volume resuscitated, for example a cardiac tamponade which presents with refractory hypotension in the patient on the intensive care unit. Indications that cardiac injury may have been sustained are listed in Table 23.1.

Emergency care

As with any trauma, the initial approach is based on the principles of advanced trauma life support (ATLS), and starts with the primary survey. This ABCDE assessment identifies life-threatening complications of the primary insult and corrects them as they are found.

The primary survey and its adjunctive treatment is followed by a detailed head-to-toe secondary survey. This allows a reassessment of the issues identified in the primary survey, unearthing of other apparent injuries and formulation of a plan for definitive management, including further investigation if indicated.

Finally a tertiary survey may be performed as a delayed procedure. The tertiary survey reviews the entire resuscitation, investigation and

Table 23.1 Pointers to underlying cardiovascular injury.

Mechanism of injury
Bruising or deformity of chest wall
Thoracic entry or exit wound
Painful sternum
Muffled heart sounds, narrow pulse pressure and distended neck veins
CXR – 1st rib fracture, widened mediastinum, left-sided haemothorax, deviation of gastric tube
Arrhythmias on electrocardiogram (ECG)
Shock with no obvious site of haemorrhage

management of the patient to ensure that nothing has been overlooked or ignored in the initial stages of treatment.

There is classically a trimodal distribution of death in trauma. The initial peak occurs at the scene, and no medical treatment affects the outcome at this point. Only primary prevention, for instance firearms legislation or the compulsory wearing of seatbelts in cars, has an effect on this. The second peak occurs over the ensuing minutes or hours. Here the ability to intervene in a timely manner is crucial, and the success of the 'chain of survival' is of paramount importance in reducing mortality. Getting the patient alive to an appropriate healthcare facility is the primary aim of the emergency medical services, although there is considerable debate as to how this is best done. Once in a resuscitation room an organised trauma team has the opportunity to provide life and limb saving measures and to prevent further harm. Decisions made at this point have huge consequences – this is the 'golden hour' of resuscitation. Failure to resuscitate the patient thoroughly, investigate appropriately and provide first-line treatment at this point may jeopardise the outcome of that patient. The third peak occurs over days to weeks, often from sepsis or multi-organ failure. Many factors affect the magnitude of the third peak, but the approach taken early in the course of the patient's treatment has perhaps the biggest impact.

Investigation

The need for investigation has to be weighed against the risk of delayed treatment. The case presented below illustrates the need for timely action in certain situations. In others, where time is not so pressing, considered investigation is optimal.

23.2 Blunt cardiac injury

The myocardium is susceptible to damage in relatively low velocity injuries [1]. Post-mortem evidence suggests that myocardial contusion is present in 14% of immediate fatalities from blunt trauma [2], although the true incidence is likely to be significantly higher. Compression of the myocardium results in cellular necrosis and intra- or trans-mural haemorrhage, which may, if extensive, result in septal or free wall rupture [3]. Other complications include arrhythmias, which may be fatal [3], ventricular dysfunction, acute valvular regurgitation and aneurysm formation [4]. Due to the orientation of the heart, the right ventricle is predominantly affected. Ventricular dysfunction was demonstrated by transoesophageal echocardiography (TOE) in 42% of patients with suspected myocardial contusion, with the right ventricle affected in more than 60% [5].

Diagnosis
Cardiac enzymes

Few tests are sensitive or specific for myocardial contusion. Creatine kinase (CK)-MB measurements are non-specific for myocardial injury as some skeletal CK contains the MB fraction. Cardiac troponins are specific for myocardial injury, and are released through loss of myocyte membrane integrity. Troponin I measurement has shown a sensitivity of 63%, a specificity of 98%, a positive predictive value of 40% and a negative predictive value of 98% for the diagnosis of myocardial contusion [6]. These data suggest that measurement of cardiac troponin is useful for excluding myocardial contusion, but a positive result is not diagnostic on its own. The study was limited by the use of electrocardiogram (ECG) criteria to diagnose myocardial contusion, but the low sensitivity and high specificity seems to be consistent across other studies. Elevated cardiac troponin may also be caused by transient low flow states resulting in cardiac ischaemia, making its interpretation difficult.

ECG

Forty to 83% of patients with myocardial contusion have ECG abnormalities, but most ECG changes are non-specific and are poorly predictive of outcome [7]. ST segment changes, extra-systolic beats, tachyarrhythmias, atrial fibrillation (AF) and bundle branch block may all occur. Non-cardiac conditions may impact on the ECG as well as pre-existing cardiac disease. However, the negative predictive value of an ECG has been reported at 90% [8] and may be used to exclude myocardial injury. When significant arrhythmias do develop it is usually within the first 24–48 hours after injury.

Echocardiography

Echocardiography allows the rapid assessment of cardiac function and detection of associated injuries, but is dependent on the availability of equipment and a skilled operator.

In a series of 131 patients with blunt chest trauma, TOE detected 14 aortic ruptures, 40 pericardial effusions, 34 para-aortic haematomas and 45 myocardial contusions [9]. In the same patient group transthoracic echocardiography (TTE) provided suboptimal images in 83 patients, and it detected only 15 myocardial contusions.

Radionucleotide scans

High false negative rates and the expense and difficulty obtaining scans immediately preclude use of this imaging modality in blunt chest trauma [10].

Management

In the absence of ECG abnormalities and elevated plasma troponin concentrations no further investigation is necessary. If no other injuries exist these patients may be discharged after 24 hours of monitoring. Those with ECG or troponin changes should be investigated with TOE and further management directed as appropriate.

Invasive monitoring of right-sided filling pressures and of cardiac output may be necessary to guide fluid and inotrope management. If adequate cardiac output cannot be maintained, the use of intra-aortic balloon pump

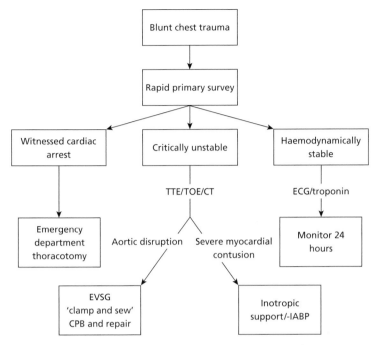

Figure 23.1 Algorithm of management of blunt cardiac injury. TTE, Transthoracic echocardiogram; TOE, transoesophageal echocardiogram; CT, computed tomography; ECG, electrocardiogram; EVSG, endovascular stent graft; CPB, cardio-pulmonary bypass; IABP, intra-aortic balloon pump.

counterpulsation should be considered [11]. An algorithim for the management of blunt cardiac trauma is presented in Figure 23.1.

Outcome

In a prospective study of 118 patients with manifest or suspected blunt thoracic trauma, 56.8% were admitted to a surgical intensive care unit. Of the intensive care group, 19.8% were diagnosed with myocardial contusion on ECG, CK-MB and echo criteria. There were no deaths due to cardiac causes in this series, and no long-term sequelae at long-term follow up [12].

23.3 Aortic injury

Blunt aortic injury is frequently lethal, with an estimated pre-hospital mortality of around 85%. In a series of 387 fatalities from blunt trauma, aortic injury was the second most common cause of death after head injury [13]. In a review of 242 cases of fatal blunt aortic injury, 68% involved motor vehicle accidents [14], with the isthmus of the aorta involved in 58% – a lower figure than that classically quoted, but one which perhaps reflects the greater lethality of other sites of injury.

Diagnosis
Chest X-ray
This is rarely diagnostic of aortic or cardiac injury but is still a useful investigation. Widening of the mediastinum, obliteration of the aortic knob, deviation of the trachea to the right, obliteration of the space between the aorta and the pulmonary artery, deviation of the gastric tube to the right with depression of the left main-stem bronchus, an apical cap, a left-sided haemothorax and first rib or scapula fractures are all associated with injury to the great vessels after blunt injury.

A widened mediastinum is defined as having a width of over 8 cm, or a mediastinal/chest width ratio of > 0.38 [15]. However, the finding is often subjective and non-specific, especially in the supine film taken in the emergency department.

Chest computed tomography
The advent of helical and spiral computed tomography (CT) scanners has enabled rapid diagnosis of aortic injury with high sensitivity and a negative predictive value of 100% [15]. If the scan is equivocal and the patient is haemodynamically stable, an angiogram may then be helpful.

Transoesophageal echocardiography
TOE is 93% and 98% sensitive and specific for detecting aortic rupture. In addition, the delay before committing to surgery was significantly reduced from 71 to 30 minutes. However, TOE requires local expertise which may be lacking in many centres [9].

Management
The mainstay of management is emergency surgical intervention, with or without cardio-pulmonary bypass (CPB). In a retrospective analysis of 65 patients who underwent surgery for blunt aortic injury over a 12-year period, there was no difference in mortality between those managed with 'clamp and sew' and those managed on cardio-pulmonary bypass. However, 12% treated with a 'clamp and sew' approach developed paraplegia, compared with none in the CPB group. This occurred in those with complex injuries or repairs, defined as extension proximal to the subclavian artery or involvement of branch vessels or requiring manoeuvres that interfered with anastamosis construction [15].

Since the early 1990s, endovascular stent grafting (EVSG) has become an accepted treatment for abdominal aortic aneurysm repair, and this technique has been used successfully in the repair of blunt aortic injury. In a series of 16 patients treated with EVSG for blunt aortic injury all survived, with only one complication [16]. Although the outcome with EVSG appears to be better than open repair, there are as yet no long-term data on outcome.

When patients with suspected aortic disruption are unstable, intervention may need to be performed in the emergency department. Indications for emergency thoracotomy in penetrating chest injury are

Table 23.2 Indications for emergency department thoracotomy.

Blunt trauma
- Unresponsive hypotension
- More than 1500 ml blood loss from chest drain

Penetrating trauma
- Witnessed traumatic cardiac arrest
- Unresponsive hypotension

Adapted from Brohi [17], with permission of Trauma.org.

unresponsive hypotension, rapid exsanguination from a chest drain
(> 1500 ml) and traumatic cardiac arrest with previously witnessed cardiac
activity (Table 23.2). Survival is not as good as for penetrating chest trauma,
with rates varying between 0 and 2.5% [17].

Outcome

The multicentre trial of the American Association for the Surgery of
Trauma involves the largest number of cases (274) of blunt aortic injury
reported. All of those who arrived in extremis and those with a ruptured
pseudoaneurysm subsequently died. Overall the mortality rate was 31% [18].

23.4 Penetrating cardiac and great vessel injury

Most patients with penetrating cardiac injuries die before arriving in
hospital. In a review of 1198 cases from the University of Natal only 6%
were alive on arrival at hospital [19], and those who did survive tended to
have either stab wounds or cardiac tamponade. The cardiac injuries may
be single or multiple and may affect either single or multiple chambers.
Injury may also involve the intrapericardial great vessels and clinical
differentiation between the two is impossible. In a series of 117 patients
with penetrating cardiac injury, 13 had vascular injuries, most of whom
presented with cardiac tamponade [20].

Entry wounds are often precordial, but adjacent wounds may produce
cardiac or great vessel injury if the penetrating weapon is long enough and if
the trajectory is directed towards the heart [20].

Investigation

For the most part this is confined to identifying immediately life-
threatening injuries in the primary survey. Further, detailed investigations
are only appropriate in those who are haemodynamically stable and in
whom there is doubt as to the underlying injury.

Chest X-ray

This is the standard first-line investigation. Its advantages lie in the relative
speed in acquiring an image, and the ability of many to interpret the results.

However, a small volume haemothorax may be missed on a supine film, and it is likely that thoracic ultrasound performed in the emergency department improves the sensitivity and specificity of detecting small pleural effusions [21].

Echocardiography

Echocardiography is now considered a front-line investigation in trauma, and is part of a Focused Assessment with Sonography for Trauma (FAST) scan. A subcostal view gives an assessment of the pericardium and of gross cardiac function in the hands of a non-expert. Indeed, ultrasound performed by surgeon-sonographers on 238 patients with penetrating truncal injuries and possible haemopericardium resulted in 100% sensitivity, 96.7% specificity and 97% accuracy [22]. These results were similar to those of emergency physicians trained in FAST scanning [22].

Computed tomography

CT has a role in evaluating the stable patient in whom cardiac tamponade and significant haemothorax have been ruled out either clinically or by ultrasound.

Management

An algorithm for the management of penetrating chest injury is presented in Figure 23.2. Aggressive fluid resuscitation should be delayed until thoracotomy to prevent hydraulic disruption of effective thrombus with secondary fatal haemorrhage. Delayed fluid resuscitation improved survival and showed a trend to reduced postoperative complications [23]. If the patient has actually had a cardiac arrest, CPR is not indicated and may only serve to exacerbate the situation. The only life-saving intervention is immediate thoracotomy to relieve tamponade and gain haemostasis [18].

Operative intervention is the mainstay of treatment, with thoracotomy or sternotomy performed in either the emergency department or the operating theatre depending on the clinical state of the patient. Emergency department thoracotomy is only indicated in those who had some evidence of cardiac activity at the scene of the accident and who subsequently arrest or deteriorate. The shorter the time between cardiac arrest and thoracotomy, the better the outcome. In a retrospective review of 302 patients presenting to Detroit Receiving Hospital, none of the 43 patients who arrested on scene survived. In contrast, 19% of the 27 patients who arrested in the emergency department survived [24].

In those who are haemodynamically stable after initial resuscitation, thoracotomy or sternotomy can be carried out in the operating theatre, with midline sternotomy being advocated as the better approach. Sternotomy allows better access to the right side and posterior aspects of the heart, and thoracotomy often needs to be extended across the midline to achieve similar exposure [20].

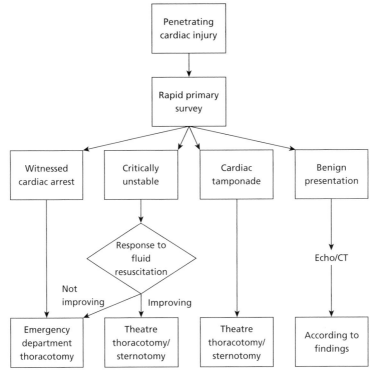

Figure 23.2 Algorithm of management of penetrating cardiac injury. (Modified from Degiannis [19].)

Outcome

Comparison between hospitals and countries is difficult as many factors impact on outcome. Hospital mortality may indeed be worse with better access to pre-hospital care, as patients may be brought in alive but sicker than in areas with poor pre-hospital care.

Patients suffering gunshot wounds are more likely to be critically unstable at presentation (65% vs 35%) and have a higher mortality (82% vs 35.5%) than those with cardiac stab wounds [20]. The presence of cardiac tamponade was found to be protective, but only in those with stab wounds, with an 8% mortality in this group. The reason for this is that those sustaining great vessel wounds outside of the pericardium rapidly exsanguinate and die on scene due to lack of containment of the resulting haemorrhage. Emergency department thoracotomy for stab wound had a survival rate of 43%, but in those who had been shot there were no survivors. Other injuries associated with poor outcome include left ventricular and multi-chamber wounds and great vessel injury. Late sequelae, mainly valvular or septal defects, were found in 19% of patients with penetrating cardiac injury [25], and long-term echocardiographic follow-up is needed to diagnose these lesions.

23.5 Summary

Cardiac trauma presents the clinician with time-sensitive diagnostic and therapeutic challenges. Maximising the chances of survival requires good team working and early decisive intervention in a centre capable of managing the critically injured patient. Access to appropriate imaging, especially TOE, is critical to the diagnostic work-up, to ensure that injuries are found and treated appropriately. Surgical intervention must be available from the earliest point of contact to ensure that those who require thoracotomy in either the emergency department or the operating theatre get it. The use of interventional techniques such as stent grafting is increasingly important to further improve outcome.

Hand-in-hand with surgical developments is the constant need for improved safety, both on the roads and in the workplace, to reduce the burden of blunt cardiac trauma, and the imperative to tackle the use of the knives and guns that play such a devastating part in the lives of many young men living in the inner city.

Case study

An inner-city teenager was assaulted with a knife, and received a solitary stab wound to the front of his chest. He collapsed to the ground and a bystander called for help. The Helicopter Emergency Medical Service was mobilised and on scene within 10 minutes. The doctor found him to be obtunded, but with a pulse. He performed a clamshell thoracotomy and found the pericardium ballooning out. He incised the pericardium and relieved the tamponade, and cardiac activity resumed. He was then intubated and ventilated, and cardiac massage was performed to maintain an output. The patient was transferred to the trauma centre where his thoracic cavity was explored by the emergency physician on the trauma team. A 1-cm incised wound was found in the intrapericardial aorta, along with a small iatrogenic pulmonary incision from the thoracotomy. Both of these were closed with sutures, haemostasis was secured and the clamshell was then closed with chest drains inserted. The patient was transferred to ITU for ongoing monitoring and support. There was no further bleeding and the patient remained haemodynamically stable. He developed a simple right-sided pneumothorax following removal of his chest drains, which required insertion of a further intercostal drain, but his progress was otherwise uneventful and he was extubated on day 2. The following day he was transferred to the ward with an epidural for analgesia and after 1 week was discharged home, fit and well.

References

1. Feghell N, Prisant L. Blunt myocardial injury. *Chest* 1995;108:1673–77.
2. Wisner D, Reed W, Riddick R. Suspected myocardial contusion. Triage and indications for monitoring. *Ann Surg* 1990;212:82–6.
3. Sakka SG, Huettemann E, Giebe W, et al. Late cardiac arrhythmias after blunt chest trauma. *Intensive Care Med* 2006;26(6):792–5.
4. Tenzer M. The spectrum of myocardial contusion: a review. *J Trauma* 1985;25:620–7.
5. Garcia-Fernandez M, Lopez-Perez J, Perez Castellano N, et al. Role of transoesophageal echocardiography in the assessment of patients with blunt chest trauma: correlation of echocardiographic findings with electrocardiogram and creatinine kinase monoclonal antibody measurements. *Am Heart J* 1998;135:476–81.
6. Edouard A, Felten M-L, Herbert J-L, et al. Incidence and significance of cardiac troponin I release in severe trauma patients. *Anesthesiology* 2004;101:1262–8.
7. Potkin R, Werner J, Trobaugh G, et al. Evaluation of non-invasive tests of myocardial damage in suspected cardiac contusion. *Circulation* 1982;66:627–31.
8. Healey M, Brown R, Fleizer D. Blunt cardiac injury: is this diagnosis necessary? *J Trauma* 1990;30:137–46.
9. Chirillo F, Totis O, Cavarzerani A, et al. Usefulness of transthoracic and transoesophageal echocardiography in recognition and management of cardiovascular injuries after blunt chest trauma. *Heart* 1996;75:301–6.
10. Kaye P. Myocardial contusion: emergency investigation and diagnosis. *Emerg Med J* 2002;19:8–10.
11. Demas C, Flancbaum L, Scott G, et al. The intra-aortic balloon pump as an adjunctive therapy for severe myocardial contusion. *Am J Emerg Med* 1987;5(6):499–502.
12. Lindstaedt M, Germing A, Lawo T, et al. Acute and long-term clinical significance of myocardial contusion following blunt thoracic trauma: results of a prospective study. *J Trauma* 2002;52(3):479–85.
13. Smith R, Chang F-C. Traumatic rupture of the aorta: still a lethal injury. *Am J Surg* 1986;152(6):660–3.
14. Bukhart H, Gomez G, Gerardo G, et al. Fatal blunt aortic injuries: a review of 242 autopsy cases. *J Trauma* 2001;50:113–5.
15. Miller P, Kortesis B, McLaughlin C, et al. Complex blunt aortic injury or repair: beneficial effects of cardiopulmonary bypass use. *Ann Surg* 2003;237(6):877–83.
16. Dunham M, Zygun D, Petrasek P, et al. Endovascular stent grafts for acute blunt aortic injury. *J Trauma* 2004;56(6):1173–8.
17. Brohi K. *Emergency Department Thoracotomy*. Trauma.org 2006. www.trauma.org/index.php/main/article/361/.
18. Fabian T, Richardson J, Croce M, et al. Prospective study of blunt aortic injury: multicenter trial of the American Association for the Surgery of Trauma. *J Trauma* 1997;42(3):374–83.
19. Degiannis E, Loogna P, Dietrich D, et al. Penetrating cardiac injuries: recent experience in South Africa. *World J Surg* 2006;30:1258–64.
20. Altun G, Altun A, Yilmaz A. Hemopericardium-related fatalities:a 10-year medicolegal autopsy experience. *Cardiology* 2005;104:133–7.
21. Brooks A, Davies B, Smethhurst M, et al. Emergency ultrasound in the acute assessment of haemothorax. *Emerg Med J* 2004;21:44–6.

22. Rozycki G, Feliciano D, Ochsner G, et al. The role of ultrasound in patients with possible penetrating cardiac wounds: a prospective multicenter study. *J Trauma* 1999;46(4):543–52.

23. Bickell W, Wall M, Pepe P, et al. Immediate versus delayed fluid resuscitation for hypotensive patients with penetrating torso injuries. *New Engl J Med* 1994;331(17):1105–9.

24. Tybursky J, Astra L, Wilson R, et al. Factors affecting prognosis with penetrating wounds of the heart. *J Trauma* 2000;48(4):587–91.

25. Demetriades D, Charalambides C, Sareli P, et al. Late sequelae of penetrating cardiac injuries. *Br J Surg* 1990;77(7):813–4.

24 Hypertensive Crises

Liao Pinhu[1,2] and Mark J.D. Griffiths[3]

[1]National Heart and Lung Institute, Imperial College London, UK
[2]Youjiang Medical University for Nationalities, Baise, PR, China
[3]Royal Brompton & Harefield NHS Foundation Trust, London, UK

Take Home Messages

- Hypertensive crises are defined by a systemic blood pressure of at least 180/110, although the significance of the level of hypertension varies greatly between patients.
- The diagnosis of a hypertensive emergency requires the presence of a new organ failure, most frequently renal dysfunction or encephalopathy.
- Management is determined by the cause of hypertension and by the associated risks, usually in terms of organ function and haemorrhage.
- There is a dearth of evidence to guide the choice of individual agents used to treat hypertensive emergencies.
- Treating hypertensive emergencies is fraught with danger for the unwary.

24.1 Introduction

A minority of hypertensive patients in intensive care units (ICU) are admitted with hypertension as their primary problem (Table 24.1). In the majority of cases, systemic hypertension is a complication of a medical condition or a reaction to medical intervention. Nevertheless, early recognition of injurious hypertension and its appropriate management may prevent organ failure and death. As in the more common scenario of hypotension and shock, these cases may require full invasive monitoring and the support of multiple organ systems.

In this chapter we discuss these issues, concentrating on cardiovascular complications of hypertension and systemic hypertension as a complication of cardiovascular conditions.

Cardiovascular Critical Care. Edited by M. Griffiths, J. Cordingley and S. Price.
© 2010 Blackwell Publishing Ltd.

Table 24.1 Causes of hypertensive crises.

Essential hypertension – interruption of, incompliance or interaction with
antihypertensive medication
Renal disease, e.g. glomerulonephritis, renal artery stenosis
Collagen vascular disease or vasculitis, e.g. scleroderma
Drug abuse, e.g. cocaine, amphetamine
Drugs, e.g. erythropoietin, monoamine oxidase inhibitors, cyclosporin
Tumour – phaeochromocytoma, renin secreting tumour
Pregnancy – pre/eclampsia and HELLP syndrome
Intracranial trauma
Aortic coarctation
Cushing's or Conn's syndrome
Guillain–Barré syndrome

HELLP Pregnancy-related syndrome of haemolysis, elevated hepatic enzymes and
thrombocytopaenia.

24.2 Hypertensive crises

Definitions

The definition of hypertensive crises generally requires the systolic blood
pressure (SBP) to be greater than 179 mmHg or the diastolic blood pressure
(DBP) to be greater than 109 mmHg. The classification of hypertensive
syndromes was reviewed by the Joint National Committee (JNC) on the
Prevention, Detection, Evaluation and Treatment of High Blood Pressure
in 2003, producing the JNC7 report [1]. Hypertensive emergencies and
urgencies are distinguished by the presence and absence respectively of
acute organ dysfunction (Table 24.2). The term malignant hypertension,
requiring the co-existence of encephalopathy or acute nephropathy, has
been superseded by hypertensive emergency.

Table 24.2 Organ dysfunction associated with hypertensive emergency.

Organ/system failure	Symptoms	Signs	Differential diagnosis
Encephalopathy	Headache, altered conscious level	Focal signs uncommon, retinopathy	Subarachnoid haemorrhage, stroke, epilepsy, meningitis, encephalitis, intoxication
Cardiac	Angina, dyspnoea	Pulmonary oedema	Aortic dissection, myocardial infarction
Renal	Dyspnoea	Oedema, oliguria, haematuria	Primary renal disease (e.g. acute nephritic syndrome), acute intermittent porphyria
Blood: micro-angiopathic haemolytic anaemia Thrombocytopaenia	Mucosal bleeding, epistaxis, haematuria, dyspnoea	Pallor, bruising, petechiae	Disseminated intra-vascular coagulation

Epidemiology

Prior to the introduction of effective antihypertensive agents, 7% of hypertensive patients suffered hypertensive emergencies (HE), which conferred approximately an 80% 1-year mortality. It has been recently estimated that 1–2% of hypertensive patients will suffer HE and despite efforts to improve therapy the incidence of HE has risen over the last 40 years. The risk factors for HE parallel those of essential hypertension: increased age, male gender, Afro-Caribbean origin and poor control of essential hypertension [2, 3].

Pathophysiology

At an organ level, damage occurs when the level of blood pressure exceeds the upper limit of autoregulation to control blood flow. In normotensive individuals, normal arteries can maintain relatively normal flow rates over a wide range of mean arterial pressure (MAP), usually 60–150 mmHg. Chronic hypertension causes compensatory functional and structural changes in the arterial walls and alters the relationship between blood flow and MAP (Figure 24.1). In HE autoregulatory capacity is impaired, particularly in the cerebral and renal beds. At autopsy, cerebral oedema, acute and chronic inflammation of the medium and small arteries and arterioles, fibrinoid necrosis and microthrombi (often associated with necrosis) have been demonstrated [4]. An understanding of autoregulation is critical for therapy because sudden lowering of blood pressure into a range that would otherwise be considered normal may reduce it below the autoregulatory capacity of the hypertensive circulation and lead to inadequate tissue perfusion.

The mechanisms that underlie the increase in vascular resistance that precedes the acceleration of hypertension towards a crisis are poorly

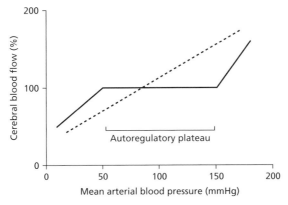

Figure 24.1 Autoregulation is a characteristic of certain organs including the brain, heart and kidney, which maintain an even blood flow over a wide range of blood pressures (the autoregulatory plateau) owing to a compensatory mechanism in afferent arteries. During hypertensive crises this capacity of afferent arteries is lost (dotted line) so that rapidly lowering the blood pressure may cause organ hypoperfusion.

understood. Endothelial injury associated with dysregulated coagulation and increased permeability is associated with fibrinoid necrosis of arterioles and consequent tissue ischaemia. The release of vasoconstrictors is encouraged by hypovolaemia and organ hypoperfusion. For example, the renin-angiotensin system is typically activated, and the resultant increased release of angiotensin 2 mediates endothelial damage and the production of reactive oxygen species and inflammatory mediators such as interleukin-6 [5].

Presentation

Organ dysfunction associated with hypertension is uncommon when DBP is less than 130 mmHg. Patients with chronic hypertension are relatively protected, whereas pregnant women and children may develop encephalopathy at a DBP of 100 mmHg [6]. The rate of increase in blood pressure may be as important as the absolute value in terms of causing organ dysfunction; similarly, very high MAP levels are often well tolerated by chronically hypertensive patients. It is crucial to measure blood pressure accurately in both arms as a consistent discrepancy is suggestive of aortic coarctation or dissection. The use of a cuff that is too small for the patient's arm will produce an artificially elevated measurement.

In patients presenting with left heart failure, it is important to distinguish between diastolic dysfunction often associated with chronic hypertension in the elderly and systolic dysfunction that may be associated with mitral regurgitation.

24.3 Hypertension complicating cardiovascular conditions

Following cardiac surgery and acute coronary syndromes

A meta-analysis of 30 studies has shown that hypertensive patients are only 1.3-fold more likely to experience adverse cardiac events than normotensive patients after general surgery. There is little evidence to support the practice of delaying procedures because of a raised blood pressure, unless further evaluation of organ damage is required or organ function may be improved or protected as a result of the delay. In the perioperative period, beta-blockers or alpha-2 agonists may help to maintain haemodynamic stability and prevent major cardiac complications [7]. Whilst it is accepted that patients who are established on beta-blockers should continue their medication through the peri-operative period for non-cardiac surgery, the results of the recent POISE trial have curbed the enthusiasm for commencing beta-blockade for patients with a variety of risk factors [8]. In the trial, 8351 patients received either high-dose controlled-release oral metoprolol or placebo. Beta-blockade was associated with a significant reduction in non-fatal myocardial infarctions, but an increased incidence of total mortality and stroke [9].

Systemic hypertension is common after cardiac surgery and even minor degrees of hypertension may be dangerous in circumstances where suture

Table 24.3 Causes of hypertension in patients after cardiac surgery.

Inadequate sedation or analgesia
Hypothermia and shivering
Inappropriate cardiovascular support
Abnormal arterial blood gases
Withdrawal of antihypertensive medication
Perioperative acute brain injury
Hypoglycaemia
Altered baroreceptor function after carotid endarterectomy
Post-coarctation repair

lines are vulnerable or where bleeding has been difficult to control. Good communication at handover of the patients from the theatre to the ICU team is key to optimising individual management plans. In most cases the risk of bleeding recedes within hours of the end of the operation and it is possible to achieve relative hypotension and prevent bleeding whilst maintaining adequate end-organ perfusion.

Common causes of post-operative hypertension are listed in Table 24.3. Alternating hypo- and hypertension should raise the possibility of a technical issue with an infusion pump or associated intravenous line or less commonly may indicate that the patient is hypovolaemic.

The same causes of sympathetic overactivity cause hypertension in patients suffering myocardial ischaemia. Systemic vasoconstriction increases left ventricular afterload and myocardial stroke work, whilst increasing the left ventricular wall tension. Both factors increase myocardial ischaemia and decrease cardiac output. The haemodynamic features are exacerbated in patients with severe left ventricular hypertrophy. Patients with acute myocardial infarction and a history of hypertension or elevated blood pressure on admission have a greater risk of intracranial haemorrhage after thrombolysis. It is generally recommended that SBP is lowered below 180 mmHg before thrombolysis is administered, but this relative contraindication may prompt the use of percutaneous intervention [10].

Rarely, in patients immediately after coronary artery bypass grafting or with severe coronary artery disease there appears to be a direct relationship between systemic blood pressure and cardiac output. This may result from pressure-dependent flow in a partially obstructed coronary circulation, such that decreased MAP is associated with ischaemia and a reduction in cardiac output. If this phenomenon is associated with regional wall motion abnormality on echocardiography or increased cardiac enzymes, then coronary angiography may be indicated.

Aortic dissection

This condition is associated with a high immediate mortality and the management of blood pressure is therefore different from other conditions. The objective is to decrease SBP to below 120 mmHg within 20 minutes and to reduce the force applied to the aortic dissection flap by left ventricular ejection (Chapter 22). Consequently, beta-blockers are the

Table 24.4 Agents used in hypertensive emergencies according to the causative condition or resulting organ failure.

Condition	Vasodilator	Beta-blocker	Other
Acute myocardial ischaemia	Nitrates Calcium antagonist	+++	Analgesia
Aortic dissection	Calcium antagonist Nitroprusside	+++	Analgesia
Acute pulmonary oedema	Nitrates ACE inhibitor	+ (diastolic dysfunction)	Loop diuretic Opiate
Encephalopathy	Calcium antagonist	Labetolol	Magnesium*
Pregnancy	Calcium antagonist	Labetolol	Benzodiazepine
Catecholamine excess (phaeochromocytoma, Guillian-Barré syndrome, cocaine overdose)	Calcium antagonist Phentolamine	**	Sedation
Post-operative	Nitrate Calcium antagonist	Labetolol	Analgesia

ACE, Angiotensin converting enzyme.
+++ Recommended as first-line agent.
* Magnesium may potentiate the effects of calcium antagonists.
** Unsuitable as first-line agents because blocking β receptor mediated effects without first blocking α1 receptors may exacerbate hypertension and precipitate heart failure.

mainstay of treatment, used in combination with vasodilators and adequate analgesia (Table 24.4) [11].

24.4 Management

Strategy

Patients diagnosed with hypertensive urgencies do not require intensive care management and, depending on the presence of chronic organ dysfunction and other parameters, may not need to be admitted to hospital if they respond well to oral agents. The aim of treatment is to lower MAP into the normal range over days. Combination oral therapies can be used; in general two or three agents are required. The choice of agents will depend on patients' comorbidities and the potential adverse effects of individual drugs. Removal of triggering factors is an important adjunct to drug treatment, for example moving a patient into a stress-free environment may be as effective as drug treatment in the short term.

By contrast, patients with established or evolving organ failure should be admitted to intensive care for continuous invasive blood pressure monitoring using an arterial line, organ support and treatment with intravenous antihypertensive medication. The immediate aims are to decrease MAP by no more than 20% in the first hours of treatment and to prevent organ failures. For example, the use of vasodilators may expose hypovolaemia and too rapid a decrease in MAP may exacerbate encephalopathy. Exceptions to these rules include cases where hypertension puts the patient at risk of fatal haemorrhage (e.g. aortic dissection and selected cases after cardiac surgery) and hypertension associated with cerebrovascular accident. Stroke is almost invariably associated with hypertension and affects cerebral autoregulation, resulting in perfusion to the penumbral zones being dependent on high MAP. Conversely there is no evidence to suggest that hypertension adversely affects the course of stroke recovery and the tendency is for the MAP to decrease spontaneously over subsequent days.

Antihypertensive agents

There is very little evidence to support using one drug over another in hypertension in general and the overwhelmingly important determinant of outcome is the achievement of the target blood pressure. There is an even greater paucity of evidence in the area of hypertensive crises, where randomised controlled trials have not clearly demonstrated that drug treatments improve morbidity or mortality, let alone showing which drugs are most efficacious [12]. The choice of drug should be determined by the aetiology of hypertension and co-existent organ failures (Table 24.4); in practice, local availability or licensing of drugs may be a major determinant. For example, intravenous preparations of the calcium antagonist Nicardipine and the dopamine-1 receptor antagonist Fenoldopam are unavailable in the UK, despite being mainstays of treatment elsewhere [13–15].

Beta-blockers

Beta-blockers that are suitable for use intravenously in emergency situations include Esmolol, Metoprolol and Labetolol; the latter has some alpha-blocking activity in a ratio of approximately 7:1, $\beta{:}\alpha$. The effect of Esmolol is extremely short-lived, the onset of action being within 60 seconds, with a duration of action of 10–20 minutes. The metabolism of Esmolol is not dependent on renal or hepatic function.

The effects of beta blockade are particularly beneficial in the management of hypertension associated with aortic dissection, myocardial ischaemia and diastolic heart failure. Patients with chronic hypertension and left ventricular hypertrophy are particularly susceptible to diastolic heart failure associated with a stiff myocardium that fills slowly, and may experience left ventricular outflow tract obstruction in systole, both of which are benefited by negative chronotropy and inotropy. Where absolute contra-indications to beta-blockers prevent their use, calcium antagonists with a negative chronotropic effect, such as Verapamil or Diltiazem, may be substituted.

Sodium nitroprusside

This is a potent arterial and venous vasodilator with a rapid onset of action and a short duration of effect (minutes) on discontinuation. In patients with ischaemic heart disease, a significant reduction in regional myocardial blood flow can occur as a result of 'coronary steal' and nitroprusside administration early after acute myocardial infarction was associated with a doubling of mortality [16]. Nitroprusside decreases cerebral blood flow while increasing intracranial pressure, effects that are particularly disadvantageous in patients with hypertensive encephalopathy or following a cerebro-vascular accident.

Nitroprusside contains 44% cyanide by weight, which is released non-enzymatically in a dose-dependent manner. Cyanide metabolism and removal requires intact liver and renal function, and adequate bioavailability of thiosulphate. Cyanide toxicity may result in cardiac arrest, coma, encephalopathy, convulsions and irreversible focal neurologic injury. The current methods of monitoring patients to detect cyanide toxicity are insensitive and the development of metabolic acidosis is usually a preterminal event. The recommended dose of nitroprusside (up to 10 μg/kg/min) results in cyanide formation at a rate that exceeds the capacity for detoxification. Therefore, nitroprusside should only be used in emergencies when alternatives are unavailable or inappropriate, the duration of treatment should be as short as possible and the infusion rate should not exceed 2 μg/kg/min [17].

Nitrates

These agents are potent venodilators that cause arterial dilation only at high doses [18]. Their hypotensive effect depends upon decreasing preload and cardiac output. Nitrates cause reflex tachycardia. Tachyphylaxis decreases the effect of nitrates after 24–48 hours of continuous infusion. Glyceryl trinitrate is indicated in treating hypertension associated with myocardial ischaemia and pulmonary oedema; it is commonly used to treat hypertension after cardiac surgery. Particular care is required in managing hypertension with nitrates in patients with left ventricular hypertrophy, for example after aortic valve replacement. In this setting excessive venodilatation can result in decreased venous return and cardiac output. The resultant fall in coronary blood flow can precipitate myocardial ischaemia because the demand of the myocardium is high as is the left ventricular end-diastolic pressure.

Miscellaneous antihypertensive agents

Phentolamine is a rapidly acting non-selective alpha-blocker that is most often used to treat hypertension caused by catecholamine excess, for example that induced by drugs or in a patient with a phaeochromocytoma [19].

Hydralazine is a directly acting vasodilator that increases uterine blood flow. It is rarely used except to treat hypertensive crises affecting pregnant patients because intravenous administration may be followed by dramatic and long-lived (hours) hypotension. However, even this indication should probably be abandoned owing to an associated increased risk of adverse maternal and neonatal outcomes [20]. Similarly, oral and sublingual Nifedipine should not be used because it has caused precipitous decreases in blood pressure and the drug is not absorbed by the buccal mucosa.

The effects of angiotensin converting enzyme (ACE) inhibitors are difficult to titrate in hypertensive crises and the intravenous agent enalaprilat is not available in the UK. ACE inhibitors are contraindicated in pregnancy. Oral ACE inhibitors are safe and effective second-line agents in hypertensive crises that have beneficial long-term effects in patients with cardiovascular disease. Most patients with hypertensive crises are volume depleted and therefore diuretics should be used with caution except in patients with associated pulmonary oedema.

24.5 Conclusions

The management of hypertensive crises should be determined by the underlying cause and by associated risks to the patient including organ failure and haemorrhage. A small minority of patients require intensive care admission to monitor the treatment of a hypertensive emergency and associated organ failures. There is very little evidence to guide the choice of antihypertensive agents, but the available drugs have serious adverse effects and may be lethal if used inappropriately.

Case study

A 28-year-old woman with no significant past medical history presented to Casualty with a 10-day history of fever, headache and vomiting. She had recently taken paracetamol and ibuprofen, was a non-smoker and drank moderate amounts of alcohol. The patient was uncooperative and drowsy. It was not possible to visualise her fundi but there were no focal neurological signs. The blood pressure was repeatedly measured from both arms non-invasively at around 240/130 mmHg. The skin examination showed a telangiectatic rash on the face and neck, sclerodactyly and a red, scaly rash on both upper arms. Computed tomography (CT) scan of the head was normal; otherwise initial investigations can be summarised as the electrocardiogram (ECG) showing left ventricular hypertrophy, there was borderline cardiomegaly on a frontal chest X-ray, anaemia (Hb 9 g/dl) and thrombocytopaenia (70×10^9/l). Renal biochemistry was normal although urinalysis was strongly positive for blood and protein. The pregnancy test was negative.

During transfer to the medical admissions unit, the patient had an episode of desaturation to 89% on air, which responded to stopping her intravenous fluids, a bolus dose of frusemide and oxygen via a face mask. She was instead transferred to intensive care, where a repeat chest X-ray was suggestive of pulmonary oedema. A transthoracic echocardiogram revealed left ventricular hypertrophy, mild mitral and aortic regurgitation and no pericardial effusion. Ventricular function was globally impaired with an ejection fraction of 20%. Pulmonary artery systolic pressure was estimated as being 40 mmHg. The patient's cardiac

Continued

output was monitored continuously by pulse contour analysis calibrated by lithium dilution. The systemic hypertension was initially treated with intravenous prostacyclin and sodium nitroprusside. The patient's blood pressure decreased by the target of 30% in the first 24 hours, but she became increasingly hypoxic and confused without evidence of pulmonary oedema, culminating in her pulling out her central venous catheter. Whilst her blood pressure rapidly returned to pretreatment levels the oxygen saturation also increased to 95% on air, indicating an adverse effect of intravenous vasodilators on ventilation-perfusion matching. The antihypertensive medication was changed to prostacyclin and esmolol, and subsequently to oral metoprolol when it was clear that the patient tolerated beta adrenoceptor blockade. The patient's blood pressure came under control and the signs of end organ dysfunction subsequently improved. She was ultimately discharged on an ACE inhibitor, long-acting calcium antagonist and a beta-blocker.

A skin biopsy of the upper arms revealed extensive fibrosis and perivascular lymphocytic infiltrate consistent with scleroderma. A history of 2–3 years of facial telangiectasias, severe Raynaud's phenomenon and mild heartburn was elicited, suggesting the diagnosis of systemic sclerosis. Renal ultrasound was unremarkable and magnetic resonance imaging of the renal arteries showed no evidence of stenosis. The thrombocytopenia and microangiopathic haemolytic anaemia were felt to be secondary to hypertension. Pheochromocytoma, multiple endocrine neoplasia and thyroid disease were excluded.

Comment

Systemic sclerosis is a connective tissue disease characterised by fibrosis of the skin, blood vessels and visceral organs. Antinuclear antibodies are present in 95% of patients, including anti-Scl-70 antibodies (20% of cases), antinucleolar antibodies (20–30%) and anticentromere antibodies (10%) [21]. Females are affected three times as often as males and even more during childbearing years. Cardiac involvement includes pericarditis, heart failure, heart block and cardiomyopathy, and can also lead to heart failure secondary to systemic or pulmonary hypertension. Fibrosis affecting small coronary arteries or the conduction system may cause angina and dysrhythmia. Historically, renal crisis was the leading cause of death in patients with scleroderma, but this has been dramatically reduced by the use of ACE inhibitors [22].

References

1. Chobanian AV (Chairman). The seventh report of the Joint National Committee on Prevention, Detection, Evaluation, and Treatment of High Blood Pressure: the JNC 7 report. *JAMA* 2003; 289, 2560–72.
2. Elliott WJ. Clinical features in the management of selected hypertensive emergencies. *Prog Cardiovasc Dis* 2006; 48, 316–25.

3. Zampaglione B, Pascale C, Marchisio M, et al. Hypertensive urgencies and emergencies. Prevalence and clinical presentation. *Hypertension* 1996; 27, 144–7.
4. Strandgaard S, Paulson OB. Cerebrovascular consequences of hypertension. *Lancet* 1994; 344, 519–21.
5. Patel HP, Mitsnefes M. Advances in the pathogenesis and management of hypertensive crisis. *Curr Opin Pediatr* 2005; 17, 210–4.
6. Rey E, LeLorier J, Burgess E, et al. Report of the Canadian Hypertension Society Consensus Conference: 3. Pharmacologic treatment of hypertensive disorders in pregnancy. *CMAJ* 1997; 157, 1245–54.
7. Hanada S, Kawakami H, Goto T, et al. Hypertension and anesthesia. *Curr Opin Anaesthesiol* 2006; 19, 315–19.
8. Fleisher LA, Poldermans D. Perioperative beta blockade: where do we go from here? *Lancet* 2008; 371, 1813–14.
9. Devereaux PJ, Yang H, Yusuf S, et al. Effects of extended-release metoprolol succinate in patients undergoing non-cardiac surgery (POISE trial): a randomised controlled trial. *Lancet* 2008; 371, 1839–47.
10. Maggioni AP, Franzosi MG, Santoro E, et al. The risk of stroke in patients with acute myocardial infarction after thrombolytic and antithrombotic treatment. Gruppo Italiano per lo Studio della Sopravvivenza nell'Infarto Miocardico II (GISSI-2), and The International Study Group. *N Engl J Med* 1992; 327, 1–6.
11. Ouriel K. Descending thoracic aortic dissection: clinical aspects and anatomic correlations. *Semin Vasc Surg* 2002; 15, 83–8.
12. Perez MI, Musini VM. Pharmacological interventions for hypertensive emergencies. *Cochrane Database Syst Rev* 2008; CD003653.
13. Feldstein C. Management of hypertensive crises. *Am J Ther* 2007; 14, 135–9.
14. Marik PE, Varon J. Hypertensive crises: challenges and management. *Chest* 2007; 131, 1949–62.
15. Slama M, Modeliar SS. Hypertension in the intensive care unit. *Curr Opin Cardiol* 2006; 21, 279–87.
16. Cohn JN, Franciosa JA, Francis GS, et al. Effect of short-term infusion of sodium nitroprusside on mortality rate in acute myocardial infarction complicated by left ventricular failure: results of a Veterans Administration cooperative study. *N Engl J Med* 1982; 306, 1129–35.
17. Robin ED, McCauley R. Nitroprusside-related cyanide poisoning. Time (long past due) for urgent, effective interventions. *Chest* 1992; 102, 1842–5.
18. Bussmann WD, Kenedi P, von Mengden HJ, et al. Comparison of nitroglycerin with nifedipine in patients with hypertensive crisis or severe hypertension. *Clin Investig* 1992; 70, 1085–8.
19. Pacak K. Preoperative management of the pheochromocytoma patient. *J Clin Endocrinol Metab* 2007; 92, 4069–79.
20. Magee LA, Cham C, Waterman EJ, et al. Hydralazine for treatment of severe hypertension in pregnancy: meta-analysis. *BMJ* 2003; 327, 955–60.
21. Mitchell H, Bolster MB, LeRoy EC. Scleroderma and related conditions. *Med Clin N Am* 1997; 81, 129–49.
22. Steen VD. Scleroderma renal crisis. *Rheum Dis Clin N Am* 2003; 29, 315–33.

25 Pregnancy

Lorna Swan

Royal Brompton & Harefield NHS Foundation Trust, London, UK

Take Home Messages

- Pregnant or peripartum women should be considered as a high-risk intensive care admission despite their age.
- Cardiac disease is now the commonest cause of maternal mortality.
- Ischaemic heart disease, aortic dissection, cardiomyopathy and pulmonary hypertension are the commonest causes of death.
- Specialist multidisciplinary team care is essential to direct complex decision making.
- In life-threatening situations investigation and treatment should not be withheld because of concerns over foetal outcome (rare exceptions depending on maternal wishes).

25.1 Introduction

Pregnancy is associated with significant changes in the cardiovascular system, which may predispose the vulnerable patient to haemodynamic instability. Despite being relatively rare, cardiac disease is now the commonest cause of maternal mortality in the UK [1].

Although much of the literature in this area focuses on pre-existing valvular and congenital structural heart disease the majority of deaths are due to newly acquired disease – including ischaemic heart disease and aortic dissection. Thus, although many of these deaths are sudden and unpredictable, up to 40% are potentially preventable [2].

25.2 General principles

The nursing and medical care of pregnant women are specialist roles. It is therefore imperative that a critically ill pregnant woman with cardiac disease is cared for within a multidisciplinary team, including intensivists, anaesthetists, obstetricians, midwives, cardiologists, cardiac surgeons, neonatologists and haematologists.

Cardiovascular Critical Care. Edited by M. Griffiths, J. Cordingley and S. Price.
© 2010 Blackwell Publishing Ltd.

Traditional critical care scoring systems, such as APACHE II, are inadequate to describe risk and all such pregnant or peripartum women should be assumed to be at high risk [3].

Cardiovascular factors
During pregnancy there is a significant expansion in blood volume in response to the requirements of the uterus and developing feto-placental unit [6]. In addition there is an increase in baseline heart rate and a fall in peripheral vascular resistance. In contrast, central venous pressure and pulmonary vascular pressures remain fairly constant. The net result is a 50% increase in cardiac output. During labour each contraction, in the absence of analgesia, is associated with a further 30% increase in cardiac output [7]. Uterine contraction and bleeding are additional factors that may lead to unpredictable fluctuations in cardiac output posing particular difficulties for an already compromised circulation.

Cardiac arrest
Cardiac arrest in a pregnant woman is uncommon (1 in 30,000 pregnancies) but rarely associated with survival. Bag-and-mask ventilation is often ineffective and early intubation is vital to deliver effective ventilation and to avoid aspiration [8]. The important issue of aorto-caval compression in the supine position leading to a significant drop in cardiac output must not be forgotten in the acute setting [9]. Manually moving the uterus or using a wedge to achieve an oblique position can counteract these effects. In the event of a maternal cardio-respiratory arrest the foetus only stands a reasonable chance of survival if it is delivered as soon as possible [10]. This is by emergency caesarean section via a longitudinal mid-line incision if the foetus is at a potentially viable gestation.

Respiratory factors
In the third trimester important changes affect the respiratory system: diaphragmatic elevation by the gravid uterus leads to a reduction in functional residual capacity, associated with a compensatory increase in respiratory rate. Oxygen uptake increases and there is a mild respiratory alkalosis. Tracheal intubation of the pregnant women is a time of increased risk, with an eight-fold increase in the incidence of failure [4]. This is thought to be due to increased intra-abdominal pressure, mucosal oedema, soft tissue swelling and difficulties in positioning. Pregnant women poorly tolerate prolonged attempts at intubation and are at high risk of rapid desaturation and gastro-oesophageal reflux [5].

Thrombosis
The risk of thrombosis is significantly elevated in pregnancy and the puerperium. Pulmonary embolism, for example, is up to 20 times more common in the puerperium [11]. Sepsis, cyanosis, left ventricular dysfunction and pulmonary hypertension further exacerbate this risk. Prophylaxis with low molecular weight heparin should be considered for all

pregnant women in hospital. A review of deep venous thrombosis is outside the scope of this chapter.

Peripartum haemorrhage

Normal peripartum bleeding should not excede 500 ml at the time of vaginal delivery or 1000 ml at caesarean section. Although this is usually tolerated well, in a patient with cardiac disease or other co-morbidity it may be associated with instability. Most cases are caused by uterine atony. Manual compression, uterine massage, compression sutures and oxytocin may all be used to prevent catastrophic bleeding [12]. Boluses of oxytocin should be avoided in women with haemodynamic instability as it may lead to life-threatening hypotension [13]. Ergometrine increases the blood pressure, and thus the combination of ergometrine and oxytocin (syntometrine) has unpredictable effects and is not recommended in cardiovascularly unstable patients.

Foetal issues

Although care of the mother is the main priority, the ICU team also have a duty of care to the unborn child. The balance of maternal and foetal priority is a difficult issue and depends on gestation and the wishes of the mother/family. Foetal growth scans may be required during a long intensive care unit (ICU) admission and regular cardiotocography (CTG) is required near term. Many of the interventions required for the mother's survival may adversely impact on the foetus, including exposure to potentially teratogenic drugs, the haemodynamic effects of cardiovascular support, repeated irradiation, surgical procedures and cardiopulmonary bypass.

On occasion, the underlying maternal condition may necessitate early delivery of a premature child. Where advanced neonatal services are available a baby born at 30 weeks gestation has a 95% chance of survival [14]. Again priority is almost always given to the maternal well-being, but each of these decisions will need to be considered in full and discussed with the family.

25.3 Specific cardiovascular disorders in pregnancy

Ischaemic heart disease

The incidence of ischaemic heart disease complicating pregnancy is increasing, at least in part due to an increase in maternal age and body mass index. A mother presenting with an acute coronary syndrome will require care very similar to a non-pregnant individual. Ideally this should involve early coronary angiography with stenting. A bare-metal rather than a drug-eluting stent may avoid the need to use additional antiplatelet agents in the peripartum period. Aspirin and beta-blockers should also be prescribed in most circumstances. If primary percutaneous coronary intervention is not possible then thrombolysis should be considered.

Thrombolysis is utilised in several conditions that may occur during pregnancy – these include massive pulmonary embolism, acute thrombotic stroke and thrombosis of a metal valve. Although bleeding from the placental bed may occur (miscarriage, early foetal loss, placental abruption or peripartum haemorrhage) thrombolysis is highly effective in mitigating the effects of potentially life-threatening disorders. Streptokinase and alteplase do not appear to cross the placenta [15].

Patients presenting with acute cardiogenic shock secondary to infarction will require standard ICU support, including inotropic therapy and intra-aortic balloon pumping where indicated. The mortality in this setting is high. Spontaneous coronary dissection is also seen in pregnancy, although this accounts for only a minority of cases. The majority of patients with acute coronary syndromes during pregnancy have traditional atherosclerotic risk factors.

Aortic dissection

Pregnancy is associated with an increased risk of aortic dissection, particularly in the third trimester or in the first month post-partum. Marfan syndrome, coarctation of the aorta, collagen vascular disorders, hypertension and atherosclerosis all predispose to dissection. Chest or back pain in a pregnant woman requires urgent assessment and imaging, particularly in patients with an underlying condition associated with increased risk of dissection. In the ICU setting, early involvement of cardiac surgeons and interventional cardiologists is vital. Blood pressure must be meticulously controlled, usually using intravenous agents such as beta-blockers. If urgent cardiopulmonary bypass is required prior to foetal maturation, then it is proposed that high-flow, normotensive techniques may improve foetal outcome [16].

Pulmonary oedema

The causes of pulmonary oedema in the pregnant patient include those of the non-pregnant patient, and those related to pregnancy, its complications and its management (Table 25.1). Thus, in a patient presenting with clinical symptoms and signs of pulmonary oedema, there should be a very low threshold for electrocardiography, chest X-ray and echocardiography.

Table 25.1 Causes of pulmonary oedema during pregnancy and the peripartum period.

Mitral stenosis
Aortic stenosis
Coarctation of the aorta
Hypertensive heart disease
Left ventricular dysfunction
Tocolytic use
Fluid overload
Acute respiratory distress syndrome
Amniotic fluid embolism
Neurogenic pulmonary oedema (cerebral haemorrhage)

Treatment should be directed towards the cause and cardiorespiratory support given in the interim. This includes the use of diuretics, vasodilators, inotropes, mechanical ventilation, haemofiltration, intra-aortic balloon pumping or even urgent cardiac intervention.

The most classic cause of pregnancy-associated pulmonary oedema is rheumatic mitral stenosis. The incidence of rheumatic heart disease is again increasing due to an enlarging immigrant population. This can present with arrhythmia, profound effort intolerance, orthopnoea and systemic thrombosis. The presence of elevated pulmonary artery pressures indicates severe disease, and diuretics, control of the heart rate, anticoagulation and percutaneous balloon valvuloplasty may all be required [17]. A similar clinical picture can also be seen in patients with congenital heart disease with prior left atrio-ventricular valve surgery (for example in those with atrio-ventricular septal defects).

Pregnancy-associated hypertension

Systemic blood pressure usually falls in the first and second trimesters and then rises again towards term. In 1 in 8 pregnancies this secondary rise is exaggerated, resulting in pregnancy-induced hypertension. In a subset of patients this develops into a multisystem disorder, with proteinuria, renal dysfunction and abnormal coagulation (pre-eclampsia). Occasionally the disease progresses with liver and cerebral involvement. Any hypertension in pregnancy should be urgently assessed and treatment established early. When pre-eclampsia is combined with other disorders – for example pre-existing valvular heart disease – morbidity and mortality rise. The treatment of pregnanacy-associated hypertension is beyond the scope of this chapter, and is usually the remit of specialist obstetricians in the context of a multidisciplinary team.

Pulmonary embolism

The incidence of pulmonary embolism during pregnancy is between 10 and 15 per 100,000. There are multiple predisposing factors, including multi-parity, obesity, age and pre-existing thrombotic tendencies (e.g. lupus anticoagulant). In the ICU setting the priority is to achieve stabilisation of haemodynamics and prevention of further clot formation and embolism (anticoagulation and possibly deployment of an inferior vena cava filter). When there is haemodynamic instability thrombolysis is the treatment of choice. Manual (catheter) fragmentation of the pulmonary artery clot may be used in the critically unwell patient, as may surgical embolectomy. If the patient survives, a full assessment including a thrombophilia screen should be performed.

Amniotic fluid embolism

Small amounts of amniotic fluid are often present in maternal blood after a normal delivery. Rarely there is a more substantial embolism, often associated with abruption or vigorous uterine contractions. Amniotic fluid embolism very quickly results in left ventricular dysfunction, pulmonary hypertension, pulmonary oedema, shock, seizures and cardio-respiratory arrest. Treatment is supportive but, despite this, mortality remains high at approximately 80%.

Congenital heart disease

There are multiple congenital heart defects that may lead to major adverse cardiovascular events during pregnancy. The most problematic are those with cyanosis, pulmonary hypertension, ventricular dysfunction and severe obstructive lesions. Maternal cyanosis provides an additional risk to the foetus and foetal survival is uncommon with maternal saturations less than 85% on air. The management of pregnant patients with congenital heart disease should be within a specialist centre, allowing liaison between experts in congenital heart disease and obstetrics, in order to balance the risks and benefits of any treatment for both mother and child [18].

Peripartum cardiomyopathy

Peripartum cardiomyopathy is defined as the new presentation of heart failure between the last month of pregnancy to the first 6 months post delivery in the absence of other causes of ventricular dysfunction. When a pregnant (or peripartum) patient presents with breathlessness, abnormal blood pressure or arrhythmia there should be a very low threshold for performing a chest X-ray and echocardiogram. Any ventricular dysfunction should be discussed with a cardiologist and therapy instituted early. The critically unwell patient with peripartum cardiomyopathy should be treated aggressively (diuretics, inotropes and intra-aortic balloon pump). A left ventricular or biventricular assist device may be used as a bridge to transplantation [19].

Pulmonary hypertension

Pulmonary hypertension of any aetiology is associated with a significant maternal mortality [20]. Expert multidisciplinary care is required. Anticoagulation and the use of pulmonary vasodilators (sildenafil, inhaled nitric oxide, oxygen, prostacyclin) are key. These agents appear to be relatively safe during pregnancy. Bosentan is usually avoided but may be utilised post delivery. The post-partum period is often the most dangerous and patients may require ICU care for several weeks post delivery.

25.4 Delivery in a critically unwell patient

If the patient is critically ill, delivery will usually be by caesarean section. When the patient is already mechanically ventilated, at risk of pulmonary oedema or arrhythmia, then this is usually performed under general rather than regional anaesthesia. Great care must be taken over effective haemostasis, particularly if the use of oxytocin is contraindicated.

If semi-urgent cardiac surgery is required then ideally this should be delayed until 2–3 days post delivery. This is to ensure that the anticoagulation of cardiopulmonary bypass does not re-trigger further post-partum bleeding. Clearly, this delay will not be possible in life-threatening situations such as an unstable aortic dissection.

25.5 Conclusion

The critically ill pregnant woman with cardiovascular disease presents many additional challenges in the intensive care setting. Care needs to be individualised and multidisciplinary to provide the best possible outlook for both mother and child.

Case study

A pregnant 23-year-old woman with significant primary pulmonary hypertension presented at 33 weeks with a deterioration in her exercise capacity accompanied by an increase in brain natriuretic peptide (BNP). Transthoracic echocardiography revealed features consistent with the diagnosis (Figure 25.1): a high pulmonary vascular resistance (Figure 25.2), poor right ventricular function and supra-systemic right ventricular pressures, which again reflected a further deterioration. Prior to this planned pregnancy she was in NYHA class II heart failure on bosentan, sildenafil and nebulised iloprost. Bosentan was stopped at 7 weeks gestation owing to concerns regarding embryopathy. During her pregnancy she had been on therapeutic doses of low molecular weight

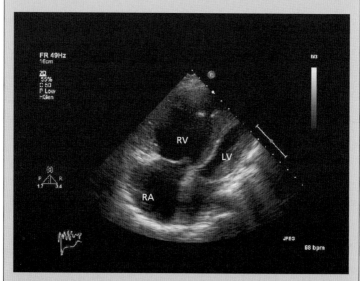

Figure 25.1 Four-chambered view from trans-thoracic echo demonstrating a very dilated right heart (RA and RV) and squashed left ventricle (LV). The ventricular septum is pushed over to the left due to the high right heart pressures. RA, right atrium; RV, right ventricle.

Continued

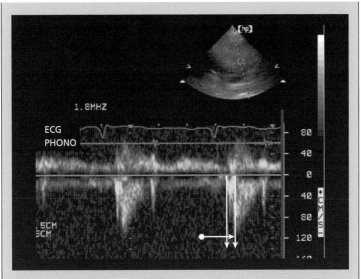

Figure 25.2 Trans-thoracic echocardiogram across the pulmonary valve in a patient with systemic pulmonary artery pressures. Here, the Doppler (pulse wave, PW) is positioned at the level of the pulmonary valve leaflets (see minaturised 2D figure), and the amount of time from onset of pulmonary flow to peak pulmonary velocity is measured (arrowed). In conjunction with pulmonary artery systolic pressures measured using tricuspid regurgitation which enables non-invasive measurement of pulmonary artery systolic pressures, this measurement (pulmonary acceleration time) gives an indication of the pulmonary vascular resistance. A value of < 80 msec indicates a high pulmonary vascular resistance (PVR). ECG, electrocardiogram; PHONO, phonocardiogram.

heparin (LMWH) and aspirin which replaced her pre-pregnancy warfarin. Elective caesarian section was planned under general anaesthesia at 34 weeks as it was felt induction of labour at this gestation was unlikely to be successful. General anaesthesia was chosen rather than regional anaesthesia due to maternal anxiety and to assist with the administration of inhaled nitric oxide should that be needed.

Following delivery the patient was transferred to the cardiac intensive care. At this point the patient had already been extubated; she was, however, acidotic and hypoxic. On arrival in the ICU the patient was relatively bradycardic (heart rate 56 bpm), partly due to long-standing beta-blocker and amiodarone therapy. A Swan–Ganz was not placed due to the concern of inducing arrhythmia, but there was invasive assessment of venous pressure and arterial blood pressure. The patient's nebulised iloprost schedule was increased from 8 to 14 doses on the day of delivery. A further echo suggested that an increase in heart rate may improve cardiac output. A lithium dilution cardiac output monitoring (LiDCO) continuous non-invasive assessment of cardiac output was used to guide the use of small doses of isoprenaline, which improved cardiac output and symptoms.

Continued

There was no significant post-partum bleeding (a uterine compression suture had been placed) and the LMWH was restarted 6 hours after delivery. Intravenous pulmonary vasodilators and inhaled nitric oxide were not required. Given that the most critical time period for these patients is the 2 weeks following delivery, this patient remained in intensive care for 10 days. Bosentan was restarted on day 3. At the time of discharge to the cardiology ward there had been no improvement in the echocardiography findings and the BNP was still 177 pmol/l. Discharge home followed 16 days later.

References

1. *Confidential Enquiry into Maternal and Child Health. Saving Mothers' Lives. Reviewing maternal deaths to make motherhood safer – 2003–2005.* December 2007. The Seventh Report of the Confidential Enquiries into Maternal Deaths in the United Kingdom. Centre for Maternal and Child Enquiries, London.
2. Steinberg WM, Farine D. Maternal mortality in Ontario from 1970 to 1980. *Obstet Gynecol* 1985;66:510–12.
3. Utility of Acute Physiology, Age, and Chronic Health Evaluation (APACHE III) score in maternal admissions to the intensive care unit. *Am J Obstet Gynecol* 2006;194(5):e13–5.
4. King TA, Adams AP. Failed tracheal intubation. *Br J Anaesth* 1990;65:400–14.
5. Rizk NW, Kalassian KG, Gilligan T, et al. Obstetric complications in pulmonary and critical care medicine. *Chest* 1996;110:791–809.
6. Robson SC, Hunter S, Boys RJ, et al. Serial study of factors influencing changes in cardiac output during human pregnancy. *Am J Physiol* 1989;256:H1060–65.
7. Hendricks CH, Quilligan EJ. Cardaic output during labour. *Am J Obstet Gynecol* 1956;71:953–72.
8. Nolan J (ed). *Advanced Life Support* (5th edition). 2006. Resuscitation Council (UK), London.
9. Andrews PJ, Ackerman WE, Juneja MM. Aortocaval compression in the sitting and lateral decubitus positions during extradural catheter placement in the parturient. *Can J Anaesth* 1993;40(4):320–4.
10. Katz V, Balderston K, DeFreest M. Perimortem cesarean delivery: were our assumptions correct? *Am J Obstet Gynecol* 2005;192(6):1916–20.
11. Heit JA, Kobbervig CE, James AH, et al. Trends in the incidence of venous thromboembolism during pregnancy or postpartum: a 30-year population-based study. *Ann Intern Med* 2005;143(10):679–706.
12. Hayman RG, Arulkumaran S, Steer PJ. Uterine compression sutures: surgical management of postpartum hemorrhage. *Obstet Gynecol* 2002;99:502–6.
13. Weis FR Jr, Markello R, Mo B, et al. Cardiovascular effects of oxytocin. *Obstet Gynecol* 1975;46(2):211–14.
14. Stoelhorst GM, Rijken M, Martens SE, et al. Changes in neonatology: comparison of two cohorts of very preterm infants (gestational age < 32 weeks): the Project On Preterm and Small for Gestational Age Infants 1983 and the Leiden Follow-Up Project on Prematurity 1996–1997. *Pediatrics* 2005;115(2):396–405.
15. Leonhardt G, Gaul C, Nietsch HH, et al. Thrombolytic therapy in pregnancy. *J Thrombo Thrombolysis* 2006;21(3):271–6.

16. Parry AJ, Westaby S. Cardiopulmonary bypass during pregnancy. *Ann Thorac Surg* 1996; 61(6):1865–9.
17. Sivadasanpillai H, Srinivasan A, Sivasubramoniam S, et al. Long-term outcome of patients undergoing balloon mitral valvotomy in pregnancy. *Am J Cardiol* 2005;95(12):1504–6.
18. Steer PJ, Gatzoulis MA, Baker P. *Heart Disease and Pregnancy*. 2006. RCOG Press, London.
19. Rasmusson KD, Stehlik J, Brown RN, et al. Long-term outcomes of cardiac transplantation for peri-partum cardiomyopathy: a multiinstitutional analysis. *J Heart Lung Transplant* 2007;26(11):1097–104.
20. Weiss BM, Zemp L, Seifert B, et al. Outcome of pulmonary vascular disease in pregnancy: a systematic overview from 1978 through 1996. *J Am Coll Cardiol* 1998;31(7):1650–7.

26 Vasculitis

Lorna Swan

Royal Brompton & Harefield NHS Foundation Trust, London, UK

Take Home Messages

- Vasculitis is a rare but potentially life-threatening cause of cardiac disease.
- Vasculitis should be considered when there is an unusual cardiac presentation in the setting of a systemic illness.
- There needs to be a high index of suspicion as there are few clear diagnostic features.
- Expert rheumatological advice should be sought early (do not wait for the autoimmune screen results).
- There should be a low threshold for coronary angiography.
- Treatment will be associated with increased risks of sepsis.

26.1 Introduction

Significant cardiovascular vasculitis is rare and requires a high index of suspicion to make the diagnosis in a timely manner. The majority of patients presenting with acute vasculitis with cardiovascular involvement will have been previously diagnosed. For those presenting with a first episode there are unfortunately few pathognomic features [1]. Cardiovascular involvement is usually a component of a more generalised multi-system presentation with renal, skin, respiratory and neurological manifestations. In this context systemic vasculitis is associated with a significant mortality [2]. Failure to make the correct diagnosis will lead to treatment delays, or the administration of inappropriate immunosuppressive therapy to a critically unwell individual. Care in this setting should be multidisciplinary, involving rheumatologists, intensivists, interventional cardiologists, cardiac surgeons, vascular surgeons and renal physicians.

The classification of vasculitides, and their presenting features, depends on the size of the vessels involved [3]. There is, however, a degree of overlap between and heterogeneity within these groups. In the intensive care setting

---

Cardiovascular Critical Care. Edited by M. Griffiths, J. Cordingley and S. Price.
© 2010 Blackwell Publishing Ltd.

the patient with cardiovascular vasculitis can present with a number of distinct clinical syndromes.

26.2 Cardiovascular system involvement

Aorta

Aortic inflammation can lead to a range of clinical manifestations, from obstructive lesions to aneurysm formation and dissection. These changes can either be seen acutely – for example perioperative management of an acute thoracic aortic dissection – or with chronic sequelae. Hypertension may occur if there is significant narrowing of the aortic lumen or renal involvement. Proximal aortitis with vessel wall inflammation and dilatation may lead to aortic regurgitation even in the absence of direct leaflet involvement with valvulitis.

Other large vessels

Classically arteries in the upper body are most affected. Arterial occlusion, distal ischaemia, vessel dissection and aneurysm formation can all be seen. Neurological and opthalmological manifestations may complicate carotid and temporal vessel involvement. Bruits, vessel tenderness and diminished pulses may be found on clinical examination.

Coronary arteries

Both the large epicardial and small subendocardial vessels are potentially involved. When ischaemia occurs it may be widespread and not corresponding to any specific epicardial arterial territory. The clinical manifestations of this will be troponin positive coronary events, acute ST segment elevation infarction, ischaemic valve dysfunction and ischaemic heart failure. In this setting there should be a low threshold for invasive assessment, although difficult arterial access and contrast-nephropathy add to the risks of angiography. Prior to cardiac catheterisation, renal function should be assessed and renal-protective strategies applied.

Pericardium

Acute or chronic involvement of the pericardium have several different presentations. Acutely patients present with chest pain, rhythm upset, breathlessness, haemodynamic instability and/or tamponade. In the chronic setting pericardial constriction and chronic effusion are more common. There should be a very low threshold for performing echocardiography. Usually a transthoracic scan will suffice and it is rare that a transoesophageal approach is needed. Of note, when diagnosing pericardial tamponade, where involvement is localised, classical echocardiographic features may be absent. Furthermore, both constriction and restriction may occur together, further complicating the haemodynamic diagnosis. Finally, where the patient is supported with positive pressure mechanical ventilation, some echocardiographic features will differ from those in the spontaneously ventilating patient.

Myocardium

Acute myocarditis presents with right, left or bi-ventricular failure, arrhythmia and an elevation in cardiac enzymes. The presence of significant lung involvement may mask the diagnosis of pulmonary oedema and again there should be a low threshold for formal physiological echocardiography, measurement of brain natriuretic peptide (BNP) and invasive haemodynamic assessment.

Valves

There may be primary valve involvement with a valvulitis, but this is rare. Most frequently valvular regurgitation occurs secondary to myocardial ischaemia or to disruption and dilatation of the aortic root.

26.3 General features

Many of these presentations will be accompanied by non-specific features such as pyrexia and elevation of various biomarkers including the white cell count, erythrocyte sedimentation rate (ESR) and C-reactive protein (CRP). Purpuric rashes, skin ulceration, renal impairment and proteinuria are also common.

Specific vasculitides are also associated with particular symptoms, e.g. asthma occurs in 90% of those with Churg–Strauss and the majority of patients with Wegener's granulomatosis have sinus involvement. Specific serology may be helpful, including anti-nuclear antibody (ANA), complement and anti-neutrophil cytoplasmic antibody (ANCA). The characteristic features of the major vasculitides with cardiovascular involvement are shown in Table 26.1. In the setting of an acutely unwell patient a classic history of vasculitis may be absent. There should therefore be a thorough examination to identify rashes, splinter haemorrhages, nail-fold infarcts and retinal lesions. Proteinuria, haematuria and red cell casts on urinary microscopy should also be sought (Table 26.2).

26.4 Specific vasculitides

Giant-cell arteritis

Giant-cell arteritis affects medium- to large-sized arteries and tends to be more prevalent in elderly women. Granulomatous inflammation of the head and neck vessels is more common than direct cardiac involvement. This tends to be an endarteritis rather than a cause of mural involvement. Aortic involvement occurs in 15% of cases and occlusive episodes are not a feature [4].

Behcet's disease

Most commonly seen in young males of Asian, Mediterranean and Middle Eastern origin, Behcet's disease presents with mouth and genital ulcers,

Table 26.1 Clinical features of the vasculitides.

Syndrome	Giant-cell arteritis	Behcet's	Polyarteritis nodosum	Churg–Strauss	Takayasu	Kawasaki
Vessel	Medium–large	Large	Small–medium		Large	
Population	Elderly, female	Young, male	Elderly	Middle aged	Young, Asian, female	Children
Mechanism	Endarteritis	Endarteritis obliterans	Arteritis	Eosinophilic granulomatous infiltration	Granulomatous inflammation	
Vascular	Granulomatous involvement of head and neck vessels; 15% aortitis (not occlusive) [4]	Head and neck vessels, aorta (abdominal and thoracic), carotid aneurysms, aortic regurgitation, venous thrombosis [5]	Subepicardial coronary arteritis (50%)	Coronary arteritis	Arterial stenoses (wall thickening and fibrosis) interspersed with aneurysm formation. Aorta, renal and mesenteric vessels	Coronary artery aneurysm formation. Later coronary stenoses
Cardiac	Uncommon	Uncommon	Myopericarditis (19%)	Pericarditis, myocardial infarction, arrhythmia, cardiomyopathy, endomyocardial fibrosis, heart failure. Causes 50% of deaths	Hypertensive heart failure, myocarditis	Pericarditis, vavlulitis, myocarditis, myocardial infarction, sudden death
Other	Headache, weight loss, depression	Mouth and genital ulcers, conjunctivitis, arthralgia	Stroke, polyneuropathy	35–60% ANCA positive [6], asthma	Systemic upset, hypercoagulable state, hypertension	Systemic upset, rash, lymphadenopathy

Table 26.2 Baseline investigations of suspected vasculitis.

Bloods
Renal function
Biochemical profile including proteins and liver function
Full blood count (including eosinophil count)
C-reactive protein
ANCA, ANA, rheumatoid factor
Complement, immunoglobulins
Thrombophilia screen
Anti-endothelial antibodies
ESR
Cardiac enzymes (troponin, creatine kinase)
Pro-NT BNP
Blood cultures

Urinalysis, urinary protein levels, GFR
ECG, CXR
Cardiac imaging – echocardiography (TTE or TOE)

ENT assessment
Biopsies including skin, renal, vascular (e.g. temporal artery)
Invasive assessment and more complex imaging will be required dependent on the scenario

ESR, Erythrocyte sedimentation rate; BNP, brain natriuretic peptide; Pro-NT BNP, pro-N-terminal brain natriuretic peptide; ANCA, anti-neutrophil cytoplasmic antibody; ANA, anti-nuclear antibody; GFR, glomerular filtration rate; ECG, electrocardiogram; CXR, chest X-ray; TTE, transthoracic echocardiogram; TOE, transoesophageal echocardiogram; ENT, ear, nose and throat.

conjunctivitis and arthralgia. Large vessel involvement is well recognised and associated with occlusion of head and neck vessels (endarteritis obliterans), carotid artery aneurysms and involvement of the arch and abdominal aorta [5]. Aortic regurgitation secondary to aortic root dilatation can occur and venous thrombosis is also a feature.

Polyarteritis nodusum
Cardiac involvement is more common in this small to medium vessel arteritis. The coronaries, usually at the small subepicardial level, are affected in 50% of cases. Myopericarditis may also be present (19%). Neurological manifestations include stroke and polyneuropathy.

Churg–Strauss
Churg–Strauss, also called allergic granulomatosis, is most common in middle-aged adults. There is an eosinophilic granulomatous infiltrate and 35–60% of patients are ANCA positive [6]. Cardiac disease accounts for 50% of deaths [7]. There are multiple potential cardiac manifestations including pericarditis, pericardial constriction, myocardial infarction (eosinophilic coronary arteritis) and arrhythmia. A restrictive cardiomyopathy, endomyocardial fibrosis and heart failure also occur.

Rheumatoid vasculitis

This small to medium vessel vasculitis occurs in only a minority (approximately 5%) of those with chronic rheumatoid arthritis [8]. Sub-clinical coronary vasculitis is more common and is present in up to 20% of post mortem specimens [9]. There are other significant associations between rheumatoid arthritis and the cardiovascular system that are outside the scope of this chapter.

Relapsing polychondritis

This disease attacks non-cartilaginous tissues including vessel walls, valve leaflets and the pericardium. Aortic regurgitation is seen in 5% of cases.

Wegener's granulomatosis

Cardiac involvement is rare in Wegener's. Lung, nasal, sinus and renal disease predominate. Isolated case reports describe complete heart block, pericarditis, coronary inflammation and heart failure. The majority of patients are ANCA positive [10].

Takayasu's disease

Takayasu's disease is classically a disease of young Asian females. At presentation systemic upset is common. A granulomatous inflammation affects large vessels, particularly the aorta. Arterial stenoses are common with vessel wall thickening, fibrosis and wrinkling. Lesions are patchy and stenotic areas are interspersed with areas of dilatation and aneurysm. The mesenteric and renal arteries are frequently involved. In the long term, hypertension and hypertensive heart failure occur and signs can mimic those of coarctation of the aorta. Myocarditis and hypercoagulable states are also recognised.

Kawasaki's disease

Kawasaki's disease initially presents in childhood with a self-limiting systemic upset including rashes and lymphadenopathy. Coronary artery aneurysms then appear but may be reduced by the early use of intravenous immunoglobulin [11]. Pericarditis, valvulitis and myocarditis are also common. Later in life, coronary aneurysm, coronary stenoses, acute infarction, heart failure and sudden death are all recognised. Aspirin with or without warfarin, anti-anginal medication, percutaneous coronary intervention and bypass grafting are all utilised in the treatment of coronary lesions.

26.5 Treatment

The mainstays of treating the vasculitis are high-dose corticosteroids and immunosuppressives – usually cyclophosphamide as a first line [12]. Mycophenolate, anti-TNF-α modulators, plasma exchange, plasmapheresis and multiple cytotoxic agents have also been used [13–15]. These treatments require very early specialist input from a rheumatologist and immunologist with a special interest in the vasculitides to ensure timely, but appropriate, care. Care of the patient receiving high-dose immunosuppression includes the standard approach to the immunocompromised.

The management of the other cardiac manifestations of the vasculitides is as for the general population. Treatment of acute coronary syndromes requires standard treatment, up to and including percutaneous coronary intervention and/or coronary artery bypass grafting. Management of heart failure is also standard, including intra-aortic balloon pumping and ventricular assist devices when there is severe myocardial involvement.

26.6 Summary

Although uncommon, patients with systemic vasculitis may present with cardiac manifestations. Scrupulous patient examination and a high index of suspicion are required to make the diagnosis, which may be particularly challenging when a history is not obtainable in a critically ill patient. Although immunosuppressive therapy is often successful, the mortality for those with vasculitis resulting in intensive care admission from cardiac complications remains high.

Case study

A 27-year-old patient with an unclassified lupus-like syndrome presented to the rheumatologists with an exacerbation of arthritis and a recent history of central chest pain. A resting ECG showed minor flattening of the lateral ST segments and an initial creatine kinase (CK) was negative. The C-reactive protein and white cell count were elevated, but there was no evidence of focal infection and blood cultures were negative. Joint pain limited exercise and therefore a thallium myocardial perfusion scan was performed using pharmacological stress (adenosine). During the thallium scan the patient developed severe crushing cheat pain and widespread deep T wave inversion. The patient was admitted to the cardiac care unit where antiplatelet, beta-blocker and low molecular weight heparin were commenced. Pain was ongoing and required large doses of opiates.

Four hours later the patient developed hypotension (systolic blood pressure of 76 mmHg), requiring transfer to the ICU for intra-aortic balloon pumping, invasive monitoring and inotropic support. An urgent coronary angiogram did not reveal any proximal lesions amenable to percutaneous intervention. There was, however, sluggish flow in the epicardial vessels and the suspicion was of diffuse small vessel disease. Cardiac enzymes confirmed significant myocardial necrosis (troponin > 50 µg/l) and a bedside transthoracic echo revealed global left ventricular dysfunction and moderate functional mitral regurgitation. There was no pericardial effusion.

Continued

Pain did not completely settle and increasing cardiovascular support was required to maintain the blood pressure and diminishing urine output. The patient was given a pulse of methyprednisolone (1 g i.v.) and the rheumatologists were discussing the addition of cyclophosphamide and alternative immunosuppressants. However, later that evening despite increasing doses of inotropic support the patient had a pulseless electrical activity cardiac arrest and resuscitation was unsuccessful. Post-mortem examination revealed extensive sub-endocardial infarction and an obliterative small vessel vasculitis.

References

1. Semple D, Keogh J, Forni L, et al. Clinical review: vasculitis on the intensive care unit – part 1: diagnosis. *Crit Care* 2005; 9: 92–7.
2. Griffith M, Brett S. The pulmonary physician in critical care illustrative case 3: pulmonary vasculitis. *Thorax* 2003, 58:543–6.
3. Hunder GG, Arend WP, Bloch DA, et al. The American College of Rheumatology 1990 criteria for the classification of vasculitis. Introduction. *Arthritis Rheum* 1990, 33:1065–7.
4. Evans JM, O'Fallon WM, Hunder GG. Increased incidence of aortic aneurysm and dissection in giant cell (temporal) arteritis. A population-based study. *Ann Intern Med* 1995;22(7):502–7.
5. Morelli S, Perrone C, Ferrante L, et al. Cardiac involvement in Behçet's disease. *Cardiology* 1997;88(6):513–17.
6. Conron M, Beynon HL. Churg–Strauss syndrome. *Thorax* 2000, 55:870–7.
7. Hasley PB, Follansbee WP, Coulehan JL. Cardiac manifestations of Churg–Strauss syndrome: report of a case and review of the literature. *Am Heart J* 1990, 120:996–9.
8. Turesson C, Jacobsson L, Bergström U. Extra-articular rheumatoid arthritis: prevalence and mortality. *Rheumatology* 1999;38(7):668–74.
9. Leibowitz WB. The heart in rheumatoid arthritis. *Ann Inter Med* 2963;58:102.
10. Savige J, Davies D, Falk RJ, et al. Antineutrophil cytoplasmic antibodies and associated diseases: a review of the clinical and laboratory features. *Kidney Int* 2000, 57:846–62.
11. Tse SM, Silverman ED, McCrindle BW, et al. Early treatment with intravenous immunoglobulin in patients with Kawasaki disease. *J Pediatr* 2002;140(4):450–5.
12. Tervaert JW, Huitema MG, Hené RJ, et al. Prevention of relapses in Wegener's granulomatosis by treatment based on antineutrophil cytoplasmic antibody titre. *Lancet* 1990;336:709–11.
13. Hellmich B, Lamprecht P, Gross WL. Advances in the therapy of Wegener's granulomatosis. *Curr Opin Rheumatol* 2006;18(1):25–32.
14. Antoniu SA. Treatment options for refractory Wegener's granulomatosis: a role for rituximab? *Curr Opin Investig Drugs* 2007;8(11):927–32.
15. Takeshita S, Nakamura H, Kawakami A, et al. Hepatitis B-related polyarteritis nodosa presenting necrotizing vasculitis in the hepatobiliary system successfully treated with lamivudine, plasmapheresis and glucocorticoid. *Intern Med* 2006;45(3):145–9.

27 Endocrine Problems and Cardiovascular Critical Care

Philip Marino[1] and Susanna Price[2]
[1]Kingston Hospital, Kingston-Upon-Thames, UK
[2]Royal Brompton & Harefield NHS Foundation Trust, London, UK

Take Home Messages

- Endocrine disorders are common in ICU patients and are associated with significant morbidity and mortality.
- Intensive insulin therapy can reduce morbidity and mortality in patients staying in the ICU for more than 3 days.
- Setting a low glycaemic control target (4.4–6.1 mmol/l) is associated with significant risk of hypoglycaemia and adverse events.
- Low-dose hydrocortisone therapy should be considered in patients with septic shock refractory to fluid resuscitation and vasopressors.
- A short synacthen test is not required prior to starting therapy.
- Hypothyroidism is associated with increased cardiovascular risk and replacement therapy should be introduced cautiously in elderly patients and those with severe coronary artery disease.

27.1 Introduction

Endocrine dysfunction and disease commonly occur in the critically ill, with a broad spectrum of presentation. Endocrine disorders may either cause or result from cardiovascular illness, requiring intensive care unit (ICU) admission. This chapter reviews the presentation, investigation and management of these disorders where relevant to cardiovascular critical care.

Hyperglycaemic states

Diabetes mellitus affects 2.3 million people in the UK [1]. The diabetic emergencies diabetic ketoacidosis (DKA) and hyperosmolar non-ketotic state (HONK) are the most commonly seen endocrine disorders in the ICU, although acute illness may precipitate hyperglycaemia in any patient

---

Cardiovascular Critical Care. Edited by M. Griffiths, J. Cordingley and S. Price. © 2010 Blackwell Publishing Ltd.

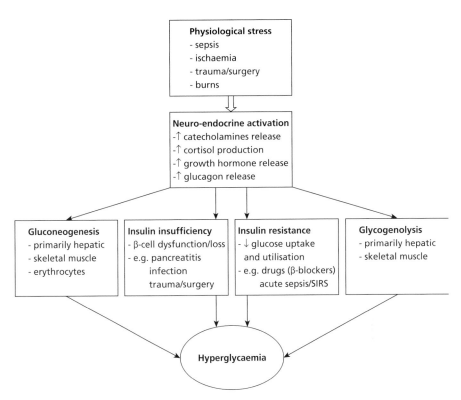

Figure 27.1 Development of hyperglycaemia in critical illness. SIRS, Systemic inflammatory response syndrome.

by stimulating catecholamine, cortisol, growth hormone and glucagon release (see Figure 27.1). This increases hepatic gluconeogenesis, glycogenolysis and peripheral insulin resistance, raising glucose production and decreasing peripheral utilisation [2]. These changes are associated with increased mobilisation of free fatty acids from adipose tissue, promoting gluconeogenesis, fatty acid oxidation and ketoacidosis. The resultant hyperglycaemia and increased levels of free fatty acids consequently cause end-organ dysfunction through various mechanisms, including direct impairment of cellular function and reduced tissue perfusion due to decreased cardiac output, and intravascular blood volume through osmotic diuresis [3].

The chronic cardiovascular consequences of diabetes mellitus relate to microvascular disease and accelerated atheroma, resulting in premature coronary artery disease and renovascular disease.

Management
The diabetic patient

Diabetes is associated with a high incidence of cardiovascular disease, leading to myocardial infarction and requirement for revascularisation either surgically or percutaneously. In such patients, significant hyperglycaemia (either DKA or HONK) may accompany any significant cardiac insult. In particular, myocardial infarction in the diabetic patient may be 'silent' and should be actively excluded and aggressively treated. In diabetic patients, ICU management may be complicated by renovascular disease, difficulties in peripheral arterial access and intra-aortic balloon pump (IABP) insertion. Furthermore, the microvascular disease associated with diabetes can result in myocardial ischaemia and ventricular dysfunction seemingly disproportionate to the angiographically detectable coronary artery disease. In such patients undergoing cardiac surgery, requirement for IABP should be anticipated and, where required, insertion performed, preferably under angiographic or ultrasound guidance and by an experienced operator.

As diabetic patients are at increased risk of post-operative infection, scrupulous asepsis must be observed with all invasive procedures, and careful glycaemic control post-procedure is essential – in avoidance of both hyper- and hypoglycaemia.

In parallel with standard management of the underlying medical condition, where hyperglycaemia occurs the principles of treatment include: fluid resuscitation, careful glycaemic control and correction of serum electrolytes and acid-base balance. Appropriate fluid resuscitation restores intravascular volume, cardiac output and tissue perfusion, improving renal function, acid-base status and insulin resistance. Isotonic saline is preferred, with the first litre administered rapidly, then a continuous infusion depending on clinical response and cardiac function [5]. Care must be taken in patients at risk of developing pulmonary oedema, in whom invasive haemodynamic monitoring and echocardiography may be required to guide fluid replacement. Fluid replacement and insulin therapy may cause electrolyte disturbance through intracellular shift, haemodilution and diuresis, precipitating cardiac arrythmias due to hypokalaemia. Both potassium and magnesium levels should be monitored and treated accordingly.

Non-diabetic patient: stress hyperglycaemia

Hyperglycaemia often occurs in critical illness and is associated with significant morbidity and mortality, even in the non-diabetic patient. Studies in patients with hyperglycaemia after myocardial infarction or cerebrovascular event have shown a reduction in morbidity and mortality in patients who received insulin therapy to improve glycaemic control [6, 7]. More recent studies in surgical and medical ICU patients have also shown improved morbidity (e.g. infections, renal failure, neuropathy) and mortality with intensive insulin therapy (IIT), aiming for a target blood glucose between 4.4 and 6.1 mmol/l [8, 9]. The first study in cardiothoracic surgical patients showed a significant reduction in mortality from 8% to 4.6% in patients receiving IIT for more than 5 days [8]. In addition, the duration of mechanical ventilation, ICU and hospital length of stay were reduced in both studies, whilst mortality fell in patients receiving IIT for more than 3 days in the medical patients (43% vs 52%). However, there was a trend to higher mortality in medical patients receiving IIT for less than 72 hours, thought to be due to recurrent hypoglycaemia.

The risk of hypoglycaemia has been attributed to the relative low blood glucose range targeted in these studies and may be compounded when the symptoms of hypoglycaemia are disguised by sedation and mechanical ventilation. The potential harm of tight glycaemic control has been highlighted by two further studies. The first compared intraoperative IIT (target glucose 4.4–5.6 mmol/l) with conventional therapy (treat if glucose > 11.1 mmol/l) in patients undergoing elective, on-pump cardiac surgery [10]. There was no difference in total adverse events (e.g. deaths, sternal infections, arrhythmias, renal failure), but more strokes and deaths occurred in the ITT group. The more recent VISEP (Volume substitution and Insulin therapy in severe SEPsis) trial investigated IIT (glucose range 4.4–6.1 mmol/l) and pentastarch resuscitation in patients with severe sepsis [11]. Hypoglycaemia occurred in 17% of patients with IIT compared to 4% in the conventional therapy group and was an independent risk factor for death. Subsequent studies have confirmed the benefits of glycaemic control at higher target glucose levels (8 mmol) to avoid potentially harmful hypoglycaemia and are now advocated in the current surviving sepsis guidelines [12, 13].

27.2 Adrenal failure and insufficiency

Acute adrenal failure is an acute medical emergency associated with significant morbidity and mortality. It may be primary or secondary, due to hypothalamic-pituitary disorders or long-term corticosteroid therapy (see Table 27.1). Recent studies in the critically ill have also recognised the development of relative adrenal insufficiency in severe sepsis and its effects on morbidity and mortality. Although an acute Addisonian crisis may be precipitated by an acute illness, as in hyperglycaemia (above), heparin administration (common in cardiothoracic critical care) may cause acute adrenal insufficiency, presenting as an Addisonian crisis. This particular condition may occur through direct adrenal haemorrhage or in the context of heparin-induced thrombocytopaenia, where the development of a coagulopathy may precipitate bilateral adrenal haemorrhage and subsequent insufficiency [14]. This association has been reported with heparin administration at both treatment and prophylactic doses, and in both unfractionated and low molecular weight preparations. The major relevance of adrenal insufficiency to cardiovascular critical care is, however, in the administration of corticosteroids for relative adrenal insufficiency.

Relative adrenal insufficiency

Endogenous corticosteroids help to maintain normal metabolic, immune and haemodynamic function. Relative adrenal insufficiency has been identified in the critically ill and those who have previously received etomidate. The condition, now referred to as 'critical illness related corticosteroid insufficiency' (CIRCI), is associated with a worse prognosis,

Table 27.1 Causes of adrenal insufficiency.

Primary adrenal insufficiency
Autoimmune (Addison's disease)
Infection (tuberculosis, histoplasmosis, cytomegalovirus, HIV)
Haemorrhage (ITP, TTP, SLE, Waterhouse–Friderichsen syndrome)
Tumour (metastasis, lymphoma)
Amyloidosis
Genetic (congenital adrenal hyper- or hypoplasia)
Secondary adrenal insufficiency
Exogenous corticosteroid therapy
Hypothalamic-pituitary disease
• Tumour (adenoma, craniopharyngioma)
• Infiltrative disease (sarcoidosis, haemochromatosis, amyloidosis, histiocytosis)
• Surgery
• Trauma
• Radiotherapy
• Haemorrhage
• Post-partum pituitary necrosis (Sheehan's syndrome)
• Autoimmune
• Empty Sella syndrome

ITP, Idiopathic thrombocytopaenic purpura; TTP, thrombotic thrombocytopaenic purpura; SLE, systemic lupus erythrematosus.

particularly in patients with septic shock [15]. It is thought to occur through a combination of reduced production of endogenous corticosteroid and inflammation-induced glucocorticoid receptor resistance. As a consequence, there has been considerable debate regarding the diagnosis and treatment of this condition.

Initial studies using high or supra-physiological dose corticosteroid therapy showed no benefit or increased mortality, primarily due to super-infection [16]. Further studies using physiological steroid doses (low-dose hydrocortisone with/without fludrocortisone) found reduced vasopressor use and mortality in patients with septic shock who had a low baseline cortisol level (< 21 μg/dl) and poor response to ACTH on short synacthen test (< 9 μg/dl) [17]. However, many patients received etomidate which is known to cause adrenal suppression, thereby questioning the clinical significance of the short synacthen test (SST) and the potential benefits of low-dose replacement therapy.

The recent CORTICUS (corticosteroid therapy of septic shock) study sought to determine whether 'non-responders' to the SST would indeed benefit more from low-dose hydrocortisone therapy (11 day course) and to determine the validity of the SST in diagnosing CIRCI [18]. The trial demonstrated faster reversal of septic shock refractory to fluid resuscitation and vasopressor therapy with steroid therapy, irrespective of whether the patient was a 'responder' or 'non-responder' to the SST. There was a non-significant trend to lower mortality in patients with a low baseline cortisol (< 9 μg/dl) and poor SST response (< 10 μg/dl). The risk of super-infection may account for these findings, although a shorter duration of treatment and improved immuno-surveillance may reduce such complications.

In cardiothoracic intensive care, 'physiological' steroid therapy should be considered in patients with profound vasoplegia and hypotension requiring high (and increasing) levels of vasopressor support and where a SST shows a poor response. If the post-operative hypotension and vasoplegia is catastrophic, the first dose of corticosteroids may be required before results from the SST are known. Here, if an optimal result is found, corticosteroids may be withdrawn. The new surviving sepsis guidelines advocate that low-dose hydrocortisone therapy be considered in patients with septic shock responding poorly to fluid resuscitation and vasopressors without prior SST [12].

Alternative measures of adrenal insufficiency in critical illness are being investigated in view of the limitations of the SST. This may also help to determine which patients may potentially benefit from corticosteroid therapy. Most circulating cortisol (> 95%) is bound to coritsol-binding globulin (CBG), but it is the free cortisol that is biologically active. CBG levels fall during critical illness, potentially raising free cortisol levels [19]. Therefore, it may be possible to determine adrenal insufficiency by measuring the free cortisol and identify patients who may require replacement therapy. Another potentially useful measure may be the plasma cortisol (active):cortisone (inactive) ratio. In health, microsomal enzymes catalyse the conversion of cortisol to cortisone and vice versa, with a normal ratio of 6:8. This ratio is increased in sepsis and a poor response may be used as a diagnostic tool for identifying CIRCI, although further studies are required [20].

27.3 Thyroid dysfunction

Hypo- and hyperthyroidism are relatively common medical conditions, but the extremes (myxoedema coma and thyroid crisis) are rarely seen in the ICU (see Table 27.2). By contrast, abnormalities of measured thyroid function tests (TFTs) are often seen in the critically ill, and are associated with significant mortality that increases with disease severity [21]. These abnormalities may arise through reduced T4 and T3 production and release, decreased thyroid stimulating hormone (TSH) secretion and peripheral tissue resistance to T4 and T3 [22]. Three main patterns of disease have been described:
- Low T3 syndrome (70% of cases)
- Low T4 syndrome (50% of cases)
- Low T3, T4 and TSH syndrome

Drugs frequently used in cardiothoracic intensive care such as corticosteroids, dopamine, amiodarone and iodinated radio-contrast agents may exacerbate these syndromes. Specifically, in patients with congenital heart disease, thyroid dysfunction is commonly seen in association with amiodarone therapy. Serial TFTs aid diagnosis, as single readings are difficult to interpret. Thyroid hormone replacement is not

Table 27.2 Thyroid disease in the critically ill.

Hypothyroidism
Autoimmune (primary, Hashimoto's thyroiditis)
Drugs (carbimazole, amiodarone, radio-iodine)
Tumour (adenoma, carcinoma)
Post thyroidectomy
Post radiotherapy
Goitre
Iodine deficiency
Juvenile hypothyroidism
Congenital hypothyroidsm
Ectopic or absent thyroid
Hypothalamic-pituitary failure

Hyperthyroidism
Autoimmune (Grave's disease, Hashimoto's syndrome)
Multi-nodular goitre
De Quervain's thyroiditis (post-viral syndrome)
Post-partum thyroiditis
Tumour (adenoma, carcinoma)
Drugs (amiodarone)
TSH-secreting pituitary adenoma
Ectopic TSH production (trophoblastic tumour, terotoma)
TSH hypersecretion syndrome

Sick euthyroid syndrome
Low T3
Low T4
Low T3, T4, TSH

TSH, Thyroid stimulating hormone.

currently advocated, unless true primary hypothyroidism is present, as previous studies in the critically ill have produced conflicting results.

Hypothyroidism and cardiac disease

Thyroid hormone activity is required for maintaining normal cardiac function. There is an increased incidence of cardiac disease in patients with hypothyroidism, specifically coronary artery disease, left ventricular dysfunction and arrhythmias. This is primarily due to a combination of functional cardiac abnormalities, particularly ventricular systolic and diastolic dysfunction, and impaired endothelial function with progressive atherosclerosis [23]. These risks are present even in individuals with sub-clinical disease. Newly diagnosed patients are at potential risk of myocardial ischaemia and dysfunction if thyroxine replacement therapy is introduced too rapidly owing to an increase in myocardial oxygen demand. Clinical studies have shown reduced morbidity using low doses initially (e.g. thyroxine 25 μg od) with increments every 4–6 weeks until adequate replacement is achieved [24].

However, there remain concerns regarding the initiation of thyroxine replacement in elderly patients and those with advanced coronary artery disease. In high-risk cases evaluation with cardiac catheterisation and subsequent coronary revascularisation with bypass surgery has reduced mortality [25]. Thyroxine replacement may then be introduced as previously outlined.

Myxoedema coma

Myxoedema coma is associated with high mortality (> 20%) unless recognised early and treated immediately [26]. The most common precipitating factors are acute illness (sepsis, trauma, burns, surgery), hypothermia and drugs (β-blockers, amiodarone, diuretics, opiates) [27].

Clinical presentation

Most patients have known hypothyroidism, though occasionally myoxedema coma may be the first presentation. The reasons a patient may present to a cardiac ICU include bradycardia, hypotension and cardiomyopathy and/or pericardial collection.

Clinical investigations

In addition to routine investigations, creatine kinase should be measured to exclude rhabdomyolysis. Arterial blood gas analysis may demonstrate hypoxia, hypercapnia and respiratory acidosis. TFTs confirm the diagnosis. Echocardiography should be performed to demonstrate any cardiac dysfunction (either incidental or due to hypothyroidism) and pericardial collection, although these require drainage only rarely.

Management

Treatment involves thyroid hormone replacement and general supportive measures. The type and route of thyroid hormone therapy depends on disease severity [27, 28]. Oral therapy is preferred, typically T4 (50–100 μg/day), with smaller doses in patients with ischaemic heart disease to avoid myocardial ischaemia or arrhythmias. Intravenous therapy may be required in severe cases, giving a T4 bolus (200 – 500 μg iv), then 50–100 μg daily thereafter. Whilst T3 has a more rapid onset of action, its use has been associated with an increased mortality.

Supportive therapy includes intravenous fluid replacement and electrolyte correction, particularly in those with arrhythmia. Intravenous dextrose is used to correct hypoglycaemia and sodium bicarbonate considered in severe metabolic acidosis (pH < 7), although caution should be used with severe ventricular dysfunction, as pulmonary oedema may result. Intravenous corticosteroids may be used as adrenal insufficiency often occurs, but a baseline cortisol level and SST should be performed beforehand. Vasopressor and inotropic support may be required in persistent hypotension and cardiac failure, with appropriate haemodynamic monitoring, though the response may be blunted due to adrenergic receptor down-regulation. Active warming is indicated in moderate to severe hypothermia (< 32°C) until core temperature exceeds 34°C. Precipitating factors should be actively sought and broad-spectrum antibiotics considered unless infection can be excluded.

Thyroid crisis or 'storm'

Thyroid storm is characterised by a hypermetabolic state with multi-organ dysfunction and is associated with significant morbidity and mortality (20–30%) [29]. Most patients have pre-existing hyperthyroidism and the condition is most commonly triggered by thyroid surgery, radio-iodine therapy and withdrawal of anti-thyroid drugs. Other precipitating factors include sepsis, myocardial infarction, DKA, trauma and drugs (amiodarone, iodinated radio-contrast dyes).

Clinical presentation

The cardiovascular manifestations of thyroid storm include tachycardia, arrhythmia (atrial and ventricular), hypertension, hypotension, tachypnoea and dyspnoea. Where cardiac failure and tachy-arrhythmias are associated with a low systemic vascular resistance and abnormally warm peripheries, particularly in patients treated with amiodarone, the diagnosis should be entertained.

Clinical investigations

Routine tests may identify possible precipitating factors such as sepsis, and TFTs confirm the diagnosis. TSH may also be reduced by dopamine or corticosteroid therapy, so TFTs must be interpreted with caution.

Management

Treatment comprises controlling thyroid hormone activity, supportive measures and treating any underlying cause. Propylthiouracil (PTU), iodine therapy (e.g. potassium iodide) and intravenous corticosteroids should be started to prevent further thyroid hormone production and release [28]. β-blockers (e.g. propanolol 40–80 mg 4- to 8-hourly) help control adrenergic symptoms. Supportive therapies include oxygen therapy, intravenous fluid replacement and active cooling measures (cold fluids, antipyretics, cooling blankets) for hyperthermia [28]. Vasopressor and inotropic support may be needed in circulatory collapse and cardiac failure; however, tachyarrhythmias may preclude their use. Here, emergency ablation in parallel with specific treatment of the thyrotoxicosis may be considered. Plasmapheresis and plasma exchange have been used successfully in life-threatening cases, whilst emergency thyroidectomy has been undertaken [30, 31]; however, where patients present with profound cardiovascular collapse, their haemodynamic status may preclude this.

27.4 Conclusion

Endocrine disease or dysfunction is common in cardiothoracic ICU patients, most commonly as the result of long-term diabetes resulting in coronary artery disease. On occasion, however, abnormalities in the endocrine system may cause profound cardiovascular dysfunction, in which case treatment of the underlying disease is crucial, whilst continuing to support the cardiovascular system.

Case study

A 51-year-old man with recently diagnosed pulmonary stenosis was admitted for elective balloon valvuloplasty. He had been diagnosed with thyrotoxicosis a month earlier (free thyroxine 5 1IU, TSH below 0.05 IU) and was started on carbimazole. In addition, he was hypertensive and suffered from recurrent palpitations. An electrocardiogram (ECG) showed sinus rhythm with first-degree heart block, right bundle branch block and ventricular hypertrophy, whilst a 24-hour Holter study showed frequent multi-focal ventricular ectopics with occasional 2-second pauses and a few brief runs of a junctional rhythm.

The patient was clinically and biochemically euthyroid prior to admission. During the pulmonary valvuloplasty under general anaesthesia, he developed acute pulmonary oedema and subsequently required transferred to the ICU for invasive ventilation. A trans-oesophageal echocardiogram showed good left and right ventricular function with a residual pulmonary valve gradient of 28 mmHg. The chest radiograph confirmed bilateral peri-hilar shadowing consistent with pulmonary oedema.

Soon after admission the patient became pyrexial (38.1°C) and hypotensive (MAP 55–60) with recurrent episodes of junctional bradycardia and third-degree atrio-ventricular block. A vasopressor infusion was started to maintain the MAP above 70 and an isoprenaline infusion introduced to prevent further bradycardia. Broad-spectrum antibiotics and enteral feeding were added.

Subsequent septic screen and synacthen test were unremarkable, but repeat TFTs showed a significantly raised free thyroxine level of 75 IU and a TSH less than 0.05 IU. On day 4 an endocrinology review was sought and the diagnosis of 'hyperthyroid crisis or thyroid storm' was made. The carbimazole dose was increased and both intravenous corticosteroids and oral β-blockers commenced, whilst Lugol's solution (oral iodine and iodide) could be considered if there was no response to therapy. By the following day he was haemodynamically stable and the pulmonary oedema was beginning to resolve, allowing the noradrenaline and isoprenaline infusions to be stopped.

Over the next 48 hours both the pyrexia and agitation gradually resolved, though the patient remained mildly disorientated. The free thyroxine level had fallen to 47 IU, but the patient continued to experience junctional bradycardia with third-degree atrio-ventricular block, causing 2- to 3-second pauses. The β-blocker was stopped and a temporary pacing wire inserted as some episodes caused significant hypotension (MAP 45–55). A permanent dual chamber pacemaker was inserted and the β-blocker reintroduced. The patient was successfully extubated after the procedure but required intermittent continuous positive airway pressure (CPAP) initially with an FiO_2 of 0.4. The free thyroxine and TSH levels had fallen to 32 IU and 0.12 units respectively.

By the following day, the patient was fully orientated and was both clinically and biochemically euthyroid. He was discharged from the unit to the care of the cardiology team with appropriate endocrine follow up.

References

1. *Diabetes Prevalence 2007*. Diabetes UK, London.
2. McGarry JD. Lilly Lecture 1978: new perspectives in the regulation of ketogenesis. *Diabetes* 1979; 28: 517–23.
3. Kitabachi AE, Umpierrez GE, Murphy MB, et al. Technical review: management of hyperglycaemic crises in patients with diabetes. *Diabetes Care* 2001; 24: 131–53.
4. Ennis ED, Stahl EJVB, Kreisberg RA. The hyperosmolar hyperglycaemic syndrome. *Diabetes Rev* 1994; 2: 115–26.
5. American Diabetes Association. Position statement: hypergylcaemic crises in patients with diabetes mellitus. *Diabetes Care* 2001; 24: 154–61.
6. Malmberg K, Norhammer A, Wedel H, et al. Gly-cometabolic state at admission: important risk marker of mortality in conventionally treated patients with diabetes and acute myocardial infarction: long term results from the Diabetes and Insulin-Glucose in Acute Myocardial Infarction (DIGAMI) study. *Circulation* 1999; 99: 2626–32.
7. Gray CS, Taylor R, French JM, et al. The prognostic value of stress hyperglycaemia and previously unrecognized diabetes mellitus in acute stroke. *Diabet Med* 1987; 4: 237–40.
8. Van den Berghe G, Wouters P, Weekers F, et al. Intensive insulin therapy in critically ill patients. *N Eng J Med* 2001; 345: 1359–67.
9. Van den Berghe G, Wilmer A, Hermans G, et al. Intensive insulin therapy in the medical ICU. *N Engl J Med* 2006; 354(5): 449–61.
10. Gandhi GY, Nuttall GA, Abel MD, et al. Intensive intraoperative insulin therapy versus conventional glucose management during cardiac surgery. *Ann Intern Med* 2007; 146: 233–43.
11. Brunkhorst FM, Engel C, Bioos F, et al. Intensive insulin therapy and pentastarch resuscitation in severe sepsis. *N Eng J Med* 2008; 358: 125–39.
12. Dellinger RP, Levy MM, Carlet JM, et al. Surviving Sepsis Campaign: international guidelines for the management of severe sepsis and septic shock 2008. *Crit Care Med* 2008; 36: 296–327.
13. Finney SJ, Zekveld C, Elia A, et al. Glucose control and mortality in critically ill patients. *JAMA* 2003; 290(15): 2041–7.
14. Kurtz LE, Yang S. Bilateral adrenal hemorrhage associated with heparin induced thrombocytopaenia. *Am J Hematology* 2007; 82(6): 493–4.
15. Marik PE, Pastores SM, Annane D, et al. American College of Critical Care Medicine. Recommendations for the diagnosis and management of corticosteroid insufficiency in critically ill adult patients: consensus statement from an international task force by American College of Critical Care Medicine. *Crit Care Med* 2008; 36(6): 1937–49.
16. Bone RC, Fisher CJ Jr, Clemmer TP, et al. A controlled clinical trial of high dose methyl-prednisolone in the treatment of severe sepsis and septic shock. *N Eng J Med* 1987; 317: 653–8.
17. Annane D, Sebille V, Charpentier C, et al. Effect of treatment with low dose of hydrocortisone and fludrocortisone on mortality in patients with septic shock. *JAMA* 2002; 288: 862–71.
18. Sprung CL, Annane D, Keh D, et al. Hydrocortisone therapy for patients with septic shock. *N Eng J Med* 2008; 358: 111–24.
19. Hamarahian AH, Oseni TS, Arafah BM. Measurements of serum free cortisol in critically ill patients. *N Eng J Med* 2004; 350: 1629–38.
20. Voseger M, Felbinger TW, Roll W, et al. Increased ratio of serum cortisol to cortisone in acute-phase response. *Horm Res* 2002; 58: 172–5.

21. Plikat K, Langgartner J, Buettner R, et al. Frequency and outcome of patients with nonthyroidal illness syndrome in a medical intensive care unit. *Metabolism* 2007; 56(2): 239–44.

22. Chopra IJ. Clinical review 86. Euthyroid sick syndrome: is it a misnomer? *J Clin Endocrinol Metab* 1997; 82: 329–34.

23. Biondi B, Klein I. Hypothyroidism as a risk factor for cardiovascular disease. *Endocrine* 2004; 24(1): 1–13.

24. Feldt-Rasmussen U. Treatment of hypothyroidism in elderly patients with cardiac disease. *Thyroid* 2007; 17(7): 619–24.

25. Ellyin F, Fuh CY, Singh SP, et al. Hypothyroidism with angina pectoris. A clinical dilemma. *Postgrad Med* 1986; 79(7): 93–8.

26. Yamamoto T, Fukuyama J, Fujiyoshi A. Factors associated with mortality of myxoedema coma: a report of eight cases and literature survey. *Thyroid* 1999; 9: 1167–74.

27. Wartofsky L. Myxoedema coma. In: Braverman LE, Utiger RD, editors. *Werner & Ingbar's The Thyroid: A Fundamental and Clinical Text*, 8th edn. Philadelphia: Lippincott Williams & Wilkins: 2000; pp. 843–7.

28. Young R, Worthley LI. Diagnosis and management of thyroid disease and the critically ill patient. *Crit Care Resusc* 2004; 6(4): 295–305.

29. Tietjens ST, Leinung MC. Thyroid storm. *Med Clin N Am* 1995; 79: 169–84.

30. Tajiri J, Katsuya H, Kiyokawa T, et al. Successful treatment of thyrotoxic crisis with plasma exchange. *Crit Care Med* 1984; 12: 536–7.

31. Goldberg PA, Inzucchi SE. Critical issues in endocrinology. *Clin Chest Med* 2003; 24: 583–606.

28 Haemodynamic Monitoring and Therapy: A Personal History 1961–1994

Ronald Bradley

Intensive Care Medicine, St Thomas' Hospital, London, UK

In the beginning it became apparent that there was a need for measurement in the care of those who were grievously sick. Yet in this country the notion of a special unit in which to look after such people remained in 1961 but an idea. This meant that any equipment needed to make the measurements had to go to the patient, wherever that might be in the hospital. As a very junior lecturer in Peter Sharpey Schafer's medical unit at St Thomas' Hospital, with nought but a basic medical degree and a degree in physiology, my prospects were limited. When Schafer asked what ideas I had if any, my answer was that when really sick people arrived in the casualty department, the cardiologists' attitude was – 'make him better, and then I'll catheterise him' – I thought that this seemed illogical, indeed that the chances of making such patients better might be improved if some measurements could be made whilst disaster still hovered in the air. Remarkably, after what seemed an immensely long pause, this brief discussion was concluded with 'take three years, and see what you can do'.

So it was that I set about sawing up lengths of steel piping to construct a scaffold mounted on wheels that would fit into any lift, and then busied myself mounting on it four pressure transducers, their preamplifiers, an electrocardiogram (ECG), a set of gas electrodes and a pH meter. There was room also for a small centrifuge for measuring haematocrits; that and a four-channel recorder completed the initial steps as I set out upon a road full of fascination that was to last for the next 33 years. Kindly disposed hospital carpenters plated the skeleton with formica, making the whole rather more acceptable to the Nightingale Sisters who would have to countenance this juggernaut in their scrupulously clean wards. Whatever they truly thought of it, the 'buggy', as it became known, was received with good humour and a deal of banter, which was as well, for in those days nothing could happen within the hospital without the acquiescence of the nursing staff (Figure 28.1).

As I look at this illustration I am reminded that bits were added to the initial array as fresh ideas came to mind; notably an oxygen electrode made by David Band that was linear in its performance to very high oxygen

Cardiovascular Critical Care. Edited by M. Griffiths, J. Cordingley and S. Price.
© 2010 Blackwell Publishing Ltd.

(a)

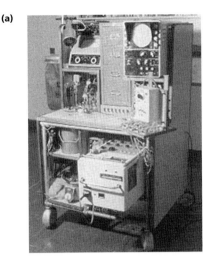

(b)

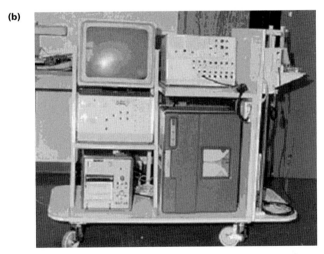

Figure 28.1(a) and (b) The first and second mobile investigation carts. Both had four pressure transducers and the thermal dilution system. The first (**a**) also had a set of gas electrodes, a centrifuge for haematocrits and a four-channel writer. The second (**b**) had a 14-channel tape recorder.

tensions, which allowed the measurement of the oxygen content as well as tension in samples of blood, without recourse to the infinite tedium of Van Slyke's method, which was so demanding of skill, patience and time. The rapid measurement of oxygen content with an electrode [1], when combined with the ability to float miniature catheters into the pulmonary artery [2], opened the door to the then gold standard of cardiac output measurement by Fick's principle. Peter Korner, a deft Australian physiologist, published details of a method of measuring cardiac output in rabbits using what was essentially the indicator dilution technique with a slug of cold fluid as the indicator [3]. If the technique could be made to work in an animal as small as a rabbit, it cried out to be attempted in a human. Strangely the most difficult part of making the technique work in a human proved to be preserving the coldness of the indicator bolus on its way to the point of mixing in the circulation. The principle involved was the release of a measured bolus of coldness into the right atrium, mixing of that cold signal with the blood flow through the right heart, and the detection of the diluted coldness as a function of time as it passed up the pulmonary artery.

If the indicator was delivered to the right atrium through a catheter in the arm, a considerable portion of the cold signal was lost across the catheter into the tissues of the arm. The problem was solved by looking up the anatomy of the internal jugular vein, and the discovery that it was usually relatively easy to locate the vein with a needle just lateral to the carotid artery. Delivery of the cold indicator through a small catheter in the internal jugular vein meant that any coldness lost through the catheter into the blood in the internal jugular and the superior vena cava was swept into the blood flow through the right heart and was therefore included. Also loss of coldness into the wall of the right heart proved not to matter, for, in as much as the muscle warmed up again, much of the coldness must have returned to the blood flowing through the cavity of the ventricle. All this, and the fact that satisfactory mixing of the cold bolus with the blood must have occurred, is implicit in the remarkably good correlation of the results with the measurements made by the direct Fick method.

When, later, the thermal technique was commercialised in the United States, its most remarkable asset was wantonly squandered. A thermal indicator does not recirculate; it is entirely lost in a single passage around the systemic circulation. The mass of muscle and all the solid organs supplied by the systemic circulation are immensely effective as a heat sink. Release of a cold bolus into the root of the aorta produces no detectable cold signal in the pulmonary artery. This being so, calculation of the flow through the pulmonary artery is better made by integrating the entirety of the cold signal with respect to time. In contrast to the classic Hamilton dye curve, there is no recirculation hump to be removed, and the mathematical abstractions relating to its removal are superfluous.

The development of these techniques happened to coincide with the opening of the purpose-built ICU at St Thomas' Hospital, and with it the provision of one–to-one nursing around the clock. The unit was almost entirely designed by Dr Geoffrey Spencer [4] and proved over many years to be ideal in its conception. It provided large open areas, unconstrained by dividing walls, which could be adapted to meet almost any need, together with a few partitioned areas that could be used when isolation was important. The open plan areas had enormous advantages over the small cubicalised units that appeared in other hospitals, which limited the amount of apparatus that could be deployed around any one patient (Figure 28.2) and limited the ability of nursing staff to keep an eye on the patient next door for short periods.

Far from obviating the need for the original mobile investigative cart, further updated versions appeared. The first of these had at its heart a

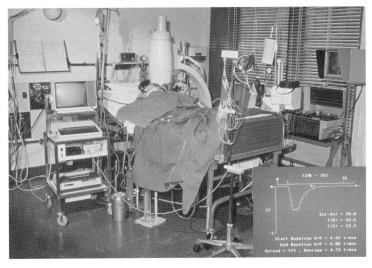

Figure 28.2 This figure shows the extent of investigative effort that could be brought to bear if necessary. On the left is the small trolley with the BBC microcomputer, monitor screen and printer, which dealt with the outputs of the four pressure transducers and the thermal dilution system, in the middle a mobile image intensifier, and on the right a video recorder on which angiograms could be recorded. Inset is the print-out of the cardiac output system showing that there is no recirculation. The temperature time function was integrated using the starting and finishing baselines, and cardiac output was the average of the two values.

14-channel tape recorder to collect signals from the pressure transducers and thermal dilution systems. It was a hand-built masterpiece of miniature electronic engineering produced by Terry Cowell and Barry Waldron entirely within the hospital's very remarkable bioengineering department. This second investigative cart was so effective that there came a suggestion that yet another should be built. That suggestion triggered an intellectual storm amongst the bioengineers, out of which came a most fundamental and remarkable technical innovation. Unaccountably it was never exploited anywhere outside St Thomas', and for the quite extraordinary reason that it was too cheap to produce.

Cowell and Waldron wrote programmes for the BBC microcomputer, which at that time cost a mere £350, allowing this small basic computer to function as a preamplifier for all four pressure transducers, and at the same time to accept and integrate the thermal signals and provide immediate printouts of measurements of cardiac output. This same computer unit was later programmed to control the home-made haemofiltration apparatus that preceded those that were yet to become commercially available. No manufacturer could be persuaded to take up this brilliant concept. All those in the business of manufacturing conventional pressure preamplifiers and then thermal dilution systems at the time pointed out that the only part of such a system that they could market would be the software, which would be relatively easy to pirate or even reproduce from scratch. There was no hardware for them to manufacture, and the general adoption of such systems would lead to their bankruptcy. In price, it undercut anything that could provide the same functions by a factor of at least times ten – a bizarre reason for its failure to be accepted! Had the NHS had the wit to run its own research and development organisation, with the flair of the Thomas's bioengineering department, all might have been different.

In the same vein, it seemed entirely reasonable to make measurements to discover how the human circulation was behaving under extreme conditions of failure. It seemed obvious that we would be better able to make rational decisions about the control of such situations in individual patients if we understood their physiology. Thus we set about to analyse circulatory behaviour in the sickest of patients with all manner of acute circulatory problems [5, 6] – massive myocardial infarction, massive acute pulmonary embolism, and indeed patients suffering from extremes of circulatory derangement for reasons that we did not necessarily understand initially.

The nature of our analysis was based on that so brilliantly and exhaustively worked out in normal dogs by Stanley Sarnoff and his associates in the 1950s, observing the relation of both stroke volume and stroke work to changes in filling pressure for both sides of the heart. Fortune smiled upon us in that by chance we elected to make the observations starting at the highest filling pressures, then measuring the changes in stroke volume, and work following the rapid removal of volume from the circulation. If the measurements are made the other way about, in response to an increase in volume, the fluid infused is likely to have had the wrong pH, the wrong calcium and potassium concentrations and to have been at the wrong temperature. Certainly measurements made in such a way show a much greater degree of scatter and far less consistency.

Having been brought up with the notion of the 'Starling curves' that pervade physiology text books, it was a surprise to discover that, when measured in the intact human, the relation between filling pressure and both stroke work and stroke volume was a straight line function over the range that we were able to follow it. It also emerged that the equations of stroke volume in relation to filling pressure were arranged in two fans, one for each side of the heart. It followed from this that measurements providing a single value of stroke work in relation to filling pressure could be used to predict the entire linear equation, and from this in turn the value of stroke work at zero filling pressure could be predicted. The useful work generated by the heart at this standardised filling pressure – the intercept on the ordinate – was a measure of each ventricle's ability to generate pressure and flow, which was independent of the 'fullness' or 'emptiness' of the circulation. The left-sided intercept proved to be of considerable practical clinical value for it served as a measure of contractility to all but the purists. With a normal value in excess of 50 g m, it was found that left ventricular intercepts of less than 13 sustained for any length of time were not compatible with survival, and that patients with intercepts less than 20 required mechanical ventilatory support to relieve them of the work of breathing (Figure 28.3a–c).

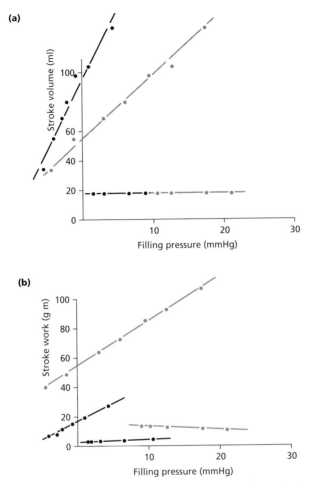

Figure 28.3(a) and (b) All left heart functions are in red and right in blue. (**a**) Changes in stroke volume as filling pressure varies in a normal patient are contrasted with those in a patient with heart failure sufficiently severe to produce a fixed low stroke output. (**b**) Relation of stroke work to filling pressure in the same two patients.

The other unlooked-for by-product of these investigations was a clinically useful measure of venous compliance, the units in which it was measured being millilitres of volume change per millimetre of mercury change in right atrial pressure. The right atrial pressure response to rapid volume removal from the circulation in different clinical states showed that the venous capacity bed could become less compliant than the normal by a factor of 10 following extensive myocardial infarction or major pulmonary embolism. A healthy volunteer giving blood to a bank shows a compliance of 300–350 ml volume change for a fall in right atrial pressure of 1 mmHg. Removal of as little as 30 ml from a 'tight' circulation will produce the same fall in right atrial pressure. In addition to these observations, the response

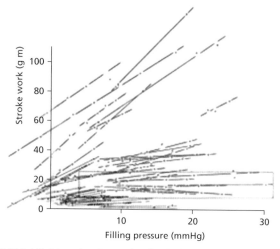

Figure 28.3(c) All left heart functions are in red and right in blue. The figure shows equations of stroke work of the left and right hearts measured in 70 patients, varying from normality to extremes of failure, from which the general equations below were derived:

$$WL = \frac{(b-13)PL + 10b - 130}{a + 10} + 13$$

and the intercept on the ordinate

$$IL = \frac{10b - 130}{a + 10} + 13$$

$$WR = \frac{bPR + 10b}{a + 10}$$

and the intercept on the ordinate

$$IR = \frac{10b}{a + 10}$$

where WL and WR are the stroke work of the left and right heart respectively in gram metres, PL and PR are its filling pressure in millimetres of mercury related to the sternal angle, I R is the intercept on the ordinate, and a and b are the x and y co-ordinates of any single point on the equation.

of the pulse pressure to Valsalva's manoeuvre provided an alternative, less invasive method of discovering the relation between the stroke volume equations – a normal rapid drop in pulse pressure suggesting normality of the relation between left and right atrial pressure, and a 'square wave' response, by indicating an abnormally large volume in the pulmonary venous bed, suggesting that the stroke volume equation of the left heart was displaced to the right.

The total patterns of venous compliance, stroke work and stroke volume pumped by both left and right hearts, and in particular the relation of the left- and right-sided stroke volume equations, together with the measurements of systemic and pulmonary resistance obtained in the presence of extremes of circulatory derangement gave a 'feel' for the way that the circulation would behave and how it might be manipulated. In general, six patterns of behaviour were identified that were more or less repeatable. An enormously important seventh group with major circulatory derangement due to sepsis were less predictable in their behaviour, in that their systemic and pulmonary resistances might be raised or lowered, and most commonly in opposite directions, and who also might have myocardial failure or normal functioning hearts.

The likely patterns of the equations of function, being known, it was found possible by clinical examination, using nothing more invasive than clinical observation of the response to a Valsalva manoeuvre, to place patients on the equations predicted for their group. Central to this clinical analysis was an estimate of cardiac output. Clinicians are not normally trained to estimate in litres a minute the flows being generated by the heart of the patient they are examining. Yet in the limiting case of flows dwindling toward the point of death, the matter is fairly obvious, and by employing some unfamiliar physical signs, it is possible to estimate the flow or cardiac output in considerably less time than it takes to make measurements (Figure 28.4). There is a common misapprehension that this system depends overmuch upon the observation of skin flows, but it does take account of those patients who 'would seem to mislead' about the state of their systemic resistance. Those who dissemble in this way most commonly in fact prove to be suffering from sepsis, and are using the constriction of their skin circulation to raise a fever.

As the years passed and confidence in the reliability of the system of clinical assessment increased, offering as it does numerical values for the systemic and pulmonary resistance, and for the left- and right-sided intercepts, so the emphasis passed from invasive measurement to such

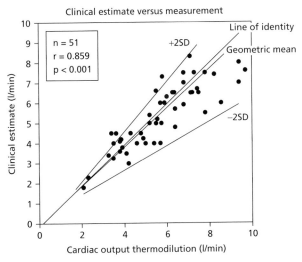

Figure 28.4 A comparison of clinical estimation of cardiac output and simultaneous measurement using thermal dilution in 51 patients. Although there is quite a scatter at higher values, errors at this end are of less consequence to the system of non-invasive analysis that was devised within the unit for use with programmable pocket calculators.

measures only being deployed where there was difficulty and doubt, of either diagnosis or management. In the mid 1970s a lady of 66 with pulmonary emboli taught us about the importance of volume change upon the resistance of vascular beds. Twice in her history, sitting up with her legs dependent had produced syncope and cardiac arrest. With an RAP of 3 mmHg and a left ventricular end-diastolic pressure (LVEDP) of 1 mmHg, the stroke volume was 21 ml (cardiac output (CO) 1.9 l/min) and the pulmonary vascular resistance (PVR) 14 times normal. Infusion of 0.5 l of dextran raised the right atrial pressure (RAP) to 13 mmHg, the LVEDP to 6 mmHg and the stroke volume to 36 ml (CO 3.1 l/min) and the PVR was then only 9 times normal. Whilst the volume load lifted the work produced by the right heart from 7 to 11 g m, this modest increase in work done

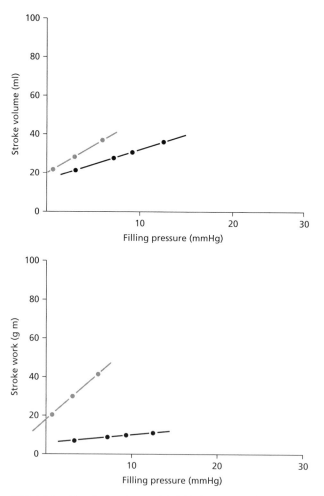

Figure 28.5 Left heart functions are in grey, right in black. Equations of stroke volume and stroke work related to filling pressure measured in a patient with a massive pulmonary embolus.

against pulmonary resistance was insufficient to increase the cardiac output by a similar margin (Figure 28.5). It is the proportion of the volume expander that is distributed within the pulmonary bed and the 'expansion of the bed around the emboli' which causes the reduction in resistance and increases the flows so markedly. That the expansion of a vascular bed with an incompressible fluid of necessity drops the resistance across the bed is an important practical truth about the circulation; so also the opposite, that removal of volume must increase the resistance, and this was the mechanism of the patient's syncope. The erect posture, haemorrhage, morphine, the induction of anaesthesia, the injection of contrast material during angiography and tying of the inferior vena cava (IVC) all reduce the right atrial pressure and drop the stroke volume pumped into the pulmonary bed. Transiently the output of the right heart drops before that of the left, and volume is lost from the pulmonary bed into the systemic. It is this shift of volume from the pulmonary bed, and the inevitable critical rise in pulmonary resistance, which makes all of these things potentially lethal in the presence of large pulmonary emboli.

Such then were a few of the insights that our measurements offered in fulfilment of the idea that the chances of making such patients better might be improved if some measurements could be made whilst disaster still hovered in the air. It remains immeasurably sad that Schafer died so prematurely, unable to enjoy the harvest of circulatory insights that he had begun.

References

1. Branthwaite MA, Bradley RD. Measurement of cardiac output by thermal dilution in man. *J Appl Physiol* 1968; 24: 434–8.
2. Bradley RD. Diagnostic right heart catheterisation with miniature catheters in severely ill patients. *Lancet* 1964; 2: 941–2.
3. Korner PI. The effect of section of the carotid sinus and aortic nerves on the cardiac output of the rabbit. *J Physiol London* 1965; 180: 266–78.
4. Bell JA, Bradley RD, Jenkins BS, et al. Six years of multidisciplinary Intensive Care. *BMJ* 1974; 2: 483–8.
5. Bradley RD, Jenkins BS, Branthwaite MA. The influence of atrial pressure on cardiac performance following myocardial infarction complicated by shock. *Circulation* 1970; 42: 827–37.
6. Bradley RD. *Studies in Acute Heart Failure*. Edward Arnold, London, 1977.

Index

Page numbers in *italics* represent figures, those in **bold** represent tables.